Dental Anesthesia and Analgesia

(Local and General)

Third Edition

Dental Anesthesia and Analgesia

(Local and General)

Third Edition

G. D. Allen, M.B., F.F.A.R.C.S.

Diplomate, American Board of Anesthesiology
Professor, Department of Anesthesiology and Oral Surgery
Center for the Health Sciences
University of California, Los Angeles
Los Angeles, California

Lecturer, Oral Surgery, Department of Oral Surgery
Loma Linda University
Loma Linda, California

Four Contributors

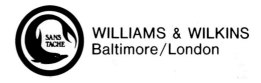

WILLIAMS & WILKINS
Baltimore/London

Editor: James L. Sangston
Associate Editor: Jonathan W. Pine, Jr.
Copy Editor: Leilani Ellison
Design: Joanne Janowiak
Illustration Planning: Lorraine Wrzosek
Production: Carol L. Eckhart

Accurate indications, adverse reactions, and dosage schedules for drugs are provided
in this book, but it is possible that they may change. The reader is urged to review
the package information data of the manufacturers of the medications mentioned.

*The Publishers have made every effort to trace the copyright holders for borrowed
material. If they have inadvertently overlooked any, they will be pleased to make the
necessary arrangements at the first opportunty.*

Made in the United States of America

First edition, 1972
Second edition, 1979
  Reprinted 1981

Library of Congress Cataloging in Publication Data

Allen, Gerald D., 1924–
  Dental anesthesia and analgesia.

  Includes bibliographies and index.
  1. Anesthesia in dentistry. I. Title. [DNLM: 1. Anesthesia, Dental. 2. Analgesia.
WO 460 A425d]
RK510.A44 1984   617′.9676   83-16735
ISBN 0-683-00068-3

Composed and printed at the
Waverly Press, Inc.
Mt. Royal and Guilford Aves.
Baltimore, MD 21202, U.S.A.

Preface

The previous editions of the text were developed following publication by the National Institute of Dental Research of "Target for the 70s," which promised major advances and prospects for pain control in dentistry. In the guidelines for the teaching of comprehensive control of pain and anxiety in dentistry published by the American Dental Association, Council on Dental Education, May 1971, and the Commission on Accreditation, February 1975, the recommended teaching for general anesthesia was to include a didactic course in general anesthesia for one hour per week for 10 weeks. In addition, two hours per week of lectures on oral, intravenous, and inhalation techniques of sedation and analgesia for one quarter were suggested. Both courses were to be supplemented by demonstrations and practical experience. It is apparent that such extensive teaching of pain control has not been achieved in the majority of dental schools. The teaching of the details of general anesthesia is not accorded the importance suggested in the 1975 guidelines. Course directors indicate that greater significance is attached to the teaching of local anesthesia and conscious sedation. It has therefore become necessary to reduce the general anesthesia sections in this edition and direct the basic sciences content to conscious sedation. This edition is an attempt to accord more with the realities of current teaching. While increasing numbers of dentists and oral surgeons are performing general anesthesia, their formal training allows reading beyond the scope of a text useful for the dental student. The newer curricula, however, place a greater emphasis on spe-

cial patient care, wherein general anesthesia has an important role. Therefore, some features of the previous editions have been retained in order to allow understanding of general anesthesia by the dental student, and perhaps to emphasize the historical role that the dentist has played in the development of general anesthesia.

The development of an American Board of Dental Anesthesiology is recognition of the need for unique training of the dentist in anesthesiology. It will accord with the certification required by many states for the administration of general anesthesia in the office for dental procedures. Indeed many states now recognize the ability of the dentist to perform anesthesiology for all procedures. It is an acknowledgment of the continuum of anesthesiology throughout the whole field of pain control.

An aspect of dental pain control frequently neglected is the ability of many of the drugs and techniques to produce general anesthesia, intentionally or inadvertently. Whether "sedation," "twilight sleep," "ultralight anesthesia," or other terminology is used, the major problems that have occurred with such techniques are related less to the techniques themselves than to the administrator's failure to recognize the complications that may occur. Such hazards are usually related to depression of protective pharyngeal and laryngeal reflexes, with loss of airway integrity, or impairment of cardiorespiratory function. If general anesthesia is considered essential for the patient, then general anesthesia should be used deliberately. Attempts to circumvent general anesthesia should not obscure the activity of the drugs administered. Most drugs used for conscious sedation may, if given in sufficient dose, produce analgesia and general anesthesia but may not be particularly suited for general anesthesia as the margin for safety in anesthetic dosage is low. If only for this reason the general dentist should understand general anesthesia, its implications, its modalities and its techniques. As newer drugs are developed and newer techniques arise with older drugs, the definition between analgesia and anesthesia becomes obscured and nomenclature is significant. Analgesia has been used throughout the text as synonymous with conscious sedation. The term has historical significance as it describes the action of the agents used and has the advantage of being applicable to all health care services, not only dentistry.

Relevant basic science material has been included in each section in order to illustrate the practical application of such knowledge, even if the relevance is not evident. Ignorance of, or disregard for, basic scientific principles have resulted in the perpetuation of some of the unsound techniques and unsafe equipment in addition to the failure to develop valid research in the past and present practice of dental anesthesia and analgesia. The practice of fitting all patients into a stereotypical technique is no longer appropriate or acceptable, if indeed it ever was. Selection of the appropriate pain control method should be based on an assessment of the patient's physical status, the training and experience of the operator, the pain control requirements of the operative procedure, the availability of drugs and safe equipment. Dental pain control is founded upon scientific knowledge gained from carefully controlled research and the application of previously known principles of physics, chemistry, and pharmacology. The goal of pain control is safe alteration of the patient's perception of pain and state of consciousness so that dental treatment becomes a pleasurable, acceptable experience. Anecdotal experience as the method of evaluating drugs, equipment, and techniques has been replaced by well-designed clinical research as the basis for reproducible and predictable results in the hands of many varied clinicians.

The section on pain has been revised in accord with the advanced scientific knowledge on stimulation-produced analgesia (SPA). Expansion of this section has replaced what were considered psychological effects. The section on hypnosis is included with preoperative preparation, as it is often a part of sedation, albeit unwittingly. The sections on evaluation present the principles that apply to all patient care for local anesthesia, conscious sedation, or anesthesia. Local anesthesia is an essential part of dental pain control. It involves an understanding of anatomy, physiology, and pharmacology that is not confined to the local area, but involves total patient evaluation, examination, and understanding. Much of the material in the sections on emergency care is now a replication of information taught in mandatory CPR courses, while the details of medical emergencies form the basis of separate texts. Therefore only such features of emergency care relevant to sedation and anesthesia are retained and included as part of the overall management of the patient under sedation or anesthesia.

Reference

Editorial: Time for an honest look at basic sciences. *J Am Dent Assoc* 94:795, 1977.

Acknowledgments

In the previous editions Drs. G. B. Everett, R. A. Meyer, and A. G. Tolas contributed both to the concept and material aspects of the text. Much of their work remains, and I gratefully acknowledge their contribution. Additional material was provided by the Audio-Visual Department of the Dental School at UCLA, under the direction of Irene Petravicius, with artwork by William Bishop and the late Charles Wishowski; and C. Teare-Richardson of the University of British Columbia. In addition, the photograph reproductions were by Richard Friske and Catherine Boris. The changes in the text were reproduced by the Word Processing Center of the Dental School at UCLA under the direction of Rhoda Freeman; Barbara Mersini and Michele Kirsch of UCLA and Sue Daniels of Southern Illinois University contributed significantly in the preparation of the manuscript.

Contributors

Joseph Barber, Ph.D.
Los Angeles, California

**David Donaldson, B.D.S., F.D.S.R.C.S.,
M.D.S.**
Professor
Director of Clinics
University of British Columbia
Vancouver, Canada

William M. Goebel, D.D.S., M.S.D.
Professor and Head
Section of Oral Diagnosis/Oral Medicine
School of Dental Medicine
Southern Illinois University
Alton, Illinois

Richard J. Kroening, M.D., Ph.D.
Associate Professor
Director, Pain Management Center
Schools of Medicine and Dentistry
University of California, Los Angeles
Los Angeles, California

Contents

Preface   v

Acknowledgments   vii

Contributors   ix

 1. Preoperative Care   1

 2. Physiology and Pharmacology of Local Anesthesia   48

 3. Local Anesthetic Agents   60

 4. Local Anesthetic Armamentarium   77

 5. Techniques of Local Anesthesia   98

 6. Complications of Local Anesthesia   163

 7. Management Problems of the Anesthetized and Sedated Patient   178

 8. Gases   218

 9. Equipment for Inhalation Analgesia   233

10. Inhalation Analgesia (Sedation)   254

11. Intravenous, Intradermal, Subcutaneous, and Intramuscular Injection   267

12. Oral, Intramuscular, and Intravenous Sedation   284

13. General Anesthesia in Dentistry   300

14. Postoperative Care   344

15. Selection of Pain Control Modality   360

16. Accidents   387

17. Pain   400

Index   423

CHAPTER 1

Preoperative Care

Thorough preoperative evaluation of the patient is essential prior to general anesthesia, but not this type of service exclusively. Local anesthesia, analgesia, and comedication all demand that the patient be evaluated prior to administration of a drug. These same principles are evident regardless of the procedure or the method of pain relief and form part of the overall aspect of total patient care. Each drug administration is an individual and unique experiment. The object, as in all good experiments, should be to decrease the physiological and pharmacological variables and reduce the physiological upset to a minimum.

The major use of general anesthesia for dentistry in the past has been for outpatient oral surgical procedures, but recently it has been extended to restorative dentistry. The low mortality rate seen with this form of anesthesia should be related to the surgery performed. Trauma is minimal; therefore, we should not be satisfied until the mortality and morbidity are reduced to zero. The physical status of the patient who submits to outpatient general anesthesia is significant, in that only relatively healthy patients are considered for outpatient practice. Thus, the satisfactory results can in part be attributed to the careful preoperative evaluation which dentists accord to their general anesthesia patients.

Ideal treatment would dictate the delay of any general anesthetic until the optimal physical condition of the patient is achieved. In recent years, however, patient convenience has increased as a contributing factor in the decision to operate under outpatient general anesthesia. Therefore, it is imperative to perform the preoperative preparation of the patient with even greater care, for in anesthetizing patients for whom general anesthesia may not be essential but is based on humanitarian motives only, no additional risk can be accepted. Without this service, however, many would not avail themselves of dental treatment.

Careful preparation is pertinent to all aspects of dental practice.

PATIENT EVALUATION

It is important to establish good rapport with the patient, and the preoperative evaluation provides an opportunity to develop this communication. Following evaluation, a standard physical status, as recommended by the American Society of Anesthesiologists' Classification, can be applied. In this fashion, patients can be categorized in the correct physical status for purposes of comparison and assessment of risk.

P.S. 1: A patient without systemic disease, a normal, healthy patient.

P.S. 2: A patient with mild systemic disease.

P.S. 3: A patient with severe systemic disease that limits activity, but is not incapacitating.

P.S. 4: A patient with incapacitating systemic disease that is a constant threat to life.

P.S. 5: A moribund patient not expected to survive 24 hours with or without operation.

P.S. E: Emergency operation of any variety which precedes the number.

General Physical Characteristics

These can be noted on the chart by the receptionist at the first visit of the patient.

AGE

The extremes of age pose problems in analgesia and anesthesia. In those under 3 years of age establishment of contract with the patient, maintenance of a patent airway, and a stormy induction are significant management problems. At the other end of the spectrum, the disease processes of the aged are more numerous and of greater clinical significance. Many electrocardiographic and cardiovascular abnormalities may be present in those over 40 years of age. Delayed complications can develop following general anesthesia.

RACE

The black patient can present specific problems in sedation and anesthesia because of various hemoglobinopathies, such as sickle cell disease and thalassemia and its various manifestations. In those individual cases where a broad nose is present, the nasal mask may be a poor fit, requiring the use of a nasopharyngeal tube during outpatient anesthesia to ensure a patent airway and delivery of gaseous agents.

SEX

For the female patient a chaperone is mandatory. Also, the question of pregnancy should always be posed. The teratogenic effects of anesthetic agents and drugs and the induction of abortion with general anesthesia must be considered in the first trimester. The induction of premature labor in the last 3 months should be a feature for consideration. The second trimester is the most desirable period for general anesthesia, if surgery is necessary. The female, generally, is more relaxed than the male and requires less general anesthesia. The teenage female may respond to analgesia with agitation and hysteria.

WEIGHT

Recent changes in weight, especially loss, pose problems. A recent weight loss will often indicate a more than corresponding reduction in blood volume, with subsequent difficulties in the maintenance of normal blood pressure.

The obese patient presents numerous unique anesthetic problems. The prolonged anesthetic induction and recovery, decreased functional residual capacity, and possible upper airway obstruction contribute to the development of arterial hypoxemia.

PERSONALITY

The response of the intelligent patient is often useful, as the adjuvant of hypnotic contact with a patient is possible. However, many intelligent people do not like to sense the loss of contact with reality which analgesia and premedication will produce.

OCCUPATION

There are many occupations in which exposure to the various elements in the atmosphere predispose to respiratory disease. These are especially evident in mining areas and the fiberglass industry. Many of the industrial pollutants and their metabolites are capable of inducing hepatic microsomal changes which may have significant clinical effects on the patient and the biotransformation of the anesthetic drugs utilized.

HABITS
Cigarette Smoking

It is important to stress that cigarette smoke should be avoided for at least 2 weeks or longer prior to general anesthesia. The irritation of the respiratory tract by cigarette smoke predisposes to coughing and an uneven anesthetic level. There is a greater increased risk of postoperative pulmonary complications.

Alcohol

The habitual drinker will require larger doses of drugs. The concept of enzyme induction, now established, places this on a rational basis. Alcohol stimulates the metabolic pathways in the liver, and in consequence anesthetic drugs are more rapidly metabolized. The habitual drinker will require a larger dose of intravenous agent for induction of anesthesia, and the effect is more transitory than in the normal patient due to enzyme induction.

Drug Dependence

The drug-dependent patient usually has hepatitis or hepatic dysfunction. The effect of these diseases on anesthesia or analgesia depends on the drug. Alcoholism will produce cross-tolerance to other drugs, and fluid balance is altered depending upon the state of the alcoholic. Thus with a rising alcohol level, diuresis occurs; with a stable alcohol level antidiuretic activity is evident; and on withdrawal the patient becomes overhydrated. In addition, hypoglycemia, myocardial depression, myopathies and the adverse effects of alcoholism on nutrition are noted. The sedatives also will produce drug dependency, and delirium tremens can be seen on barbiturate withdrawal, while a central anticholinergic syndrome is noted with over-the-counter sedatives such as belladonna derivatives. Prolonged excitement is noted during induction. Narcotic dependency will manifest itself with respiratory depression and sensitivity to other drugs. Hypertension, hyperpyrexia and convulsions are common accompaniments to dependence on amphetamines, whereas hallucinogens such as LSD potentiate the narcotics and succinylcholine.

Previous and current drug habits pose problems to the anesthetist as often there is denial of the habit or refusal to admit the problem. The hazards of anesthesia are greatly increased. The margin of safety is reduced and there are major responses to minimal changes in concentration of the administered drug. An additional hazard is posed by the difficulty in finding a suitable vein, as many are thrombosed from self-administration.

History

Genuine interest while the history is being recorded will improve patient response.

CHART REVIEW

This should be done before the patient is seen, to indicate awareness of the patient as an individual.

Record

It is often tedious to review the patient's medical record, but it is essential to assure good patient care to review all the notes in the record.

Treatment Record

A prior anesthetic record may explain the patient's behavior during surgery and anesthesia. In addition, the response to prior drugs and the amounts used provide valuable data in the conduct of the procedure.

CURRENT ILLNESSES

There may be more than one illness as a presenting feature. The dental disease may not be primary.

Presenting Disease

If the patient is presenting with the dental problem, ensure that it is not complicated by another disease process.

Coexisting Medical Disease

The presence of coexisting disease has a profound effect, both on the choice and technique selected. Drug inserts are noteworthy for their wide disclaimers of responsibility for complications which may arise from the drugs in the presence of concomitant disease.

Renal disease highlights the need for care in the choice of relaxant drugs, and cardiovascular disease indicates avoidance of factors which increase myocardial oxygen consumption, such as increased heart rate, myocardial tension, and myocardial contractility. In the presence of glaucoma, anticholinergic drugs, such as atropine, are a danger to the patient.

Upper Airway Infection (Common Cold)

Anesthesia should be postponed for 3 weeks in any nonurgent case when a cold is detected. Apart from the possible transmission to operator and anesthetist, the morbidity suffered by patients who have anesthesia while suffering from a cold is greatly enhanced.

Previous Anesthesia

Additional information can be obtained from the patient, through previous management of anesthesia. The anesthetist should not ignore the patient's description of a previous anesthetic experience. In the majority of cases, it is an inaccurate version and an exaggeration of the normal symptomatology of local and general anesthesia. However, there are, on rare occasions, instances of reactions to anesthesia which will be a valuable guide to the subsequent anesthetic choice. Even the reactions of the patient's relatives may be evidence of a genetic trait which is significant in the subsequent anesthetic. A failed local anesthetic in the dentist's office is the usual previous anesthetic problem described. The failure may be due to poor knowledge of anatomy or pharmacology. If it is the latter, it may be due to alterations in the local tissue which alter the pharmacodynamics of the local anesthetic. The question can readily be re-

solved by communication with the previous administrator of anesthesia.

Pyrexia

Fever is a frequent complaint of dental patients. It will increase the oxygen and anesthetic requirements because of increased rate of metabolism. The increased pulse rate with diminished stroke volume poses a hazard to subsequent anesthesia. In addition, hyperventilation may develop to eliminate the excess carbon dioxide produced by increased metabolism. A high fever under general anesthesia can develop into malignant hyperthermia or can cause central nervous system convulsions. Prolonged fever can cause excess sweating and subsequent decreased blood volume.

Fever may be the only presenting symptom of an undiagnosed disease.

Pain

The patient in pain preoperatively will probably have taken analgesics which will modify the pharmacological effect of the anesthetic agents. Presence of pain is an indication for an analgesic premedication. In order to eliminate pain with minimal dosage of analgesic, it is better to give the analgesic before the requirement is imperative.

Vomiting

Prior history of vomiting following general anesthesia or nitrous oxide-oxygen sedation can often alert the anesthetist to a subsequent postoperative problem, and he can modify his technique accordingly. A certain number of patients, probably 5 per cent, will always vomit following general anesthesia. The problem is complicated in dentistry because of the presence of blood and secretions in the mouth which will in themselves induce nausea and vomiting. The major hazard of prolonged preoperative vomiting is the change in electrolyte and fluid balance consequent to the loss of gastric and intestinal contents. Low blood volume should be suspected with a history of vomiting.

Specific Systems

Following the general review of the patient's history and nonspecific evaluation, it is imperative to evaluate certain specific systems which are uniquely related to the problems of outpatient general anesthesia and analgesia.

CARDIORESPIRATORY SYSTEM

It is difficult to delineate the symptomatology of cardiovascular and respiratory disease. Dyspnea, chest pain, and cough, together with decreased activity, can all be attributed to both systems.

Dyspnea

Dyspnea is difficult or labored breathing. Dyspnea at rest and nocturnal dyspnea, which awakens the patient during sleep, are indications of cardiovascular disease. They can be distinguished from dyspnea due to respiratory disease as they are not associated with cough.

Cough

Three types: wet, dry, or paroxysmal. The wet cough with production of sputum can be due either to left ventricular failure or to a respiratory problem. Inspection of the sputum produced will often distinguish the main problem and indicate the principal area of disease. A dry or paroxysmal cough is usually due to irritating foci in the upper airway passages. Chronic cough indicates that anesthesia should be delayed until the afternoon, in order that the patient clear the secretions from the tracheobronchial airway; this will facilitate general anesthesia. Often local anesthesia will be aided by delay in scheduling so the patient will not interrupt the

operation with his coughing. A chronic cough is not necessarily indicative of smoking and should not be passed over as such.

Chest Pain

Chest pain can be due to either cardiovascular disease, respiratory disease, or chest wall pain. A distinguishing feature of cardiovascular involvement is that the chest pain (angina pectoris) relates to activity, meals, or cold and disappears with rest or nitroglycerine. Chest pain related to respiration indicates an intrapulmonary problem.

Limitation of Activity

The patient with cardiovascular disease limits activity because of either dyspnea or cough. In consequence, exercise tolerance is diminished, and activity becomes more limited. It is a vicious circle in which the patient does not develop the necessary physical activity to revascularize the myocardium. It may be an early symptom of incipient cardiovascular disease.

Exercise Tolerance

The inability to perform exercise or activity is a useful index of cardiovascular reserve. The patient who can climb a flight of stairs without shortness of breath is usually in reasonable physical condition and has adequate cardiopulmonary reserve for general anesthesia.

Edema

Presacral or ankle endema is indicative of right-sided cardiac failure, a late symptom, which indicates that the patient is not suitable for any form of outpatient treatment.

LIVER AND KIDNEY

Specific questions related to liver and kidney diseases are worthy of mention during the preoperative history as these organs are intimately involved in the metabolism and excretion of parentally administered agents.

Genitourinary disease is indicated by polyuria or nocturia. Although these have no deleterious effect on anesthesia, it is well not to give fixed agents in the presence of urinary disease lest drug excretion be impaired.

METABOLIC
Adrenal

In this group the problem is the hazard of therapy. As will be discussed later, the suppression of normal adrenal secretion requires that excess supplementation be given prior to, during, and after general anesthesia.

Thyroid

The patient is usually aware of a thyroid condition. The major aspect is the presence of excess circulating thyroid hormone, which could lead to cardiac irregularities during anesthesia. Diminished thyroid secretions (hypothyroidism) result in slow metabolism with greater sensitivity to anesthetic agents and narcotic analgesics. In addition, these patients have an increased incidence of an early onset of arteriosclerotic vascular disease and cardiomyopathy.

Pancreas

In evaluating the patient for diabetes, selection of site of operation, either in the hospital, on an outpatient basis, or in the office, is of paramount importance. Fasting, a prerequisite for general anesthesia, upsets the control of diabetes mellitus. Marked postoperative edema, trismus, and pain following certain complex oral surgical procedures may impair fluid and caloric intake. Optimal patient care may dictate hospitalization of the diabetic patient for this reason.

CENTRAL NERVOUS SYSTEM

The patient with central nervous system disease is often referred for general anesthesia for dentistry. It is imperative that the degree of neurologial deficit be delineated prior to the administration of the anesthesia. Although the general anesthetic and drugs will not affect the subsequent course of the disease, medicolegal involvement can be a prominent feature.

A history of epilepsy would indicate preference for barbiturate premedication and/or the administration of thiopental. Excessive changes above or below the norm of carbon dioxide level and the lowering of oxygen tension may initiate convulsive seizures. Hyperventilation with hypocarbia and hypoventilation with hypercarbia can produce stimulating foci which will induce epileptic seizures. The incidence of abnormal EEG activity in certain animal studies when methohexital was used should alert the dentist to possible central nervous system sequelae. The choice of another anesthetic induction agent should be considered.

ALLERGIES

Allergic manifestations to common drugs should always form part of the history and evaluation of the patient. It is useful to indicate allergic reactions on the front of the patient's chart in large letters. The common agents and materials about which inquiry should be made are adhesive tape, codeine, aspirin, and local anesthetics. A particular hazard is an allergic reaction to the materials or agents used to wash the rubber goods which form part of the armamentarium for the administration of analgesia and anesthesia.

A history of hay fever of bronchial asthma may indicate that a new allergy can develop. The atopic patient and asthmatic, as well as the individual with a hyperactive airway (such as chronic bronchitis or smoker), does not have a greater probability of developing an allergic or anaphylactic reaction, but rather when adverse reactions do occur, they are of a greater magnitude and complexity than in the normal patient. In such patients, it is useful to include an antihistamine in the premedication.

MEDICATIONS

The medications prescribed or administered by physicians are probably the greatest hazard for those who administer both local and general anesthesia, or those who administer any drugs for pain control by either intravenous or inhalation analgesic techniques. It is a problem for all who administer any medication. A known factor is interaction of drugs in the individual. The increasing complexity of active drugs has compounded the problem. Combinations of drugs are rarely studied, and as polypharmacy is popular, the hazard will continue and increase. It will be reduced only when the problems of polypharmacy are appreciated. The problem in outpatient practice is worse as the patient has an unknown background and drug pattern, and interaction of drugs can occur with any of the agents administered for the relief of pain. The responsibility for administering a drug is serious. The gravity of the problem should be noted in the context that 5 per cent of all admissions to hospitals are for drug reactions, and 10 per cent of all patients have a reaction to drugs while in the hospital.

The *PDR* (*Physicians' Desk Reference*) *Diary* in the United States or *Compendium of Pharmaceuticals and Specialties* in Canada are valuable references available for the identification of the drugs which the patient is receiving.

Pharmacodynamics

Understanding of the side and toxic effects and methods of drug inactivation is necessary in order that the influence of medication upon subsequent anesthesia and analgesia can be understood.

SIDE EFFECTS

Side effects are defined as the proper action of a drug in an improper place. The more potent the agent, the more widespread the pharmacological and physiological activities. The lists of side effects noted in drug inserts are usually there for the protection of manufacturer, not to help the administrator of the drug. The widespread activity of current potent drugs is such that the list could be identical for the majority of drugs in use today. However, understanding of the activity and the basic pharmacology of the drug gives the best chance of protection for the patient.

Some side effects are useful in anesthesia. The side effects of the phenothiazines are often used for their ability to potentiate general anesthetics. However, they can cause severe hypotension or confusion and neurological disturbances in the elderly.

TOXIC EFFECTS

Toxic effects are defined as an improper action of a drug. Drugs with grave toxic effects have no place in anesthesia where they can do immense harm. The triple response—wheal, line, and flare—is the classic triad of histamine release and is best seen with narcotics. Blood dyscrasias and the toxic effects of radiation therapy are often evident in dental treatment, where full mouth odontectomy is a necessary preliminary to radiation therapy of the jaw.

The hepatotoxic and nephrotoxic activity of anesthetics has been highlighted recently—in particular, halothane and methoxyflurane. The activity of these agents is discussed in the chapter devoted to anesthesia.

Drug Inactivation

METHODS OF INACTIVATION

The routes of inactivation of a drug are metabolic, redistribution, and excretion.

The pharmacodynamics of the drug determines its route of inactivation and biotransformation. Physiological factors may also affect the distribution, metabolism, and excretion of anesthetic agents. The duration and magnitude of the response will depend primarily upon the pharmokinetics of the drug, but the response is modified by various factors such as site of action, local tissue condition, pH, and tissue perfusion.

These principles are well demonstrated by the several barbiturates, where the uptake, distribution, metabolism, and excretion vary. The short acting barbiturate is rapidly redistributed and metabolized in the liver. The long acting barbiturate is normally excreted by the kidney. The influence of physiological factors is seen in the blood levels of thiopental and its distribution. Not only does hypercarbia or hypocarbia influence the peripheral blood flow and in consequence the distribution, but hypercarbia increases the thiopental in the cell and decreases the level of thiopental in the plasma, and hypocarbia results in a lowering of thiopental in the cell with an increase in the plasma thiopental. As intracellular action determines effective action of a drug, hypercarbia results in increased activity of thiopental, whereas hypocarbia results in decreased activity of thiopental. Hypercarbia lowers the plasma level, and hypocarbia increases the plasma levels; thus, plasma levels with barbiturates must be critially evaluated if they are to be used as an index of depth of anesthesia.

The rate of metabolism can be affected by other drugs, and enzyme induction is a potent factor in determining the rate of metabolism of a drug. Classically, the barbiturates, alcohol, and DDT are agents which promote enzyme induction, and thus, they, as well as other drugs, are metabolized more rapidly.

It must be appreciated that, teliologically, metabolism is only to aid the excretion of a drug. Often, metabolites of the active drug are themselves active. A metabolite of diazepam, oxazepam, is itself a hypnotic.

PHARMACOLOGICAL FACTORS

Enzyme induction is an important mechanism by which the speed of inactivation has been hastened. As previously mentioned, some agents (DDT, alcohol) increase the rate of metabolism of themselves and, in addition, increase the rate of metabolism of other concomitantly administered drugs. It explains the short action of barbiturates when administered to alcoholics and the brevity of action of subsequent doses of drug after initial induction doses. The acute tolerance described with thiopental can be attributed to self-induction.

Alternative explanations of tolerance are that the route of metabolism is altered, there is an increase in the threshold affector site reactivity which decreases the response, or there are changes in the permeability of the blood barrier either to the drug itself or to the drug's metabolic breakdown products.

Analeptics may be another pharmacological method of drug inactivation. An ideal analeptic acts by decreasing the cell concentration of the drug, or by direct chemical stimulation of the cell. Apart from naloxone there are only physiological antagonists which stimulate the patient and can cause convulsions, thereby increasing the oxygen requirements of the cells.

Physiological Factors Affecting Drug Metabolism

RACE

This is not well demonstrated in humans but in animals there are well demarcated species and strain differences. It is a reminder that it is important not to extrapolate results obtained from animals to the human.

AGE

The young do not have as many metabolic enzymes as the mature adult. The neonate is approximately twice as sensitive to curare as the adult. This is probably related to inadequate plasma protein binding power in the neonate.

HORMONES

The effect of drugs varies with the sex hormonal cycle. The gestational hormones affect the levels of insulin, thyroid, and adrenocortical hormones, which in turn profoundly influence drug metabolism. As the excretion of those hormones is stimulated by anesthesia, the effect is compounded. The barbiturates show profound or pronounced sex differences, the female being extremely sensitive to overdosage with barbiturates.

NUTRITIONAL STATE

A patient who has been starved for over 24 hours shows a decreased ability to metabolize drugs, and with a lowered serum protein there is less active protein for combining power. These factors account for the unpredictable and exaggerated response to the barbiturates in the presence of reduced serum plasma proteins.

TEMPERATURE

Metabolism increases 7 per cent for every degree Fahrenheit rise in temperature.

ROUTE OF ADMINISTRATION

The best example of the influence of route of administration on drug metabolism is seen in barbiturates, which can be given orally, rectally, or intravenously. The large dosage required to achieve anesthesia when given rectally indicates that metabolism probably occurs in the portal circulation; large doses are necessary in order to achieve satisfactory anesthetic levels.

STATE OF CONSCIOUSNESS

A patient who has had little sleep before treatment will require less sedation and recovery may be delayed.

OXYGEN TENSION

A lowered oxygen tension decreases the rate of metabolism as the cellular enzymes are particularly sensitive to oxygen lack.

pH

Metabolic acidosis or alkalosis produces changes which parallel those of respiratory acidosis and alkalosis noted with barbiturates. The pH is of great clinical significance as it is related to the pK_a of a drug. The pH will determine the degree of ionization of the drug at its respective pKa. Thus, the ionized portion of the drug in the active portion of the drug will be determined by the pH of local tissue and the pK_a of the agent.

DRUG CATEGORIES WHICH ARE ANALGESIC AND ANESTHETIC HAZARDS

This section discusses drugs which may pose unique problems.

SEDATIVES

Synergism of sedatives with anesthetics must be stressed. Barbiturates are not protective for toxic reactions to local anesthetics.

TERATOGENIC DRUGS

Anesthesia could be blamed for abnormalities of the fetus; thus, if drugs of known toxicity are given at the same time, note should be made of their presence. Drugs which are frequently teratogenetic in activity are the thyroid inhibitors, the anticoagulants, the antibiotics, and the antihistamines. The drug insert for methohexital gives a warning regarding administration to pregnant women. To date the barbiturates have a long history of successful use, and there has been no incrimination of local anesthetics in teratogenesis.

ANTIHYPERTENSIVE AGENTS

The patient on antihypertensive therapy should be maintained on his medication since withdrawal from drug ther-

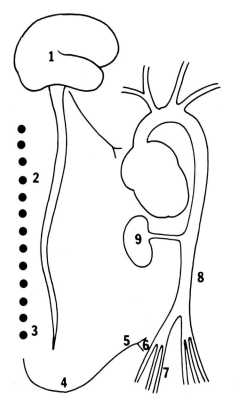

Figure 1.1. The numerous sites at which antihypertensive drugs may act are illustrated.

apy is very dangerous and may precipitate uncontrolled hypertension with its attendant sequelae. This is particularly evident when clonidine is withdrawn. The major problem with the antihypertensive agents is the combined central and peripheral action of the drugs in altering the adrenergic nervous system. The agents are used in combination with diuretics to reduce the blood volume, alter serum electrolytes, and have a direct relaxing effect on vascular smooth muscle to reduce blood pressure (Fig. 1.1 and Table 1.1). These drugs are often administered in combination with the ataractics or sedatives, further compounding the problem.

Many articles indicate that there is no need for delay in administration of anesthesia with the hypotensive drugs. The problems are those of hypertension itself, in that a labile blood pressure is a feature of the disease. There are many hazards of stopping the medication, and possibly the most satisfactory solution is to proceed with the anesthesia. There are, however, rare instances of failure to respond to vasopressors when on antihypertensive drugs. In dentistry, it is suggested that care be taken in approaching these patients.

CARDIAC GLYCOSIDES AND DIURETICS

These drugs have a low therapeutic index, which in itself is a major hazard. They do, however, produce hypovolemia, low sodium levels, and low potassium levels with subsequent decreased muscle

Table 1.1.
The Sites of Action of Some of the Antihypertensive Drugs

2	Clonidine	Central α-adrenergic block
4	Guanethidine (Ismelin)	Adrenergic neuron block
8	Hydralazine (Apresoline)	Smooth muscle relaxation
5	L-Dopa (Levo-Dopa)	Decreased sympathetic nerve
3	Methyldopa (Aldomet)	Decreased sympathetic outflow
6	Monoamine oxide inhibitors	Accumulation false transmitters
5	Propranolol (Inderal)	β-Adrenergic block
1	Reserpine (Serpasil)	Depletion central catecholamines
7	Thiazides (Diuril)	Peripheral vascular
9		Decrease blood volume
1	Tricyclic antidepressants	Depletion catecholamine stores

response. In addition, they have a profound effect on drug distribution as acid-base balance is affected. The associated changes in metabolic acid-base balance indicate a need for care, in adding another factor to the altered acid-base balance, that of a respiratory component. Determination of preoperative electrolyte level is indicated.

ANALEPTICS

These drugs usually lower the response of the patient to the anesthetic, though occasionally there may be an exaggerated response. The latter is noted particularly if the patient has been on amphetamines or methylphenidate (Ritalin). The narcotic antagonist, naloxone (Narcan) is effective in reversing the pharmacological effects of the narcotic. The short half life of naloxone may require repeat administration to completely reverse the longer duration of the narcotic agent. Naloxone alone has no direct stimulating or depressing action on the cardiac or respiratory functions. If other narcotic antagonists are used in overdose, they can produce respiratory depression.

PSYCHOACTIVE DRUGS

Currently, psychoactive drugs are of critical importance. The widespread use of drugs for sedation and mood elevation produces major hazards for the person administering anesthesia (Table 1.2). There has been a resurgence in the use of MAO inhibitors together with tricyclic antidepressants.

The actions of tricyclic antidepressants and the phenothiazine drugs on the cardiovascular system are complex. These agents have a combined direct effect on the heart and blood vessels and an indirect effect mediated by way of the autonomic system and reflexes. The hypotension produced by the phenothiazines is by inhibition of centrally mediated pressor responses and direct adrenergic blockade of the peripheral vasculature. The drugs also have a direct negative ionotropic action on the myocardial and papillary muscles. The tricyclic antidepressant drugs appear to have a greater effect on the cardiovascular system than the phenothiazines. Anesthesia in the patient who is maintained on tricyclic medications is a greater clinical risk than those on the phenothiazines. The primary problems associated with anesthesia and the tricyclic drugs are related to the quinidine-like action of the drugs on the conduction system and blockage of norepinephrine uptake. The net effect of the electrophysiological alteration on the action potential is to decrease membrane responses and decrease the velocity of conduction throughout the specialized tissue of the myocardium.

The electrophysiological alteration explains the electrocardiographic changes seen with these agents. Prolonged P-R and Q-T intervals, wide QRS, and S-T segment depressions are seen in 20 per cent of

Table 1.2.
The Three Major Groups of Psychoactive or Ataractic Drugs

MAO Inhibitors	Tricyclics	Phenothiazines
Isocarboxazid (Marplan)	Amitriptyline (Elavil)	Chlorpromazine (Thorazine)
Pargyline (Eutonyl)	Desipramine (Norpramin)	Fluphenazine (Prolixin)
Phenelzine sulfate (Nardil)	Imipramine (Tofranil)	Perphenazine (Trilafon)
Tranylcypromine sulfate (Parnate)	Nortriptyline (Aventyl)	Thioridazine (Mellaril)
	Protriptyline (Vivactil)	Triflupromazine (Vesprin)

patients receiving therapeutic doses of the tricyclic antidepressants. Thus, there is facilitation of re-entrant excitation which is the primary mechanism in the production of serious cardiac arrhythmias in such patients. In addition, any factor which would further decrease conduction velocity, such as vagal stimulation, will further aggravate the condition and increase the probability of serious cardiac dysrhythmias. The blockade of norepinephrine uptake is of great clinical significance for the primary mechanism of terminating adrenergic stimulation is by reuptake of norepinephrine into the axon. Thus, those factors which tend to increase adrenergic stimulation and release catecholamines will markedly exaggerate adrenergic response. Any exogenous epinephrine administered, as in a local anesthetic with a vasopressor, may produce severe adrenergic stimulation leading to cerebral hemorrhage.

It is strongly recommended that a patient receiving therapeutic doses of tricyclic antidepressants not be operated upon until a 2-week period has passed without medication, though not if this endangers the patient's psychic welfare. Consultation with the physician during this period is imperative to ensure good patient care.

MONOAMINE OXIDASE (MAO) INHIBITORS

An explanation of the activity of MAO is of value. MAO catalyzes the deamination of the amines, dopamine, tyrosine, and 5-hydroxytryptamine (serotonin), which are the precursors of norepinephrine and epinephrine. Thus, momoamine oxidase inhibitors increase the 5-hydroxytryptamine in the tissues. The 5-hydroxytryptamine level is maximal in the brain and all sympathetic tissues. The MAO inhibitors therefore stimulate the reticular activating system, the cortex, and the sympathetic nervous system. The direct hazards are production of edema, hypotension, and blood dyscrasis.

The tissues are sensitized to excess amines either injected in local anesthetics, or present in food rich in tyramine (Stilton cheese and Chianti), producing hypotension or hypertension. The hypotension is a reversal action often seen in receptor sites which have been sensitized.

It is important to realize that injected epinephrine and norepinephrine are not the major hazard in the presence of monoamine oxide inhibitors as the adrenergic nerves and liver contain catecholomethyltransferase, which metabolizes epinephrine and norepinephrine. However, indirect sympathomimetic drugs, which cause release of epinephrine and norepinephrine, such as amphetamine and ephedrine, and mixed acting drugs like phenylephrine are greatly potentiated by monoamine oxidase inhibitors. The hazard of monoamine oxidase inhibitors to locally injected epinephrine and norepinephrine has been overstressed, as MAO is not the mechanism of metabolism of these two pharmacologically active tissue products.

The great hazard is the effect of MAO inhibitors on other enzyme systems. Potentiation of other drug activity is the major hazard in anesthesia, and it is imperative that the anesthetist be aware of these interactions. Drugs which react or are affected are: 1) barbiturates, 2) meperidine (potentiation of morphine has not been reported), 3) codeine, 4) chloral hydrate, 5) phenothiazines, 6) anti-parkinsonian drugs, 7) cocaine, 8) reserpine, 9) sympathomimetics, 10) succinylcholine, 11) thiazides, 12) insulin. The problem is that not only is the activity of drug potentiated but the action is prolonged. The potent narcotic analgesics may interact, producing severe systemic reactions. Hypotensive crises, hypertension, tachycardia, convulsions, and severe respiratory depression with apnea and coma may occur. Meperidine is contraindicated in the patient receiving MAO inhibitors. The toxic action may be due to elevated levels of breakdown products. Caution and close observation of the patient is recommended when potent narcotic analgesics are used in the presence of these drugs.

If possible, 3 weeks should be allowed for the drug to clear the system prior to administration of anesthesia. Premedicate with chlorpromazine or propriomazine, which are adrenolytics, and anesthetize the patient with isoflurane as an adjuvant to nitrous oxide-oxygen. For hypertensive responses an α-adrenergic blocker, phentolamine (Regitine), 5 mg intravenously, and a β-adrenergic blocker, propanolol (Inderal), 5 mg intravenously, should be available. For a hypotensive response, hydrocortisone, 100 mg intravenously, followed by epinephrine infusion, 1 μg per ml, should be available.

LITHIUM SALTS

This drug is used in the treatment of manic depression. Its activity is related to the replacement of sodium within the cell. There is a decrease of norepinephrine at receptor sites, which reduces the presumed mood elevating effects of norepinephrine. Due to the effect on nervous conduction, muscular rigidity and hyperactive reflexes with tremor can occur. In combination with muscle relaxants prolonged apnea can develop. Toxicity will cause blurred speech, ataxia and tremor of the hands. As these patients are at risk if they cease taking medications, the drug should not be discontinued.

ENDOCRINES

Those endocrines which cause problems in anesthesia are the steroids, insulin, and, rarely, thryoid.

Steroids

A method for remembering whether steroids will cause a problem under anesthesia is the 2/2/2 method: if the patient has been on cortisone (or equivalent) in excess of 20 mg a day for 2 weeks within the last 2 years, then adrenal suppression must be suspected. The hazard posed is that it is not possible to detect whether the patient who has had adrenal suppression by medication will ever respond adequately to stress. It is questionable as to whether these patients will ever be suitable for outpatient general anesthesia. When such patients present for anesthesia, soluble hydrocortisone must be available. If adrenal suppression is expected, the patient should be premedicated with 25 mg the night before anesthesia followed by 25 mg intramuscularly b.i.d. the day of operation. Twenty-five milligrams b.i.d. should be given orally for the next 2 days.

Duration of action of cortisone:

	Peak	Duration
oral	60 min	4 hr
intramuscular	12 hr	16 hr

Duration of action of hydrocortisone:

	Peak	Duration
intramuscular	3 hr	6 hr

It may be preferable to avoid premedication in outpatients and have available hydrocortisone hemisuccinate, 100 mg, and a certain intravenous route, for the following reasons: the hypotensive reaction is rare and depends on the degree of depression, and it is preferable not to depress the adrenals once more if it unnecessary. Psychic effects of cortisone can potentiate the barbiturates and phenothiazines, and indeed a steroid has been developed as an anesthetic agent.

Insulin

The mild or moderate diabetic, those who are controlled with oral antidiabetic medications (tolbutamide) or diet, can be controlled by not administering the medication the morning of operation and starving the patient. During the period of operation, an IV dextrose infusion, 5 to 10 per cent, can be given to prevent development of acidosis. If the patient is a severe or juvenile diabetic, he should not be treated on an outpatient basis for general anesthesia. If the patient is on nonprotein hagedorn (NPH), lente, semilente, or ultralente, it is safer to change to regular insulin twice a day. On the morning of operation he would then receive regular insulin and glucose and be followed by blood sugar and urine sugar levels, with regular insulin and IV glucose being administered as required. Hypoglycemia is the critical problem; the brain requires 60 mg per 100 ml of glucose to survive, and therefore a period of hyperglycemia is preferable as it is tolerated by the brain.

Thyroid

Good control of patients lacking thyroid hormone has now been achieved. The influence of thyroid on the metabolism must be considered. Excessive secretion with a thyroid storm is an event not seen now in clinical practice.

HEMOTOXIC

The problem of drugs which inhibit production of red blood cells and platelets is that, in addition to anemia, they promote a bleeding problem. It can cause problems if a nasopharyngeal tube is used. Continuous nasal bleeding throughout an operation is a hazard to the anesthetist in his maintenance of a satisfactory airway, and the bleeding will interfere with the operative field. The reduction in red blood cells is such as to interfere with the oxygen-carrying capacity of the blood. Frequently these patients are on recurring courses of therapy, and there is reluctance to transfuse unless urgent, in order to avoid multiple transfusions.

BUTAZOLIDIN

Given for antiarthritic properties, Butazolidin enhances the toxicity and activity of the majority of other drugs. It has an affinity for protein, and protein binding is increased. Thus, there is less free protein to combine with any other drug given while the patient is receiving Butazolidin.

PHYSICAL EXAMINATION

With good clinical judgment and ability on the part of the examiner, the physical examination can be rapidly performed and should form part of the evaluation of every prospect for outpatient dental anesthesia and analgesia.

Obesity

Obesity is a unique hazard in general anesthesia. The development of a fatty myocardium, peripheral vascular disease, and increased work of the heart are only a few examples of the significant pathophysiogical sequelae of obesity. Adrenal insufficiency, diabetes mellitus, and other endocrine and metabolic disorders should be suspected in the obese individual and may further complicate the surgical anesthetic management.

The prevention of hypoxemia is one of the principle problems associated with the anesthetic management in obesity. Patency of the upper airway is frequently compromised secondary to the large mass of tissue, the short neck, and inability to attain the ideal sitting position in the dental chair. The reduction in the functional residual capacity (FRC) and tidal volume leads to an increase in air trapping and development of arterial hypoxemia. In addition, the increased work of respiration contributes to the decrease in respiratory reserve. Venipuncture can present a problem.

During anesthesia, the uptake and distribution of general anesthetic agents are affected by obesity; the large storage depot requires great amounts of anesthetic to achieve equilibration; and excretion is delayed.

This does not indicate larger amounts of anesthetic are required to induce or maintain anesthesia. Anesthetic requirement is determined by a metabolic requirement and correlates best with surface area and lean body mass, rather than total body weight. Thus, care should be exercised not to overdose the obese patient or further decrease cardiac and respiratory reserve which will contribute to further arterial hypoxemia.

Stature

The larger the patient, the more difficult general anesthesia, as the margin of safety is reduced. Greater amounts of administered drugs are needed to achieve equilibration, with the subsequent hazard of overdosage. Short, thick-necked patients indicate problems in maintenance of the airway under general anesthesia. The humpbacked patient with stooping posture suggests pulmonary problems which arise during general anesthesia.

Gait

As the patient walks into the room, indications of incipient or overt neurological disease are often evident. Joint or musculoskeletal disease may be evident and should alert the dentist to the possibility of cortisone therapy not listed in the history.

Eyes

Exophthalmus is now rare and may indicate hyperthyroid activity. Evidence of drug activity can be seen in the pinpoint pupil of the patient taking narcotics.

Skin

Color is no index or quantitative measure of anemia. It may, however, indicate anxiety and vasomotor instability in the anxious patient with impending syncope.

Cyanosis

Cyanosis is a quantitative measure of 5 g per 100 ml or more of reduced hemoglobin in the circulation. It is not necessarily an indication of the oxygen content, oxygen carrying capacity, or hypoxemia. The plethoric patient with an increased red cell mass or the polycythemic patient may exhibit cyanosis because of the larger amount of reduced hemoglobin, particularly in the periphery. Cyanosis does suggest, however, that treatment be deferred until the etiology has been ascertained.

Jaundice

Jaundice is an obvious indication for postponement of anesthesia.

Petechiae

Petechiae require investigation and suggest blood dyscrasias.

Sweating

Sweating is usually due to anxiety, although pyrexia must be suspected.

Skin Turgor

Skin turgor or elasticity of the skin does give an indication of the adequacy of fluid balance. This is particularly evident in the elderly, where it must not be confused with the normal loss of elasticity in the aging process.

Hands

Sweating and tremor are indications of anxiety and often normal concomitants of dentistry. Tremor may indicate chronic cerebrovascular insufficiency such as parkinsonism. Clubbing of the fingers indicates pulmonary disease and requires further investigation.

Temperature

The measurement of temperature should be a part of the office routine. Pyrexia results in an increase in metabolic rate with consequent increase oxygen in demand. A rise in temperature produces a rise in pulse rate; anesthesia often produces an increase in heart rate, and the combination could produce inadequate coronary filling.

Respiratory System

ANATOMICAL AND PHYSIOLOGICAL CONSIDERATIONS IN RELATION TO PREOPERATIVE EVALUATION

Gas passes through the nose in an anteroposterior direction over the superior middle and inferior turbinate bones. The area is rich in blood vessels and is covered by a ciliated glandular epithelium. The large surface is capable of great vascular engorgement and humidifies the air adequately even if dry gases are used. During normal sleep, the dependent nostril is congested, and resistance to respiration varies with the posture of the patient. Resistance to nasal aspiration is twice that of mouth breathing. The nose leads to the nasopharynx and thence to the oropharynx, which is covered with squamous epithelium as both air and food pass through the area.

The larynx forms below the oropharynx, the glottis being that area between the vocal cords. During inspiration the cords abduct, and during expiration they return to the midline.

The trachea commences at the sixth cervical vertebra and extends to the carina at the level of the fourth thoracic vertebra, where it divides into the two main bronchii. It is formed of incomplete rings of cartilage and is lined, as is the remainder of the bronchial tree, by ciliated epithelium, rich in glands and goblet cells. The area in which tracheostomy should be performed is below the second tracheal ring in order to avoid subsequent tracheal stenosis.

The bronchial tree subdivides progressively up to the terminal bronchioles where the respiratory unit begins and active interchange of bases occurs. The respiratory unit is composed of respiratory bronchioles, alveolar ducts, and alveoli. The air in the alveoli is separated from the capillaries by two thin layers of cells: the capillary and alveolar wall. The total area of respiratory epithelium in the adult is 55 sq. m. The bronchi are rich in elastic tissue and surrounded by muscle fibers. The parasympathetic supply *via* the vagus constricts the bronchi, and sympathetic stimulation produces dilatation. Sensory innervation is by the vagus. Constriction of the bronchi occurs with expiration. If anesthesia is not sufficiently deep, reflex responses can occur which produce bronchoconstriction. Stimulation occurs when irritant gases are admitted to the tracheobronchial tree, with vagal stimulation, or pain, or subsequent to morphine, barbiturates, physostigmine, and neostigmine.

CONTROL OF RESPIRATION

Respiration is regulated both by voluntary (cortical) and involuntary (brainstem) mechanisms. The respiratory control mechanism consists of a sensing unit (central and peripheral chemoreceptors), integrating unit (cortical and brainstem), and an effector unit. The brainstem respiratory system consists of three distinct anatomical areas located in the pons and medulla. The pneumotaxic and apneustic areas are located in the pons, and two centers are located in the medulla, the ventral respiratory group (VRG) and the dorsal respiratory group (DRG). The medullary centers are not distinct centers but designated neural aggregates of tissue. The DRG is primarily inspiratory in function and located in the ventrolateral portions of the tractus solitarius. The VRG contains both inspiratory and expiratory cells and is associated with the nucleus ambiguous and the nucleus retroambigualis. The major function of the VRG neurons is to project to distant sites and drive spinal respiratory motor neurons primarily intercostal and abdominal.

The DRG possesses only inspiratory neuron function and projects primarily to the contralateral spinal cord and serves as the principal rhythmic respiratory drive of the phrenic motor neurons. The DRG also project to the VRG but not *vice versa*; thus the VRG is driven by the DRG.

The DRG constitutes the initial intracranial processing station for many visceral reflexes affecting respiration, and is the site of origin of the rhythmic drive to the VRG as well as many spinal respiratory motor neurons. The primary site of respiratory rhythm generation may be synaptically close to the DRG or may be one and the same.

The sensors of the respiratory system are located both centrally as well as peripherally. The central and peripheral chemoreceptors are sensitive to alterations in arterial PCO_2 and pH. In addition, the peripheral chemoreceptors are sensitive to reductions in PaO_2. Thus, in normal man, ventilation is stimulated by hypercarbia, hypoxemia, and acidemia. Respiration may be influenced by cortical impulses, changes in arterial carbon dioxide and oxygen, acidemia and alkalemia, changes in body temperature, carotid body reflexes, proprioceptive impulses from muscle and joints, talking and swallowing reflexes, and the Hering-Breuer reflex. The Hering-Breuer reflex, which inhibits respiration, is particularly affected by anesthetic agents. The reflex relayed from the alveolar walls can be stimulated by increased intrathoracic pressure and various irritants.

Carbon dioxide is the principal factor which controls respiration. The primary functions of respiration or ventilation are oxygenation and the elimination of carbon dioxide. Oxygen tension is an important stimulus to ventilation only when severe hypoxemia occurs (arterial PO_2 50 mm Hg). Excess oxygen does not depress respiration, and the addition of carbon dioxide to oxygen to stimulate ventilation in asphyxial attacks is a dangerous practice. Oxygen and carbon dioxide mixtures should not be given.

LUNG VOLUMES

The following are the average adult volumes: total lung capacity, 6 liters; vital capacity, 5 liters; functional residual capacity, 2.5 liters; inspiratory reserve volume, 3 liters; expiratory reserve volume, 1.5 liters; tidal volume, 500 ml; anatomical dead space, 150 ml; and physiological dead space, 600 ml (Fig. 1.2).

Total lung capacity is the gas content of the lung after a maximum inspiration. Vital capacity is the maximum (volume of gas that can be expelled from the lung

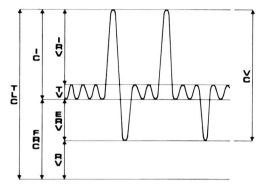

Figure 1.2. The lung volumes and capacity represented diagrammatically are given in the text.

by a forceful effort after a maximum inspiration. Functional residual capacity is the volume of air in the lung at resting expiratory level, the sum of expiratory reserve volume and residual volume. Inspiratory reserve volume is the maximum amount of gas inspired from the normal end inspiratory position. Expiratory reserve volume is the maximum amount of gas that can be expired from the end expiratory position. Tidal volume is the total volume of inspired and then expired gas during each respiration. Anatomical dead space extends from the nostrils and mouth to the respiratory unit and does not include the alveolus. It is estimated as about 1 ml per lb of body weight (150 ml). It is reduced by intratracheal intubation to half (75 ml).

Physiological dead space can be derived from the following equation:

$$PDS = V_t \left(\frac{PaCO_2 - PeCO_2}{PaCO_2} \right)$$

where V_t = tidal volume, $PaCO_2$ = tension of CO_2 in arterial blood, and $PeCO_2$ = tension of CO_2 in expired air.

Dead space is that volume of gas which is not available for respiratory exchange because of anatomy or when alveoli have no capillary blood flow or have become distended; it thus varies with ventilation.

Apparatus dead space may be a negative feature of some equipment design. Attention should be given to recent antipollution devices, introduced into dental practice, wherein no consideration has been given to this feature.

Effective tidal volume is diminished by any increase in dead space. Rapid shallow breathing is less efficient than slow deep breathing as the dead space remains the same for each type of ventilation. As tidal volume approaches dead space volume, respiratory exchange is diminished.

Factors affecting physiological dead space are: 1) tidal volume and respiratory rate, 2) the pattern of respiration, 3) lung volume, 4) pulmonary blood flow, 5) body position, 6) alveolar PCO_2, 7) changes in bronchomotor tone, 8) atropine, 9) general anesthesia, and 10) hypotension.

MECHANICAL ASPECTS OF RESPIRATION

Although inspiration is an active process (the walls of the thoracic cage expand during inspiration and relax during expiration), the flow of air into the lungs is passive. During inspiration, the thoracic cage is increased in all dimensions. The anterior diameter is increased by the sternum and upper ribs moving forward, and the transverse diameter is increased by the shape of the ribs and subcostal angle of the diaphragm and the lower ribs, while the length of thoracic cavity is increased by descent of the diaphragm. Expiration is passive owing to the elastic recoil of lung tissue which equals 5 mm Hg on expiration and 10 mm Hg on inspiration. The abdominal musculature aids in expiration, raising the diaphragm while the intercostal muscles depress the ribs. The diaphragm is the main muscle of respiration and accounts for 60 per cent of ventilation. It is innervated by the phrenic nerve (C4 with twigs from C3 and 5). It receives sensory fibers from the lower six intercostal nerves.

The internal and external intercostal muscles act by elevating the ribs during inspiration and also prevent recession during deep breathing. They aid inspiration but take no part in expiration.

Each lung is enclosed in a closed sac of pleura. The potential space is at a negative pressure of about −5 mm Hg. During the inspiratory cycle, the pleural pressure becomes more negative and the flow of fresh inspired gas fills the alveoli. The greater negative pressure generated, the greater the velocity of airflow and the potential volume of inspired air.

Compliance is the volume change produced by each unit of pressure increase. It is expressed in terms of liters per cm H_2O change. It is a volume-pressure relationship and varies from 0.1 to 0.25 liter per cm H_2O. Two factors which are responsible are thoracic cage compliance and pulmonary or lung compliance. Compliance evaluation is used in pulmonary function studies and is expressed in graphic form. Mitral stenosis decreases lung compliance through increase in the volume of the lung or decrease of elasticity. Anesthetics in lighter planes of anesthesia increase compliance due to pulmonary dilatation.

The importance of chest wall and parenchymal (lung) compliance is related to the work of ventilation. Any decrease in compliance, a stiff lung or chest, make it more difficult to breathe. This may not only effect alveolar ventilation but may greatly increase the work of ventilation.

Shunt. In the normal patient, about 8 per cent of the blood entering the lung is not aerated, that is, it bypasses or is shunted passed the alveolar air spaces. The blood passes through bronchial arteries or through arteriovenous shunts. In disease, the degree of shunting is increased, and contributes to the fall of oxygen tension. It can be roughly calculated by the use of the shunt equation (Table 1.3). It may also be affected by anesthesia and profoundly affect the course of anesthesia.

PHYSICAL EXAMINATION

Examination of the respiratory system can be accomplished simply, and much information can be gained from inspec-

Table 1.3.
Simplified Shunt Equation

$$\frac{P_b - 47 - P_{aCO2} - P_{aO2}}{20}$$

$$\frac{760 - 47 - 40 - 513}{20} = 8\%$$

A simplified shunt equation derived from an arterial oxygen sample taken with the patient breathing 100 per cent oxygen will estimate the degree of shunt. P_b represents the atmospheric pressure; from it are subtracted standard values for arterial water vapor and carbon dioxide tension. The arteriovenous oxygen consumption is an assumed value.

tion. Rate of respiration should be noted. Inspection of the chest wall reveals any abnormalities of anatomy, distortion indicating the likelihood of pulmonary problems. The trachea should be central, and the movements of the chest wall equal. The stethoscope is useful in the detection of bronchial constriction, and moist sounds indicate the presence of fluid in the alveoli. If auscultation reveals a problem, the outpatient should be deferred for further evaluation. The chest X-ray may be of immeasurable diagnostic value, although it will not diagnose bronchospasm.

A useful evalation of the respiratory system can be made by asking the patient to cough. It is our practice to have the patient cough when he sits in the chair prior to anesthesia. It has two functions: it eliminates loose mucus in the upper airway which could predispose to laryngeal stridor and respiratory problems following induction, and, secondly, it serves as a diagnostic measure to detect if the patient has developed a recent respiratory infection. A paroxysm of coughing following the cough indicates the need for reevaluation.

The air necessary to produce an effective cough is estimated to be twice the tidal volume. Close observation of the effectiveness of the cough gives important clinical information regarding the pulmonary status of the patient. Alterations and reduction of the cough are positive clinical signs of reduced lung function and an indication for more definitive pulmonary function evaluation.

Breath Holding Test

When this test is performed, the patient should not be allowed to hyperventilate before evaluation is made. It will othewise increase the ability to hold the breath. The patient is asked to hold his breath; the normal length is for 30 seconds. Twenty seconds indicates a decrease in reserve and 15 seconds or less indicates pulmonary disease.

Match Test

The patient attempts to blow out the flame of a standard match held 6 inches away from his open mouth. It is important to emphasize the open mouth as the emphysematous patient purses the lips to produce expiratory resistance, decrease trapping, and increase the airway flow. Patients who cannot blow out the match require further evaluation. It is a good index of airway lower obstruction but not a test to compare against other data, but against personal standards.

Peak Expiratory Flow

Peak expiratory flow is evaluated with a peak flow meter, normally 400 to 600 liters per minute, and is a useful evaluation of autonomic effects as change with bronchospasm is evident. It is unaffected by central depression, which should be appreciated in postoperative evaluation of ventilation, when the patient has received narcotics.

Clinical evaluation of peak expiratory flow rate can be accomplished by requesting the patient to take a breath to full inspiratory capacity and then blow out all the air as fast as possible. Any time greater than 5 seconds should increase the suspicion of pulmonary dysfunction and require further pulmonary evaluation.

Forced Expiratory Volume

This is the volume exhaled in a unit of time, normally 1 second from the start of expiration. Seventy-five per cent of the vital capacity can be expired in the normal patient, and less than 70 per cent indicates airway obstruction.

Timed Vital Capacity

It is important that vital capacity be measured over a unit of time, as the patient with emphysema can expire all the gas in the lung if sufficient time is allowed for expiration.

Maximum Breathing Capacity

This is the maximal volume of air that can be breathed per minute. It is measured over a 15-second period and expressed as flow per minute. The average is 120 liters per minute. It is an exhausting test and of little practical value, but it is noted as a concept of measurement of ventilatory performance.

Cardiovascular System

SIGNIFICANT CARDIOVASCULAR ANATOMY AND PHYSIOLOGY RELATIVE TO PREOPERATIVE EVALUATION

The heart is a muscular organ which, under resting conditions, has tremendous reserve capacity. The resting cardiac output may be 3 to 5 liters per minute, and during severe exercise it can rise to 16 to 20 liters per minute. The left side of the heart is required to push blood over long distances into a vascular bed with a high resistance. The right ventricle, however, is required to generate flow only against slight vascular resistance in the pulmonary bed.

The cardiac muscle possesses special properties, unique in that spontaneous contraction can occur at rapid rates. It also conducts impulses over the muscle without nerves.

The greater the initial or resting stretch of a muscle, the greater will be the strength of contraction. In other words, the longer the diastole, the greater the filling, the more myocardium is stretched and the greater the next contraction. The Starling curve is used to evaluate cardiac activity (Fig. 1.3). The effects of anesthetic agents on contractility have been measured and the Starling curves are often used by pharmacologists to illustrate the direct effects of these agents on isolated heart muscle. All anesthetic agents depress the function of the isolated heart and in general are dose-related responses. There is inherent rhythmicity in special areas of the heart. The normal pathway of conduction for the heart is from the sinoatrial node over the atrial wall to the atrioventricular node, from thence to the ventricular septum and walls of the ventricle to cause a pattern of excitation which initiates the organized contraction of the ventricle. This electrical activity can be measured by the electrocardiogram. Abnormalities of conduction are significant as they can indicate possibilities of an impaired blood supply, changes in the excitability of the myocardium, or irregularities of the normal electrical sequence of depolarization. Cardiac output can be affected by arrythmias, as the stroke volume can be reduced by the shortened diastolic filling time, or if there is a fixed heart rate. In the preoperative evaluation, the electrocardiogram provides a useful baseline. However, many patients with severe myocardial disease exhibit a normal electrocardiogram. The heart muscle is supplied by coronary blood flow. The right and left coronary arteries show collateral circulation as aging proceeds. The coronary blood flow is related to pressure differences between aorta and right atrium and the resistance to flow in the arteries. Thus, flow is controlled by the effective pressure and resistance in the vessels. The resistance in the extramuscular portion of the coronary arteries is negligible compared to that in

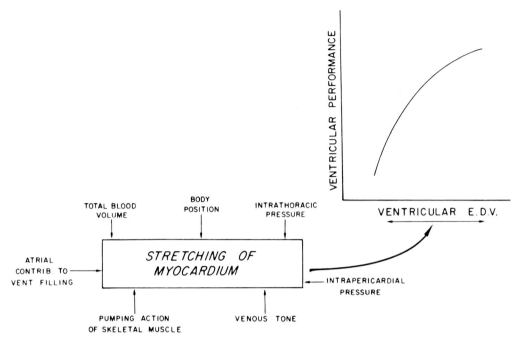

Figure 1.3. The Starling curve relates end-diastolic volume to ventricular performance. The influences which determine the degree of myocardial stretching or end-diastolic volume are shown. (Reprinted with permission from Braunwald, E., Ross, J., Jr., and Sonnenblick, E.H.: *Mechanisms of Contraction of the Normal and Failing Heart*, vol 277. Boston, Little, Brown, 1968, p 1012.)

the intramuscular portion. The resistance is controlled by active changes in the smooth muscle in the walls of the vessel and the mechanical effect on flow exerted during systole by the large massive muscles around the coronary vessels. Mean arterial pressure may also be important in maintaining flow during stress. The greatest flow occurs during diastole when coronary pressure is greatest and isometric relaxation of the muscles has begun. Thus coronary flow during the resting stage is related to diastolic pressure.

The arterial system serves to conduct blood to the tissues and to store the pressure generated by the left ventricle. There is a tendency of the arterial tree to return to its normal capacity. Elasticity allows the pressure to remain well above the capillary pressure throughout the cardiac cycle and allows regulation of the flow to various tissues by the arterioles. The driving pressure forcing blood across tissue beds is the mean arterial pressure. The

diastolic pressure contributes most of the mean pressure; mean arterial pressure is approximately equal to the diastolic pressure plus one third of the pulse pressure.

In the arteriolar bed, vessels change from passive elastic tubes to muscular active tubes. The largest resistance to flow is found in the arteriolar system. The total peripheral resistance can be altered by the vessels constricting or dilatating. It is important to appreciate that different arteriolar beds constrict or dilatate simultaneously and changes in total peripheral resistance do not mean equal constriction of all arterioles.

The arterioles change to the microcirculation: the metarterioles, the precapillary sphincter, the true capillary, and the small venules. The microcirculation system is independent of the central and autonomic nervous system controls, being regulated solely by the local factors O_2 and CO_2 tension and pH. The flow in the majority of the capillaries, however, is intermittent, as precapillary sphincters open and close. Anesthetics affect the vasomotor activity. The veins serve as the return system from the periphery. There is a pressure gradient, highest at the venous end of the capillaries and the lowest in the right atrium. The driving force is the remnant of the arterial pressure, transmitted through the capillary beds. In addition, negative intrathoracic pressure aids this driving force. The venous system serves as a volume reservoir with 70 per cent of the blood volume being contained in the veins at any time. Normal right atrial pressure of 4 to 6 cm H_2O is due to this value. The venous tree is not passive, as a considerable quantity of smooth muscle is present within the walls and can readily contract.

Coronary Circulation

The coronary circulation normally receives 5 per cent of the cardiac output, i.e., 200 ml, which can expand to 1500 ml. The flow is particularly affected by blood pressure, anoxia, and increased resistance in the aorta.

Pulmonary Circulation

Pulmonary circulation receives the majority of the cardiac output. The pulmonary vessels are a low pressure system which only offer 1/10 of the resistance to flow of the systematic circulation; thus, pressure is 25/8 mm Hg. There is a great increase in cardiac work if this pressure is increased. The vasomotor control is primarily dependent on local factors, tissue hypoxia and hypercarbia. The arterioles constrict to shunt blood to areas where gas exchange can occur. The distribution of blood flow in the lungs is affected by gravity in that higher lobes have smaller blood flow. A 400- to 600-ml reservoir of blood is contained in the lungs.

CEREBRAL BLOOD FLOW

Cerebral blood flow amounts to 15 per cent of the cardiac output or 800 ml. In addition to mean arterial pressure, a major control of cerebral blood flow is carbon dioxide tension. In neurosurgical anesthesia, advantage is taken of this by lowering the tension by hyperventilation and thus decreasing cerebral blood flow, and consequently shrinking the brain. Excess carbon dioxide tension results in vasodilatation and subsequent headache.

RENAL BLOOD FLOW

Thirty per cent of the cardiac output, or 1600 ml, passes through the kidney. The critical closing pressure in the kidney is 60 mm Hg. The pressure at which the arterioles to an organ close is of great significance, as it is an important homeostatic mechanism to preserve an adequate blood pressure in selected organs during hypotension and shock. The kidney is the only organ in which this can be measured routinely by presence or absence of urine flow. During shock the adequacy of perfusion is related to urine output, an acceptable minimum being 50 ml of urine per hour.

PORTAL CIRCULATION

The liver receives 40 per cent of the cardiac output or 2000 ml. An important feature is the low PaO_2 (40 mm Hg) in the blood supplying the liver. The liver is thus uniquely sensitive to hypoxia and hypercarbia. Hepatotoxicity develops when there is decreased oxygen or increased carbon dioxide tension.

Control of Circulation

Cardiac and vasomotor centers are in the midbrain. They have a spontaneous activity which can be detected in the floor of the fourth ventricle, and they relay impulses via the sympathetic and vagal nerves to the heart. The right vagus supplies the sinoatrial node, the left vagus the atrioventricular node. The parasympathetic impulses are inhibitors.

The sympathetics are accelerators and augment heart action. The fibers arise in the lateral horn cells in segments T3 and T4. Some fibers pass directly to the heart as thoracic cardiac nerves, the others to the inferior, middle, and superior cervical ganglia whence the cardiac nerves pass to the heart. Activation of the sympathetic nervous system is a nonspecific response from anywhere in the body. It results in tachycardia, hypertension, hypercarbia, hyperglycemia, and increased free fatty acids. Sympathetic stimulation may increase myocardial oxygen consumption and the electrophysiological alterations in the cellular level may produce alterations in cardiac function and rhythmicity. It is also known to decrease the threshold for ventricular fibrillation. These can be prevented by β-adrenergic blocking agents or adequate anesthesia. Reflex vagal stimulation can occur when specific areas of the body are stimulated. It results in bradycardia and hypotension. Cardiac arrest can occur from vagal activity in the presence of hypoxia and hypercarbia. Specific areas which give rise to vagal effects are the eyeball and ocular muscle, the larynx, lung, mesentery, and peritoneum. In addition, stimulation of the anus, bladder, and periosteum may occasionally give rise to vagal activity. Vagal effects are nearly complete within 1 second, but sympathetic effects are only 90 per cent complete in 30 seconds; thus, given maximal simultaneous activation of both systems, vagal effects will predominate early with balance achieved later.

The effects of blood gases on the vascular system are complicated by the fact that direct effects can be overridden by reflex effects. Thus, hypoxia will directly depress the vascular system and central nervous system, but hypoxia stimulates the chemoreceptors and reflexly stimulates the heart and vascular system. The effects of CO_2 and pH changes are even more complex; thus, metabolic acidosis depresses the vascular system. However, respiratory acidosis results in myocardial stimulation and peripheral vasodilation. The stimulatory effects of CO_2 can be overwhelmed by other agents such as

deep anesthesia and a severe depression of pH.

PHYSICAL EXAMINATION

The patient's exercise tolerance is by far the most helpful single criterion for the evaluation of his cardiovascular status. An excellent evaluation of exercise tolerance is to escort the patient on a short walk up a flight of stairs, checking blood pressure and heart rate before and after, and looking for evidence of fatigue, dyspnea, and anginal pain. There is no indication for any further physical evaluation of the patient's exercise tolerance in dental anesthetic practice.

Peripheral edema, ascites, engorgement in neck veins, and hepatomegaly are indicative of right-sided heart failure, some of which can be noted on superficial examination of the patient.

An examination of the pulse reveals many features. Cardiac rate in excess of 180 beats per minute can produce cardiac failure due to inadequate filling (Fig. 1.4). A resting pulse in the normal adult male is in the range of 70 beats per minute. A rate below 50 or above 90 after rest indicates possible disease and necessitates further evaluation. The character of the pulse is important. A full and pounding pulse indicates fever and/or evidence of peripheral vasodilation. Rhythm should be noted, and cardiac irregularities are

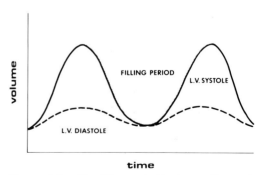

Figure 1.4. The filling period in the cardiac cycle occurs during ventricular diastole. If the cardiac rate is increased, then cardiac filling may be inadequate. It demonstrates tachycardia as a cardiac arrhythmia.

readily detected. Palpation of the vessel wall detects thickening or hardening.

It is important to check the position of apex beat and heart size before auscultation of the heart sounds. The vibrations produced in the heart during this contraction are heard as sounds. The sounds are produced by contractions of the ventricle, the closure of the aortic and pulmonary valves, and the vibrations in the chorda tendineae. Irregularity of closure of the valves can produce split sounds, which indicate imbalance between the right and left sides of the heart. Triple rhythm is due to the sound of atrial contraction as in a diseased heart there is actual contraction of the atrium to allow explosive filling of the ventricle. Triple rhythm is an early index of cardiac disease. It is difficult to compare patients, but changes in the same patient are obvious and have considerable significance; hence the importance of preoperative assessment.

The anesthetist can be expected to recognize some classical murmurs, but any murmur which is unusual would be better referred to a cardiologist for an opinion.

A systolic murmur unrelated to any pathology is a frequent finding. If all other symptoms and signs of the cardiorespiratory system are normal, it is reasonable to assume that the systolic murmur is functional and of no significance. It may, however, indicate mitral valve prolapse, a cause of fainting or cardiac arrhythmia occurring prior to or during treatment. Similarly, split heart sounds, indicative of right and left imbalance, are of no clinical significance in the conduct of routine dental anesthesia and, if detected prior to induction of anesthesia, only merit notation in the case report.

Blood Pressure

Blood pressure estimation should be evaluated in every patient presenting for any form of dental treatment and pain control, be it local or general anesthesia, sedation or inhalation analgesia. In the patient's record a note should be made of the blood pressure and the arm on which it was recorded as the variance between arms is considerable (e.g., 120/80 R).

The blood pressure is usually determined by auscultation determining systolic and diastolic blood pressure by the Korotkov sounds. Another useful alternative is by oscillometer, but this may give a false high reading.

Blood pressure develops from the product of cardiac output and peripheral resistance. Anesthesia can affect both factors, and thus blood pressure is a significant measurement if drugs are to be administered to patients.

Cardiac Output

Cardiac output is dependent upon adequate venous return. The negative intrathoracic pressure aids venous return, and thus alteration by intermittent positive pressure ventilation may reduce venous return. The tone in the walls of the vein, vasomotor tone in the arterioles, the influence of muscular contractions, the muscle pump, and gravity all affect venous return and are liable to be influenced by the drugs used in pain control. The legs can contain 500 ml of blood, a convenient reservoir for return of blood to the heart. Force of contraction of the heart affects cardiac output and is dependent upon the initial length of the myocardial fiber. Adequate venous return and blood volume influence the stretching of muscle fibers and thus are influenced by preoperative dehydration and blood loss in multiple odontectomy. If the cardiac rate is increased, the cardiac output is increased, as with the adminstration of methohexital or atropine.

The falls in blood pressure seen with the drugs used for pain control are usually due to falls in total peripheral resistance. The elasticity of the vessels is decreased as age advances, and the rigid vessel causes rises in blood pressure. Viscosity of the blood affects the total peripheral resistance, and it can be reduced by intravenous fluids and increases in temperature.

Special Tests

It should be noted that many diseased hearts have a normal electrocardiogram, and preoperative assessment of the electrocardiogram may only be indicated as a routine in those patients over 40 years of age, who is to have general anesthesia, or if there are indications of a cardiac problem.

SPECIAL PROBLEMS

Cardiorespiratory evaluation is indicated in all patients prior to therapy. There are, however, circumstances when other systems should be examined and evaluated.

CENTRAL NERVOUS SYSTEM

The patient may be referred for restorative dentistry or for multiple odontectomy under general anesthesia, because of neurological problems. A complete work-up will have been recorded by a neurologist, but some attempt should be made by the anesthetist to define the area and limitations of the disease. It should be stressed that all neurological deficits which have occurred and have been attributed to subarachnoid block have been noted with general anesthesia.

Simple tests are 1) the pupillary response to light and conversion, 2) the presence or absence of nystagmus, 3) reflexes readily elicited, such as triceps, biceps, knee jerk and plantar response, 4) motor function of arms, hands, legs, and feet.

MUSCULOSKELETAL SYSTEM

Limited movement is significantly of note, especially when a musculoskeletal disorder is present. Under general anesthesia, especially if muscle relaxants have been given, stretching of the ligaments can occur. Thus, the protective contractures are lost and the patient suffers extreme pain in the joints following the anesthetic. Trismus of masticatory muscles or ankylosis of the temporomandibular joint limit mouth opening, a potential problem in direct laryngoscopy. A disease of the musculoskeletal system which produces hazard in general anesthesia is kyphoscoliosis or lordosis as restriction of respiratory excursion occurs.

Specific Evaluations for General Anesthesia, Sedation or Analgesia

INTRAVENOUS

It is important at the first examination to check the patient for good veins. If necessary, it is usually possible to dilatate veins on the back of the hand, the most useful location for intravenous medication. If none is readily available, warming of the hands will often display veins previously recognized. Occasionally a vein in the foot needs to be used, in which case an intravenous should be set up before induction of anesthesia. The more difficult the venous system for intravenous technique the more is it imperative that anesthesia not be induced until an open vein is available.

TEETH

The presence of loose teeth, loose fillings, and calculus should be noted in order that they not be dislodged prior to treatment. The critical time is during induction when the loose tooth can be dislodged.

NOSE

Deformities of the nose and nasal septum present hazards in the passage of a nasopharyngeal or nasoendotracheal tube. The fitting of the nasal mask over the nares is an important feature, and one may decide prior to induction of anesthesia whether nasal mask or nasopharyngeal tube should be used. A nasal vasoconstrictor spray as 0.5 per cent Neosynephrine nasal spray can be used prior to induction to determine if the patient can breath through the nose.

NECK

Airway maintenance is often difficult in the short bull-necked patient, as the larynx is attached close to the mandible, and it is difficult to maintain the jaw in a forward position. Such patients are best approached with caution.

Deviation of the trachea can also present problems during intubation.

CONGENITAL FEATURES

The patient with retrognathia, temporomandibular joint arthrosis, ankylosis, or fixed cervical spine is one of the greatest hazards for outpatient oral surgery.

In the black patient, a low hematocrit suggests that the sickle cell test be performed to preclude homozygous sickle cell disease or heterozygous hemoglobins (sickle trait). These individuals are extremely sensitive to hypoxia. It is imperative during anesthesia to ensure that no hypoxic incident occurs.

PSYCHOLOGICAL FEATURES

Many anesthetists consider that this aspect of the patient evaluation is grossly neglected. The psychological status of the patient is readily evaluated at interview. In the context of outpatient anesthesia this is adequate. If any psychological disorder is evident, a note is made on the chart.

MINIMAL LABORATORY WORK

The outpatient should be no less well treated than the inpatient, and minimal laboratory work is an essential part of preoperative evaluation. If the patient is admitted to the hospital prior to general anesthesia, it is a requirement that he have laboratory evaluation of hematocrit and urinanalysis. It is not indicated for analgesia and sedation unless specific indications are evident, but prior to outpatient general anesthesia this is essential. Meyer evaluated 1349 patients further with blood and urine tests after they had been judged fit for office general anesthesia for oral surgery. Nearly 11 per cent had abnormalities of the blood or urine which were significant. Another 1.8 per cent had previously undetected disease which was a direct contraindication to general anesthesia: diabetes mellitus, anemia, infectious mononucleosis, and leukemia. In addition, a significant service was provided to the dental patient in that occult diseases were referred for early treatment.

Hematocrit or Hemoglobin Level

A 30 per cent hematocrit or 10 g per 100 ml hemoglobin is the limiting amount for general anesthesia. Any result below these requires further evaluation prior to general anesthesia. It is imperative to have a predetermined limit, as it covers the range of error in the test. A repeat of the test and perhaps red blood cell count is indicated at the next evaluation if any abnormality is detected.

In the second trimester of pregnancy, there is an increase in blood volume with subsequent low hematocrit, but as nonurgent outpatient anesthesia is not essential at this time, it is not a problem to the dental anesthetist.

Urine

The presence of sugar or albumin in the urine is not a direct contraindication to anesthesia. It is necessary to evaluate these items, however (Fig. 1.5).

If sugar is detected, diabetes must be suspected and glycosuria be investigated by an internist. If the patient is found to have diabetes, it is more readily controlled prior to general anesthesia as a baseline therapy can be established.

If albumin is found, general anesthesia

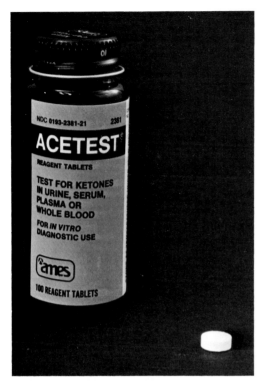

Figure 1.5. Laboratory tests can be readily performed by assistants with the aids available for the principal blood and urine reactions.

can proceed, and the patient is evaluated after operation.

Additional Laboratory Tests

These are not indicated for routine outpatient anesthesia. They may be necessary for major oral surgery, or if a bleeding diathesis is suspected, or if the patient has purpura. It may also be necessary to do these additional laboratory tests if the patient is on anticoagulant therapy, and if extensive regional blocks are to be performed.

BLOOD GROUP

It is important to remember that 1 in 1000 patients reacts to a blood transfusion. If it is possible to have accurate grouping and cross-matching before the need becomes urgent, it will be of benefit to the patient.

PROTHROMBIN TIME

A time of 12 to 15 seconds is normal for the control period but the control varies in different laboratories. The aim is to have a prothrombin time at least 60 per cent of control prior to anesthesia.

BLEEDING AND CLOTTING TIMES

These are useful if the patient has a bleeding diathesis or has been on anticoagulant therapy. A partial thromboplastin time (PTT) is a more accurate test of clotting time.

Bleeding time may be in excess of 10 minutes in those patients taking aspirin. Platelets become bound to aspirin, and it takes about 5 days to restore one third of the platelets after ceasing to take aspirin. In such cases, PTT and PT are normal.

SICK CELL SCREENING TEST

About 10 per cent of American blacks and 6 per cent of the Puerto Rican population have a sickle cell trait. If anemia is detected in this population, a simple diagnostic test should be performed which is positive to the abnormal hemoglobin.

PERMIT AND CHARTING

Prior to any procedure it is mandatory that the permit and signatures on the permit be checked and signed copies of both permit and postoperative instructions be retained in the chart.

It is a useful practice to have the patient sign the form on which his history has been recorded. There are many patients who deny problems in order that they may be treated without delay, or even some who consider that related medical problems are of no concern to anesthesia. Emphasis on the serious nature of pain control procedures does not have to frighten the patient; rather it can be an enlightening and educational process. All data both negative and positive should be noted, but it should be stressed that one should not neglect the patient in order to complete the chart. It is no excuse, however, not to have all data charted, as in the postoperative period data can be recorded which have been collected throughout the operative procedure. The record should be to protect the patient and anesthetist, not provide data for litigation.

There are many fine examples of preoperative evaluation cards, such as that of the American Dental Society of Anesthesiology, or that in *Accepted Dental Therapeutics*, 37th ed., by the Council on Dental Therapeutics of the American Dental Association, but as each operator's situation varies, his aim should be to develop his own card (Fig. 1.6). The advantage of this is that his secretary will accord with his wishes. A card or questionnaire which indicates the salient features saves time and prevents omissions.

Permit

The permit should indicate that informed consent has been obtained. The anesthetist should discuss the procedure with the patient, explaining the salient features of the technique. We consider it never advisable to persuade a patient to have any form of anesthesia which he does not consider suitable or safe. This does not mean that the patient will dictate his anesthetic, but that given a choice the patient's preference is important, especially if he exhibits anxiety over the type of anesthesia to be administered.

The signatures on the permit should be legible, if necessary printing the name under the signature.

The qualifications of any witnesses are essential, as they validate the informed consent. The doctor must be a witness, emphasizing that the patient has been informed and consented after discussion.

The patient must appreciate and have given permission for any anesthetic and medications considered necessary. It is useful not to restrict choice of anesthetic, as it may not be possible to fulfill the promised anesthetic technique. If there

are no veins available, it is not sensible so suggest that intravenous anesthesia will be used.

At this time explain and indicate any type of monitors which will be used on the patient. The sphygmomanometers, electrocardiographic leads, or chest stethoscopes may cause a problem if the patient has not been informed that they will be used for his safety.

The operation should be detailed and a notation made that there is freedom for any operative procedure that the surgeon considers necessary for the patient's well-being.

In any particular area it is imperative that the anesthetist be aware of the definition of the emancipated minor, and that he understand the responsibility of the accompanying adult who signs for a minor.

Chart

The following items should be listed on every chart:

Name: Sex: Referring doctor:
Age:
Current history:
Previous medical history:
Medications: Steroids
             Agents affecting blood pressure
             Monoamine oxidase inhibitors
             Tranquilizers
             Anticoagulants
             Others

If some index such as the above is used, it will give the individual anesthetist the opportunity to add other drugs to the list as the drug industry expands.

ORDERS AND PROCEDURES

It is imperative that instructions be given to the patient in the preoperative evaluation, not in the operating room after the patient has received premedication. Neither is it useful to give the patient instructions in the recovery room.

It is useful to develop a printed order sheet which is given to the outpatient—an essential in outpatient anesthetic practice as it alerts other doctors to problems.

MEDICAL HISTORY

Date_____

Name_____
Last   First   Middle

Address_____
Number & Street

City   State   Zip Code   Home & Business Phone

Date of Birth_____ Sex_____ Height_____ Weight_____ Occupation_____

Married_____ Spouse_____   Single_____

Closest Relative_____   Phone_____

If you are completing this form for another person, what is your relationship to that person?_____

PLEASE ANSWER EACH QUESTION

Check One
Yes No

1. Have you been a patient in a hospital during the past 2 years? .... ☐ ☐
2. Have you been under the care of a physician during the past 2 years? .... ☐ ☐
3. Have you taken any kind of medicine or drugs during the past year? .... ☐ ☐
4. Has anyone in your family been advised of difficulties during anesthesia? .... ☐ ☐
5. Are you allergic to penicillin, codeine or any other drugs or medicine? .... ☐ ☐
6. Have you ever had any excessive bleeding requiring special treatment? .... ☐ ☐
7. Circle any of the following which you have had:

heart trouble	asthma	arthritis
congenital heart lesions	cough	stroke
heart murmur	diabetes	epilepsy
high blood pressure	tuberculosis	psychiatric treatment
anemia	hepatitis	sinus trouble
rheumatic fever	jaundice	

8. (Women) Are you pregnant now? .... ☐ ☐
9. Have you had any other serious illnesses? .... ☐ ☐

   TO BE ANSWERED ONLY BY PATIENTS RECEIVING
   SEDATION OR GENERAL ANESTHESIA:

10. Have you had anything to eat or drink within the last 4 hours? .... ☐ ☐
11. Are you wearing a removable dental appliance? .... ☐ ☐
12. Are you wearing contact lenses? .... ☐ ☐
13. Who is to drive you home today?

    a. Name_____

Chief Dental Complaint:

Reviewed by_____   Signature_____

Figure 1.6. The chart suggested in *Accepted Dental Therapeutics* illustrates the principal features of an adequate medical history. Note family history to highlight the possibility of malignant hyperpyrexia.

If endotracheal intubation is used, this is noted.

A useful practice for the dentist who has evaluated the patient and found abnormalities is to refer him for evaluation by an internist. Not only is this good patient care, but it also establishes good rapport in the health care community.

Preoperative Orders

The patient should be NPO after midnight for a morning operation; for an afternoon operation, a light breakfast is indicated. In the case of general anesthesia there should be no compromise with the established rule that 4 hours elapse between oral intake of food or fluid and the administration of general anesthesia. Even an emergency operation in oral surgery practice can wait this period of time.

In the case of conscious sedation or analgesia, a light meal is indicated as nausea is more likely to develop with the empty stomach, and the risk of regurgitation with analgesia is slight and that of aspiration negligible.

It is mandatory that a responsible adult accompany the patient after outpatient anesthesia and some intravenous sedative techniques. It is useful to stipulate that the companion not be accompanied by other young children as they could interfere with patient care.

Make-up should not be used the day of operation, as it not only alters color changes in the patient, but often makes for difficult jaw maintenance. Eye make-up can produce conjunctivitis. The recent increase in use of false lashes is an additional hazard to outpatient anesthetic practice. Contact lenses should be removed.

The patient should void before anesthesia, and loose, nonconstrictive clothing be worn.

The patient should not be allowed to drive an automobile after the administration of general anesthesia. Driving after sedation or analgesia may be hazardous, and the dentist should indicate that there may be some mental impairment and that it is advisable not to drive. It is not yet clear as to how analgesia or influences recovery. Trieger's investigation of nitrous oxide-oxygen analgesia with the Bender-Gestalt test indicates that there is complete neurological recovery from nitrous oxide analgesia; however, it has been shown that traces of nitrous oxide are present in the blood up to 4 hours after brief exposure.

Postoperative Orders

A patient who has been intubated should receive a note to this effect, with necessary additional details. A return date should be indicated for postoperative assessment. If the patient is a referral, the procedure and medications should be indicated.

The patient should be instructed to avoid large meals the day of operation as these may induce vomiting. Alcohol or sedatives additional to those prescribed on the day of operation must be avoided as they may produce reversion to sedative levels. This is a particular hazard with diazepam. For surgical therapy we advo-cate cold compresses for treatment of the surgical problem. It is important, if possible, to maintain fluid balance by oral intake of fluids.

Special Orders

NURSING ORDERS

Medications for pain relief should be detailed, cortisone therapy noted, and for the diabetic the insulin requirement prescribed. Intravenous insulin is not recommended to correct hypoglycemia unless in the acute and emergent diabetic coma when continuous blood sugar samples can be evaluated. The use of regular crystalline insulin for the surgical patient via the subcutaneous route still remains the ideal method of administration. During long surgical procedures, if IV insulin is used, the electronegative particles adhere to the glass; thus the effect may be diminished. If this is appreciated, with an understanding that only small amounts of active insulin are required, then it can be an effective method of controlling the blood sugar.

TIME OF OPERATION

If possible, the first operation on the schedule should be reserved for diabetics, as there is less liability to disturbance of the pattern of glucose and insulin requirement early in the day. Children should be scheduled as early as possible to avoid starvation and dehydration. Children, with their relatively small blood volume, develop changes more rapidly than the adult.

If premedication is ordered, then it is critical that the exact time of the premedication be noted and that the nurse who administers the premedication write the time it was actually given on the chart.

FLUID REPLACEMENT

Intravenous fluids are recommended for operations which last longer than 15 minutes. The normal starved oral surgery outpatient has a 5 per cent blood volume deficit. These patients can all benefit from 500 cc of Ringer's lactate solution as it prevents orthostatic hypotension. No purgatives should be given.

Premedication

The relative value of patient consultation prior to administration of a drug is well illustrated by Egbert's work. The value of the preoperative assessment, evaluation, and discussion is incomparably greater for the patient than any possible drug combination. This is typified by the pediatric patient, where the careful establishment of rapport by the anesthetist is of immense value. Drug response is completely unpredictable in children, unless they are overmedicated. The danger of an unsupervised drug response should be stressed in the outpatient. If the outpatient is given oral premedication in an unsupervised situation, the anesthetist is responsible for any untoward reaction, and if for no other reason than medicolegal, the practice of giving oral premedication at home prior to an appointment should be avoided.

Frequently the premedication is not given at the time ordered. The problem is then worse than if none were given, as either the premedication has ceased to act if given too early, the patient is now alert without having had the operation, or cardiorespiratory depression is exaggerated during anesthesia.

Dosage of medication is usually weight related. There are individuals in whom it is not possible to predict the response, and consequently overmedication occurs or undermedication does not produce the desired effect.

USES OF PREMEDICATION

Premedication is used to decrease apprehension and fear, to facilitate induction of anesthesia, to produce amnesia, to decrease the basal metabolic rate, to decrease the oxygen requirement, to decrease the amount of anesthesia required, to decrease the possible toxic reaction to local anesthesia, to decrease reflex excitability, and to decrease secretions.

DISADVANTAGES OF PREMEDICATION

There may be an increase in anxiety in patients who prefer to be alert, often evident in either very intelligent people or those who have never had alcohol. Some of the disadvantages of premedication are delay of induction of anesthesia if inhalation methods are used, decrease in the metabolism of the patient when it should be increased to cope with the anesthetic problems, decrease in oxygenation of the patient due to respiratory depression, if a potent agent is used, the combined effect could give severe cardiorespiratory depression; the concept that the toxic reactions to local anesthetics are reduced by barbiturates is fallacious; it requires 100 times the average dose of anticholinergic drugs to block vagal reflexes totally (dry secretions can lead to atelectasis, and a dry mouth is a frequent patient complaint); recent studies have shown that the minimal anesthetic requirement is reduced minimally be premedication.

SPECIAL INDICATIONS

Premedication should be given only when a finite indication exists. For pain, analgesics prior to the operation, although they do not reduce the anesthetic requirement, do make the patient more comfortable. If an intravenous induction is to be used, there is no indication for withholding of analgesics.

In the asthmatic patient diphenhydrazine (Benadryl) is often a useful sedative producing sleep. It allows the anesthetist to avoid opiates which are not indicated in the asthmatic because of histamine release.

The use of atropine to decrease oral secretions may be indicated.

Agents

The pharmacology of these agents is also discussed in the section on intravenous agents (Table 1.4).

Narcotics

These agents are given for their mood-elevating properties rather than for the production of analgesia. Prolonged respiratory depression can occur with such agents. Vomiting is a frequent side effect occurring in up to 50 per cent of those who receive a narcotic. The narcotics used principally are: 1) morphine, in the dose of 0.15 mg per kg, the average adult dose being 10 to 15 mg; and 2) meperidine, 1.0 mg per kg, the average dose for an adult male being 50 to 100 mg. There is little cardiovascular depression with morphine, but meperidine frequently causes severe falls in blood pressure. It offers little advantage over morphine, as the mood-elevating property is not great. The advantages of meperidine are its useful side effects: an atropine-like action, decreasing secretions, and a quinidine-like action on the myocardium, reducing the incidence of arrhythmias.

Another major problem with narcotics is that they may release histamine, possibly resulting in circulatory collapse in addition to producing urticarial wheals and bronchiolar constriction.

Table 1.4.
Sedative Hypnotic Equivalents

Drug	Oral Dose
	mg
Alcohol (100 proof)	90 ml (3 oz)
Chloral hydrate (Noctec)	1000
Chlordiazepoxide (Librium)	25
Diazepam (Valium)	10
Diphenhydramine (Benadryl)	50–100
Ethchlorvynol (Placidyl)	750
Flurazepam (Dalmane)	30
Glutethimide (Doriden)	500
Hydroxyzine (Vistaril)	50–100
Meprobamate (Equanil)	400
Methaqualone (Quaalude)	300
Pentobarbital (Nembutal)	100
Secobarbital (Seconal)	100

Barbiturates

With pentobarbital (1.0 mg per kg) the average adult dose is 50 to 150 mg (Nembutal). Other similar drugs are secobarbital in 100- to 200-mg doses and amylobarbitone, 200-mg doses. They may make the patient restless as they are only sedative without analgesic properties and are therefore often combined with a narcotic. These medium acting barbiturates are useful preanesthetic sedatives as they induce sleep and allay anxiety without depressing the central nervous system as much as opiates. They are of especial value if given orally the night before operation for sleep. The intravenous dose is effective and certain if given immediately prior to anesthesia but oral premedication along with 1.5 oz of water is often used 1½ hours before operation. Overdose of the drug can produce coma and cardiorespiratory depression.

Nonbarbiturate Sedatives

With chloral hydrate, the dosage is 0.5 to 1.0 g orally, and with glutethimide (Doriden) it is 250 to 500 mg orally. Chloral hydrate is a useful hypnotic which has an onset in less than 1 hour and lasts for about 8 hours. It leaves no hangover and is extremely safe. It is supplied in tablet form which causes less gastric irritation than solutions. Glutethimide is an analog of bemegride, a central nervous stimulant. It is a useful nonbarbiturate hypnotic similar in action to the medium acting barbiturate. Onset occurs within 45 minutes and the duration of action is for about 6 hours. Flurazepam (Dalmane) can be included in this group as a hypnotic that is useful for sedation the night before operation. Induction of sleep is rapid in the dose of 15 to 30 mg.

Ataractics

These drugs have potent effects. The principal ones are chlorpromazine (50 mg or 0.5 mg per kg), hydroxyzine (Atarax, Vistaril) (0.5 mg per kg; dose 25 to 50 mg), promethazine (Phenergan) (0.5 mg per kg;

25 to 50 mg). These drugs are given for their ataractic action and have potent antiemetic actions. Fall in blood pressure is an effect which is undesirable, and hydroxyzine is probably the least culpable in this respect. These drugs have an onset of 20 to 25 minutes if given intramuscularly and a duration of 3 hours. They can be given alone or in combination with other agents for preoperative sedation.

Benzodiazepines

The use of 10 mg of diazepam either orally or intravenously as premedication is a well established technique for adults. Relief of anxiety is a major feature. Lorazepam (Ativan), 2 to 4 mg, has recently been introduced into practice as an oral premedication. It is most useful for the production of a profound amnesia. It is also readily absorbed after intramuscular injection in contrast to diazepam, which has a slow and uncertain absorption by the intramuscular route.

Anticholinergic Drugs

The administration of these drugs for children should be related to weight. For the average adult, the dose range for atropine is 0.6 to 0.4 mg and for scopolamine, 0.4 mg. They have differing spectra of activity, and selection should be made for the unique property required. Atropine produces better vagal block while scopolamine is the better drying agent. Administered intramuscularly in normal clinical dosage, these drugs cannot be relied upon to eliminate all possible sources of arrhythmia, especially succinylcholine-related arrhythmias.

Atropine has no effect on the psyche and produces no sedation. There is an increase in respiratory dead space because of bronchial dilatation. Tachycardia occurs because of partial vagal blocking, and there is a drying effect on the mouth. Atropine is contraindicated in glaucoma, as it closes the drainage of aqueous through the canals of Schlemm. Eye signs for indication of depth of anesthesia cannot be used because of action on the iris.

Scopolamine is a central nervous system depressant causing drowsiness, sleep, and amnesia. This latter is the most useful property. It is not indicated in old patients as they become agitated. Scopolamine is a better antisialogogic than atropine. After an initial dose of scopolamine, tachycardia develops, but a secondary bradycardia which lasts up to 3 hours can develop.

Glycopyrrolate is a synthetic quaternary ammonium anticholinergic agent which has been shown to be superior to atropine and scopolamine in antimuscarinic activity. It will not cross the blood brain barrier and therefore does not produce delirium as does scopolamine. It is twice as potent as atropine in antisialagogue activity, and has three times the duration. Significant is the reduction in the incidence of dysrhythmias, and less initial tachycardia is produced. When used with neostigmine, it decreases the incidence of bradycardia. It may be of significant value in reducing the gastric pH which usually is above 2.5 when glycopyrrolate is used as a premedicant.

Combinations of Drugs

The usual combination of drugs is to prescribe a barbiturate the night before operation. The morning of operation it is usual to give an opiate plus an ataractic and an anticholinergic drug. These combinations have proven most satisfactory for those who advocate routine heavy premedication. The ataractic, together with an analgesic and an anticholinergic like scopolamine, results in a tranquil, relaxed patient. They must be given 45 minutes to 60 minutes preoperatively to be effective.

ROUTE OF ADMINISTRATION OF PREMEDICATION

Intramuscular

The disadvantage of the intramuscular injection is that it is painful for the child but has the advantage that the child may then only dislike the nurse and not the anesthetist. If the dosage is accurately predicted, the result is excellent. Onset of sedation occurs within 20 minutes and lasts for up to 1½ hours.

Subcutaneous

The disadvantage of subcutaneous injection is lack of predictability of onset of action. Although it can be given by less skilled personnel, absorption may be delayed for up to 1½ hours. Duration of action, of course, is then correspondingly increased.

Intravenous

This is a simple and rapid method of giving premedication. In some respects it is the most valuable method, as not only can the effect be sure, but the dose can be titrated to produce the required effects. It is the method of choice for the outpatient, as responsible premedication cannot be given until the patient reaches the office. Hydroxyzine should not be given intravenously as thrombophlebitis has been shown to be a frequent complication.

Oral

The oral route produces uncertain reactions, and the patient will be taking the oral medication prior to leaving the house. It has been shown that, provided absorption is satisfactory, there is little hazard of regurgitation. Absorption is unpredictable in the anxious patient.

Rectal

Barbiturates can be given rectally and are useful sedatives in children and the handicapped. The suppository may be inserted under the guise of taking the temperature.

Children

Dosage is based on weight and varies between heavy and complete sedation to use of only anticholinergic drugs. It is difficult to predict the right dose; the best method is to win the confidence of the child.

The dose range for parenteral premedicant drugs is: morphine, 0.1 mg per lb to a maximum of 10 mg; meperidine, 0.5 mg per lb to a maximum of 75 mg; pentobarbital, 2 mg per lb to a maximum of 150 mg; chloral hydrate, 10 mg per lb to a maximum of 500 mg; atropine or scopolamine, 0.01 mg per lb to a maximum of 0.4 mg.

Procedures

The following pattern should be followed for all patients when they present for outpatient general anesthesia for oral surgery or restorative dentistry. If the patient has had a failed local anesthetic that day, then it is advisable to postpone the procedure until the following day as there is a high level of circulating endogenous catecholamines in addition to the drugs containing epinephrine already administered for local anesthesia. It is an additional hazard predisposing to cardiac arrhythmias.

The chart and permit should be checked. The patient should be spoken to and name checked. The operation should be reviewed briefly with the patient and the chart reviewed in order to ensure that preoperative orders have been performed.

The patient should then be checked for spectacles, contact lenses, false eyelashes, dentures (in particular partial dentures), and, in children, it is advisable to check the cheek for chewing gum and the nose for foreign bodies. Prior to the administration of the anesthetic a check should be made to ensure that a responsible adult is available to accompany the patient home. The operation can then proceed.

HYPNOSIS IN DENTISTRY
Why Hypnosis Is Relevant to Dentistry

Though this idea may surprise some dental patients, most dentists want their patients to be comfortable and relaxed.

Chemical anesthetics cannot accomplish that comfort for every patient in every situation. Some patients are frightened and tense and their attitudes create a painful experience, no matter how well anesthetized are the nerves of their teeth. Some patients present difficulties, either biochemical or anatomical, that prevent successful local anesthetic blocks. In both cases, the patient needs the psychological support of the dentist. That is, the patient needs to know that the dentist can still take care of the patient, that the patient is not being "uncooperative," and that the patient does not need to anticipate suffering from pain. One of the most powerful tools of psychological support the dentist has is the skillful use of hypnosis.

Hypnosis has a wide range of therapeutic applications in dentistry, among which are the following:

PATIENT RELAXATION

A tense patient can be rapidly relaxed through hypnosis, preventing the difficulties that tension can bring (including headache, backache, and facial pain).

ANXIETY REDUCTION

An anxious patient can create potential behavior problems, thus actualizing their fears about pain. The skillful use of hypnosis can prevent this and can also result in the re-education of the patient, creating an unusually "good" patient.

ORTHODONTURE

Some patients have unnecessary objections to orthodontic or prosthodontic appliances, or to the proper care of them. Hypnotic education can result in proper acceptance and care of such appliances.

MAINTENANCE OF COMFORT DURING EXTENSIVE TREATMENT

During long periods of dental work, patients can become overly fatigued. Prior use of hypnosis can prevent this, thereby potentially increasing the efficiency of dental appointments.

MODIFICATION OF NOXIOUS DENTAL HABITS

Dental habits such as thumb sucking, tongue thrusting, and bruxing can all be effectively treated with the proper use of hypnosis.

The operative use of hypnosis in dentistry include:

REDUCTION OF THE NEED FOR ANESTHESIA OR ANALGESIA

Use of hypnotic suggestions for pain control can significantly reduce, even eliminate, the need for chemoanesthesia or analgesia.

POSTOPERATIVE ANALGESIA

Patients who undergo operative procedures need suffer no postoperative discomfort if hypnosis is used prior to or during the procedure.

SUBSTITUTION FOR PREMEDICATION IN GENERAL ANESTHESIA

Premedication can be reduced, even eliminated, if hypnosis is used to promote relaxation and quiescence.

CONTROL OF REFLEX AND AUTONOMIC PROCESSES

Hypnosis can be used to eliminate gagging and nausea and can be used to control salivary flow and bleeding. The effectiveness of this is demonstrable and dramatic.

MANAGEMENT OF DIFFICULT PATIENTS

Emotionally disturbed or mentally retarded patients, or those with motor spasticity, can be effectively managed if the use of hypnosis is integrated with proper dental care.

History, In Brief

We are in the midst of an explosive increase in the use of hypnosis in dentistry, an increase that began in the middle of the 19th century, when in 1837 a case of tooth extraction using hypnosis as the sole anesthetic was first reported. While dentistry has always pioneered in the clinical development of hypnosis, clinicians from psychology and medicine have also contributed to our current knowledge. Anton Mesmer may have been the first physician to widely demonstrate the clinical efficacy of hypnosis (though he conceived of it as animal magnetism). Throughout the 19th century, however, Braid, Charcot, Liebeault, and Bernheim demonstrated that hypnosis was a phenomenon of widespread occurrence and could be utilized for a wide variety of medical and psychological treatments. In the early 20th century, Freud and then McDougall and Hull elucidated more fully the psychological nature of hypnosis and its use as a tool in psychoanalysis, and it became progressively widespread until in the 1930s when Milton Erickson, a psychiatrist, developed an innovative integration of hypnosis into non-Freudian psychotherapy—a radical and effective departure.

Currently, hypnosis is used throughout the world by skilled clinicians in dentistry, psychology, and medicine, and its basis as a natural human experience is becoming better understood. In many many medical and dental schools throughout the country, hypnosis is taught as a treatment of pain and anxiety, as well as a tool for resolving those problems discussed previously.

Modern Conception of Hypnosis

Although hypnosis has at various times been explained as a mystical event, or a magnetic one, or one involving imagination, the modern and most widely accepted conceptualization of hypnosis is as an altered state of consciousness characterized by narrowed, heightened attention, and the capacity for producing alterations in memory and perception. Professor Ernest Hilgard has recently provided a theoretical basis for understanding hypnotic control of pain. Briefly, his neo-dissociation theory suggests that the special state of consciousness created by hypnosis creates interruption in the usual afferent flow of information to consciousness and that, while the information (sensory pain) may be appreciated at lower levels of consciousness, even at an "unconscious" level, this interruption prevents conscious awareness of the information.

It is difficult to measure physiological correlates of the hypnotic state that differ from those of the normal waking state. Recently, however, Saletu and colleagues reported that there are significant features of the EEG that characterize the hypnotic state, features that differ from the normal waking EEG. Further, these investigators found that the sensory evoked potential (SEP)—the electrical event in the brain that reflects awareness of a sensory stimulus—is modified when the individual is made hypnotically analgesic to the stimulus. No other physiological correlate has been demonstrated to uniquely characterize the hypnotic state, however. (This is not surprising when you consider that a state as dramatically different from waking consciousness as sleep also does not have uniquely different autonomic characteristics.)

There are no dangers intrinsic to the hypnotic state, even though myths still abound about people who "never wake up," or people who have been coerced through the power of hypnosis to do outrageous or illegal acts. There is no demonstrated case of an individual being made to do something through hypnosis that the individual could not have been made to do in the absence of hypnosis.

Obstacles to Use in Clinical Dentistry

Considering the apparent value of hypnosis in dentistry, associated with no danger, one may wonder why it is not even more widely used. If you were to survey clinicians who do not integrate the use of hypnosis into their practices, you would probably hear three prominent reasons why:

1. *"Hypnosis is too time consuming."* It is believed by some that in order to use hypnosis with a patient, significant time must be taken for doing so. This creates a problem of practicality, since, for the clinician, time is money.

The question, however, is: What is the alternative when hypnosis is needed? When a patient is too anxious to behave cooperatively, or who gags excessively, or who is an anesthetic risk, what low-risk alternative is there? Hypnosis provides the most effective treatment for these problems.

And the fact is that, if used appropriately, hypnosis can be a *time-saver.* Time that otherwise would be taken up with continually coping with the difficult patient is time that can be invested in teaching that patient, through hypnosis, how to be comfortable throughout the dental appointment. Used skillfully, hypnosis need not be time consuming at all.

Some dentists like to use nitrous oxide sedation as an efficient adjunct to the use of hypnosis. We have found experimentally what dentists have reported anecdotally for years: that nitrous oxide sedation produces a remarkably hypnotic-like state characterized by high receptivity to suggestion, including suggestion for analgesia. Consequently, rapid sedation with nitrous oxide can sometimes appropriately substitute for a more usual hypnotic induction.

Finally, dentists do need to communicate with patients. An understanding of the principles of hypnosis and suggestion can make that communication far more effective, even if no "formal" use of hypnosis is made.

2. *"Hypnosis is unethical because it leads to control of the patient's mind and personality."* This belief proceeds from the ancient myths that hypnosis can be used to control people's minds by "implanting" suggestions that will alter their behavior inappropriately and is perpetuated by the silly antics of stage hypnotists. There is no demonstrable evidence, either clinical or experimental, that suggests that hypnosis can be used to control someone's mind. On the contrary, there is ample evidence that shows that hypnosis does not create an automaton-like state; instead, it is clear that the deeply hypnotized person remains autonomous and quite able to reject any suggestions that would ordinarily be rejected in the waking state. It is important to understand that a *hypnotized person does not necessarily respond to hypnotic suggestion.* Whether or not a particular suggestion evokes a response depends upon the context of the situation and whether or not the person's needs will be met by such a response.

3. *"Most people are not susceptible to hypnosis."* If the treatment you use is not effective for most people, it will be impractical to use it often. The notion of "hypnotic susceptibility" is an important one and requires some discussion. Susceptibility refers simply to the idea that some people respond more readily to hypnosis than others. Data from many investigations reveal that the trait of susceptibility is distributed in a statistically normal fashion throughout the population. It is also widely reported that the ability to respond to pain control suggestions, in particular, is a function of susceptibility: the probability is that if an individual is not susceptible, they will not develop analgesia. Reports suggest generally that hypnotic analgesia is successful in about 25 per cent of the population.

If this is the case, then the use of hypnosis in dentistry has practical limitations. No clinician feels encouraged to use a tool that will be successful only 25 per cent of the time.

Recent evidence, however, both from the experimental laboratory and the clinical dental setting, suggests that this need not be the case. Barber and Mayer, using a hypnotic induction called Rapid Induction Analgesia (RIA), demonstrated that each of their experimental subjects was able to dramatically alter their awareness of experimental dental pain, irrespective of hypnotic susceptibility. We also found that this has clinical significance: 99 per cent of unscreened dental patients were able to undergo normally painful dental procedures using only hypnosis, as induced by RIA. These included "difficult" patients and patients who had been previously labeled "nonsusceptible."

James Fricton now at the University of Minnesota School of Dentistry found that RIA produced analgesia to experimental pain significantly more effectively than a conventional hypnotic procedure and was particularly effective for individuals of measured low susceptibility. RIA will be discussed more later.

It appears from this recent evidence, then, that susceptibility may not be the important factor in determining successful hypnotic analgesia; instead, it appears that virtually every individual can benefit from a particularly effective use of hypnosis.

Although these three reasons might be found to account for the limited use of hypnosis, we would like to offer a further one: Many dentists have the reputation, for instance, of being technically competent but of never looking at their patients when talking to them, and of perceiving the patient as an "oral cavity," or as a "root canal procedure," or "an extraction," rather than as a person with a dental problem.

Although virtually any dentist can readily learn the skillful use of hypnosis, those dentists who do feel comfortable being with people tend to learn more readily and later tend to use hypnosis more than those who find it awkward to look at and deal with patients as people.

Principles for Effective Hypnosis

Hypnosis is a naturally occurring altered state of consciousness characterized by a narrowed, heightened level of attention and the enhanced ability to utilize suggestions for the alteration of memory or perception. There are three psychological principles relevant to the effective induction of hypnosis:

1. The Law of Concentrated Attention suggests that whenever a person's attention is concentrated on an idea repetitiously, the idea tends to spontaneously realize itself. For example, one might suggest: "I wonder which of the fingers of your right hand will move first? Just notice them, one by one, and pay attention to how easily they can move, and notice them and how easily they can move, and wonder which will move first . . . just notice which will move first." It is probable that the person will be surprised to notice that at least one finger begins to twitch.

2. The Law of Reversed Effect suggests that trying *hard* to accomplish something makes the accomplishment more difficult, and the harder one tries, the more impossible does it become. A common and destructive application of this principle is demonstrated by people who develop insomnia by chronically *trying* to sleep—the harder they try, the more wide awake they become. You can demonstrate this principle for yourself. It is not ordinarily difficult for a person to hold their eyes open. However, if you say to someone: "Try *hard* to keep you eyes from closing, even momentarily. Try *hard*. Try *harder*!" it is probable that their eyes will close, if momentarily. Trying implies the possibility of failure. Maintained attention to trying distracts from the actual behavior, and the feedback of this fact creates increased doubt, increased trying, and a cycle of ever more probable failure.

3. The Law of Dominant Effect suggests that the stronger of two emotions tends to replace the weaker one. For instance, if a person's fear that they will not be able to successfully complete a particular thing is stronger in their experience than the confidence and enjoyment of doing so, the experience of fear can become dominant and result in failure. This can be utilized

by the subtle use of physiological cues to strengthen psychological suggestions. The physiological cues tend to strengthen the particular experience and increase the probability of its being the stronger emotion.

The above are well-known principles, first described by Emile Coué, and are fundamental to an understanding of effective hypnosis.

There are more sophisticated principles, however, that have been described by Milton Erickson. Their understanding and competent integration into one's skills of hypnosis can make the difference between therapeutic success and failure, particularly with difficult patients.

OBSERVATION

Careful observation of the patient can reveal subtle needs that require gratification in order to succeed at hypnosis. For example, you may notice that the patient site with hands gripping the arm rests. This may well indicate considerable apprehension on the part of the patient— even if, upon query, the patient indicates otherwise.

UTILIZATION

Accept whatever behavior the patient offers and utilize that behavior in the furtherance of your therapeutic goals. "Resistant" behavior can in this way be inverted toward cooperative behavior. For instance, if a patient would benefit from eye closure, but the patient continues to hold the eyes open, even after repeated suggestions that they close, the effective clinician can, without hesitating, begin offering suggestions for maintaining the eyes open, as if that were the goal from the beginning. Now, if the patient continues to hold the eyes open, this is being done *cooperatively*, since that is what has been suggested. If, on the other hand, they now close their eyes, it can be suggested again that now the eyes can remain comfortably closed, and this be-

havior, too, has been *reframed* as being cooperative. Resistance has been utilized to create cooperation.

Short of violence there is virtually no behavior that a patient may offer that cannot be turned to therapeutic advantage. If a patient continues to gradually close the jaw while clinical treatment is being administered, the effective clinician can suggest that the jaw will close a bit more, and then a bit more, and now, since the behavior has been implicitly defined as under the cooperative control of the dentist, suggestions for opening wider can be more readily accepted, since the previous behavior was also cooperative. The concept of "resistance" becomes virtually nonexistent when the clinician becomes proficient at utilization procedures.

INDIRECT SUGGESTION

Traditionally, hypnotic suggestions have taken the form of authoritarian commands. Hypnotic suggestions are sometimes even referred to as "hypnotic commands." A subject is told, for instance, "Your eyes are getting heavier..." Such a sentence implies that the hypnotist has some special knowledge about the subject, and some special power over the subject to be able to *make* the subject's eyes become heavy. Direct suggestion of this sort is the most common kind of suggestion, and is the kind, in fact, that is used in tests of hypnotic susceptibility. Empirically, then, a majority of the population does not respond well to direct suggestion.

An alternative to directly suggesting something is to use *implicit communication*. An indirect, implicit way of suggesting that eyes are getting heavier might be: "I wonder if you'll enjoy the comfort you can feel as you watch your eyelids close?" In this case, there is no connotation of power of one person over another. The clinician is not saying something about the patient's feelings, but about their own: "I wonder..."—and it is implied, then, that the eyes will close.

There are two fundamental advantages to using indirect suggestion over direct suggestion:

1. Indirect suggestion is not threatening or offensive to the patient. There is not potentiation of defensiveness. The subject has no reason to resist; no commands are given.

2. Since there are no direct commands, there is no indication to the subject of possible failure, no matter what the subject does. If, for instance, the suggestion is given: "I wonder if you'll enjoy the comfort you can feel as you watch your eyelids close," and the subject's eyes do not close, there is no problem created. The hypnotist never said they would close. There was no command given, so there is no command to fail to obey. Therefore, if for any reason the subject does not respond to a suggestion, the induction can continue to proceed. This is in contrast to the situation created by failure to obey a direct suggestion: the subject is not cooperating, the hypnotist has made a mistake, and the possibility for rapport and continued induction has been reduced.

These principles were incorporated into the development of a hypnotic induction technique specifically designed for use in clinical dentistry. Rapid Induction Analgesia (RIA), as the technique is called, was found to be effective in 100 per cent of experimental subjects, and in clinical trials it was effective in 99 per cent of cases. We subsequently determined that RIA is successful in hypnotically low susceptible subjects as well as hypnotically high susceptible subjects in the control of dental pain.

The purpose of RIA is to gently and nonthreateningly elicit the cooperation of the patient to develop a hypnotic state and learn posthypnotic cues for analgesia so that present and future dental work can be done without chemical anesthesia and with control of autonomic processes (i.e., salivation and bleeding). Because the language of RIA is indirect, many patients do not realize that they were hypnotized, even after a comfortable experience of dental treatment.

The text of a sample utilization of RIA is included at the end of this chapter. You may wish to use this transcript to help create an experience of comfort for a patient: to reduce anxiety, induce relaxation, and promote analgesia.

Hypnotic Training

Many dental schools include courses in hypnosis as part of the curriculum. In addition, clinical hypnosis can be learned through the auspices of the American Society of Clinical Hypnosis and the Society for Experimental and Clinical Hypnosis. Both professional organizations offer clinical training workshops throughout the United States. The student should be critical in considering any organizations that offer training in hypnosis since many do not offer adequate training and many offer training based on unscientific notions and myth. Some, in fact, teach hypnosis as if it were part of a 19th century magic show.

Hypnosis is a clinical tool that can be essential to the treatment of the patient as a whole person. Hypnosis can effectively treat various behavioral problems related to the patient's dental needs (such as gagging, bruxing, poor hygiene, difficulty in wearing ortho- or prosthodontic devices, etc.) and can be valuable in operative dentistry by creating pain control either by itself or as an adjunct to chemical anesthesia or analgesia. It is also a valuable tool in controlling bleeding, salivation, and muscle tension.

The dentist should be cautious, however, in limiting such treatment to the context of dentistry. When a patient's psychological problems extend beyond the context of dentistry and, therefore, beyond the competence of the dentist, it is appropriate to refer that patient to psychological treatment.

Rapid Induction Analgesia Procedure

The purpose of the following procedure is to develop complete analgesia and muscular relaxation in as short a time as possible (approximately 10 minutes).

Elicitation of cooperation

I'd like to talk with you for a moment to see if you'd like to feel more comfortable and relaxed than you might expect. Would you like to feel more comfortable than you do right now?

Initiation of deep relaxation

I'm quite sure that it will seem to you that I have really done nothing, that nothing has happened at all. You may feel a bit more relaxed, in a moment, but I doubt that you'll notice any other changes. I'd like you to notice, though, if you're surprised by anything else you might notice. OK, then ... the really best way to *begin feeling more comfortable* is to just begin by sitting as comfortably as you can right now ... go ahead and adjust yourself to the most comfortable position you like ... that's fine. Now, I'd like you to notice how much more comfortable you can feel by just taking one very big, satisfying deep breath. Go ahead ... big, deep, satisfying breath ... That's fine. You may already notice *how good that feels* ... how warm your neck and shoulders can feel ... Now, then ... I'd like you to take four more very deep, *very comfortable* breaths ... and, as you exhale, notice ... just notice how comfortable your shoulders can become ... and

Eye closure

notice how comfortable your eyes can feel when they close ... and when they close, just let them stay closed ... that's right, just notice that ... and notice, too, how, when you exhale, you can just *feel that relaxation beginning to sink in* ... Good, that's fine ... now, as you continue breathing comfortable and deeply and rhythmically, all I'd like you to do is to picture in your mind ... just imagine a staircase, any kind you like ... with 20 steps, and you at the top ... Now, you don't need to see all 20 steps at once, you can see any or all of the staircase, any way you like ... that's fine ... Just notice yourself,

Saying each number with the initiation of subject's exhalation, watching for any signs of relaxation and commenting on them

at the top of the staircase, and the step you're on, and any others you like ... however you see it is fine ... Now, in a moment, but not yet, I'm going to begin to count, out loud, from 1 to 20, and ... as you may already have guessed ... as I count each number I'd like you to take a step down that staircase ... see yourself stepping down, feel yourself stepping down, one step for each number I count ... and all you need to do is notice, just notice, how much more comfortable and relaxed you can feel at each step, as you go down the staircase ... one step for each number that I count ... the larger the number, the farther down the staircase ... the farther down the staircase, the more comfortable you can feel ... one step for each number ... all right, you can begin to get ready ... now, I'm going to begin ... One ... one step down the staircase ... Two ... two steps down the stair case ... that's fine ... Three ... three steps down the staircase ... and maybe you already notice how much more relaxed you can feel ... I wonder if there are places in your body that feel more relaxed than others ... perhaps your shoulders *feel more relaxed* than your neck ... perhaps your legs feel more relaxed than your arms ... I don't know, and it really doesn't matter ... all that matters is that you feel comfortable ... that's all ... Four ... four steps down the staircase, perhaps feeling already places in your body beginning to relax ... I wonder if the deep relaxing, restful heaviness in your forehead is already beginning to spread and flow ... down across your eyes, down across your face, into your mouth and jaw ... down through your neck, deep restful, heavy ... Five ... five steps down the staircase ... a quarter of the way down, and already beginning, perhaps, to really really enjoy your relaxation and comfort ... six ... six steps down the staircase ... perhaps beginning to notice that the sounds which were distracting become less so ... that all the sounds you can hear become a part of your experience of comfort and relaxation ... anything you can notice becomes a part of your experience of comfort and relaxation ... Seven ...

Confusingly, permissively eliciting arm heaviness

seven steps down the staircase ... that's fine ... perhaps noticing the heavy, restful, comfortably relaxing feeling spreading down into your shoulders, into your arms ... I wonder if you notice one arm feeling heavier than the other ... perhaps your left arm feels a bit heavier than your right ... perhaps your right arm feels heavier than your left ... I don't know, perhaps they both feel equally, comfortably heavy ... It really doesn't matter ... just letting

Each number, each suggestion of heaviness enunciated as though the hypnotist, too, is becoming intensely relaxed

Integration of sighing with enunciation is helpful . . . watch for responsiveness . . .

Suggestion to pay attention

More and more directly suggesting enjoyment of the experience . . . more taking for granted the fact of the relaxation . . .

Naming of the excitement of being near the bottom

yourself become more and more aware of that comfortable heaviness . . . or is it a feeling of lightness? . . . I really don't know, and it really doesn't matter . . . Eight . . . eight steps down the staircase . . . perhaps noticing that, even as you relax, your heart seems to beat much faster and harder than you might expect, perhaps noticing the tingling in your fingers . . . perhaps wondering about the fluttering of your heavy eyelids . . . Nine . . . nine steps down the staircase, breathing comfortably, slowly, and deeply . . . restful, noticing that heaviness really beginning to sink in, as your continue to notice the pleasant, restful, comfortable, relaxation just spread through your body . . . Ten . . . ten steps down the staircase . . . halfway to the bottom of the staircase, wondering perhaps what might be happening, perhaps wondering if anything at all is happening . . . and yet, knowing that it really doesn't matter, feeling so pleasantly restful, just continuing to notice the growing, spreading, comfortable relaxation . . . Eleven . . . eleven steps down the staircase . . . noticing may be that as you feel increasingly heavy, more and more comfortable, there's nothing to bother you, nothing to disturb you, as you become deeper and deeper relaxed . . . Twelve . . . twelve steps down the staircase . . . I wonder if you notice how easily you can hear the sound of my voice . . . how easily you can understand the words I say . . . with nothing to bother, nothing to disturb . . . Thirteen . . . thirteen steps down the staircase, feeling more and more the real enjoyment of this relaxation and comfort . . . Fourteen . . . fourteen steps down the staircase . . . noticing perhaps the sinking, restful pleasantness as your body seems to just sink down, deeper and deeper into the chair, with nothing to bother, nothing to disturb . . . as though the chair holds you, comfortably and warmly . . . Fifteen . . . fifteen steps down the staircase . . . three-quarters of the way down the staircase . . . deeper and deeper relaxed, absolutely nothing at all to do . . . but just enjoy yourself . . . Sixteen . . . sixteen steps down the staircase . . . wondering perhaps what to experience at the bottom of the staircase . . . and yet knowing how much more ready you already feel to become deeper and deeper relaxed . . . more and more comfortable, with nothing to bother, nothing to disturb . . . Seventeen . . . seventeen steps down the staircase . . . closer and closer to the bottom, perhaps feeling your heart beating harder and harder, perhaps feeling the heaviness in your arms and legs become even more clearly comfortable . . . knowing that nothing really

18–20 said more slowly, as though in increasing anticipation of being at the bottom

matters except your enjoyment of your experience of comfortable relaxation, with nothing to bother, nothing to disturb ... Eighteen ... eighteen steps down the staircase ... almost to the bottom, with nothing to bother, nothing to disturb, as you continue to go deeper and deeper relaxed... heavy ... comfortable ... restful... relaxed... nothing really to do, no one to please, no one to satisfy ... just to notice how *very comfortable* and heavy *you can feel*, and continue to feel as you continue to breathe, slowly and comfortably ... restfully ... Nineteen ... nineteen steps down the staircase ... almost to the bottom of the staircase ... nothing to bother, nothing to disturb you as you *continue to feel more and more comfortable*, more and more relaxed, more and more rested ... more and more comfortable ... just noticing ... and now ... Twenty ... bottom of the staircase ... *deeply, deeply relaxed* ... deeper with every breath you take ... as I talk to you for a moment about something you already know a lot about ... remembering and forgetting ... you know

Amnesia suggestions

a lot about it, because we all do a lot of it ... every moment, of every day you remember ... and then you forget, so you can remember something else ... you can't remember everything, all at once, so you let some memories move quietly back in your mind ... I wonder, for instance, if you remember what you had for lunch yesterday ... and yet ... I wonder if you remember what you had for lunch a month ago today ... I would guess the *effort is really too great* to dig up that memory, though of course *it is there* ... somewhere, deep in the back of your mind ... no need to remember, *so you don't* ... and I wonder if *you'll be pleased* to notice that the things we talk about today, with your eyes closed, are things which you'll remember tomorrow, or the next day ... or next week ... I wonder if you'll decide to let the memory of these things rest quietly in the back of your mind ... or if you'll remember gradually, a bit at a time ... or perhaps all at once, to be again resting in the back of your mind ... perhaps you'll be surprised to notice that the reception room is the place for memory to surface ... perhaps not ... perhaps you'll notice that it is more comfortable to remember on another day altogether ... it really doesn't matter ... doesn't matter at all ... whatever you do, however you choose to remember ... is just

The amnesia isn't necessary, though

fine ... absolutely natural ... doesn't matter at all ... whether you remember tomorrow or the next

Analgesia suggestions

day, whether you remember all at once, or gradually . . . completely or only partially . . . whether you let the memory rest quietly and comfortably in the back of your mind . . . really doesn't matter at all . . . and, too, I wonder if you'll notice that you'll *feel surprised* that you visit here today is so much *more pleasant* and comfortable than you might have expected . . . I wonder if you'll *notice that surprise* . . . that there are *no other feelings* . . . perhaps you'll *feel curious* about that surprise . . . surprise, curiosity . . . I wonder if you'll be *pleased* to notice that today . . . and any day . . . whenever you feel your head resting back against the headrest . . . when you feel your head resting back like this . . . you'll feel reminded of how very comfortable you are feeling right now . . . even more comfortable than you feel even now . . . comfortable, relaxed . . . nothing to bother, nothing to disturb . . . I wonder if you'll be reminded of this comfort, too, and relaxation, by just noticing the brightness of the light up above . . . perhaps *this comfort and relaxation* will come flooding back, quickly and automatically, whenever you find yourself beginning to sit down in the dental chair . . . I *don't know* exactly how it will seem . . . I only know, as perhaps you also know . . . that your experience will seem surprisingly *more pleasant*, surprisingly *more pleasant*, surprisingly *more comfortable*, surprisingly *more restful* than you *might expect* . . . with nothing to bother, nothing to disturb . . . whatever you are able to notice . . . everything *can be a part* of your experience of comfortableness, restfulness and restfulness and relaxation . . . everything you notice *can be a part* of being absolutely comfortable . . . and I want to remind you that whenever [doctor's name] touches your right shoulder, like this . . . whenever it is appropriate, and only when it is appropriate . . . whenever [doctor's name] touches your right shoulder, like this . . . or whenever I touch your right shoulder like this . . . you'll experience a feeling . . . a feeling of being ready to do something . . . perhaps a feeling of being ready to close your eyes . . . perhaps a feeling of being ready to be even more comfortable . . . perhaps ready to know even more clearly that there's nothing to bother, nothing to disturb . . . perhaps ready to become heavy and tired . . . I don't know . . . but whenever I touch your right shoulder, like this . . . you'll experience a feeling . . . a feeling of being ready to do something . . . it really doesn't matter . . . perhaps just a feeling of

**Direct posthypnotic
suggestion for analgesia**

**Every sensation creates the
analgesic experience (nothing
detracts from it)**

**Posthypnotic suggestion for a
variety of behaviors, but with
purpose of developing a
trance . . . and with
implication for analgesia**

Preparation for end to this comfortable experience

Suggestion for arousal

Numbers on inhalation ... lilting, arousing intonations ... more quickly at first ... watch for responsiveness

If no apparent arousal, slow down, inject more suggestion for arousal

After 5, increasingly slowly ... repeat suggestion for arousal and positive experience

being ready to be even more surprised ... it doesn't really matter ... nothing really matters but your experience of comfort and relaxation ... absolutely deep comfort and relaxation ... with nothing to bother and nothing to disturb ... that's fine ... and now, as you continue to enjoy your comfortable relaxation, I'd like you to notice how very nice it feels to be this way ... to really enjoy your own experience, to really enjoy the feelings your body can give you ... and in a moment, but not yet ... not until you're ready ... but in a moment, I'm going to count from 20 to 1 ... and as you know, I'd like you to feel yourself going back up the steps ... one step for each number ... you'll have all the time you need ... after all, time is relative ... feel yourself slowly and comfortably going back up the steps, one step for each number I count ... more alert as you go back up the steps, one step for each number I count ... when I reach three, your eyes will be almost ready to open ... when I reach two, they will have opened ... and, when I reach one, you'll be alert, awake, refreshed ... perhaps as though you'd had a nice nap ... alert, refreshed, comfortable ... and even though you'll be alert and feeling very well ... perhaps surprised, but feeling very well ... perhaps ready to be surprised ... no hurry, you'll have all the time you need, as you begin to go back up these restful steps ... Twenty ...Nineteen ... Eighteen ... that's right, feel yourself going back up the steps ... ready to be surprised, knowing what you had for lunch yesterday, and yet ... Seventeen ... Sixteen ... Fifteen ... a quarter of the way back up, more and more alert ... no rush, plenty of time ... feel yourself becoming more and more alert ... Fourteen ... Thirteen ... Twelve ... Eleven ... Ten ... half way back up the stairs ... more and more alert ... comfortable but more and more alert ... Nine ... that's right, feel yourself becoming more and more alert ... Eight ... Seven ... Six ... Five ... Four ... Three ... that's right ... Two ... and One ... that's right, wide awake, alert, relaxed refreshed ... that's fine. How do you feel? Relaxed? Comfortable?

Since the subject has been given posthypnotic suggestions as part of the initial hypnotic experience, it is now possible to elicit an even more satisfactory hypnotic state (including development of analgesia) by utilizing one or more of the posthypnotic cues suggested. Whenever in the future cues are properly given, the subject rapidly and automatically develops a satisfactory hypnotic state and is adequately analgesic for clinical procedures.

Bibliography

Allen GD: The indiscriminate use of atropine. *Anesth Prog* 17:8, 1970.

Alper MH, Flacke W, Krayer O: Pharmacology of reserpine and its implications for anesthesia. *Anesthesiology* 24:524, 1963.

Connor JT, Katz RL, Bellville JW, et al: Diazepam and lorazepam for intravenous surgical premedication. *J Clin Pharmacol* 18:285, 1978.

Driscoll E: Anesthesia for the ambulatory patient. In American Society of Oral Surgeons, Report of 48th Annual Meeting, Chicago, ILL., 1966.

Egbert LD, Battit GE, Turndorf H, et al: The value of the preoperative visit by an anesthesiologist. *JAMA* 185:553, 1963.

Gorlin RJ, Pindborg JJ: Kippel-Feil syndrome. In *Syndromes of the Head and Neck.* New York, McGraw-Hill, 1964.

Hayward JR: The staircase test (editorial). *J Oral Surg* 28:327, 1970.

Hill GE, Wong KC, Hodges MR: Lithum carbonate and neuro muscular blocking agents. *Anesthesiology* 46:122, 1977.

List WF, Gravenstein JS: Effects of atropine and scopolamine on the cardiovascular system in man. *Anesthesiology* 26:299, 1965.

Meyer R: Preoperative laboratory screening before administration of general anesthesia in the office. *J Oral Surg* 28:332, 1970.

Perks ER: Monoamine oxidase inhibitors. *Anaesthesia* 19:376, 1964.

Plumpton FS, Besser GM, Cole PV: Corticosteroid treatment and surgery. *Anaesthesia* 24:3, 1969.

Svedmyr N: The influence of a tricyclic antidepressive agent (protriptyline) on some of the circulatory effects of noradrenaline and adrenaline in man. *Life Sci* 7:77, 1968.

Tisi GM: Preoperative evaluation of pulmonary function. *Am Rev Resp Dis* 119:203, 1979.

Wyant GM, Kao E: Glycopyrrolate methobromide: effect on salivary secretion. *Can Anaesth Soc J* 21:230, 1974.

Hypnosis

Alman, B. and Carney R: Consequences of direct and indirect suggestions on success of posthypnotic behavior. *Am J Clin Hypn.* 23:112, 1980.

Barber J: The eficacy of hypnotic analgesia for dental pain in individuals of both high and low hypnotic susceptibility. Unpublished doctoral dissertation, University of Southern California, 1976.

Barber J: Rapid induction analgesia: a clinical report. *Am J Clin Hypn* 19:138, 1977.

Barber J, Donaldson D, Ramras S, et al. The relationship between nitrous oxide conscious sedation and the hypnotic state. *J Am Dent Assoc* 99, 624, 1979.

Barber J, Mayer D. Evaluation of the efficacy and neural mechanism of a hypnotic analgesia procedure in experimental and clinical dental pain. *Pain* 4:41, 1977.

Erickson M: *Advanced Techniques of Hypnosis and Therapy.* New York, Grune & Stratton, 1967.

Hilgard E, Hilgard J: *Hypnosis in the Relief of Pain.* Los Angeles, Kaufman, 1975.

Joy E, Barber J: Psychological, physiological, and pharmacological management of pain. *Dent Clin North Am* 21:577, 1977.

Saletu B, Saletu M, Brown M, et al: Hypno-analgesia and acupuncture analgesia: a neurophysiological reality. *Neuropsychobiology* 1:218, 1975.

CHAPTER 2

Physiology and Pharmacology of Local Anesthesia

The first chemical local anesthetic came with the discovery of cocaine in 1860 by Albert Nieman, but its anesthetic properties were not realized until 1862 when Schraff noted its local effect on the tongue. General anesthesia and analgesia as entities had been known since 1842 when Crawford Long, a physician, used ether to produce euphoria and removed a tumor of the neck, and Horace Wells, a dentist, used nitrous oxide "anesthesia" to extract a tooth in 1844. Local anesthesia added a new dimension to pain control. William Halsted, M.D., carried out the first recorded inferior dental nerve block using cocaine in 1884 and Dr. Charles Nash administered the first infraorbital nerve block in the same year. By 1890, cocaine injections of the gingivae and alveolus became common for tooth extraction. Unfortunately, the drug was misused, resulting in local tissue sloughing, addiction, and death. Some of the early pioneers were well aware of the cortical stimulation potential of this new drug and they fell victim to its abusive potential.

Physical methods of local analgesia have been recorded as early as 1050 when cold water was used to reduce the discomfort of "anal surgery." the use of snow and ice and ice in salt water was also advocated in 1848 for operations including dental surgical manipulation. Pressure or compression anesthesia was advocated in 1784 for surgical pain control and a screw clamp was constructed which applied pressure to the leg in an attempt to control operative pain. All of these *with modification* are in use today, some in local anesthesia for dentistry.

Modern chemical local anesthetic agents came of age when Alfren Einhorn achieved esterification of a basic alcohol with benzoic acid to synthesize procaine in 1904–05. It remained as the basic benzoic acid ester anesthetic until the more recent discovery of the aniline derivatives. Today procaine, although not as widely used as early in the 20th century, still remains the basis of comparison for all modern local anesthetics. Lidocaine, the first popular amide anesthetic, was synthesized in 1943 by Lofgren in Sweden. This with other now available amide agents initiated a new era in safer and more efficient local anesthesia.

By definition, anesthesia refers to loss of consciousness and analgesia refers to an increased pain threshold. When anesthesia is modified with the word local, analgesia is implied and not loss of consciousness. For the purpose of discussion, local analgesia and local anesthesia are used interchangeably and in this text imply loss of sensation with no change in consciousness. The purpose of local anesthesia (analgesia) is to block a painful stimulus from being propagated from peripheral nerve endings to the central nervous system. Any number of agents and/or classes of drugs have the ability to accomplish this, but only a few are appropriate for clinical use. The requirements of acceptable local analgesic agents are as follows:

1. *Reversible.* All current agents are "self-reversing" as redistribution throughout the body and metabolism renders the agents inactive and reduces their local site concentration below physiologically

active levels. This happens without any permanent effect on the nerve so full function is regained. There is no chemical agent that safely reverses local anesthetic effects.

2. *Low systemic toxicity.* All agents have some degree of systemic toxicity but this should be below clinically detectable levels. The amount of the drug necessary for local action at a subcutaneous site must not result in blood levels which cause systemic effects.

3. *Low local toxicity.* Local irritation is produced to some extent by all agents, but this degree of irritation must not be of such magnitude to cause residual or permanent damage to the nerve. The degree of local toxicity in routinely used agents does not cause clinically perceptible tissue damage. There are agents that produce local anesthetic effects because they are chemically irritating and actually destroy the nerve. This does result in analgesia but is not reversible.

4. *Rapid onset.* Onset time, referred to as latency, varies with each agent used but must be within an appropriate period of time to be effectively used in clinical practice (2 to 10 minutes is acceptable).

5. *Sufficient duration.* Duration of action varies considerably between agents and an appropriate drug can be chosen to fit the expected time requirement of the planned procedure.

6. *Sufficient potency.* Potency, sometimes referred to as efficiency, must be adequate at a safe dose so as not to violate other qualities as listed previously. Sufficient potency must be balanced against low or negligible toxicity.

7. *Versatility.* The anesthetic agent should be applicable for use in a wide range of clinical settings and procedures. This includes use as an injectable and/or a topical agent. Certain agents meet this criteria, others are special purpose only.

8. *Free of adverse reactions.* Any agent in some predictable and unpredictable situations may produce allergic reactions, idiosyncratic reactions, or other complications, although current agents now

have a minimal history of such occurrences.

9. *Sterile.* The agent should be sterile when received from the manufacturer with packaging safeguards which insure continued sterility during storage or be capable of being sterilized at the time of use.

10. *Stable.* Stability in solution, whether free or in combination with other additives such as buffers, preservatives, and vasoconstrictors, is an absolute requirement. This stability should give a relatively long storage life (shelf life) if packages are stored properly. All agents are labeled with a storage life date so it is possible to determine the age of stored agents. Improper storage conditions reduce stability and decrease shelf life by inactivating ingredients.

11. *Readily metabolized and/or excreted.* Anesthetic solutions must not only be biocompatible at the site of use but be predictably metabolized to a nontoxic product and/or readily excreted to avoid local or systemic continued action of the agent. Liver and/or renal function normally accomplishes this. In rare circumstances, patients have diseases or genetic alterations that do not allow for the metabolism and excretion of the agents.

No local anesthetic agent absolutely meets all of these requirements. Restrictions as to total dosage and choices of different agents for specific purposes and procedures allows modern agents to be used safely, predictably, and efficiently so that minor deficiencies can be accommodated without resulting in unnecessary risk.

PHYSIOLOGY AND PHARMACOLOGY

Local anesthetics for the most part are made up of three basic components; a lipophilic aromatic portion, an intermediate chain, and a hydrophilic amine, usually a tertiary amine portion (Fig. 2.1). The linkage in the intermediate hydrocarbon chain designates whether the anesthetic compound is an ester or an

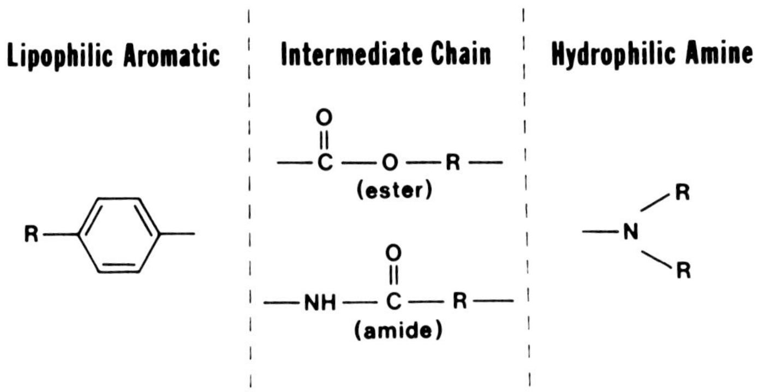

Figure 2.1. General molecular configuration of local anesthetic agents.

amide. Each of the components imparts certain properties to the agent and can be varied by synthesis to provide significant changes in potency, toxicity, duration, and diffusibility. The lipophilic aromatic portion of the local anesthetic molecule is thought to result in the anesthetic's property, which allows it to penetrate the lipid-rich nerve. The hydrophilic amine portion is responsible for the molecule's diffusibility properties so that it can diffuse through interstitial fluid to arrive at a nerve. The most successful anesthetics have balanced lipophilic, hydrophilic, potency and toxicity properties so that effective safe local analgesia is achieved. If any of these properties are lacking or are unbalanced, an agent has only limited applicability. An example of this would be those agents that lack a hydrophilic portion and are therefore not suitable for injection but are suitable to be used topically.

Ester-linked agents are formed by combining an aromatic acid and an amino alcohol and amide agents are formed by combination of an aromatic amine and an amino acid. The linkage difference accounts for two clinically distinct metabolic degradation pathways and a difference in allergic potential. These combinations result in the pure anesthetic called the *anesthetic base*. The *base* is weakly basic in pH, is not readily soluble in water, and is unstable. An agent with these characteristics would not be feasible

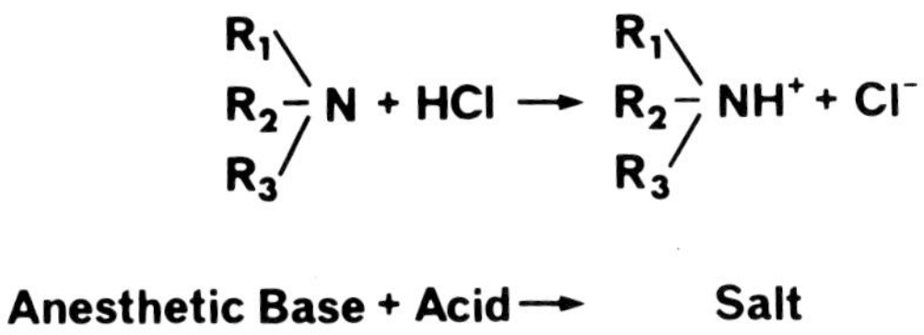

Anesthetic Base + Acid ⟶ Salt

Figure 2.2. Formation of the anesthetic salt.

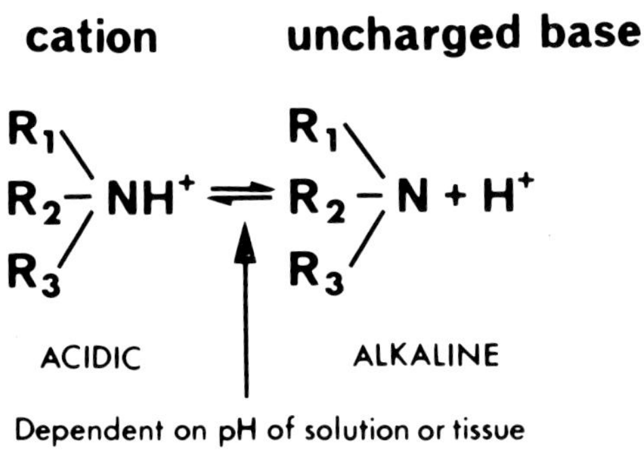

Figure 2.3. Effect of pH on dissociation of the local anesthetic agent.

for injection so the *base* is combined with an acid to form a salt which is quite soluble and stable (Fig. 2.2). This salt is diluted in a solution of water or saline to an appropriate concentration. Each different agent has a dissociation constant (pK$_a$) that is particular to itself, and when in solution has the ability to exist in equilibrium as an uncharged tertiary amine or a positively charged quaternary amine (cation), depending on the pH of the solution (Fig. 2.3).

This equilibrium changes as the pH of the solution changes. A clinical entity which alters this equilibrium is the pH of tissue fluid. Normal tissue fluid has a pH of 7.3 to 7.4, slightly alkaline compared to the adjusted pH of the anesthetic solutions, 3.8 to 6.5. At an acidic pH, most of the anesthetic exists as a charged cation. In normal tissue, at a higher pH, the amount of cation (charged form) decreases and the uncharged form increases. This uncharged form is necessary for diffusion of the agent and neural membrane penetration. Intraneural pH is relatively constant and after membrane penetration allows re-equilibration of the charged and uncharged forms so a sufficient amount of charged form again exists. It has now been demonstrated that both the charged (cation) and uncharged forms of the molecule have anesthetic potential, although the cation plays the major role in impulse blockade. If tissue pH is decreased by infection to 6.0 or lower, there is less uncharged agent to penetrate the nerve so the cation, although in abundance, cannot act. Thus the effectiveness of any agent is dependent on normal tissue pH. Recent information has shown that biochemical changes also occur along the course of a nerve in an infected area so that anesthetic deposition, even away from clinical infection and pH change, still produces less than adequate analgesia.

When the anesthetic agent is injected into tissue, it immediately starts to diffuse geometrically from the site because of its water solubility. As this diffusion begins, immediate dilution takes place so the closer the agent is deposited to the selected nerve, the greater concentration can reach the nerve (Fig. 2.4). Initial concentration of the anesthetic is important in diffusion only and not in anesthetic activity as only a small fixed dose is necessary for nerve blockade. More than this minimum dose does not produce better blockade. Increasing the concentration of an agent will aid diffusion but this must be weighed against the potential of increased toxicity as the total dose and concentration increase.

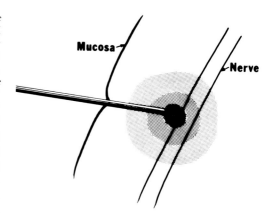

Figure 2.4. Geometric diffusion of the local anesthetic agent in tissue.

Systemic Effects

The main action of local anesthetics in dentistry is at the injection site. Rarely are actions noticed elsewhere because relatively small amounts are used and are injected only extravascularly. Although clinical systemic symptoms are not apparent, anesthetics do exert effects on many other tissues in the body. These effects can be quite varied and are summarized in the following.

After deposition at an injection site, the agent immediately starts to be absorbed and is distributed throughout the body. Absorption is a function of vascularity. Tissue blood flow varies widely and therefore alters the speed with which an anesthetic is absorbed from the site. The important factor for dental local anesthesia is that the local anesthetics are injected into the oral region which is considerably more vascular than other areas of the body. This vascularity can be expected to lead to a higher blood level for equivalent doses of the local anesthetic than injections elsewhere. Only a minimum amount of work has been done concerning blood levels of locals after dental injections, as most studies have evaluated brachial plexus, intercostal, ulnar, and epidural blocks.

The work that has been done shows that the particular drug injected is of considerable importance as there are dramatic differences among common dental local agents. Systemic effects from these are not seen with routine low dose injections because the total dose is well under the maximum allowable limit (maximum doses are discussed in Chapter 3) in an extravascular site. An intravascular or high dose injection will result in clinically detectable symptoms.

Distribution of the agent after it is absorbed from the injection site is a function of organ and tissue blood perfusion. The organs and tissues with the highest perfusion rates will receive the highest concentrations of the local agent. Drugs, however, have specific affinity for certain tissues and thus these tissues ultimately receive the largest amounts. Muscle mass probably accounts for the largest portion of the redistributed agent although muscle itself does not have a definite affinity for local anesthetics. Other tissues which do have an affinity and result in rapid accumulation of the agent are liver, kidney, salivary glands, and the brain.

All of this redistribution reduces the amount of the drug at the injection site and in the general circulation and thus reduces the amount available for clinical action. The redistributed drugs are slowly absorbed back into the blood for hydrolysis or transport to specific organs for metabolism and excretion.

The metabolism of local anesthetic agents can be categorized by their specific drug classification, ester or amide. Ester agents are metabolized chiefly by a plasma enzyme cholinesterase. This enzyme hydrolyzes the agent into *para*-aminobenzoic acid, which may be further metabolized or excreted directly in the urine. This pathway of metabolism and detoxification is rarely affected by disease and in most individuals is extremely predictable. There are rare disease states, however, that result in atypical forms of cholinesterase. This altered enzyme, not capable of rapidly detoxifying ester compounds, may result in prolonged blood levels of the agent and prolonged toxic

effects if large doses are used. Individuals with these disorders usually know of their condition since it will have been diagnosed at an early age, before dental therapy is normally necessary, and a suitable anesthetic choice can be made. If it is undiagnosed, it is not likely to be of sufficient magnitude to result in severe clinical symptoms as long as low doses of the ester anesthetics are used.

Amide local anesthetics have a much more complex metabolic pathway that involves detoxification in the liver with relatively little detoxification in the plasma. Because of this, individuals with severe liver disease may be susceptible to prolonged blood levels and prolonged toxic effects with amide agents. Fortunately, some metabolism is also accomplished by the kidney so severe clinical problems could result only rarely, even in the face of severe liver dysfunction or disease. The by-products of amide metabolism are then excreted in another complex pathway through the biliary tree to the intestinal tract. Here the products are reabsorbed and then transported *via* the blood stream to the kidneys for final urinary excretion. Both ester and amide compounds eventually require renal function for final elimination. The specific pathways of different agents are discussed in Chapter 3.

One other important consideration is redistribution of local anesthetics in the pregnant female. Virtually all agents passively diffuse across the placenta so a maternal blood level will result in a fetal blood level. As long as the maternal level is safe and low, no problem is expected in the fetus. A prolonged or toxic blood level in the mother can be equally hazardous to the unborn child. As with all drugs, care must be exercised in the administration of local anesthetics during pregnancy.

Effects on Specific Organ Systems

The central nervous system is one of the most sensitive tissues in the body to the effects of local anesthetic drugs. These effects are dose-related and clinical effects are seen when blood levels either from an overdose or an intravascular injection reach a threshold level. All local anesthetics are central nervous system depressants and have inhibitory or depressant effects on excitable membranes throughout the body. When the blood concentration is low as with most dental injections, there is virtually no effect on central nervous system tissue. As the dose and corresponding blood level increases, electroencephalographic changes occur. These changes are indicative of an approaching toxic blood level with corresponding clinical symptoms.

The initial clinical sign of a toxic reaction is excitement and/or apprehension which may include lightheadedness, dizziness, slurred speech, shivering, and tremors. In the case of a more severe reaction, and a higher blood level, convulsions appear. This cortical excitation is thought to be precipitated by the depressant effects of the anesthetic on inhibitory cortical synapses, thus allowing excess uncontrolled cortical activity of facilitory neurons. This excitation phase is followed by a compensatory period of clinical depression, as illustrated by Hiatt (Fig. 2.5), and is in relation to the degree of excitement. If the local blood level is higher yet, complete depression of inhibitory and facilitory neurons occurs with only the clinical manifestations of depres-

sion (unconsciousness) and, in severe cases, coma, flattening of the electroencephalographic recording, clinical death, and brain death.

As cortical depression is occurring, medullary function is also being affected and also manifests as initial stimulation followed by depression. During stimulation, blood pressure, heart rate, and respiratory rate increase and are compensatorily followed by some degree of depression (Fig. 2.5). The effect on these organ systems is not primary but rather secondary to the drug's effect on the central nervous system. As depression deepens, whether it is preceded by clinical excitation or not, decreased respiratory activity may proceed to arrest and death.

The severity of a toxic reaction is related to each individual's tolerance, acid-base balance, the inherent potency of the drug, and the relative dose (overdose) of the drug. It must also be noted that because amide locals are not metabolized in the bloodstream, their presence in the general circulation is of longer duration than esters so any toxic symptoms will be of corresponding longer duration. Toxic blood levels have been established for the commonly used amide local anesthetics, lidocaine, mepivacaine, and prilocaine. Five μg per ml of blood is considered the threshold for toxic reactions. For bupivacaine and etidocaine the threshold concentration is between 1.4 and 4 μg per ml.

The other major organ system that is

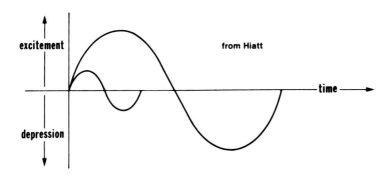

Figure 2.5. Excitation-depression curve. (Adapted from Hiatt, W.: *Dent Clin North Am* 5:243, 1961.)

directly affected by local anesthetics is the cardiovascular system. Each individual local anesthetic produces differing degrees of symptoms but all show a similar pattern of cardiovascular toxicity. The blood concentration of the anesthetic agents necessary for cardiac effects is similar to that for central nervous system effects. The effect of local agents on electrical activity of the heart is minimal at low blood levels although there is some reduction in the excitability of cardiac muscle and a prolongation of conduction through various portions of the heart muscle. This is consistent with depression of excitable membranes. With toxic blood levels, there is a definite decrease in myocardial contractility, intraventricular pressure, and a decrease in cardiac output. Conductivity and contractility of the myocardium are so disrupted that arrest may result.

The peripheral vascular bed is likewise affected to varying degrees by local anesthetic agents which may result from direct infiltration to an area or from the amount of a selected agent in the general circulation. The direct effect at the site of injection is usually one of vasodilatation as, in general, local anesthetics are vasodilators. There are some notable exceptions to this rule, however, and they are that cocaine is a strong vasoconstrictor, and prilocaine and mepivacaine are not vasodilators. There is considerable difference of opinion concerning the vasoactive properties of mepivacaine and prilocaine, probably resulting from species and target site differences of experimental models.

Systemic vascular response to all locals is always vasodilatation. This is dose dependent as virtually no effect is seen at low blood levels but a definite arteriolar vasodilatation from smooth muscle relaxation and decrease in total peripheral resistance is seen with toxic blood levels. Cocaine is the only exception and has been shown to produce vasoconstriction. It can be seen that in an overdose situation, the combination of a decrease in peripheral resistance and decrease in cardiac output resulting in severe hypotension, coupled with respiratory depression mediated through the central nervous system, could be extremely life threatening. Other miscellaneous tissues of the body such as smooth muscle of the bronchial tree and intestinal wall are affected by circulating local anesthetic agents. These effects are minor, however, when compared to the life-threatening cardiovascular and central nervous system effects.

NEUROPHYSIOLOGY

The local anesthetic agent is only one factor in the physiological and pharmacological actions of local anesthesia. The other and equally important component is the nerve itself. The main site of action of local anesthetic agents is the selected nerve. Nerves are living cells involved directly and indirectly with metabolism, protection, and nourishment of the nerve membrane. The nerve membrane propagates impulses from peripheral sites to a central point of interpretation. If the propagation of this impulse is impaired, the sensation of pain can be abolished.

Each nerve fiber is composed of an axon, the peripheral process of the more centrally located nerve cell body in the dorsal root ganglia. Each axon is surrounded by a continuous nerve membrane which separates the gelatinous axoplasm from the extracellular fluid. The axoplasm is responsible for growth, development, nourishment, and maintenance of the nerve membrane but does not play an active role in impulse propagation.

The nerve membrane is a multilayered structure, 70 to 80 Å thick, with a central core composed of lipid layers sandwiched between two layers of protein. Some of the protein molecules extend through the lipid core. The lipid component is formed by polarized cholesterol and phospholipid molecules (Fig. 2.6). The nerve membrane controls the highly different ionic concen-

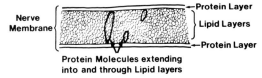

Figure 2.6. Schematic representation of components of the nerve membrane.

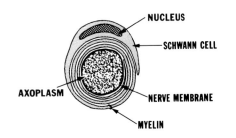

Figure 2.7. Cross-sectional depiction of a nerve fiber surrounded by a Schwann cell and myelin.

trations between the intracellular fluid of the axoplasm and the extracellular fluid of surrounding tissue. Changes in this ionic gradient result in membrane depolarization and impulse propagation.

The membrane has a high electrical resistance which prevents passage of potassium, sodium, and chloride ions which would normally flow across such a concentration gradient. The ionic concentration that is actively maintained isolates a high level of potassium in the axoplasm with relative depletion of sodium and chloride. The important ions in this process are sodium (Na) and potassium (K).

Human nerve fibers, except for very small axons, are additionally surrounded by another covering layer called myelin. Myelin surrounds the nerve fibers in a lamellar, cylindrical fashion and when present is produced by Schwann cells (Fig. 2.7). All peripheral nerve fibers are surrounded by Schwann cells but myelin is not produced in every case. The function of myelin and Schwann cells is related to maintenance and protection of the nerve fiber, as neither are actively involved in impulse propagation. Myelin, when present, presents a diffusion/absorption barrier to the local anesthetic as

these agents do not readily penetrate the myelin layer. Fortunately, the myelin layer is regularly interrupted, every 0.5 to 3.0 mm, exposing the naked nerve membrane. These interruptions are known as nodes of Ranvier. At these sites, local anesthetic solutions can easily diffuse to the nerve membrane and effect neural blockade.

Impulse Propagation

The stimulus that is propagated at peripheral sites travels along selected and isolated nerve fibers to a central point where interpretation of the impulse is accomplished. Each impulse is self-propagating once it has started as energy used for propagation arises from energy released by the nerve fiber along its length. The electrical impulse that occurs is actually a rapid change of membrane potential and is propagated as a wave of depolarization spreading away from the point of initiation. This wave is called the action potential (Fig. 2.8). Nerve fibers are subdivided by size and speed of impulse propagation, but all physiologically function in the same manner so are not separated in the following discussion.

The inside of a resting nerve membrane is negatively charged as compared to the positive outside. This potential difference is approximately −70 mV. As a stimulus occurs, the voltage slowly rises to −40 to −55 mV. This voltage is the firing threshold of the nerve fiber and once this level is reached depolarization occurs and the action potential is initiated. If this critical level is not attained, no impulse is produced. This illustrates the all-or-nothing principle of nerve impulses. After the firing threshold is reached, the voltage overshoots to +40 or +50 mV and then repolarizes and returns to the resting membrane potential. The process of depolarization and repolarization occurs along the entire length of the nerve fiber as the impulse is being propagated. Immediately after the action potential is initiated, the nerve goes through an absolute refractory

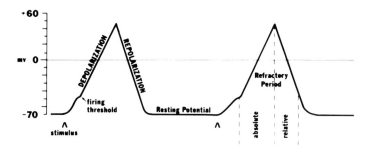

Figure 2.8.   Action potential.

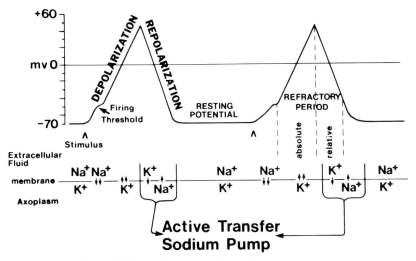

Figure 2.9.   Action potential and ion movement.

period where further stimulation is not possible. After this, but before repolarization, there is a relative refractory period where a new impulse could be generated if a stimulus were much stronger than normal (Fig. 2.8).

At rest, the inside of the nerve membrane is negatively charged compared to the positive outside. Although this is considered a resting state, it is maintained by an active process. This polarity is reversed at the height of depolarization. This change creates a flow of current between depolarized and adjacent resting segments of a nerve and, as a result, membrane potential decreases ahead of the active portion. When the membrane potential decreases, the permeability of the membrane to sodium increases and sodium ions passively start to enter the

nerve. This entry of sodium ions creates less negativity on the interior of the nerve membrane and thus generates a new action potential (Fig. 2.9). In this manner, the impulse is propagated.

The resting nerve membrane is a formidable barrier to sodium ions, as it successfully keeps these ions out against a concentration gradient and an electrostatic gradient. The nerve membrane is said to be minimally permeable to sodium ions. To maintain this, there is an active outward flow of sodium ions called the sodium pump. This results from oxidative metabolism of adenosine triphosphate (ATP). Potassium ions are maintained on the interior of the nerve membrane by two mechanisms. The most important is the electrical gradient. The negative charge of the membrane holds the positively charged potassium ions intracellularly by electrostatic attraction. Any change in electrostatic force of resting membrane potential allows the outflow of potassium ions. In addition, there may be a less important theoretical but active potassium pump.

During depolarization, sodium ions move through sodium channels in the membrane as it becomes more permeable. This initiates a new action potential and reduces the voltage difference across the membrane. The electrostatic restraint imposed by the resting membrane on potassium ions is now lost. Shortly after the membrane permeability changes to sodium and their concentration starts to increase on the interior, potassium ions start to migrate along their concentration gradient to the outside of the nerve membrane due to the loss of the electrostatic force. This process is then quickly reversed at the height of the action potential and the resting membrane potential is regained during repolarization. Figure 2.9 compares the action potential to the movement of sodium and potassium ions.

Individual ions are thought to move through channels in protein molecules extending through the nerve membrane. This has led to a *schematic theoretical* representation of channels of varying size which can selectively restrict large ions (Fig. 2.10). Resting membrane sodium

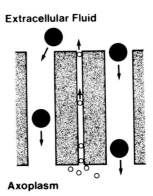

Extracellular Fluid

Axoplasm

Figure 2.11.   Depolarizing nerve membrane.

channels are too small to permit entry of these ions into the cytoplasm of the axon but during depolarization enlarge to rapidly admit sodium. Potassium channels are always open but not used until sodium ion influx reduces the charge of the membrane allowing potassium to pass through its channels (Fig. 2.11).

Theories of Local Anesthetic Action

The exact site and mechanism of action of anesthetics is still theoretical, although all available evidence points to the nerve membrane as the primary site and the control of sodium ion permeability as the primary mechanism. Local anesthetic agents decrease the maximum rate of rise of the action potential so that the threshold potential is not attained. This prevents depolarization of the nerve membrane from occurring and thus produces a conduction block. Depolarization is a function of sodium permeability and movement through sodium channels so research has concentrated on this action to investigate the site of local anesthetic action.

It is now believed that all local anesthetic agents exert their effect by altering the sodium channel of the nerve membrane. Two receptor sites plus membrane expansion are theorized. Common injectable local anesthetics such as lidocaine, mepivacaine, prilocaine, and procaine are thought to bind to receptor sites located

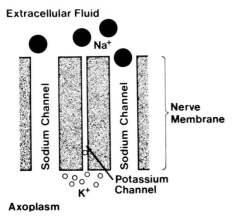

Extracellular Fluid

Na+

Sodium Channel

Sodium Channel

Nerve Membrane

Potassium Channel

K+

Axoplasm

Figure 2.10.   Resting nerve membrane.

on the internal surface of the nerve membrane at the sodium channel (Fig. 2.12). Biotoxins (biological toxins) such as tetradotoxin from the ovaries of puffer fish and saxitoxin found in dinoflagalates are thought to act by binding to receptor sites located on the external surface of the nerve membrane at the sodium channel (Fig. 2.13). These agents are 250,000 times as potent as common local anesthetic agents. They have no clinical use but are excellent research tools.

The third theory of action of local anesthetics is based on the action of agents such as benzocaine and benzyl alcohol. These agents act by penetrating into the nerve membrane and causing membrane expansion. This decreases the diameter of

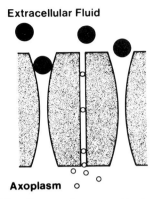

Figure 2.14. Benzocaine nerve block; molecule causes expansion of the nerve membrane.

sodium channels and prevents depolarization (Fig. 2.14).

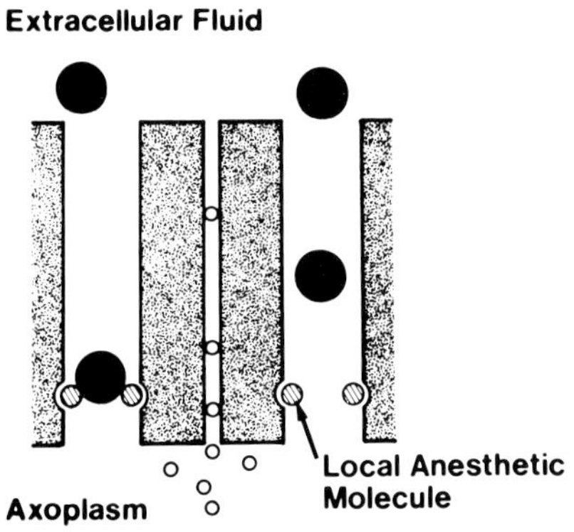

In summary, information available theorizes that the action of local anesthetic agents is related to a sequence of events which include: 1) binding to receptor sites in the nerve membrane; 2) reducing the sodium permeability of the nerve membrane; 3) decreasing the rate of depolarization so the threshold firing potential is not reached; 4) failure of an action potential to develop, which therefore leads to *neural blockade.*

The previous discussion of action potential, impulse propagation, and sites of local anesthetic action relates to individual nerve fibers. The actual conditions under which these take place is modified slightly when a myelin sheath is present. In addition to providing a maintenance function for the nerve membrane, myelin also acts as an insulator, separating the membrane from the extracellular environment. In myelinated nerves, the majority of the activity concerning conduction of impulses and ionic currents are concentrated at the nodes of Ranvier. The most excitable portion of a nerve membrane is the area exposed at the nodes. Conduction of the impulse occurs in a jumping fashion from one node to the next with relatively little activity in between. This type of conduction is known as *saltatory* conduction. The importance of this is that for a local anesthetic to act,

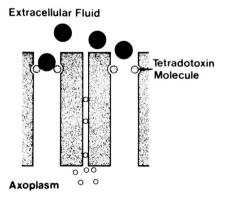

Figure 2.12. Conventional local anesthetic nerve block; molecule binds on the internal surface of membrane at sodium channel.

Figure 2.13. Biotoxin nerve block; molecule binds on the external surface.

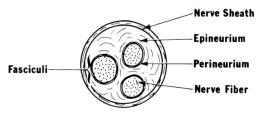

Figure 2.15. Schematic anatomy of a nerve trunk.

two or more adjacent nodes must be inactivated. The larger the nerve fiber, the farther apart the nodes. A sufficient concentration of anesthetic agent must reach several *consecutive* nodes to completely block impulse propagation. Nerve blockade is easier to accomplish in terminal, unmyelinated nerves.

The properties of local anesthetic solutions allow for them to diffuse to these nodes. All individual nerve fibers and their associated myelin sheaths are separated from each other by connective tissue (Fig. 2.15). Nerve fibers are packed together into a fasiculi or bundle and again encased by perineurium. Many fasciculi and their perineuriums are embedded in loose connective tissue called epineurium, with the outer layers of the epineurium forming the nerve sheath. This arrangement, although consisting of many parts, is highly organized and takes up very little cross-sectional area. Approximately 5,000 nerve fibers occupy only 1 sq mm of tissue. All of these various structures act to some degree as barriers to diffusion of a local anesthetic agent to each individual nerve fiber. A sufficient concentration of local solution must not only reach the nerve sheath but then penetrate each individual fiber if a complete block is to be obtained. Local anesthetic agents are successfully able to accomplish this without damage to nerves and thus the practice of local anesthesia is a successful and safe daily occurrence.

Bibliography

Cawson RA, Spector RG: *Clinical Pharmacology in Dentistry.* Edinburgh, London and New York, Churchill Livingstone, 1978.

Covino BG: Physiology and pharmacology of local anesthetic agents. *Anesth Prog* 28(4):98–104, 1981.

Covino BG, Giddon DB: Pharmacology of local anesthetic agents. *J Dent Res* 60(8):1454–1459, 1981.

Covino BG, Vassalo HG: *Local Anesthetics—Mechanisms of Action and Clinical Use.* New York, Grune & Stratton, 1976.

DeJong RH: *Local Anesthetics,* ed 2. Springfield, Ill., Charles C Thomas, 1977.

Gilman AG, Goodman LS, Gilman A: *The Pharmacological Basis of Therapeutics,* ed 6. New York, Macmillan, 1980.

Grossman LI: Local anesthesia use revisited (letter to editor). *J Am Dent Assoc* 105(4):610, 1982.

Hiatt W: Local anesthesia: history; potential toxicity; clinical investigation of mepivacaine. *Dent Clin North Am* 5:243, 1961.

Kramer SL, Milton VA: Complications of local anesthesia. *Dent Clin North Am* 17:443, 1973.

Moore DC: The pH of local anesthetic solutions. *Anesth Analg* 60(11):833–834, 1981.

Najjar TA: Why can't you achieve adequate regional anesthesia in the presence of infection? *Oral Surg* 44(1):7–13, 1977.

Rhart JP: A short history of local anesthesia. *Bull Hist Dent* 20:27, 1972.

CHAPTER 3

Local Anesthetic Agents

Local anesthetic agents are by far the most common drugs administered by the dentist, be they generalist or specialist. The frequency of these administrations and the relative infrequency of complications attest to the safety of the drugs in common use. A conservative estimate of all dental anesthetic injections given in the United States is over 50,000,000 per year, and very few of these are associated with any complications.

Today there are numerous local anesthetic compounds, most of which fall into two basic compound classes: esters and amides. The amide compounds have gained widespread approval and are the most popular because they are less allergenic than ester compounds and are more potent at a reduced concentration. They have virtually replaced the ester compounds in clinical practice and there are few, if any, reasons for using injectable ester derivatives for dentistry. The drugs in most common use by the dentist are lidocaine, mepivacaine, and prilocaine. There are other agents but these represent the most popular. A more complete list of anesthetics available for use is found in Table 3.1.

The following is a short summary of the more important and most popular local solutions.

PROCAINE

Procaine (para-aminobenzoyl-diethyl-amino ethanol) was developed by Einhorn in 1904–1905 and has served as an effective and reliable anesthetic. In the last 20 years it has been replaced by the safer and more efficient amide local anesthetics. This makes it a secondary choice for local anesthesia in dentistry. It now has major importance as the standard by which all new locals are evaluated and rated. If it is combined with other more potent agents, it can still be clinically useful but this does not circumvent the problems of using an ester-linked anesthetic. The concentrations found most clinically useful have been 2% and 4%. It is an intense vasodilator and has a relatively short duration of action. Its onset time is likewise slow and is useful for dentistry only with a vasoconstrictor (Fig. 3.1).

CHLOROPROCAINE

2-Chloroprocaine (β-diethylamino-ethyl-2-chloro-4-aminobenzoate) is a drug very similar to procaine except for the substitution of one chlorine atom in the benzine ring. As a dental anesthetic, it has a rapid onset and very short duration. Its short duration does not make it very suitable for routine dental procedures but it has been proposed to be used in combination with other slow onset, long duration anesthetics. Unfortunately, this combination has not worked as expected as the subjective onset time was very short, but the true objective onset of anesthesia was not markedly shortened. The surgical procedures could not actually be started sooner. It would seem then that its only use for dentistry is in combination with a vasoconstrictor. It is used in a 2% concentration but is not marketed in a dental cartridge (Fig. 3.1).

PROPOXYCAINE

Propoxycaine (2-diethylaminoethyl-4-amino-2-propoxybenzoate) is one of the more popular ester-linked agents, although is not used alone. It is combined with 2% procaine to achieve a good combination of onset and duration. Propoxycaine is approximately 10 times as potent as procaine and also considerably more

toxic. Therefore, it is used in a 0.4% solution in conjunction with 2% procaine (Fig. 3.2).

LIDOCAINE

Lidocaine (diethylaminoacetate-2,6-xylide) was the first popular amide local anesthetic. It was introduced in Europe by Lofgren and Lundquist in 1943. Since then, it has undergone extensive animal and clinical testing and is now the most widely used dental local anesthetic. Considerable evidence exists which supports its popularity, although there is also evidence that other locals may have equal or

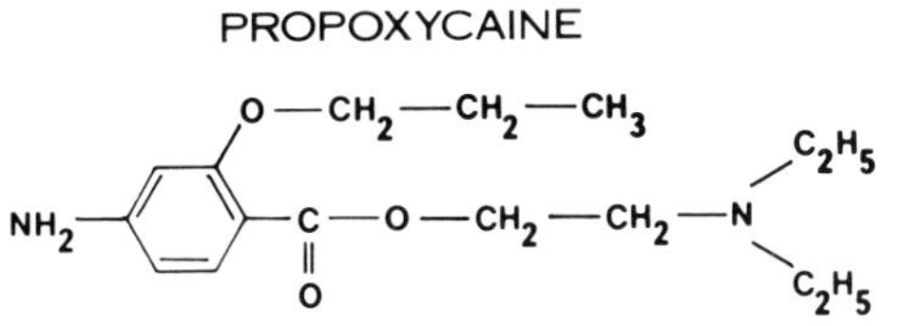

Table 3.1.
Local Anesthetics

Ester derivatives
  Procaine
  2-Chloroprocaine
  Tetracaine
  Propoxycaine
  Benzocaine (topical only)
  Cocaine (topical only)
Amide derivatives
  Lidocaine
  Mepivacaine
  Prilocaine
  Bupivacaine
  Etidocaine
Ketone-linked
  Dyclonine (topical only)
Aromatic alcohols
  Benzyl alcohol (topical only)

PROPOXYCAINE

Figure 3.2. Chemical configuration of local ester anesthetic agent.

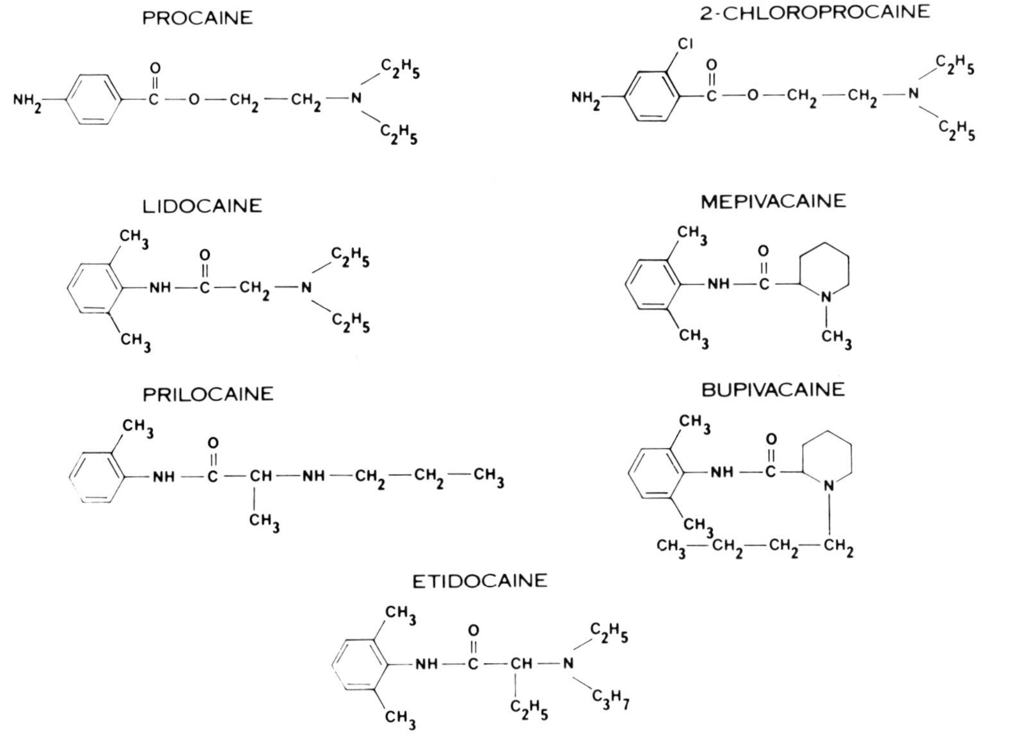

Figure 3.1. Chemical configuration of local anesthetic agents.

superior qualities. Regardless, none have been able to surpass its impressive and long clinical record for safety and effectiveness. It has approximately two times the potency of procaine and is used as a standard for comparison of other amide local agents. Lidocaine is commonly employed in a 2% solution for injection and up to a 10% concentration for topical anesthesia (Fig. 3.1). It is a potent vasodilator, so for dental anesthesia is almost always combined with a vasoconstrictor to increase efficiency and duration.

Lidocaine is also used in cardiology to control myocardial excitability in infarct and arrest situations. This cardiovascular effect is shared to some degree by other amide locals but none are as effective or used as extensively as lidocaine. The effect of lidocaine varies with the method of administration and the dose. Nerve block can be achieved with small doses. The antiarrhythmic effect is produced by 300 mg as a deltoid intramuscular injection or 50 to 100 mg as an intravenous injection. These doses should not result in bradycardia, hypotension, or serious side effects, as the expected blood level is approximately 1.8 μg/ml. This is below the 5 μg/ml threshold for CNS toxicity.

MEPIVACAINE

Mepivacaine (*dl*-N-methylpipecolic acid-2,6-xylide) was synthesized in 1956 by af Ekenstam, Egner and Petterson. It is closely related to other amide locals and is similar to lidocaine in most respects. Mepivacaine has gained acceptance because of its clinical safety and effectiveness, which are closely related to its lack of vasodilatation and low toxicity. These characteristics make mepivacaine suitable with or without a vasoconstrictor. Investigations have shown that when a vasoconstrictor is added, lidocaine and mepivacaine can be expected to act similarly in all dental applications. It is used in a 2% or 3% concentration (Fig. 3.1).

PRILOCAINE

Prilocaine (2-propylamino-*o*-propionotoluidide), chemically related to lidocaine and mepivacaine, is the newest of the popular agents. Its synthesis was reported in 1960. It combines the safety and efficiency of the amide anesthetics with a predictable short duration. It has undergone extensive clinical trials and is gaining in popularity as a suitable dental anesthetic. One of the metabolites of prilocaine is orthotoluidine which causes methemoglobin. Ten per cent methemoglobin is considered the safe limit and this limit is not reached until 1000 mg of prilocaine has been administered. Warren pointed out that in oral surgery cases where up to 600 mg are given, no dental clinical implication from methemoglobin could be found. Numerous other agents also have been reported to cause methemoglobinemia, including lidocaine. Hjelm and Holmdahl reported that the metabolism of 500 mg of lidocaine produces 1% methemoglobin while 500mg of prilocaine produces 4.5% methemoglobin.

Of the popular amide agents, lidocaine, mepivacaine, and prilocaine, prilocaine has the shortest biological half-life. This is a potential attribute when repeated doses are given as it is metabolized faster than the other two agents. It, like mepivacaine, does not produce vasodilatation so is suitable for use with and without a vasoconstrictor. Prilocaine is clinically used in a 4% concentrtion (Fig. 3.1).

BUPIVACAINE

Bupivacaine (1-butyl-2,6-pipecoloxylidide) was synthesized in 1956. It is chemically related to lidocaine and is a homolog of mepivacaine. Its main use has been as an epidural agent, but recently it has been investigated as a dental anesthetic. It has found limited specific use because of its extremely long duration. In surgical cases, where prolonged analgesia is beneficial, bupivacaine can be used to advantage. It reduces postoperative discomfort and reduces the need for other oral or parenteral analgesics. It is utilized in a 0.25%, 0.5%, and an 0.75% solution, with and without a vasoconstrictor. It was marketed in August 1983 in a 1.8-cc dental cartridge as Marcaine 0.5% with 1:200,000 epinephrine (Fig. 3.1).

ETIDOCAINE

Etidocaine (*dl*-2-(*N*-ethylpropylamino)-2,6-butyroxylidide) is the newest of the local anesthetic agents for dental use. It is chemically and pharmacologically related to lidocaine; however, its duration of action is considerably longer. It has had some dental investigation and has clinical use and promise similar to bupivacaine. It is available in 0.5%, 1.0%, and 1.5% concentrations and is used with and without a vasoconstrictor. It is not yet available in a dental cartridge (Fig. 3.1).

TOPICAL ANESTHETIC AGENTS

Topical anesthetic agents are used to decrease the sensation of an advancing needle in the upper layers of the dermis, to control superficial discomfort, and to control gagging encountered during impression taking, intraoral radiography, and examination. They are also prescribed to facilitate food and water intake in individuals with oral erosive and ulcerative diseases.

Topical anesthetic effect is exerted on free nerve endings in or just under mucous membranes. In mucous membrane, the nerve endings are close enough to the surface that only minimal diffusion is necessary for a clinical effect. Intact cutaneous epithelium is not affected by topical anesthetics because the agents will not diffuse to the nerve endings. Any of the common injectable local anesthetic agents could be used in a topical fashion, although their concentration may have to be so high that their use is impractical (15% mepivacaine and 20% procaine). Others, like 5% lidocaine and 1% tetracaine, are effective at concentrations only

slightly increased over injectable solutions. Buffering capacity of mucous membranes is low so an increased concentration of the anesthetic is always necessary.

Other anesthetic agents not previously discussed can also be used for topical application. These are agents that lack a hydrophilic portion so are unable to deeply diffuse through connective tissue or do not readily form water-soluble anesthetic salts. These include benzocaine and dyclonine. Other agents, such as benzyl alcohol, are too irritating to inject, so can only be used topically.

Lidocaine

Lidocaine is a popular and effective topical and injectable agent. A complete discussion is found earlier in this chapter. In topical usage, the concentration is increased to at least 5%. Because it is water-soluble, systemic absorption through the oral mucosa occurs, so careful attention must be paid to total dose. If utilized carefully with only a small amount placed on a cotton-tipped applicator, no problem should occur.

Tetracaine

Tetracaine (*para*-butylaminobenzoyl-2-dimethylamino ethanol) is an extremely potent and toxic anesthetic agent. It is more than 10 times as potent as procaine with an equivalent increase in toxicity. It is an ester-linked drug and is used rarely in dentistry as an injectable agent because of its extremely slow onset and toxicity. It is found frequently in topical preparations and is most commonly used as a 2% concentration in combination with other topically active anesthetics. If it were used as an injectable agent the concentration would be reduced to 0.15%. It is water-soluble so has the same potential for mucous membrane absorption as does lidocaine (Fig. 3.3).

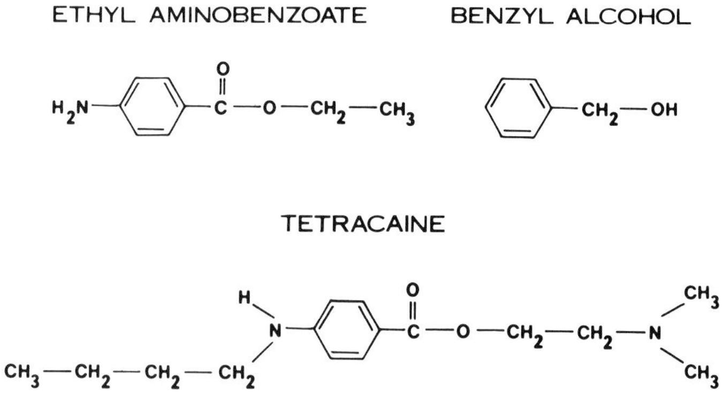

ETHYL AMINOBENZOATE   BENZYL ALCOHOL

TETRACAINE

Figure 3.3. Chemical configuration of topical anesthetic agents.

Benzocaine

Benzocaine (ethyl aminobenzoate) is an ester type anesthetic agent but lacks a basic nitrogen group so is not soluble in water and thus not suited for injection. It is an effective topical agent and is found in 10%, 15%, and 20% concentrations in many commercial topical anesthetic formulations. Ethyl aminobenzoate is quite irritating so care must be used as to the time of surface contact and used only in accordance with each manufacturer's directions. Chemical irritation of the mucous membrane can result if left in contact with tissue for more than a few minutes (Fig. 3.3).

Dyclonine

Dyclonine (4'-butoxy-3-piperidino-propiophenone) is unique compared to ester and amide type local anesthetics. It is a ketone and is quite irritating if injected, so is used only as a topical anesthetic. In addition, it is only slightly water-soluble. It is an alternative drug topical application for patients allergic to ester derivative agents (Fig. 3.4).

Benzyl Alcohol

Benzyl alcohol is an aromatic alcohol and one of numerous agents having anesthetic properties but not fitting the general chemical configuration of a local anesthetic agent. It is too irritating to be

Dyclonine

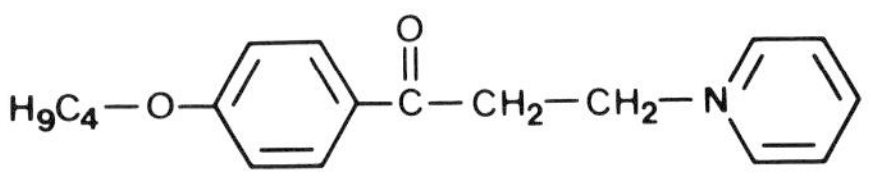

Figure 3.4. Chemical configuration of topical ketone anesthetic agent.

injected. It is used solely for topical anesthesia in dentistry in a 5% concentration. The chemical structure of this agent is depicted in Figure 3.3.

Cocaine

Cocaine, the first local anesthetic, is an excellent agent for topical application. It is also a central nervous system stimulant and a popularly abused drug. Since it is not superior in oral surface anesthesia to other anesthetics with no abuse potential, it has no dental use. Having it in an office invites abuse and theft.

VASOCONSTRICTORS

Vasoconstrictors are added to local anesthetics to reduce blood flow through the tissue into which they are injected. The results of this are to slow the absorption of the local anesthetic and decrease hemorrhage at the site of injection. If absorption of the agent is slowed, the peak blood level achieved should be reduced, the anesthetic will have more time to act, and the duration of action will be longer.

There is evidence that slowing absorption of a drug reduces its relative central nervous system toxicity because less is entering the general circulation at a given time. The effect of this is greater with a vasodilating drug such as lidocaine than with non-dilators such as mepivacaine and prilocaine. This effect differs at varying body sites and in some evaluations is very minor or nonexistent. Two oral evaluations have been conducted concerning this peak level reduction and both found non-significant reductions of lidocaine and mepivacaine blood levels when vasoconstrictors were added. The clinical implication of this is that with oral injections, the reduction in toxicity should not be overemphasized as an attribute of solutions with vasoconstrictors over those without. Indeed recent animal experiments indicate that epinephrine increases the concentration of local anesthetic in brain tissue.

The effect of increasing duration is a universally accepted phenomenon. All agents with vasoconstrictors will result in a longer duration of action. The effect of this is most dramatic in highly vascularized tissue such as the maxilla. It is less dramatic with the Gow-Gates injection and the periodontal ligament injection. The effect of "increasing potency" by adding a vasoconstrictor is also most dramatic with vasodilating agents like lidocaine. This effect is so dramatic that lidocaine is simply not effective (but available) without a vasoconstrictor while mepivacaine and prilocaine as plain solutions are excellent as short duration oral anesthetics.

Local anesthetics are not used to control or reduce hemorrhage. They are the vehicle used to inject vasoconstrictors which will decrease blood flow at the injection site. The effectiveness is in relation to the dose used. There is unfortunately a rebound vasodilatation effect, especially with higher concentrations of vasoconstrictors which can result in hemorrhage after the procedure is completed.

The vasoconstrictors used in local anesthetics commercially available in the United States are rather limited and consist basically of levonordefrin, epinephrine, and norepinephrine. In other countries, vasopressin is used as a vasoconstrictor with local anesthetics. Other vasoactive drugs are available for use, but they require the operator to mix them with the local at the time of the procedure. This would be an inconvenience for most dentists and does not offer greater safety, plus introduces the possibility of contamination of the solution and dosage errors.

All vasoconstrictors used in the United States are sympathomimetic amines (adrenergic agents) and have similar effects. There is some variation in intensity of effect but this is compensated for by differing concentrations. All produce adequate local vasoconstriction for increased duration of the anesthetic agent, and will also reduce hemorrhage at a surgical site. Chemical configurations are found in Figure 3.5. The following is a summary of those used in dentistry.

Epinephrine

Epinephrine is the most commonly used vasoconstrictor and the most potent. It is a physiological substance secreted by the adrenal medulla but it can also be synthetically produced. Its mode of action in local anesthetics is basically mediated by stimulating α-adrenergic receptors in the vessels at the site of deposition. In large doses there is a local β-adrenergic effect which involves dilatation of vessels at the site.

The amount injected in dental anesthesia will produce a β systemic effect resulting in an increase in heart rate, cardiac output, stroke volume, the rate pressure product (RPP), and cardiac oxygen consumption. These β effects are not necessarily noticeable by casual observation, but do occur. They are definitely dose-related and are seen more frequently than

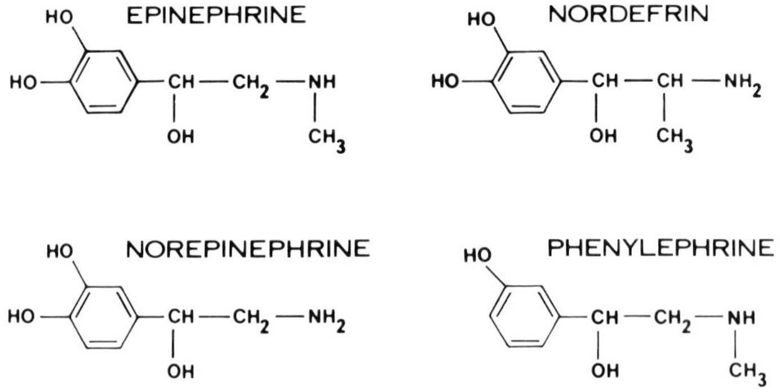

Figure 3.5. Chemical configuration of vasoconstrictor agents for local anesthesia.

one would like because of inadvertent intravascular injection. Epinephrine is commonly used in concentrations of 1:50,000, 1:100,000 and 1:200,000.

When the concentration of epinephrine is increased from 1:200,000 to 1:100,000 or 1:50,000, the α effect for local vasoconstriction and the systemic β effect increases. In addition, a rebound β effect at the injection site may produce postoperative dilatation after the initial α action has dissipated. With the 1:50,000 concentration, this can result in excellent intraoperative hemorrhage control but increased postoperative blood loss. The ideal concentration for dental practice is 1:100,000 or 1:200,000 with the minimum effective concentration being 1:200,000. The maximum allowable healthy adult dose is 0.2 mg and is attained with 5.5 cartridges of the 1:50,000 solution and 11 cartridges of the 1:100,000 solution. The anesthetic dose maximum is reached before the epinephrine maximum dose with the 1:200,000 solution.

Norephinphrine

Norepinephrine is a slightly less active vasoconstrictor than epinephrine. It acts through α receptor sites so has good vasoconstrictive properties with minimal β stimulation. Norepinephrine has been reported to cause sloughing in local infusions and consequently is not considered a primary choice for a local anesthetic

vasoconstrictor. In larger doses or in intravascular injection, just like epinephrine, it will cause a rise in blood pressure and an increase in stroke volume. It does not cause an increase in heart rate or cardiac output. It is commonly used in a 1:30,000 concentration and the maximum allowable healthy adults dose is 0.34 mg. This is reached with 5.7 1.8-ml cartridges.

Nordefrin

Nordefrin is the least active of the commonly used vasoconstrictors and is about one-fifth as active as epinephrine. It is a synthetic compound and has no physiological counterpart. The levo isomer is the active form and is one-half as active in pressor activity as epinephrine. Its clinical activity is mediated almost entirely through α receptors. This produces adequate local vasoconstriction with minimal systemic effect, as β activity is negligible. This minimizes, but does not totally eliminate, cardiac stimulation. It has not been reported to cause tissue sloughs like norepinephrine but is not quite as good for hemorrhage control as epinephrine. Levonordefrin is commonly used in a 1:20,000 concentration. The maximum allowable healthy adult dose is 1.0 mg. This constitutes 11 dental cartridges.

Phenylephrine

Phenylephrine is considered a weak vasoconstrictor and consequently rarely used in modern local anesthetic agents. It, like nordefrin, is synthetic and almost entirely α in its sympathomimetic action so has the potential for good local effect with minimal systemic cardiovascular change. It is the most stable of all the vasoconstrictors but nevertheless is the least commonly used in commercial preparations. When it is employed, it is used in a 1:2,500 concentration. The healthy adult maximum dose is 4.0 mg and this is attained after 5.5 dental cartridges.

Vasoconstrictors and Cardiovascular Disease

Because of the many reported side effects attributed to vasoconstrictors, a discussion concerning them is mandatory. The risk of a clinical reaction to the amount of vasoconstrictor used in commercial preparations is minimal if the drug is administered properly. There is no doubt that systemic changes occur when epinephrine is used, but these are rarely noted and are not detectable by casual observation. If an intravascular injection takes place, the patient will verbalize or show the effects of central nervous system and cardiovascular stimulation. These type reactions increase patient fear of dental anesthesia and intensify the magnitude of psychic reactions. Aspiration before the start of injections and repeated aspiration during the injection minimize the risk of intravascular deposition of the vasoconstrictor agents.

Considerable controversy exists as to whether patients with a history of cardiac disease should receive vasoconstrictors. For cardiac patients, a maximum dose of 0.04 mg of epinephrine, 0.14 mg of norepinephrine, and 0.2 mg of levonordefrin has been recommended. The American Dental Association guidelines recommend similar limits. Vasoconstrictors do result in a cardiovascular response, even in small doses, and are therefore used in limited doses in patients who are deemed to be a cardiovascular risk.

Determining the existence of this risk is not necessarily straightforward. Guidelines for inclusion as cardiovascular risk include *any* history of, or *any* findings of, the following: 1) resting blood pressure over 180/95; 2) rate pressure product over 12,000 (heart rate × systolic blood pressure); 3) class III status (American Society of Anesthesiology); 4) cardiovascular medication in step II antihypertensive therapy, regardless of resting controlled blood pressure; 5) over 6 months post-myocardial infarct or cerebral vascular accident. If any of the above are positive, the patient is of cardiovascular risk and the cardiovascular risk maximum vasoconstrictor dose is as follows: 0.04 mg epinephrine (1 cartridge of a 1:50,000 solution, or 2 cartridges of a 1:100,000 solution, or 4 cartridges of a 1:200,000 solution); 0.2 mg levonordefrin (2 cartridges of a 1:20,000 solution); 0.14 mg norepinephrine (2 cartridges of a 1:30,000 solution). These limits are considered safe, but 2% mepivacaine and 4% prilocaine are anesthetics which perform adequately without vasoconstrictors and these should always be considered, unless the duration of the procedure would require repeated injections.

Contraindications to Vasoconstrictors

Certain medical conditions and prescribed medications negate the use of sympathomimetic amines. Hyperthyroidism predisposes patients to cardiac arrhythmias and since vasoconstrictors produce cardiac stimulation, are contraindicated.

Tricyclic antidepressant drugs are a widely publicized contraindication to the use of amine vasoconstrictors. These drugs block the uptake of norepinephrine into sympathetic nerve terminals. There is a decreased but still existent effect with other vasoconstrictors, as increases in blood pressure and cardiac irregularities have been reported. Because of this, vasoconstrictors should not be used with tricyclic drugs.

Reports of adverse drug interaction with monoamine oxidase inhibitors (MAOI) are controversial. Monoamine oxidase (MAO) is involved with the metabolism of catecholamines but it is not the primary pathway, so vasoconstrictor use is potentially safe. Because of the numerous statements of adverse interaction of vasoconstrictors and MAOI drugs, even though they are not substantiated, their use would not be warranted, as adequate alternatives do exist.

Other Vasoconstrictors

One of the more popular vasoconstrictors available outside the United States is vasopressin, a posterior pituitary hormone and a nonsympathomimetic agent. Vasopressin, in contrast to sympathomimetic agents, has a minimal effect on coronary circulation. Unlike epinephrine, small doses, which are used with a local infiltration, act only on the venous capillary bed. Like epinephrine, large doses or higher concentrations affect the arterial side of the capillary bed. Coronary effects are noted in large doses, but in usual dental doses there is minimal or no change in blood pressure and heart rate. It would appear that vasopressin may be a good substitute for epinephrine in anesthetics for patients with coronary artery disease, especially if long duration is necessary. If duration is not a major factor, the controversy concerning safe doses of cardiovascular stimulants can still be avoided by using anesthetic agents without vasoconstrictors.

CHEMICAL ACTION RELATED TO PHYSICAL-CHEMICAL PROPERTIES

The clinical action of local anesthetics is based on potency of the agent, duration of operating action, and onset time from injection until dental therapy can begin. Each of these actions or clinical effects is in part related to physical-chemical properties of the anesthetic molecule. Potency is related to lipid solubility of the molecule, duration is related to protein binding

of the molecule, and onset time is related to the pK_a. Two other factors, inherent vasoactivity and non-neural tissue diffusibility, also affect clinical activity. These physical-chemical factors are outlined in Table 3.2.

Lipid Solubility

The lipid solubility of any of the common local anesthetics is the most important factor as a predictor or determinant of its clinical potency. The more highly lipid soluble an agent, the easier it is for it to penetrate the lipid-rich nerve membrane. A method for measuring lipid solubility is the partition coefficient. Table 3.2 lists the approximate lipid solubility of local anesthetic agents and it can be seen that as lipid solubility increases from 0.6 to 140, the relative potency also increases. The relationship is not absolute but is a good determinant of approximate comparative potency. Potency implies that the agent is able to cause conduction blockade at a very low concentration.

Protein Binding

After the anesthetic has diffused to the nerve and penetrated the lipid-rich nerve membrane, the length of time it remains in the membrane is in part related to its degree of binding to protein in the nerve membrane. As the degree of protein binding increases, the relative duration increases. Agents such as etidocaine, bupivacaine, and tetracaine are highly bound and possess a longer duration of clinical effect than procaine which is poorly bound to protein (Table 3.2).

pK_a

The pK_a of a local anesthetic is defined as the pH at which 50% of the drug exists as an unchanged base and 50% as the charged, ionized form. The uncharged base is primarily responsible for diffusion of the agent across the nerve sheath. The better the diffusion characteristics, the faster the onset. Since the anesthetic must

Table 3.2.
Comparison of Physical-Chemical Properties

Anesthetic	pK$_a$	Approximate Per Cent as Base at pH of 7.4	Onset	Approximate Lipid Solubility (Partition Coefficient)	Potency	Approximate Per Cent Protein Binding	Duration
Procaine	8.9	2	Slow	0.6	1	5	Short
Tetracaine	8.6	5	Slow	80.0	8	85	Long
Mepivacaine	7.6	40	Fast	0.8	2	75	Intermediate
Lidocaine	7.7	35	Fast	2.9	2	65	Intermediate
Prilocaine	7.7	35	Fast	1.5	2	55	Intermediate
Bupivacaine	8.1	20	Intermediate	30.0	8	95	Extended
Etidocaine	7.7	35	Fast	140.0	6	94	Extended

act in tissue which has a pH of 7.4, the lower pK$_a$ anesthetics have a quicker onset. Table 3.2 lists the pK$_a$ of common agents and the speed of onset. The percentage of an anesthetic agent existing in the unchanged base form at normal tissue pH is inversely proportional to the pK$_a$ of the agent.

Non-Neural Diffusion

Diffusion through connective tissue is a different phenomenon compared to neural sheath diffusion, as non-neural connective tissue diffusion is not directly related to pK$_a$. The concentration of the anesthetic can influence connective tissue diffusion because of the concentration gradient but all factors are not known.

Vasoactivity

Potency and duration are also affected by intrinsic vasoactivity of the agents. Agents of differing intrinsic potency and protein binding can clinically behave similarly because of the relative vasodilating and vasoconstricting tendency of the drug. All locals except cocaine are classified as vasodilators; however, mepivacaine is sometimes considered to be a slight vasoconstrictor and prilocaine is at least not a vasodilator. This vascular effect (or lack of effect) keeps the agents at the neural site longer since they are not absorbed into vascular channels as quickly as would be the case with a vasodilator such as lidocaine. This increases relative clinical potency and duration. It also explains why mepivacaine and prilocaine are effective local anesthetics without a vasoconstrictor additive, whereas lidocaine is quite inefficient (low potency and very short duration) as a plain solution.

Excellent reviews of the toxicity and potency of many local anesthetics have been made. In these comparisons, procaine is used as the standard and assigned a toxicity of one. Other anesthetics are then compared to procaine on an equiva-

Table 3.3.
Comparative Toxicities

Agent	Percentage Used in Dental Practice	Absolute Toxicity	Relative Toxicity
Procaine	2	1	2
Mepivacaine	2	2	4
Mepivacaine	3	2	6
Lidocaine	2	2	4
Prilocaine	4	1.5	6
Bupivacaine	0.25	8	2
Bupivacaine	0.5	8	4
Etidocaine	0.5	5	2.5
Etidocaine	1	5	5

lent dose basis. A comparative list of toxicity is found in Table 3.3. Relative toxicity is also important in clinical practice and is computed in Table 3.3 by multiplying the absolute toxicity by the percentage of the drug used in clinical practice. The commonly used locals, mepivacaine, lidocaine, and prilocaine, are very close in relative toxicity.

CLINICAL USE OF LOCAL ANESTHETICS

Safe use of the different local anesthetic agents in dentistry depends on many factors including patient selection, proper technique and the very important concept of minimizing the total dose. The recommended volume of anesthetic solution for each of the different dental injections is listed in Chapter 5, but these are general guidelines. The important factor is not each single injection dose but the total dose of the drug given to the patient. Any discussion of toxicity should alert practitioners that a potential risk does exist. Although in clinical practice few toxic reactions occur, there are those occasional events that do result in the death of a patient. The relative security of dental local anesthesia can make the operator passive about potential risk. This risk becomes more important as the total dose of the drug increases. The toxic blood level for the common dental local anesthetic (lidocaine, mepivacaine, and prilocaine)

is 5 μg/ml. This means that when the amount of these drugs in the general circulation reaches this level, toxic central nervous system effects start to occur. Speed of injection and site of injection affect this but the one most important criteria in controlling the blood level is the total dose of the drug administered.

Maximum allowable doses for each of the many anesthetics have been determined on the basis of milligrams of the drug and total body weight. It has been suggested that the actual weight of the patient is not as important as lean body mass, as the latter is a more clinically accurate method for assessing individual patient tolerance, but lean mass is difficult to calculate. Square surface area of the body has also been proposed as a

Table 3.4.
Lidocaine Maximum Dose

Lidocaine—maximum dose 300 mg (2.0 mg/lb) Common brand name: Xylocaine 2%	
Patient Weight in Pounds	Xylocaine 2%
20	36 mg (1 cartridge)
40	81 mg (2.25 cartridges)
60	117 mg (3.25 cartridges)
80	153 mg (4.25 cartridges)
100	198 mg (5.5 cartridges)
150	297 mg (8.25 cartridges)
175	297 mg (8.25 cartridges)

Lidocaine with vasoconstrictor—maximum dose 500 mg (3.2 mg/lb) Common brand name: Xylocaine 2% with 1:100,000 or 1:50,000 Epinephrine	
Patient Weight in Pounds	Xylocaine 2% with 1:50,000 epinephrine* Xylocaine 2% with 1:100,000 epinephrine
20	64 mg (1.75 cartridges)
40	128 mg (3.5 cartridges)
60	192 mg (5.25 cartridges)*
80	256 mg (7.0 cartridges)
100	320 mg (8.75 cartridges)
150	396 mg (11.0 cartridges)*
175	396 mg (11.0 cartridges)*

* Epinephrine limits the dose before the anesthetic maximum is reached. The limit is 5.5 cartridges of the 1:50,000 solution and 11 cartridges of the 1:100,000 solution. The maximum healthy adult dose of epinephrine is 0.2 mg.

reliable criteria but it is no better in the clinical situation than total body weight.

The maximum allowable doses and doses based on total body weight are found in Tables 3.4 to 3.7. This information is found in the drug information inserts (Fig. 3.6) that accompany every container of local anesthetic. Unfortunately it is not consistently listed in the same way and it is rarely listed as an allowable number of cartridges per body weight. It is usually listed on a milligrams per total body weight basis. To make use of the information provided and apply it logically to each patient, the practitioner must be able to convert designations such as 2%, 4%, 1:20,000, and 1:200,000 to the actual number of milligrams contained in the volume injected.

To convert percentage into total dose, % means grams per 100 cc. Example: 2% = 2 g per 100 cc = 2000 mg per 100 cc = 20 mg per cc.

To convert X:X into total dose, X:X is read X to X and means grams per cubic

Table 3.5.
Mepivacaine Maximum Dose

Mepivacaine—maximum dose 400 mg (3 mg/lb) Common brand name: Carbocaine 3% Usual vasoconstrictor is levonordefrin Common band name: Carbocaine 2% with 1:20,000 Neo-Cobefrin (in Carpules)	
Patient Weight in Pounds	Carbocaine 3%
20	54 mg (1.0 carpule)
40	120 mg (2.0 carpules)
60	180 mg (3.25 carpules)
80	240 mg (5.5 carpules)
100	300 mg (5.5 carpules)
133	400 mg (7.25 carpules)
150	400 mg (7.25 carpules)
Patient Weight in Pounds	Carbocaine 2% with 1:20,000 Neocobefrin
20	54 mg (1.5 carpules)
40	120 mg (3.25 carpules)
60	180 mg (5.0 carpules)
80	240 mg (6.5 carpules)
100	300 mg (8.25 carpules)
133	400 mg (11.0 carpules)
150	400 mg (11.0 carpules)

Table 3.6.
Prilocaine Maximum Dose

Prilocaine—maximum dose 600 mg (4.0 mg/lb) Common brand name: Citanest 4% Usual vasoconstrictor is epinephrine Common brand name: Citanest Forte with 1:200,000 Epinephrine	
Patient Weight in Pounds	Citanest 4%
20	72 mg (1 cartridge)
40	144 mg (2 cartridges)
60	234 mg (3.25 cartridges)
80	306 mg (4.25 cartridges)
100	396 mg (5.5 cartridges)
150	594 mg (8.25 cartridges)
175	594 mg (8.25 cartridges)
Patient Weight in Pounds	Citanest 4% Forte with 1:200,000 Epinephrine
20	72 mg (1 cartridge)
40	144 mg (2 cartridges)
60	234 mg (3.25 cartridges)
80	306 mg (4.25 cartridges)
100	396 mg (5.5 cartridges)
150	594 mg (8.25 cartridges)
175	594 mg (8.25 cartridges)

Table 3.7.
Bupivacaine Maximum Dose

Bupivacaine—maximum dose 90 mg (0.9 mg/lb) Common brand name: Marcaine 0.5% with 1:200,000 epinephrine	
Patient Weight in Pounds	Bupivacaine 0.5% with 1:200,000 Epinephrine
20	Not recommended for children under 12 years of age
40	
60	
80	72 mg (8.0 cartridges)
100	90 mg (10 cartridges)
150	90 mg (10 cartridges)
175	90 mg (10 cartridges)

centimeter. Example: 1:50,000 = 1 g per 50,000 cc = 1000 mg per 50,000 cc = 0.1 mg per 5 cc = 0.02 mg per cc.

The usual local anesthetic volume given is either ½ cartridge (0.9 cc) or a full cartridge (1.8 cc). The volume given must then be multipled by the number of mg per cc for each anesthetic. This must be in accordance with the weight of the patient. Tables 3.4 to 3.7 convert this in-

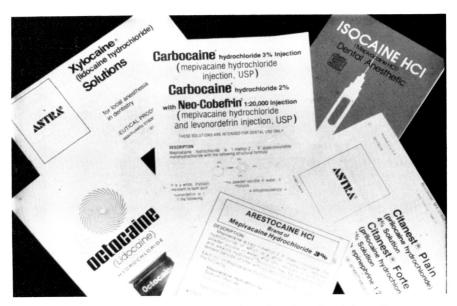

Figure 3.6. Local anesthetic package inserts—drug information.

formation into cartridges allowable. In the healthy adult, a dose of 30 to 100 mg (one to two 1.8-cc injections) of the local will be well within the allowable maximum. But in a small child it is possible to approach the maximum with only a minimum number of injections administered. For example, a 40-lb child could receive 160 mg of prilocaine, which is the maximum allowable dose. This would be achieved with slightly over two 1.8-cc, 4% injections. Three 1.8-cc, 4% prilocaine injections would be 26% more than the allowable limit (Table 3.6).

An extensive research investigation carried out by Cowan evaluated the minimum dose that is actually necessary to produce satisfactory anesthesia. This necessary minimum dose is commonly exceeded in clinical practice because of the large safety margin that exists between usual doses and toxic doses in average adults. This safety margin is much less in small individuals and pediatric patients. Age is not the important factor in the resultant blood levels of local agents. The important factor is the patient's weight.

All maximum doses are based on the assumption that proper technique has been used in administering the agent.

Dental local agents are always injected extravascularly. If they inadvertently are injected into a vascular channel, the maximum dose limitation is no longer valid because the agent is introduced into the blood stream. This creates a temporary over-dose and possible toxic reaction. Maximum doses also assume proper patient evaluation as individual tolerance alters the response to any medication.

The possibility of attaining a intravascular injection with dental injections varies with the site of the needle placement. In maxillary infiltrations vascular channels are entered in about 1% of the injections. This goes up to about 3% with zygomatic (PSA) blocks and peaks around 12% with the standard inferior alveolar block. The size of the needle lumen has also been suggested as a factor in ease of entering a vessel but in the 25-to-27-gauge size both enter at a similar rate.

The speed at which a local is eliminated from the circulation whether by metabolism or redistribution can be important in determining not only maximum single dose limits, but also the relative risk or safety of reinjection of the agent. This may occur if the length of the procedure outlasts the duration of the anesthetic. It is undoubtedly safer to administer a second dose of a local 30, 60, or 90 minutes after the first dose; however, it must be understood that detectable and relatively persistent serum levels do exist for more than 4 hours after the initial injection and reinjection of the same agent will have an additive effect to the existing blood level at the time of readministration. A safe rule of thumb is to consider maximum dose limits as 24-hour limits. Total administration during any 24-hour period should be considered cumulative and never exceed the single dose maximum. The effects of all locals are additive to each other so ½ of the maximum dose of one agent plus ½ the maximum of a second agent still results in a maximum dose. Prilocaine has been reported as being the least toxic of the common agents on a *cumulative basis*. This is because it is cleared from the blood at a faster rate than mepivacaine or lidocaine. It is not less toxic on an injection for injection basis, only on a cumulative basis.

LOCAL ANESTHETIC CHOICES

Although many different kinds and combinations of local anesthetics and vasoconstrictors are available, the dentist does not have an unlimited choice, unless mixing in the office is done. This mixing should be avoided to insure against solution contamination and dosing errors. This will not happen if commercial cartridges are used. A wide enough variety exists to satisfy virtually every general dental need. The extended duration anesthetics such as bupivacaine and etidocaine are available in multi-dose vials which, if handled properly, will remain sterile. In addition to choosing an appropriate agent that is consistent with the patient's physical and health status, a choice must be made as to vasoconstrictor content, absence and concentration.

Comparisons concerning duration and efficiency are frequently made between the three most popular locals; lidocaine, mepivacaine, and prilocaine. Concerning standard 1.8-cc dental injections when no vasoconstrictor is added, mepivacaine and prilocaine have excellent dental application. Lidocaine plain, although availble, has a very short duration and a low incidence of effective anesthesia compared to the others. The lack of vasodilatation with prilocaine and mepivacaine render these drugs suitable for dental practice without additional vasoconstrictor, where lidocaine is suitable only with a vasoconstrictor.

Mepivacaine 3% and prilocaine 4% should be considered equal in clinical activity. The onset of objective analgesia, the duration, and the efficiency are very similar. Both are considered short acting anesthetics. The onset time is in the range of 1 to 3 minutes and the duration of operating anesthesia can be expected to average 15 to 30 minutes for a maxillary infiltration and up to one hour for an inferior alveolar nerve block (Table 3.8). One must keep in mind the difference between operating duration and the duration of soft tissue subjective symptoms experienced by the patient. Operating duration refers to the time where analgesia is of sufficient profoundness that pulpal tissue or dentin can be manipulated. It could also refer to surgical operating analgesia, although this involves manipulation of periodontium and associated structures only. It is easier to achieve surgical analgesia than pulpal or dentinal analgesia. Soft tissue subjective symptoms refer to the subjective feeling on the part of the patient of paresthesia or numbness. These symptoms occur before true objective operating analgesia and persist considerably longer than operating analgesia. Subjective sensations of soft tissue analgesia last 30 to 120 minutes longer than the true operating analgesia. The duration of soft tissue symptoms *vs.* operating anesthesia can be misleading because the pulpal stimulating portion of most procedures occurs early during the course of a procedure. The true operative duration of analgesia is not realized unless this depth

Table 3.8.
Comparative Activities

Agent	Class	Maxillary Infiltration Duration	Inferior Alveolar Block Duration	Comment
		min	*min*	
Lidocaine	Amide	5–10	30	Low efficiency.
Lidocaine 2% with 1:50,000 epinephrine	Amide	60	90	Additional epinephrine is used for hemorrhage control at injection site. Routine use of this concentration is not advised.
Lidocaine 2% with 1:100,000 epinephrine	Amide	60	90	Good choice for lengthy procedure.
Mepivacaine 3%	Amide	20–30	60	Good choice for short duration procedure and when vasoconstrictor is contraindicated.
Mepivacaine 2% with 1:20,000 levonordefrin	Amide	60	90	Good choice for lengthy procedure.
Prilocaine 4%	Amide	15–20	60	Good choice for short duration procedure and when vasoconstrictor is contraindicated.
Prilocaine 4% with 1:200,000 epinephrine	Amide	60	90	Good choice for lengthy procedure.
Propoxycaine 0.4% Procaine 2% with 1:30,000 levophed	Ester	45	90	Special purpose use only as ester agents have high allergic potential.
Bupivacaine 0.5% with 1:200,000 epinephrine	Amide	120	180	Special purpose for long duration procedure. Postoperative analgesia can last 8–12 hr. Not indicated for restorative procedures, only surgical or when postoperative discomfort is expected. Contraindicated for individuals under 12 years of age and those who are mentally retarded, because of cheek and lip biting.

of anesthesia is lost while manipulating the pulp or dentin.

Prilocaine has been suggested as a drug which has a minimum duration of soft tissue symptoms after loss of operating anesthesia, although clinical studies have reported the same soft tissue duration with prilocaine 4% and mepivacaine 3%. It would seem then that similar results can be expected with either drug.

Numerous comparisons have likewise been made for prilocaine 4% with 1:200,000 epinephrine, mepivacaine 2% with 1:20,000 levonordefrin, and lidocaine 2% with 1:100,000 epinephrine. These are standard marketed and popular solutions but no studies have compared all three drugs simultaneously, therefore only averages can be listed in Table 3.8.

All three are considered long acting dental anesthetics. Onset time varies slightly with each but is within the range of 2 to 5 minutes. The duration is considerably longer with these three drug combinations than with plain mepivacaine 3% and prilocaine 4%. Operating anesthesia for a maxillary infiltration can be expected to last one hour. The soft tissue duration of analgesia experienced by the patient may last 2 to 3 hours. For inferior alveolar block injections, the operating duration is 90 minutes. The soft tissue duration of symptoms may be 3 to 4 hours. All three drug combinations can be expected to perform similarly.

Lidocaine 2% with 1:50,000 epinephrine has a duration similar to the other agents with vasoconstrictors. The increased epinephrine content does not improve efficiency or duration and is used only to control hemorrhage. Standard use of this agent for analgesia is unwarranted.

Anesthetic manufacturers list the expected duration of the respective anesthetics in their drug brochures. In almost every instance, the expected duration is underestimated, giving the operator a margin of error in choosing the appropriate drug for ech patient and procedure.

It should be noted that the frequency of satisfactory anesthesia (efficiency) will always be better for a maxillary infiltration than for an inferior alveolar neve block and will also be superior if a vasoconstrictor is added. Frequency is quite adequate with plain solutions, although the best results will be obtained with the 3 drugs containing vasoconstrictors. Average maxillary infiltration efficiency is 90 to 95%. Average inferior alveolar nerve block efficiency varies from 75 to 99%, depending on the injection technique.

Commercially prepared anesthetic solutions have agents other than the local anesthetic and vasoconstrictor incorporated into them. These include agents to adjust pH such as sodium hydroxide or hydrochloric acid, agents to control tonicity such as sodium chloride and agents to control oxidation of vasoconstrictors such as sodium bisulfite. These agents are added for specific purposes and rarely result in any problems although it must be kept in mind that pure anesthetic solutions are rarely being injected. Methyl paraben, a preservative, has been implicated as the agent responsible for most anesthetic allergies. It is now rarely found in commercial dental cartridges. This is discussed fully under complications in Chapter 6.

There are very few contraindications to the use of local anesthetic agents apart from actual drug allergy. Any component of the anesthetic solution must be considered when this is encountered. There should be only rare occasions when an ester agent would be considered the drug of choice over an amide-linked anesthetic as the amide group has virtually replaced all other chemical configurations in dental practice because of the ester allergic potential.

There are still the extremely rare occasions when it may seem appropriate to not use a local anesthetic. The only alternative may seem to be a general anesthetic but many other drugs do have local anesthetic properties. Among these are antihistamines such as tripelennamine and diphenhydramine. Other agents including meperidine, amobarbital sodium, ephedrine and chlorpromazine have also been shown to have limited local anesthetic potential. All of these, unfortunately, are very irritating when injected subcutaneously and can cause neural damage. The agent that has been used the most as a local anesthetic substitute is diphenhydramine. The success of this preparation, or any of the others, has at best been limited and is definitely a compromise. Their success, when used as an infiltration injection that requires diffusion through cortical bone, is poor. Adequate analgesia is achieved at the site of the injection only. A nerve block, where diffusion is secondary as needle tip placement carries the solution to the nerve trunk, has been more successful. The type of procedure to be undertaken also affects the success rate. The relative degree of analgesia necessary for pulpal manipulation is somewhat greater than for surgical procedures and their success decreases as painful stimulation from the procedure increases. If epinephrine is added to the solution, efficiency improves to a limited degree.

Bibliography

Aberg G, Adler R: Thermographic registrations of some vascular effects of a local anaesthetic compound. *Svensk Tandl Tidskr* 63:671, 1970.

Adler R, Adler G, Aberg G: Studies on dental blood flow in dogs. *Svensk Tandl Tidskr* 62:699, 1969.

af Ekenstam B, Egner B, Petterson G: N-alkyl pyrolidine and N-alkyl piperidine carboxylic acid amides. *Acta Chem Scand* 11:1183, 1957.

Bartlett SZ: Clinical observations on the effect of injections of local anesthetic preceded by aspiration. *Oral Surg* 33:520, 1972.

Berling C: Octapressin® as a vasoconstrictor in dental plexus anesthesia. *Odont Rev* 17:369, 1966.

Bradley DJ, Martin ND: Clinical evaluation of mepivacaine and lidocaine. *Aust Dent J* 14:377, 1964.

Cannell H, Cannon P: Intraosseous injections of lignocaine local anesthetics. *Br Dent J* 141:48, 1976.

Chilton NW: Clinical evaluation of prilocaine hydrochloride 4% solution with and without epinephrine. *J Am Dent Assoc* 83:149, 1971.

Council on Dental Therapeutics, American Dental Association and American Heart Association Joint Report: Management of dental problems in patients with cardiovascular disease. *J Am Dent Assoc* 68:333, 1964.

Covino BG: Physiology and pharmacology of local anesthetic agents. *Anesth Prog* 28(4):98–104, 1981.

Covino BG, Giddon DB: Pharmacology of local anesthetic agents. *J Dent Res* 60(8):1454–1459, 1981.

Covino BG, Vassalo HG: *Local Anesthetics—Mechanisms of Action and Clinical Use.* New York, Grune & Stratton, 1976.

De Jong RH: *Local Anesthetics*, ed 2. Springfield, Ill., Charles C Thomas, 1977.

du Mesnil de Rochemont W, Hensel H: Measurement of the blood supply of human skin under the influence of various local anesthetics. *Naunyn Schmiedebergs Arch Pharmacol* 239:464, 1960.

Foldes FF, McNall PG: Toxicity of local anesthetics in man. *Dent Clin North Am* 5(2): 257–277, 1961.

Gangarosa LP: Newer local anesthetics and techniques for administration. *J Dent Res* 60(8):1471–1480, 1981.

Gilman AG, Goodman LS, Gilman A: *The Pharmacological Basis of Therapeutics*, ed 6. New York, Macmillian, 1980.

Goebel WG, Allen G, Randall F: Circulating serum levels of mepivacaine after dental injection. *Anesth Prog* 25:52–56, 1978.

Goebel WM, Allen G, Randall F: The effects of commercial vasoconstrictor preparations on the circulating venous serum level of mepivacaine and lidocaine. *J Oral Med* 35(4):91–96, 1980.

Goebel WM, Allen G, Randall F: Comparative circulating serum levels of 2 percent mepivacaine

and 2 percent lignocaine. *Br Dent J* 148:261–264, 1980.

Gordon RA, Kerr JH, Taylor R: A laboratory and clinical evaluation of mepivacaine (Carbocaine). *Can Anaesth Soc J* 7:290, 1960.

Hjelm M, Holmdahl MH: Biochemical effects of aromatic amines. II. *Acta Anaesth Scand* 9:99, 1965.

Jorfeldt L, Lofstrom B, Pernow B, et al: The effect of mepivacaine and lidocaine on forearm resistance and capacitance vessels in man. *Acta Anaesthesiol Scand* 14:183, 1970.

Kramer SK, Milton VA: Complications of local anesthesia. *Dent Clin North Am* 17:443, 1973.

Lilenthal B: Cardiovascular response to intraosseous injections of prilocaine containing vasoconstrictors. *Oral Surg* 42:552, 1976.

Lund PC: Citanest® and methemoglobin. *Acta Anaesthesiol Scand (Suppl)* 16:189, 1965.

Luduena FP, Hoppe JE, Coulston F, et al: The pharmacology and toxicology of mepivacaine, a new local anesthetic. *Toxicol Appl Pharmacol* 2:295, 1960.

Moore DC: *Complications of Regional Anesthesia.* Springfield, Ill., Charles C Thomas, 1955.

Moore PA, Dansky JL: Bupivacaine anesthesia—a clinical trial for endodontic therapy. *Oral Surg* 55:176–179, 1983.

Reynolds F: Vasoconstrictor agents in local anesthetic preparations. *Lancet* 2:764, 1972.

Rood JP: Inferior dental nerve block. Routine aspiration and a modified technique. *Br Dent J* 132:103, 1972.

Ross N, Dobbs E: A preliminary study on Carbocaine. *J Am Dent Soc Anesthesiol* 7:4, 1960.

Sadove MS, Jobgen EA, Heller FN, et al: Methemoglobin—an effect of a new local anesthetic L-67 (Prilocaine). *Acta Anaesthesiol Scand (Suppl)* 16:175, 1965.

Stibbs GD, Korn JH: An evaluation of the local anesthetic, mepivacaine hydrochloride, in operative dentistry. *J Prosthet Dent* 14:355, 1964.

Tolas AG, Pflug AE, Halter JB: Arterial plasma epinephrine concentrations and hemodynamic responses after dental injection of local anesthetic with epinephrine. *J Am Dent Assoc* 104(1):41–43, 1982.

Ulfendahl HR: Some pharmacological and toxicological properties of a new local anesthetic, Carbocaine. *Acta Anaesthesiol Scand* 1:81, 1957.

Warren RE, Van de Mark TB, Weinberg S: Methemoglobinemia induced by high doses of prilocaine. *Oral Surg* 37:866, 1974.

CHAPTER 4

Local Anesthetic Armamentarium

A minimum amount of equipment is necessary for the safe administration of local anesthetic agents. This includes the anesthetic agent, a needle, and a syringe. The equipment is modified for use in dentistry and consequently is slightly different from comparable parenteral injection equipment. Additional items used include gauze squares, topical anesthetic, cotton-tipped applicators, and an optional antiseptic solution.

CARTRIDGES

The local anesthetic agent is commercially prepared and loaded into a single-use, single-dose dental cartridge (Fig. 4.1). In the United States, this cartridge is standardized to contain 1.8 ml of anesthetic solution. Outside the United States, the standardized cartridge contains 2.2 ml of anesthetic solution. Cartridge is the generic name for this glass container. *Carpule* is a brand name and trademark for the dental cartridge marketed by Cook-Waite Laboratories.

The cartridge is sealed on one end by a diaphragm held in place by an aluminum cap. The diaphragm is designed to be pierced by the non-injecting end of the dental needle allowing the flow of anesthetic solution. The opposite end of the cartridge is sealed with a movable rubber plunger. This plunger is designed to be engaged by the harpoon on an aspirating syringe and to slide down the internal surface of the cartridge when the piston of the dental syringe is advanced, expelling the anesthetic solution through a needle. The end seals are maintained with paraffin and the plunger is lubricated with glycerine and silicone to allow

easy movement. The plunger is color-coded; however, this coding is standard within manufacturers, not industry-wide, so cannot be relied upon for quick identification of anesthetic solution contents. Identification of contents is done by reading the painted label on each cartridge. This labeling will identify the anesthetic, volume, concentration of active components, manufacturer, manufacturer's lot number, and expiration date.

Cartridges are packaged in groups of 50 or 100 in round metal containers or in cardboard boxes (Fig. 4.2A and B). The solution in the cartridge in cans or boxes is sterile and does not require additional sterilization but the outside of the cartridge is not sterile, only clean. The sterility of the solution can be safely assumed if the aluminum cap is bright, the plunger is situated slightly below the rim of the glass cartridge, and the solution is clear. Since the outside of the cartridge is not sterile, the diaphragm should be disinfected with 91% isopropyl or 70% ethyl alcohol prior to use. The recommended methods for disinfection are to individually wipe the diaphragm before use or wipe the diaphragm in the center well of

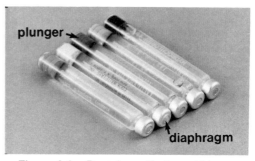

Figure 4.1. Dental anesthetic cartridges.

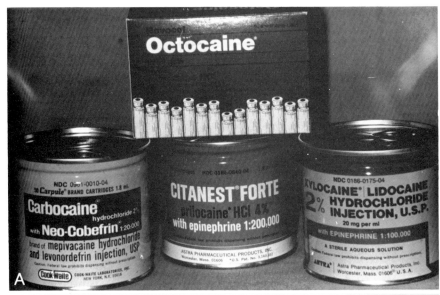

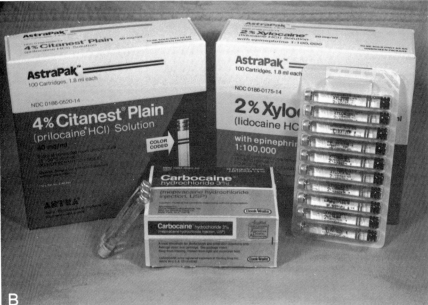

Figure 4.2. *A*, cans and boxes in which dental cartridges are packaged; *B*, box packaging of dental cartridges.

a storage container packed with alcohol gauze (Figs. 4.3 and 4.4). Under no circumstances should the diaphragm end, or the cartridge in total, be stored in disinfecting media. The storage container should not be used to submerge cartridges, as the diaphragm will leak and allow the disinfectant to contaminate the anesthetic solution. In addition, the cartridge cannot be autoclaved, as this will destroy the wax seals and may inactivate some additives. Corrosive chemicals should never be used for disinfection as these can leak into the cartridge and cause corrosion of the aluminum cap (Fig. 4.5).

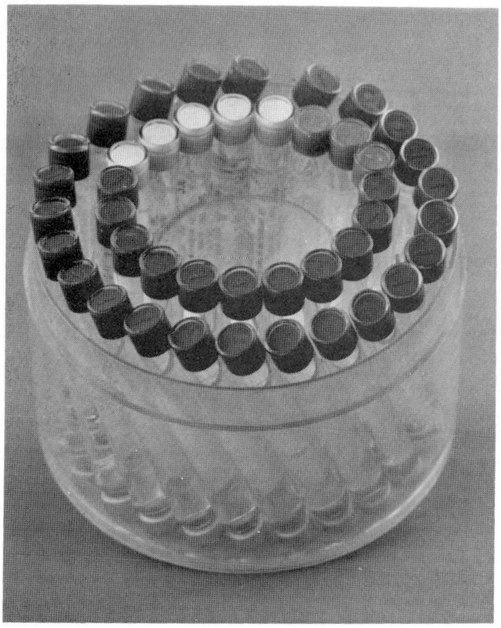

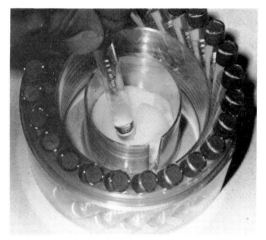

Figure 4.4. Alcohol-soaked wipe in center well of a storage container for disinfecting the diaphragm.

Figure 4.3. Storage container for anesthetic cartridges.

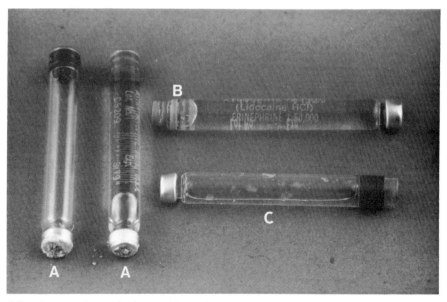

Figure 4.5. Damaged anesthetic cartridges. *A,* aluminum caps corroded from storage in disinfecting media; *B,* plunger extruded from freezing; *C,* paraffin particles floating in the solution.

It is not likely that particulate contamination of a dental cartridge will occur as the manufacturing and filling process is closely monitored, but small fragments of the rubber components and wax fragments have been known to break off and float free in the solution (Figs. 4.5 and 4.6). Any cartridge with this condition is still sterile but the cartridge should not be used because of the risk of injecting foreign debris. A fresh, sterile anesthetic solution will be absolutely clear, with no particulates floating in it. A nitrogen bubble may or may not be present in the solution. Its presence is a part of the manufacturing process but its absence can also be normal. Any cartridge should be examined before use as cracked glass can

occur during shipping. This may be almost invisible (Fig. 4.7) or easily detectable with obvious leakage and crystallization (Fig. 4.8) of the anesthetic solution. In both cases, the cartridge should not be used.

Storage of the cartridge is important in maintaining sterility of the solution and preserving shelf life. The cartridge should be stored in a cool, dry, and relatively dark environment. Heat shortens the shelf life of an anesthetic by reducing vasoconstrictor concentrations and freezing results in extrusion of the plunger and possible leakage of air (Fig. 4.5). Historically, some have advocated heating the anesthetic to body temperature before injection but this is unnecessary if the cartridge is at a reasonable room temperature. There are commercial devices available that heat the cartridges before

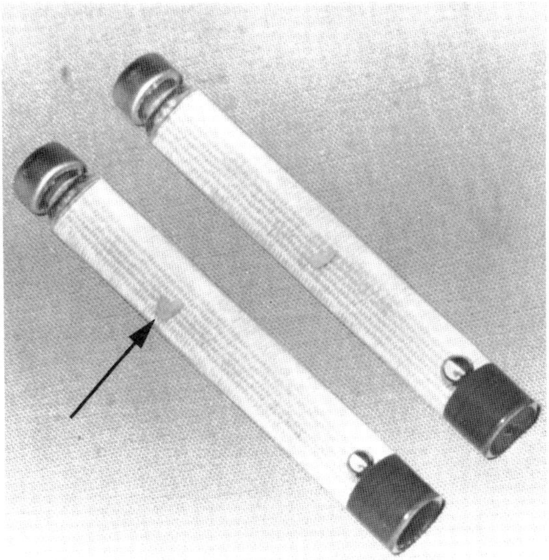

Figure 4.6. Particulate contamination in a dental cartridge.

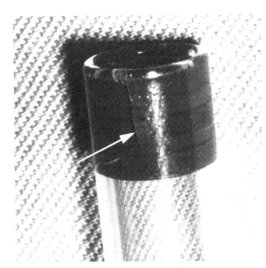

Figure 4.7. Hairline crack in dental cartridge.

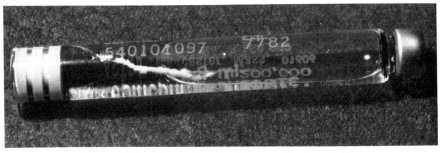

Figure 4.8. Cracked and leaking anesthetic cartridge.

use, but they use a light bulb to accomplish this and the heat created will shorten storage life (Fig. 4.9). Room temperature is more than satisfactory. If the cartridges are stored in direct sunlight, further reduction in shelf life occurs as ultraviolet light has been shown to alter the pH of local solutions and reduce the concentration of any vasoconstrictor additive.

NEEDLES

Needles for the injection of local anesthetics come in multiple lengths and gauges from numerous manufacturers. There are industry-wide standards for consistent sizing, but it has been shown that minor differences do exist. For practical purposes, these differences are clinically not detectable. The dental anesthetic needle is designed to fit specifically on the dental syringe. It is disposable and must be used for only one patient. It can be used for multiple injections on the same patient but is not designed to be sterilized and reused. This disposable feature has virtually eliminated needle breakage, cross-contamination, and spread of infection between patients which did occur with reusable equipment.

Each needle is individually packaged by the manufacturers (Fig. 4.10). If this package is not damaged, sterility is insured. The tissue insertion end of the

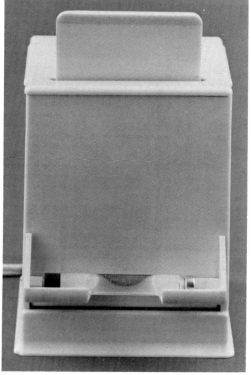

Figure 4.9. Cartridge warmer; an electric light bulb is the heat source.

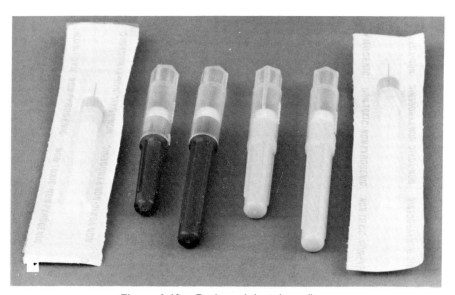

Figure 4.10. Packaged dental needles.

needle is covered with a replaceable cap called the needle cover. The diaphragm-puncturing end of the needle is exposed as soon as the sterile packaging is opened. The disposable dental needle itself consists of several parts (Fig. 4.11A). These are the tissue-penetrating (injecting) end of the *needle* (called the shank). the *hub* where the needle attaches to the syringe adapter, the *syringe adapter* which is made of either plastic or metal, and the *diaphragm-piercing* end of the needle. The end of each needle is beveled to allow for easy tissue penetration but this *bevel* also forces the needle to deflect as it passes through tissue (Fig. 4.11B).

As can be seen in Figure 4.12 there are three needle lengths available for dental use. The "long" needle is approximately 38 mm or 1½ inches in length with vari-ation among manufacturers. The "short" needle is approximately 22 mm or ⅞ inch in length with variation, and the "ultra-short" needle is 12 mm or ½ inch in length with similar variation. Different lengths are available because of different tissue penetration depth requirements. A needle should never be inserted more than ¾ of its length. If a needle breaks, it will break at the hub. If ¼ of the needle remains outside the tissue, it can be grasped and removed. Otherwise recovery is very difficult and may require surgery.

The needle diameter and lumen size are collectively referred to as gauge. Dental needles are usually limited to three gauges, the 25G, 27G, and 30G needles. Other gauges are manufactured but not routinely used. Table 4.1 lists the tubing industry standards for needle gauges but

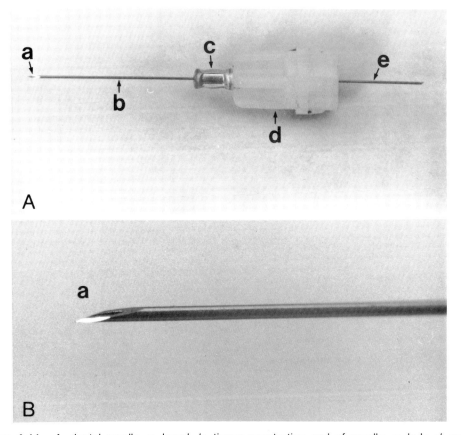

Figure 4.11. *A*, dental needle. *a*, bevel, *b*, tissue-penetrating end of needle, *c*, hub, *d*, syringe adapter, *e*, diaphragm-piercing end of needle. *B*, bevel of needle.

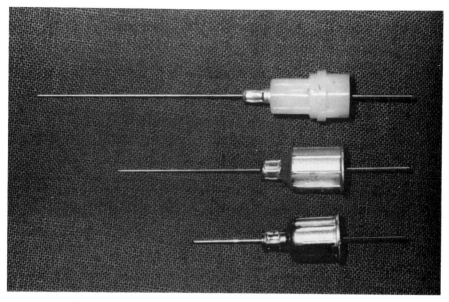

Figure 4.12. Uncovered and unpackaged dental needles.

Table 4.1.
Tubing Industry Standards for Needle Size

Size	Shank Diameter	Lumen Diameter
	inches	inches
25G	0.020	0.010
27G	0.016	0.008
30G	0.012	0.006

actual measurements have been shown to vary. The difference, however, does not present clinical problems. It can be seen that as the gauge number increases (25G to 30G) the needle shank and lumen diameter decreases. This has several clinically meaningful implications. The greater the diameter of the needle, the stronger it is and the less bevel deflection occurs when it is advanced into tissue. This means that the needle tip placement can be better controlled with the 25G needle, especially on deep injections, than with the 27G or 30G size. The greater strength of a larger shank also implies less needle breakage; however, all disposable, single-use dental needles, including the 30G needle, are sufficiently strong so that with *proper use*, needle breakage is an almost nonexistent complication.

It is a common misconception that needle gauge affects patient pain perception on tissue penetration. This myth has been propagated for years without foundation. The phenomenon has been adequately investigated by several authors and all reached the same conclusion. There is no perceptible difference in epithelial penetration discomfort among the dental 25G, 27G, and 30G needles.

Another factor which relates to lumen size of the needle is *ease of aspiration*. Aspiration is the ability to pull blood through the needle lumen as negative pressure is applied by the syringe to the cartridge. The site of anesthetic deposition must not be intravascular; therefore, *aspiration* is attempted before every dental local anesthetic injection to confirm an extravascular (subcutaneous) needle tip placement. If blood is aspirated into the anesthetic cartridge, *aspiration is positive*, and a different deposition site is sought. As a general rule, once aspiration is positive, the cartridge should be discarded and a fresh one used.

It has now been shown that aspiration of blood from human vessels is possible with the 25G, 27G, and 30G needle. However, the ease with which this can be done and the implication of positive aspiration differs and is in direct relation to the lumen size. Positive aspiration can imply needle tip placement intravascularly or in pooled blood at an extravascular site (Fig. 4.13). A 25G and 27G needle will show a stream of blood aspirated into the cartridge with an intravascular needle tip placement. The 30G needle aspirates so slowly, because of small lumen size, that this stream is not seen. Theoretically, extravascular needle tip placement produces a "cloud" of blood (Fig. 4.14) in the cartridge on aspiration and would not negate a safe injection. Practical consideration, however, would advise locating a different deposition site and confirming negative aspiration before injecting.

Considering needle strength, penetration discomfort, and aspiration reliability, it is always advisable to use the 25G or 27G needle. A 30G needle might be substituted on occasion, but its limitations must be thoroughly understood because

it could add unnecessary inaccuracies without any increase in safety. Specific exceptions for the use of a 30G needle exist and these will be discussed under the appropriate injection techniques.

After a dental needle is used it should be discarded in a manner that protects office staff from inadvertent puncture wounds and makes reuse impossible. The best way to insure this is to use a needle destruction unit (Fig. 4.15). It is designed to cut the needle shank at the hub and further cut the diaphragm-piercing portion of the needle from the adapter. The cut portions then fall into the container for later disposal. Another but less ideal disposal method is to place the used needle in a specially labeled box (Figs. 4.16 and 4.17). This does not stop unau-

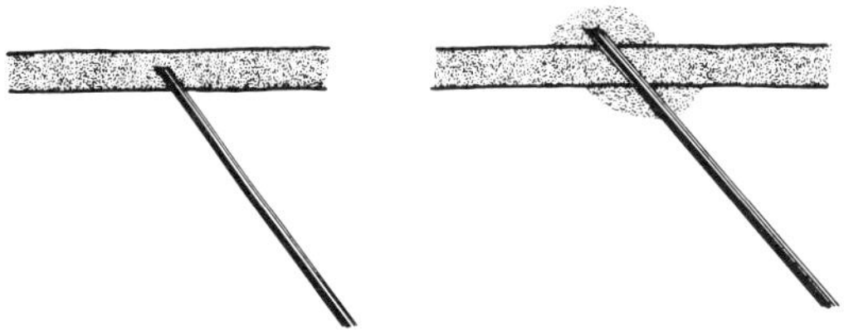

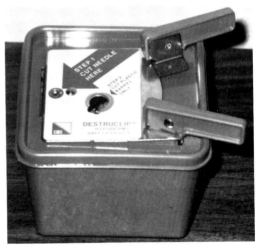

Figure 4.15.   Needle destruction unit.

Figure 4.13.   Illustration of intravascular and extravascular needle tip placement. Extravascular needle placement in pooled extravasated blood will yield positive aspiration.

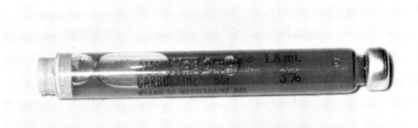

Figure 4.14.   Cloud of blood in cartridge from extravascular needle tip placement on aspiration with a 25G or 27G needle.

thorized reuse but does protect the office staff from accidental puncture wounds. Under no circumstances should a needle be placed in a wastebasket with other less hazardous waste. This invites puncture wounds with contaminated needles when the trash is emptied.

SPECIAL PURPOSE NEEDLE

There is a special purpose needle on the market designed specifically for an intraosseous injection. The needle (Fig. 4.18) consists of a 30G shank with a metal retractable sleeve and a plastic reinforcing collar to support the needle shank. The needle is used to penetrate the thick cortical bone of the maxilla or mandible. The retractable metal sleeve and the plastic collar maintain rigidity until the tip

has penetrated through the dense cortex and into the cancellous bone. Its specific use is discussed under intraosseous injection techniques in Chapter 5.

SYRINGE

The dental syringe is a device designed specifically for the convenience of dental injections. It simplifies maintenance of sterility in handling the single-use dental needle and single-dose dental anesthetic cartridge. The standard dental syringe is a metal, side-loading, autoclavable device that is sturdy enough to last years. Syringes are marketed by several companies and can be purchased as a manual aspirating, self-aspirating, or non-aspirating model. Only models capable of manual or self-aspiration should be considered. Figure 4.19 illustrates three models of aspi-

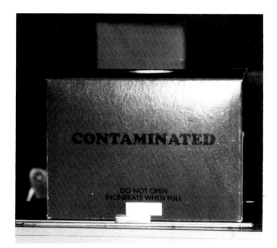

Figure 4.16. Box for storage of used needles.

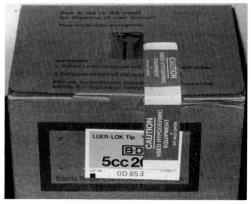

Figure 4.17. Box for storage of used needles.

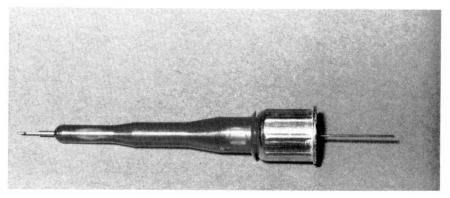

Figure 4.18. Intraosseous needle.

rating syringes and one non-aspirating breech (rear end) loading model.

The essential components of all manual aspirating syringes are illustrated in Figure 4.20. These include the *needle adapter hub*, aspiration *harpoon*, *piston*, *finger rest*, and *thumb ring*. These components are self-explanatory except for the aspirating harpoon. The barbed harpoon is seated in the rubber plunger on the cartridge prior to injection. This enables negative pressure to be applied to the cartridge by pulling back on the piston through the thumb ring (Figs. 4.21 and 4.22). A non-aspirating syringe has a flat end on the piston so the cartridge plunger can be pushed but not retracted. Therefore, reliable aspiration is not possible (Fig. 4.23).

A self-aspirating syringe is illustrated in Figure 4.24. This syringe has a flat ended piston similar to the non-aspirating syringe and is not capable of pulling the plunger back. Aspiration is achieved by a metallic sleeve in the end of the barrel of the syringe. This sleeve (Fig. 4.25) applies pressure on the cartridge diaphragm when the finger rest is squeezed toward the thumb disc (Fig. 4.26). This stretches the diaphragm and when the thumb disc is released, negative pressure is created within the cartridge, achieving aspiration. During the injection, as the piston is pushed forward with the thumb ring the diaphragm is also stretched. By releasing injection pressure, automatic aspiration again takes place. This syringe was marketed in the United States in 1981.

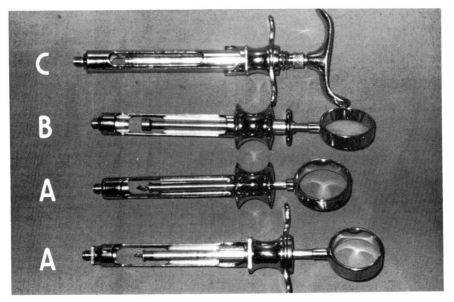

Figure 4.19. *A*, aspirating syringes; *B*, self-aspirating syringe; *C*, non-aspirating syringe.

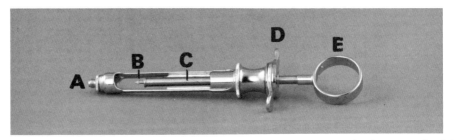

Figure 4.20. Aspirating dental syringe. *A*, needle adapter hub; *B*, aspirating harpoon; *C*, piston; *D*, finger rest; *E*, thumb ring.

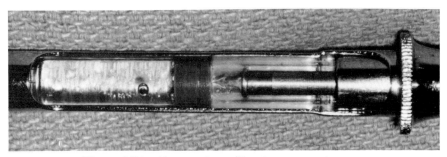

Figure 4.21. Harpoon in position to engage plunger.

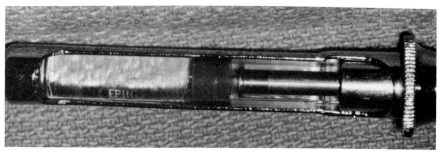

Figure 4.22. Harpoon engaged in plunger.

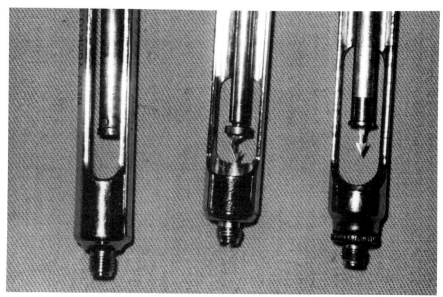

Figure 4.23. Harpoon on aspirating syringes compared to flat plunger on a non-aspirating syringe.

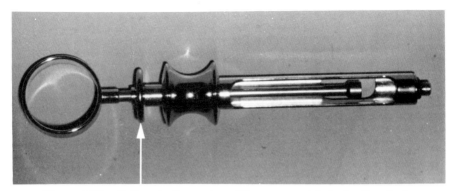

Figure 4.24. Self-aspirating syringe. The *arrow* points to the thumb disc.

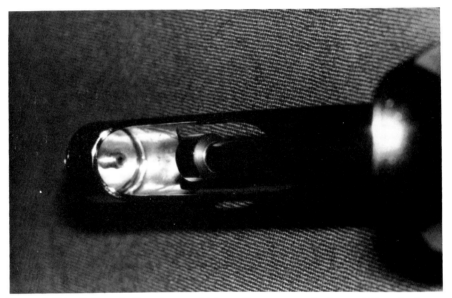

Figure 4.25. Self-aspiration sleeve which applies pressure to the cartridge diaphragm.

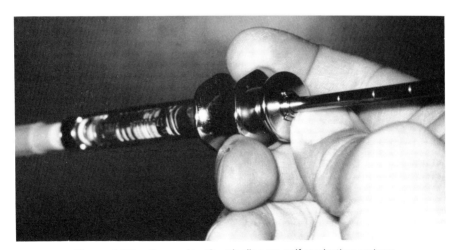

Figure 4.26. Squeezing thumb disc on self-aspirating syringe.

Plastic dental syringes are also available. These are pictured in Figure 4.27. The syringe pictured at the bottom is a combination disposable-reusable apparatus. The barbed piston and thumb ring portion of the device is autoclavable and designed for reuse. The barrel and needle of the syringe are purchased as a unit for single use. The barrel-needle assembly is loaded with a standard dental cartridge and then works as a standard dental syringe. The syringe pictured at the top in Figure 4.27 is a plastic version of the previously described metal aspirating syringe. It is reusable, sturdy, and autoclavable. It does not have the durability of the metal syringe but its cost is much less.

Standard medical parenteral injection systems can be used for dental injections (Fig. 4.28). This equipment is completely disposable but not frequently used for dental local anesthesia as the syringe will not accept the dental cartridge. It must be filled from a single or multiple dose vial.

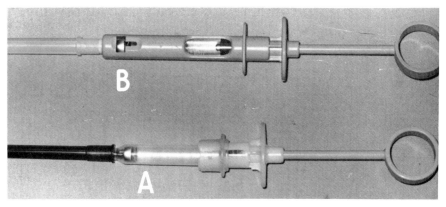

Figure 4.27. Plastic dental aspirating syringes. *A*, combination disposable-reusable syringe; *B*, plastic autoclavable syringe.

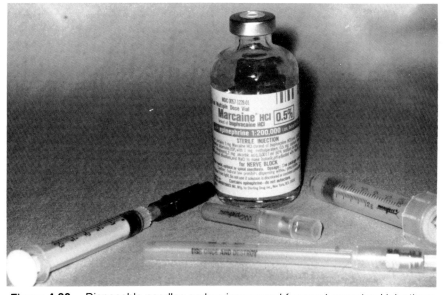

Figure 4.28. Disposable needles and syringes used for most parenteral injections.

It is used only when an anesthetic solution, or a volume of anesthetic, differs from those available in dental cartridges.

GAUZE

Gauze squares are used to dry the mucosa and remove surface debris prior to needle insertion. This improves visibility and reduces gross contamination at the injection site. To maintain asepsis, the gauze wipe should be dry and clean. The dried mucosa is then ready for topical anesthetic application, optional antiseptic application, and needle puncture.

TOPICAL ANESTHETIC

Topical anesthetics can be used just prior to needle penetration of the epithelium. Their purpose is to eliminate or at least reduce the discomfort of needle penetration. Topicals are quite effective in minimizing epithelial sensation, but they do not affect the most uncomfortable portion of any injection, which is muscle penetration, periosteal contact, and the pressure created from expanding tissue as the anesthetic solution enters the site. Topical anesthetics are not universally used by all dentists, nor are they absolutely necessary, but they do offer some advantage. The psychological advantage is that the patient perceives that the operator is doing everything possible to eliminate discomfort.

Numerous agents of differing concentrations and formulations are available from many manufacturers. All of these are not applied to the mucosa in the same manner or for the same length of time. The manufacturer's direction should be followed closely to minimize tissue damage. If the topicals are left in contact with the tissue for more than the recommended *seconds*, or *minutes*, chemical tissue injury can result. The damage is not apparent until postoperatively. Topical anesthetics are sprayed onto the tissue or applied with a cotton-tipped applicator to the site of needle penetration after the mucosa has been dried. Different topical anesthetics and cotton-tipped applicators are illustrated in Figure 4.29A and B.

TOPICAL ANTISEPTIC

The topical antiseptic is an optional part of the dental anesthetic armamentarium. In a survey of dentists it was found that less than 10% routinely used a topical antiseptic prior to needle penetration. A surface antiseptic such as Betadine or Merthiolate will aid in disinfecting the mucosa prior to injection but it should be understood that it does not sterilize the tissue. A short (15- to 30-second) application does little more than clean the area. Antiseptic application does not have to be a routine part of oral injections and is strictly the operator's choice. If the surface area is wiped of debris prior to injection, the chance of the needle carrying bacteria into the tissue is virtually nonexistent. Injection through or into an infected area is not warranted with or without antiseptic application.

SPECIAL PURPOSE SYRINGES

Recent introduction of new special purpose periodontal ligament (PDL) syringes have led to new approaches to single-tooth anesthesia in the maxilla and the mandible. Two basic designs in these syringes are available. Figure 4.30A and B illustrates these devices. They are either of the pistol grip design or of lever action design. Both are used specifically to deliver small amounts of local anesthetic solutions into the small, confined space of the periodontal ligament under considerable pressure. The technique is referred to as a "PDL" injection or intraligamentary injection. The periodontal ligament is a tightly bound, connective tissue area surrounding the root of a tooth. It does not readily allow for the diffusion of local anesthetic solutions and because it is confined by the alveolar bone and the tooth root, does not expand when solutions are injected into it. For it to accept any injected fluid, the solution must be injected under significant pressure. The "PDL sy-

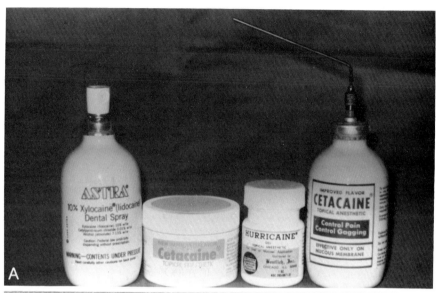

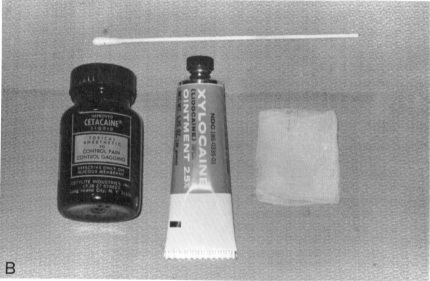

Figure 4.29. *A,* topical anesthetics; *B,* topical anesthetics.

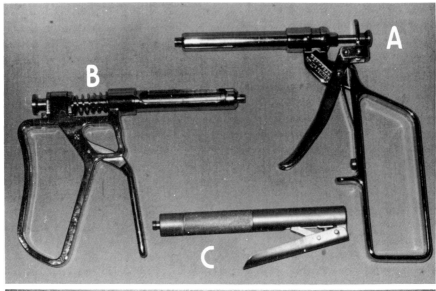

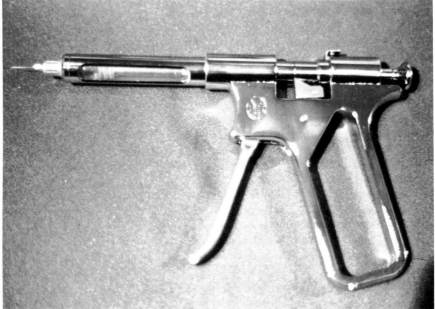

Figure 4.30. *Top*, periodontal ligament syringes. *a*, Peri-Press by Universal Dental Implements; *b*, Ligmaject; *c*, Periodontal Ligament Syringe by Special Products, Inc. *Bottom*, Henke-Ject by M.P.L. Inc.

ringes" are designed to provide a mechanical advantage to develop the necessary pressure.

This pressure is developed by squeezing the "trigger" of the pistol grip design syringes or is held automatically by squeezing the lever on the lever action design syringe which works by an internal ratchet. All of these syringes accept standard dental anesthetic cartridges and standard dental needles with plastic syringe adapters, are durable, and are autoclavable. (Some models will not accept needles with a metal syringe adapter.) Differences in design are aimed at the method of mechanical advantage and the ability to hide an emotionally threatening device from the patient's view. All work equally well for the purpose of developing anesthesia if used properly. The pistol grip design is impossible to hide from the patient because of its size. The lever action design will fit in the palm of the operator's hand.

Pressure (jet) injectors are also available that, with the release of a "cocked" spring, produce up to 2,000 psi of force, to shoot small amounts of anesthetic solution into the tissue. They do not employ a needle but work on the principle of forcing a pressurized stream of anesthetic through the epithelium. They inject small volumes (0.05 ml to 0.2 ml) so can achieve only a small superficial area of anesthesia since the stream is not forced deeply into the tissue. The best that can be expected from these jet injectors is topical anesthesia. Their use in dentistry is of minimal value and they definitely do not replace the routine needle injection.

EQUIPMENT ASSEMBLY

The assembly of the anesthetic syringe will be described in detail. The correct sequence insures proper operation of the needle-syringe-cartridge apparatus. The following description applies to the classic metal or plastic manual aspirating, side-loading syringe. Manufacturers supply detailed assembly instructions with their products and these should be followed closely when using the self-aspirating syringe, "PDL syringe," or the combination plastic disposable-reusable syringe.

The equipment is assembled in preparation for the injection in the following sequence:

1. Disinfect the cartridge diaphragm (Fig. 4.4).

2. Retract the piston on the syringe as far as possible so the harpoon withdraws into the finger grip area. This opens the barrel of the syringe for cartridge insertion (Fig. 4.31).

3. Insert the cartridge, plunger end first, into the barrel of the syringe. It should lie flat and fully inserted in the barrel. Release the piston (Fig. 4.32).

4. Engage the harpoon into the plunger of the cartridge for aspiration by firmly pushing the piston and thumb ring (Fig. 4.33). Excessive pressure is not necessary.

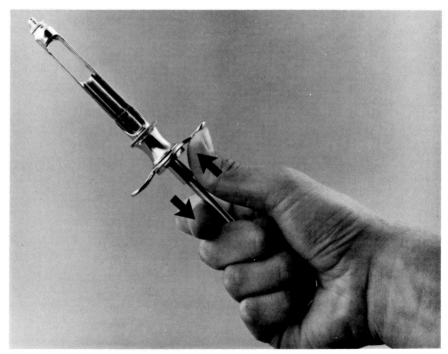

Figure 4.31. Retract the piston on the dental syringe.

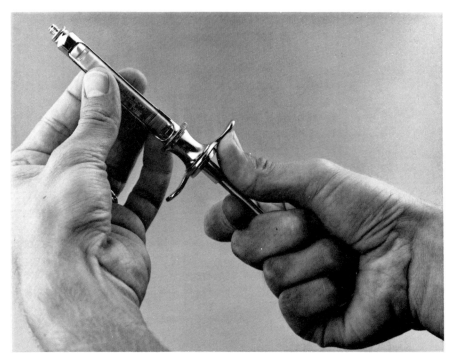

Figure 4.32. Place cartridge into barrel of syringe. After it is lying flat, release the piston.

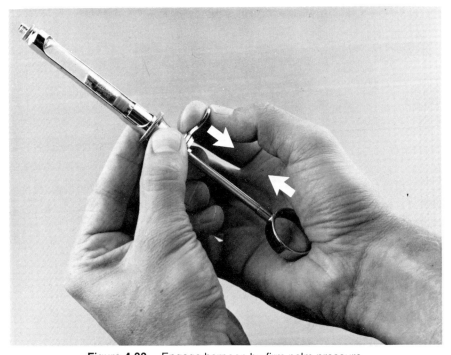

Figure 4.33. Engage harpoon by firm palm pressure.

A "stop" in piston movement will be felt when the harpoon is fully seated (Fig. 4.22).

5. Open the needle package, or remove the clear plastic cap from the diaphragm-piercing end of the needle. Do not remove the needle cover. The needle should be inserted in a straight line with the syringe to insure center puncture of the diaphragm. Screw the needle tightly to its seat on the syringe tip to firmly attach it to the syringe-cartridge assembly (Fig. 4.34). Center puncture of the cartridge diaphgram is important to insure a seal that does not leak. If the diaphragm is punctured off center, the cartridge diaphragm will leak when injection pressure is applied.

6. With the syringe in a vertical position, needle up, remove the needle cover and express the air in the needle and any nitrogen from the bubble in the cartridge until a few drops of anesthetic appear at the needle tip (Fig. 4.35). This insures proper flow and starts the plunger moving

downward in the cartridge so it can be advanced smoothly. The wax seal on the plunger is broken by doing this. If it is not moved prior to the injection it is impos-

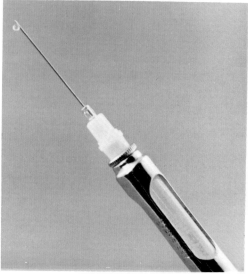

Figure 4.35. Express air from the needle and nitrogen from the cartridge.

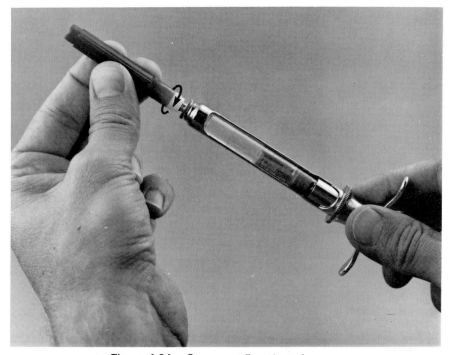

Figure 4.34. Screw needle onto syringe.

sible to create smooth injection pressure and a jerky motion will result. Replace the needle cover until the injection is ready to be given.

To unload the syringe after use, retract the piston to disengage the harpoon and invert the barrel assembly. The used cartridge will fall from the barrel of the syringe (Fig. 4.36). When removing the needle, be sure that the syringe tip is not unscrewed with the needle and inadvertently discarded (Fig. 4.37).

If more than one cartridge is needed, when the second is inserted, the needle is already in place. The diaphragm piercing end of the needle will be visible inside the barrel of the syringe (Fig. 4.38). The new cartridge is inserted as outlined in paragraph 3 above. This cartridge must lie flat and be fully in place before the piston is released. When the piston is released, the diaphragm will be forced onto the needle. The harpoon can be re-engaged into the plunger by putting gentle but quick palm pressure on the piston with the thumb ring (Fig. 4.33). Some solution will be expressed from the needle. This cannot be avoided as this breaks the wax seal on the plunger and initiates plunger movement. The piston *should not be hit*

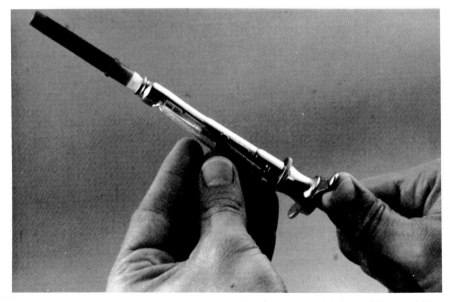

Figure 4.36. To unload a used cartridge, retract the piston completely and the cartridge will fall from the barrel.

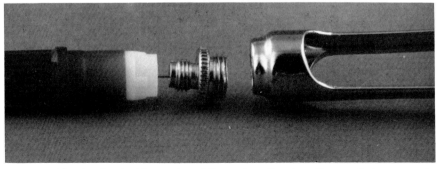

Figure 4.37. Inadvertent loosening of the syringe tip when the needle is removed.

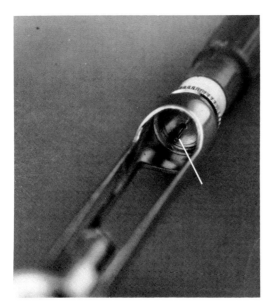

Figure 4.38. Diaphragm-piercing end of needle visible inside the barrel of the syringe.

with the palm of the hand as this can shatter the cartridge, scatter glass fragments, and injure anyone in the area.

All equipment that is to be used for the injection should be ready and assembled for use prior to initiating any aspect of the injection. If it is placed on an environmental work area, it should be covered to maintain asepsis and not in full view of the patient, as this could result in unnecessary anxiety on the part of the patient. Chapter 5 will discuss the technique of local anesthetic administration, as the equipment is now ready for use.

Bibliography

Aldous JA: Needle deflection: a factor in the administration of local anesthetics. *J Am Dent Assoc* 77:602–604, 1968.

Ciarlone AE, Fry BW: Stability of vasoconstrictors in local anesthetic solutions exposed to ultraviolet irridation. *J Dent Res* 59(6):1068, 1980.

Cooley RL, Lubow RM: Particulate contamination of local anesthetic solutions. *Oral Surg* 51(5):481–483, 1981.

Cooley RL, Lubow RM: Evaluation of ultraviolet, infrared, and fluorescent light on pH of local anesthetic solutions. *Milit Med* 146:788–791, 1981.

Cooley RL, Robinson SF: Comparative evaluation of the 30-gauge dental needle. *Oral Surg* 48(5):400–404, 1979.

Fry BW, Ciarlone AE: Storage at body temperature alters concentration of vasoconstrictors in local anesthetics. *J Dent Res* 59(6):1069, 1980.

Fuller NP, Menke RA, Meyers WJ: Perception of pain to three different intraoral penetrations of needles. *J Am Dent Assoc* 99:822–824, 1979.

Gill CJ, Orr DL: A double blind crossover comparison of topical anesthetics. *J Am Dent Assoc* 98(2):213–214, 1979.

Jacklich J: Special Products, Inc., 102 Western Ct., Santa Cruz, CA 95060 (personal communication).

Malamed SF: *Handbook of Local Anesthesia.* St. Louis, C.V. Mosby, 1980.

Mollen AJ, Ficara AJ, Provant DR: Needles, 25 gauge versus 27 gauge—can patients really tell? *Gen Dent* 29(5):417–418, 1981.

Peterson DS, Kein DR: Pain sensation related to local anesthesia injected at varying temperatures. *Anesth Prog* 25:164–165, 1978.

Trapp LD, Davies RO: Aspiration as a function of hypodermic needle internal diameter in the in-vivo human upper limb. *Anesth Prog* 27:49–51, 1980.

Watson JE, Colman RS: Interpretation of aspiration tests in local anesthetic injections. *J Oral Surg* 34:1069–1074, 1976.

CHAPTER 5

Techniques of Local Anesthesia

Local analgesia for dentistry requires complete understanding of the functional anatomy of the head and neck. Specific anatomy of the osteology, myology, vascularity, and neurology of the oral region must be reviewed and taken into consideration before introducing any foreign substances, including the needle and anesthetic agent, into tissue. The student of dentistry makes more routine use of head and neck anatomy during the administration of local anesthesia than in any other general dental procedure. This knowledge is used on virtually every patient.

This text is not meant to replace anatomy texts but rather build on basic information, putting it to practical use. The following is a pertinent review of anatomical structures that are a part of the mechanics and physiology of dental local analgesia.

The fifth cranial nerve or trigeminal nerve is the main nerve involved with oral analgesia. It has both sensory and motor roots.

Sensory components are contained in the ophthalmic, maxillary, and mandibular divisions while the motor fibers from the motor root accompany only the mandibular division. Sensory fibers carry the sensation of pain, touch, thermal response, and proprioception and the motor fibers carry impulses to the muscles of mastication. Because motor and sensory fibers are sometimes in close proximity it is not uncommon for limited motor paralysis to result from routine sensory analgesia techniques. Rarely, however, it is a problem, and when it does occur, it is not obtrusive to dental care of patient function.

Cranial nerve 5 originates in the pons and then courses to the semilunar or Gasserian ganglion in the cranium (Fig. 5.1). Three large nerve trunks then emerge from the Gasserian ganglion and exit the cranium through fissures and foramina. The smallest of these is the ophthalmic division (V_1) which courses along the lateral wall of the cavernous sinus and enters the orbit through the superior orbital fissure. From there it gives off sensory branches to the side of the nose, nasal mucosa, upper eyelid, forehead and anterior scalp. The ophthalmic nerve has no dental innervation and therefore has only minimal significance to dental anesthesia.

MAXILLARY DIVISION

The maxillary division (V_2) of the fifth cranial nerve is the second largest of the three divisions and exits the cranium through the foramen rotundum from which it enters the pterygopalatine fossa. The main nerve trunk of V_2 is accessible at this point to needle penetration and complete block of the maxillary division can be achieved at this site. The nerve is 4 to 5 cm from the lateral surface of the head in the zygomatic region and 2 to 3 cm above the posterior hard palate. The trunk is exposed in the pterygopalatine fossa for several centimeters giving off branches to the pterygopalatine (sphenopalatine) ganglion, zygomatic area, and posterior maxilla while the main nerve trunk courses into the inferior orbital fissure on its way to the infraorbital canal.

The first branches of dental interest given off from the maxillary nerve are the pterygopalatine nerves, usually two in number, which course inferiorly to the pterygopalatine (sphenopalatine) ganglion (Fig. 5.2). Numerous branches then emerge from the ganglion, some of which have synapsed in the ganglion but most which have merely passed through. Those that have synapsed provide anatomical communication for cranial nerves 5, 9, and 10 and control sensory and secretory function of the lacrimal glands and mucous glands of the nasal mucosa, hard palate, soft palate, and pharynx.

The emerging branches of dental interest which have not synapsed in the ganglion are sensory branches of V_2 coursing to the hard palate, soft palate, palatine tonsils, and maxillary gingiva. The first group of these branches are the anterior, middle and posterior palatine nerves. Although listed as three entities for purposes of discussion, they are not always identifiable as such. The fibers making up these nerves enter the pterygopalatine canal, which courses to the posterior hard palate and opens as two or more individual foramina referred to as the greater (posterior) palatine and the lesser palatine foramen (Fig. 5.3). Considerable confusion can exist because of the nomenclature of

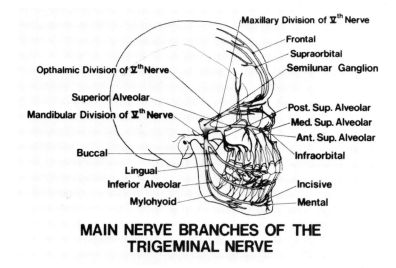

MAIN NERVE BRANCHES OF THE
TRIGEMINAL NERVE

Figure 5.1. Cranial nerve 5.

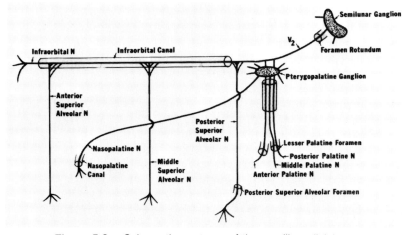

Figure 5.2. Schematic anatomy of the maxillary division.

these foramina and their respective nerves. The anterior palatine nerve (also called the greater palatine nerve) emerges from the greater palatine foramen (also called the posterior palatine foramen) and courses forward, providing sensory innervation to the mucosa of the hard palate from the foramen forward to and usually including the region of the maxillary cuspid. The middle and posterior palatine nerves emerge from the lesser palatine foramen (foramina) and course posteriorly, the middle palatine nerve providing sensory innervation to the mucous membrane of the soft palate and the posterior palatine nerve providing sensory innervation to the mucosa of the palatine tonsils and tonsilar fossa. The mucosa of the posterior hard palate and its underlying connective tissue is only a few millimeters thick, so the three palatal nerves are easily accessible for local anesthetic injection at their emergence from the associated foramina.

The next nerve of dental interest to branch from the maxillary nerve also comes from the pterygopalatine ganglion, although without synapse, as it is the second branch of the two pterygopalatine

nerves and is called the nasopalatine nerve (Fig. 5.2). This nerve enters the nasal cavity through the sphenopalatine foramen and courses down the vomer. The fibers then enter the incisive canal (nasopalatine canal) and emerge in the midline on the anterior hard palate (Fig. 5.3). Although these are bilateral nerves, they descend the incisive canal (canals) together and cannot be classified as right or left branches. These nerves innervate the mucous membrane of the palatal aspect of the premaxilla, extending posteriorly and usually including the maxillary cuspid region. Innervation of the palatal gingivae and attached mucosa in the cuspid region is shared between the nasopalatine and anterior palatine nerves. The emergence of the nasopalatine nerves on the anterior hard palate provide another access point for local anesthesia, as the canal opening is 2 to 4 mm under the mucosa.

The next aggregate of branches of the maxillary nerve are the posterior superior alveolar nerve fibers (Figs. 5.2 and 5.4). These fibers pass down the posterior surface of the maxilla and enter the posterior superior alveolar foramen to course into

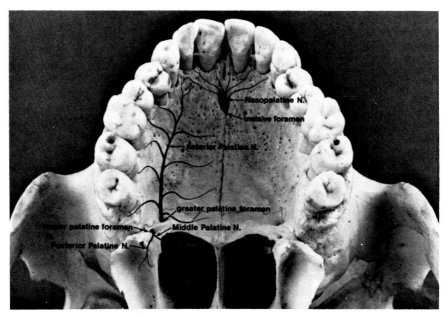

Figure 5.3. Nerves of the palate.

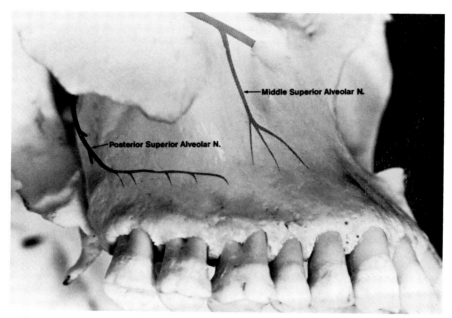

Figure 5.4. Posterior superior alveolar and middle superior alveolar nerve fibers.

the maxillary sinus and bone. Other small branches pass around the posterior lateral surface of the maxilla and innervate the buccal gingivae of the tuberosity. The fibers entering the posterior superior alveolar canal further branch in the bone to provide sensory innervation to the maxillary sinus mucosa and the pulps of the maxillary 3rd molar, 2nd molar, and distal buccal and palatal roots of the 1st molar. In addition, the fibers innervate the associated periosteum, buccal bone, and buccal gingivae of these teeth. The posterior superior alveolar nerve fibers, before entering the posterior maxilla, are within 1 cm of the height of the mucobuccal fold, above the tuberosity, providing simple access for a local anesthetic injection.

The main nerve trunk (maxillary nerve) then enters the inferior orbital groove (fissure) and the infraorbital canal, where it is called the infraorbital nerve (Fig. 5.2). This nerve trunk gives off multiple fibers known categorically as the middle superior alveolar and anterior superior alveolar nerves. These aggregates, although for discussion referred to as specific nerves, are by no means isolated

nerve trunks. In fact, all three of the superior alveolar nerves (anterior, middle, and posterior) form a superior dental plexus innervating the maxillary teeth and buccal gingivae. Specifically, the fibers of the middle superior alveolar nerve descend from the infraorbital nerve through the bone of the maxilla to innervate the mucosa of the maxillary sinus, pulps of the bicuspid teeth, the mesial buccal root of the first molar, and associated periosteum buccal bone and buccal gingivae (Fig. 5.4).

The anterior superior alveolar nerve fibers descend from the infraorbital nerve peripheral to the branching of the middle superior alveolar fibers but proximal to the infraorbital foramen (Fig. 5.5). These nerve fibers provide sensory innervation to the mucosa of the maxillary sinus, pulps of the cuspid and incisor teeth, and associated periosteum, buccal bone, and buccal gingivae.

The categorization of the three maxillary alveolar nerve aggregates comes in part from the way in which these fibers are anesthetized. Since these nerves course within bone, they are not directly accessible to local anesthetic placement.

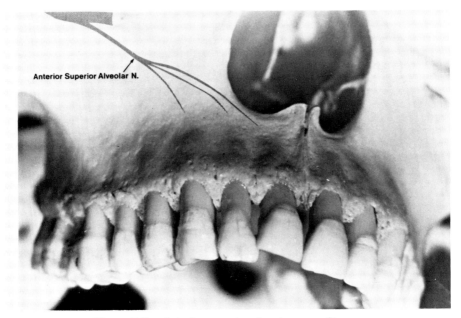

Figure 5.5.   Anterior superior alveolar nerve fibers.

The bone of the maxilla, however, is quite porous, so diffusion of anesthetic agents into the maxilla provides a pathway for anesthesia. Three maxillary injections, the anterior, middle, and posterior superior alveolar infiltrations, effectively block sensory stimulation from the maxillary teeth. This accounts for the "schematic" thinking of these isolated nerves when actually multiple fibers from the superior (maxillary) dental plexus exist (Fig. 5.6).

The infraorbital nerve continues after the branching of the anterior superior alveolar nerve and exits on the anterior maxilla through the infraorbital foramen. None of the branches from the foramen are associated with teeth but they do spread to innervate the ipsilateral lower eyelid, side of the nose, and upper lip and its associated cutaneous and mucosal surfaces. The infraorbital foramen is several millimeters under the skin of the face and approximately 1 cm above the height of the anterior mucobuccal fold, so is easily accessible for local injection from an intraoral approach.

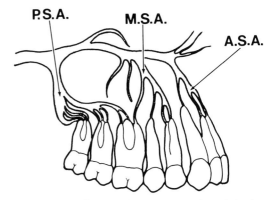

Figure 5.6.   Schematic representation of the innervation of the posterior (PSA), middle (MSA), and anterior (ASA) superior alveolar nerves of the superior dental plexus.

MANDIBULAR DIVISION

The mandibular division (V_3) of the trigeminal nerve is the largest of the three divisions. It is composed chiefly of sensory fibers with only a small but important motor component. This motor component will not be outlined in depth. The fibers of the motor component in a few cases course to their target muscles with sensory fibers so sensory block may also cause motor paralysis. Most course independently so are not affected. The muscles innervated by the motor fibers include the temporalis, the internal and external pterygoids, masseter, mylohyoid, and the anterior belly of the digastric muscle. Additional fibers innervate the small muscles of the soft palate, the tensor veli and the tensor tympani muscles. The motor fibers are rarely anesthetized with peripheral nerve block techniques but can be anesthetized with more central techniques.

The mandibular division leaves the skull through the foramen ovale and courses inferiorly on its way to the mandible (Fig. 5.7). At its exit from the skull, the nerve lies 4 to 5 cm deep to the side of the face. This centrally located site is the first location where it is accessible for local anesthetic injection. Most of the motor nerves branch quickly and proceed to their appropriate muscles or the otic ganglion, so sensory anesthesia does not always result in motor paralysis. The first branch of dental interest is the buccal nerve, also called the long buccal (Figs. 5.8 and 5.9). It branches from the main nerve trunk at the level of the external

pterygoid muscle coursing inferior and anterior. It follows the tendon of the temporalis and then downward in or on the masseter. At the level of the occlusal plane, it crosses from the inner surface of the ascending ramus to the anterior and lateral surface of the mandible, then sends terminal sensory branches to the buccal mucosa, buccinator muscle and the buccal gingivae of the mandibular molars and second bicuspid. At the point on the anterior ramus where the buccal nerve crosses from medial to lateral, it is under only a few millimeters of mucosa so easily accessible for local anesthetic injection.

The next dental branch from the mandibular nerve is the lingual nerve (Figs. 5.7 and 5.8). It descends between the ramus of the mandible and internal pterygoid muscle. At this location it is medial and anterior to the main mandibular nerve trunk, in this location called the inferior alveolar. The lingual nerve continues into the lateral lingual sulcus slightly posterior to the mandibular 3rd molar. In the sulcus it loops below the duct of the submandibular salivary gland, Wharton's duct, and then sends terminal sensory branches to the mandibular lin-

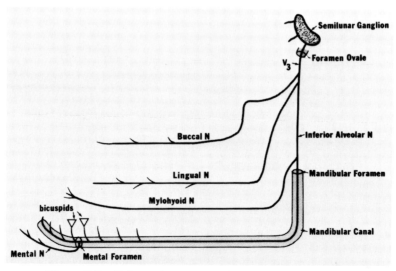

Figure 5.7. Schematic anatomy of the mandibular division.

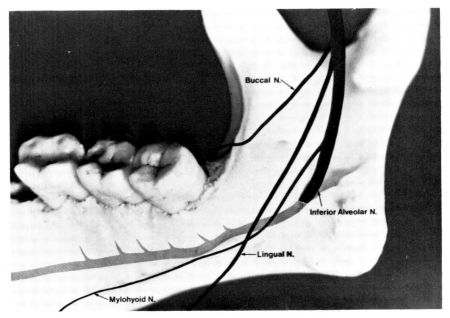

Figure 5.8.   Neuroanatomy of the mandibular sulcus.

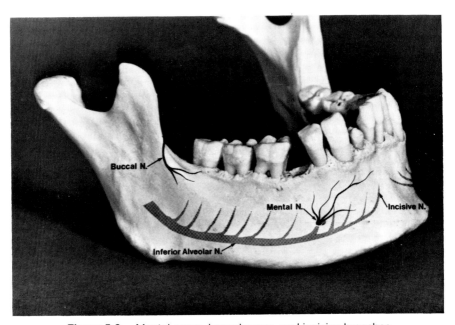

Figure 5.9.   Mental nerve, buccal nerve, and incisive branches.

gual gingivae, floor of the mouth, and anterior two-thirds of the tongue. The lingual nerve is easily reached for local anesthesia along its course as it lies from several millimeters to a centimeter deep to the mucous membrane.

At a level just below the external pterygoid muscle, the chorda tympani nerve from the seventh cranial nerve joins the lingual and courses with it to the tongue supplying secretory innervation to the submandibular and sublingual salivary glands and taste sensation to the anterior two-thirds of the tongue. Anesthesia of the lingual nerve at any point below the chorda tympani juncture will result in loss of both pain sensation and taste in the anterior two-thirds of the tongue.

The inferior alveolar nerve is the largest terminal branch of the mandibular division (Figs. 5.7 to 5.9). It courses between the internal and external pterygoid muscles down the medial surface of the ramus of the mandible to the mandibular foramen where it enters the mandibular canal. At this point the nerve is approximately 2 cm deep to the mucosa and so is easily accessible for local anesthetic injection.

At a variable distance above the canal, a terminal branch, the mylohyoid nerve, separates from the inferior alveolar nerve and courses through the sphenomandibular ligament to the mylohyoid groove. The mylohyoid nerve contains both sensory and motor fibers which go to the mylohyoid muscle and anterior belly of the digastric muscle. From the mylohyoid groove the nerve courses forward below the mylohyoid muscle and occasionally sends a few sensory branches to the mental area and mandibular incisors. The mylohyoid nerve is normally anesthetized along with the inferior alveolar because of the close approximation of the two.

In the mandibular canal, the inferior alveolar nerve supplies numerous sensory fibers to all of the mandibular teeth and their periodontal attachments. As the nerve reaches the bicuspid region it divides. One branch, the incisive, continues within the body of the mandible to the anterior mandibular teeth to the midline (Figs. 5.7 to 5.9). The other branch, the mental, leaves the mandible through the mental foramen, which is located below and generally between the first and second bicuspids. The mental nerve supplies sensory innervation to the lower lip and its associated skin and mucosa, and the

buccal gingivae of the mandibular first bicuspid, cuspid and incisors, to the midline. The mental foramen is under approximately 2 to 3 mm of tissue, so the nerve can be easily anesthetized at this point.

Certain other points of clarity must also be mentioned as they explain some occurrences during routine local analgesia. At any location where two nerves meet, there is the possibility of overlap. When working in one of the overlap areas, it is often necessary to anesthetize both nerves involved to achieve an adequate depth of operating analgesia. The most frequent sites for this phenomenon are 1) midline, maxillary or mandibular; 2) mental nerve and buccal nerve; 3) nasopalatine and anterior palatine nerve; 4) anterior superior-middle superior-posterior superior nerves.

The previous discussion of anatomy is based on anatomical dissections and by physically following the course of nerves exiting from the skull to the most terminally visible branches. Clinical practice of local anesthesia will reveal that all operative situations do not exactly fit into the neuroanatomical description.

The possibility of accessory innervation to almost any area or tooth must be considered, especially when nerve block does not result in complete sensory loss from the listed anatomical site. Anesthesia directed at "accessory" nerves in the area many times will result in complete elimination of sensation.

"Accessory" innervation is anatomically difficult to prove but has useful application. Numerous explanations exist with few proven, but theoretically the following anomalies can exist: 1) cutaneous coli (2nd cervical) innervation of mandibular teeth; 2) greater auricular innervation of mandibular posterior teeth; 3) auriculotemporal innervation of the mandibular posterior teeth; 4) high division fibers of the inferior alveolar nerve entering the mandible above the mandibular foramen; 5) supplemental sensory fibers from the mylohyoid nerve entering the lingual surface of the body of the mandible; 6) lingual nerve fibers entering the body of the mandible and innervating the mandibular teeth; 7) nasopalatine nerve branches innervating the anterior maxillary teeth; 8) anterior palatine nerve branches innervating maxillary posterior teeth.

Since the anatomical basis for these "accessory" innervations is difficult to prove, a further discussion of the clinical approach to these nerves is found in the section on supplemental injections later in this chapter.

Muscle paralysis was mentioned earlier as occurring with certain injections but rarely being a clincal problem or even clinically apparent. Most of the motor fibers of the fifth cranial nerve branch at a point central to the usual anatomical location of anesthetic deposition and are thus not affected. The one notable exception is the mylohyoid nerve, which should be anesthetized with the inferior alveolar. Clinical symptoms of digastric and mylohyoid paralysis are not usually noticed because either the contralateral muscle maintains function or other larger and stronger muscles in the area such as the intrinsic tongue muscles more than make up for the lack of function. Consequently, mylohyoid paralysis is not clinically noticed.

When anesthetic agents are deposited in soft tissue peripheral to a large nerve trunk, diffusion of the agent will also anesthetize motor nerve fibers in the area. This is common with seventh cranial nerve fibers in the lips. Thus paralysis of the area will result. Any soft tissue deposition of an anesthetic agent will anesthetize all nerves in the immediate area, so sensory, motor, and special sensory (e.g., taste) loss can occur indiscriminately. Function returns when the anesthetic action disappears.

Specific mention of myology and osteology as they relate to dentistry will be included in the techniques of local anes-

thesia. Vascularity will also be discussed in the same manner, although it should be emphasized that most nerve branches, especially those that course through bony canals, are accompanied by similarly named arteries and veins.

The foregoing discussion by no means is intended as a discussion of all nerves and their branches in the head and neck area. Only those that directly apply to dental local anesthesia have been presented.

TECHNIQUES OF LOCAL ANESTHESIA

Local anesthesia has anatomically been categorized into numerous types of nerve blocks and infiltrations which apply to anesthetic injection techniques in general. The following summarizes these (Fig. 5.10).

Nerve Block

A sensory nerve block is achieved when impulses carried by a main nerve trunk are prevented from being propagated. This is accomplished when a local anesthetic agent is deposited very close to or on the nerve trunk.

Field Block (Regional Block)

A sensory field block is achieved when impulses from macroscopically identifiable terminal nerve fibers are prevented from being propagated. This is accomplished when a local anesthetic agent is deposited very close to or on the selected nerve fibers.

Peripheral Nerve Block

A peripheral nerve block occurs when propagation of impulses is interrupted at a site peripheral to the central nervous system.

Infiltration

A sensory infiltration (nerve block) is achieved when a local anesthetic agent

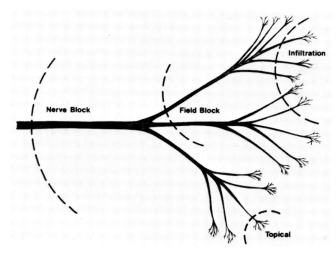

Figure 5.10. Anatomical classification of local anesthesia techniques.

prevents impulses carried by *macroscopic* and *microscopic* nerve branches from being propagated. In this instance, a small area of analgesia is produced by bathing all nerve fibers at a peripheral site with the agent rather than directing the agent at a more central, specific nerve trunk. This method relies heavily on the diffusibility of the anesthetic agent to reach all terminal fibers.

Topical

Sensory topical analgesia is produced when a local anesthetic prevents impulses from free nerve endings in the mucosa from being propagated. In this case the agent is placed on the free nerve endings.

To achieve any of the types of local analgesia, numerous methods may be used and are named by the manner in which they are produced. Topical analgesia is obviously achieved by placing the agent directly on free nerve endings. No injection is involved.

All injection analgesia relies to some degree on diffusion of the agent to the target area or nerves. Even a block injection technique relies on diffusion of the agent because it is not always possible or is it advisable in dental injections to place the needle tip directly on the nerve. Close placement is strived for so that the anes-

thetic solution easily reaches the nerve, but needle tip placement on the nerve can result in minor nerve damage. Practically, even when a block is attempted, what usually takes place is an infiltration of the area where the major nerve trunk is located. The various types of injections used for dental local anesthesia are described as follows.

Submucosal

A submucosal injection is achieved when the agent is deposited just below the mucosa (Fig. 5.11).

Paraperiosteal (Supraperiosteal)

A paraperiosteal injection is achieved when the agent is deposited on but not under the periosteum. In practical use where attached mucosa is involved, it is virtually impossible to differentiate the paraperiosteal and submucosal injection. They are easily separated where abundant connective tissue and or muscle and fat lie between the mucosa and bone (Fig. 5.12).

Subperiosteal

A subperiosteal injection is achieved when the agent is deposited into or under the periosteum. This type of injection is

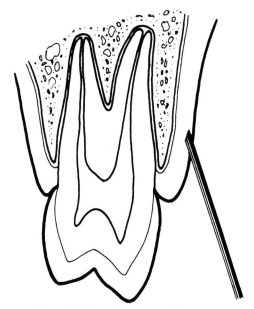

Figure 5.11.   Submucosal injection.

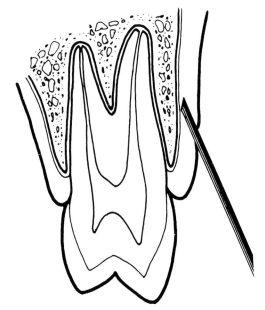

Figure 5.12.   Paraperiosteal injection.

very *painful* and cannot be done without some injury to the periosteum. There is no valid reason to use this type of injection for dental procedures (Fig. 5.13).

Intraosseous

An intraosseous injection is achieved when the agent is deposited in cancellous bone. To achieve this, the needle must be advanced through the dense cortical bone. It is a very effective method of anesthesia but potentially dangerous because the local anesthetic blood levels produced are comparable to an intravascular injection (Fig. 5.14).

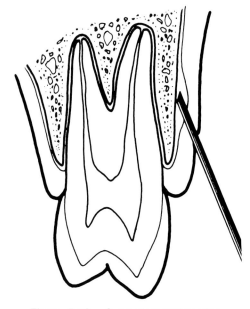

Figure 5.13.   Subperiosteal injection.

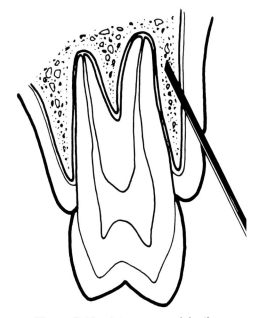

Figure 5.14.   Intraosseous injection.

Intrapulpal

An intrapulpal injection is achieved when the needle is advanced into the exposed pulpal tissue of a tooth. This injection is used during root canal therapy (Fig. 5.15).

Intrapapillary

An intrapapillary injection is achieved by advancing the needle tip into the interdental papilla. It is used as a method of injecting a hemostatic agent and/or a local anesthetic which contains a vasoconstrictor to control gingival hemorrhage and pain from periodontal procedures (Fig. 5.16).

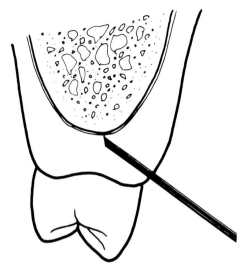

Figure 5.16. Intrapapillary injection.

Periodontal Ligament (Intraligamentary)

A periodontal ligament injection (PDL) is achieved when the needle tip is advanced into the periodontal ligament space along the root of a tooth (Fig. 5.17).

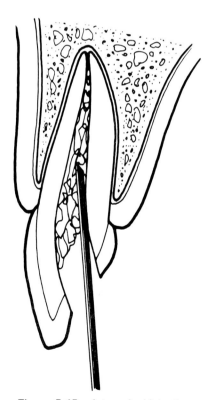

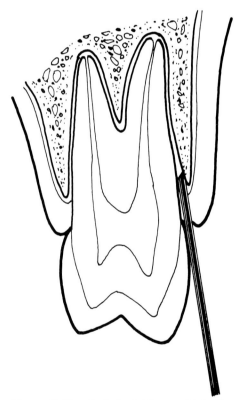

Figure 5.17. Periodontal ligament injection.

Parenteral Injections

General categories for all injections are routinely listed as intradermal, subcutaneous, intramuscular, and intravascular. The intradermal injection has no appro-

Figure 5.15. Intrapulpal injection.

priate corresponding injection in dentistry. All of the previously listed dental anesthetic injections are subcutaneous injections. Intramuscular injections are occasionally used for specific therapeutic measures and the intravascular injection (venous or arterial) is completely avoided and contraindicated. Thus a complete series of terms exist whereby each type and location of anesthetic injection used in dental therapy can be identified and discussed.

Each category of injection has a different degree of reliability, efficiency and duration (assuming equivalent doses). The closer the agent is to the fibers, the better the clinical effect. This is because as diffusion takes place, the available concentration of the drug is reduced. A nerve block has greater reliability, efficiency and duration than does an infiltration or topical epithelial application.

PATIENT PREPARATION

A specific routine for every intraoral dental injection must be developed to insure safe and effective use of the agents. A medical history and physical evaluation are an absolute necessity. The interpre-

tation of them is the subject of entire texts for dentistry and particular systemic diseases, drug interactions, and contraindications have been discussed as each agent and component of anesthetic solutions was presented in Chapter 3. The dental history has application in choosing the approach to the patient for administering a drug determined to be physiologically appropriate. The patient's emotional (psychological) response is as important as the physiological response to local anesthetic. The agents used are safe and rarely result in complications if appropriately chosen. The physical act of administering the agent, however, is the biggest reason for "reactions" to local anesthesia.

The patient is always placed in a reclined or semi-reclined chair position. Local anesthetics should never be administered with the patient in an upright or sitting position (Fig. 5.18). The reclined chair position will virtually eliminate vasovagal syncope (fainting). In this position, the trunk and legs are on the same level as the head or the legs are slightly above the head and trunk. The head should not be on a lower level than the trunk (Fig. 5.19). This reclined position

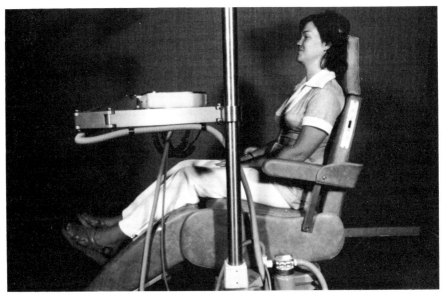

Figure 5.18. Upright chair position.

facilitates venous return and keeps the brain from being temporarily deprived of sufficient blood volume, if a vasovagal response occurs. Dilatation of vessels in the extremities and trunk therefore does not cause a relative lack of blood volume to the brain.

The semi-reclined position (Fig. 5.20)

has been shown to be the best overall position for normal homeostatic mechanisms and is satisfactory for local anesthetic administration; however, it is possible for syncope to occur in this position. Therefore, the reclined position is ideal and is recommended for all injections.

The dental history data are used to

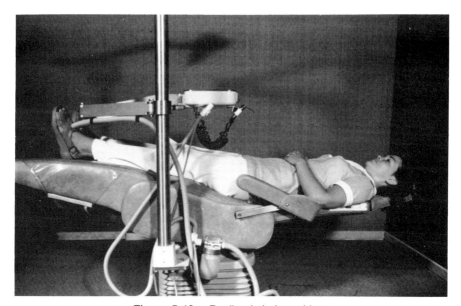

Figure 5.19. Reclined chair position.

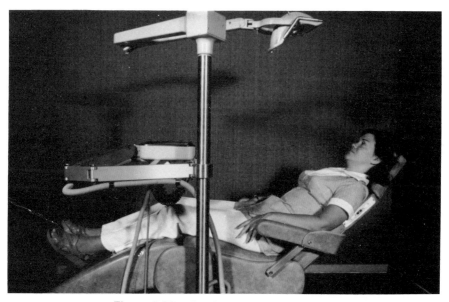

Figure 5.20. Semi-reclined chair position.

choose chair positioning as persons with a history of syncope must always be placed in the reclined position. This positioning should be verbally reinforced as "preventing you (the patient) from fainting when the anesthetic is administered." This is not to imply that non-fainting patients are treated less safely, only that historically, a reclined patient will not faint in response to the "act" of local anesthesia, whereas a non-reclined individual can faint. The upright position invites complications and should be considered physiologically and psychologically unhealthy.

The Injection

Before any injection, the site of needle puncture is identified, appropriate anatomical landmarks identified, and the end point of needle insertion (deposition site) is mentally imaged. After preparing all equipment, the mucosa is dried and the topical antiseptic is applied, if desired. The mucosa is re-dried (Fig. 5.21) and the topical anesthetic is applied to the penetration site per the manufacturer's directions (Fig. 5.22).

The non-injecting hand should be used to retract, tense the mucosa, and steady the patient's head so that inadvertent movement will not take place. The non-injecting hand should also be used in some fashion to steady the syringe (Fig. 5.23). On all injections, the barrel of the syringe should be turned so that the open part is away from the patient's teeth, making it impossible for mouth closure to break the cartridge, and in the line of sight of the operator, so the injection rate can be monitored (Fig. 5.24). The needle is than advanced to the anesthetic deposition site within the tissue. After the needle tip is in the proper location, aspiration is performed to confirm a nonvascular needle tip placement. If negative, the necessary volume of the solution is injected.

Aspiration is performed by placing gentle negative pressure on the cartridge by pulling back on the thumb ring with the thumb. Only minimal movement of the plunger is necessary and if more than several tenths of a millimeter of movement is produced at the plunger, the harpoon may disengage, negating all aspiration. Positive aspiration should be inter-

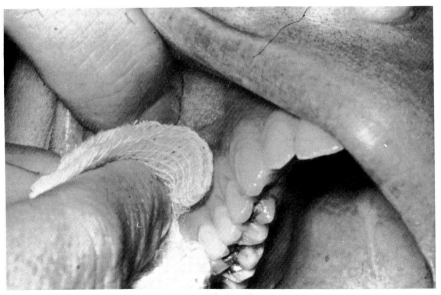

Figure 5.21. Drying the mucosa.

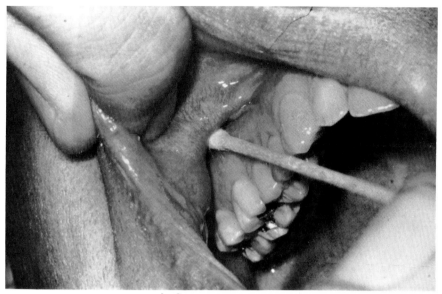

Figure 5.22. Application of the topical anesthetic.

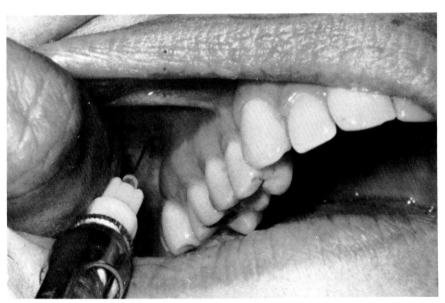

Figure 5.23. Injecting the local anesthetic.

rupted as outlined under "Needles" in Chapter 4. If extravascular needle placement can be confirmed, a small amount of blood in the solution is not a problem, although complete discoloration of the solution should be avoided. In this case, a new cartridge must be inserted and the injected sequence repeated.

The rate of injection should be *slow*; the recommended rate is *1 ml per minute.* With this rate of injection, the discomfort of injecting the anesthetic will be minimal and many times the injected area will be partially anesthetized before the needle is withdrawn. This would require almost *two* full minutes for a full cartridge and

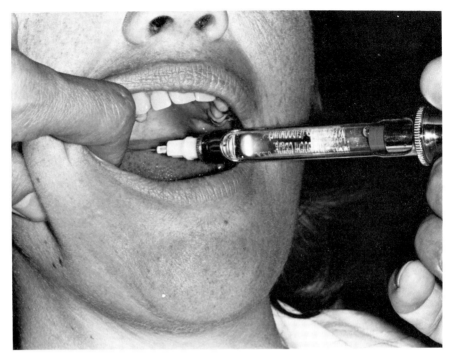

Figure 5.24. Cartridge in line of site and protected by barrel from the patient's teeth.

can be of some concern, emotionally, to the patient. A compromise of *one minute per cartridge* is acceptable. Pressure in the tissue is created by the injected volume so the tissue must be given time to expand without tearing. A fast injection rate is painful and may possibly damage the tissue. If the needle tip is inadvertently placed in a vascular channel, a fast injection will also administer a *bolus* dose of the local anesthetic, without time for circulatory dilution to reduce the toxic effect of the agent. After injecting the desired volume, the needle is withdrawn on the same line as it was inserted. Under no circumstances should needle direction be changed during or after entering the tissue. If it becomes necessary to reposition the needle tip, the syringe-needle assembly must be withdrawn to just under the mucosa and redirected. The needle should never bend. Aspiration is again necessary and should be negative after each change in needle tip position. After the injection, place the needle cover over the needle and set the syringe aside.

A summary of the injection procedure is as follows:

1. Assemble syringe-cartridge-needle apparatus.

2. Secure an adequate medical history, dental history, and physical evaluation.

3. Place patient in reclined chair position.

4. Dry the mucosa.

(4a. Optional topical antiseptic.)

5. Apply topical anesthetic.

6. Insert needle to the deposition site.

7. Aspirate.

8. Inject slowly.

9. Withdraw on line of insertion.

10. Replace needle cover.

A summary of contraindicated technique is as follows:

1. Never reuse needles or cartridge on other patients. These cannot be resterilized.

2. Never use the syringe on another patient without sterilization.

3. Never inject without aspiration.

4. Never change needle direction while

the needle is in the tissue or bend the needle.

5. Never lose finger rests or hand control of the patient during the injection.

6. Never inject with the patient in an upright position.

The foregoing assumes aseptic technique throughout. A visual display of thorough hand washing by the operator and assistant, in addition to being necessary, instills patient confidence and minimizes potential spread of infection.

DENTAL INJECTION TECHNIQUES

The success of all dental injections depends on the ability of the operator to properly deposit the anesthetic solution. There are several methods by which the needle tip is directed to the target area and each has advantages and disadvantages. In the following, methods will be presented that most consistently result in adequate analgesia and minimal side effects.

Specific angles, lines of insertion, and approaches will be presented in "dogmatic" fashion. The exact methodology is important for the novice and helpful for the experienced when difficulty is encountered. It must be understood, however, that *precise understanding of the anatomical site* is the most important aspect of all injections. Target areas deep in the tissue *must be mentally visualized* for the injection to be precise, efficient, and safe. Further, every structure the needle passes through must be known to achieve quality local analgesia. The mechanical actions are important but secondary to precise anatomical knowledge of the selected site.

Technique for Individual Tooth Analgesia by Infiltration

Infiltration analgesia of many oral structures is possible. It is easy to achieve for all soft tissues as the target area is injected directly, resulting in profound analgesia. Certain teeth may also be rendered free of pain in the same manner by an infiltration of the agent in a paraperiosteal manner, resulting in a field block. Wherever cortical bone is thin, the agent will diffuse through it to the cancellous bone and reach nerve fibers entering the apices of the teeth. Areas of the oral cavity that are amenable to "infiltration" techniques are the buccal aspects of the adult maxillary teeth and the buccal aspects of some adult mandibular incisors. (In adults, the cortical bone is too thick in all other areas to rely on sufficient diffusion.) An infiltration can be directed at any of these teeth and analgesia will be of sufficient depth to allow restorative procedures or surgical manipulation of the associated buccal gingivae. In children, all maxillary and mandibular teeth can be anesthetized because the cortical bone is thin. This technique will also provide analgesia of the buccal associated gingivae.

The technique is as follows (Figs. 5.25 and 5.26):

All following techniques presume proper patient preparation, mucosa drying and topical anesthetic application.

1. Retract the lip and/or buccal mucosa apically until the muccobuccal fold is taut. The tissue is stretched up and away in the maxilla and down and away in the mandible. This will expose the depth of the muccobuccal fold and make the outline of the convexity of tooth roots visible on the buccal alveolus.

2. Identify the area and mentally visualize where the apex of the selected tooth is located. Reasonable knowledge of tooth anatomy and average root length simplifies this procedure.

3. Needle insertion is at the greatest concavity of the muccobuccal fold and directed toward the anatomical location of the tooth apex. The angle of needle penetration to the buccal alveolus is not important as the needle can be advanced to the bone over the apex from many angles. Visibility and tissue control are of prime importance.

4. The needle is advanced until bone is

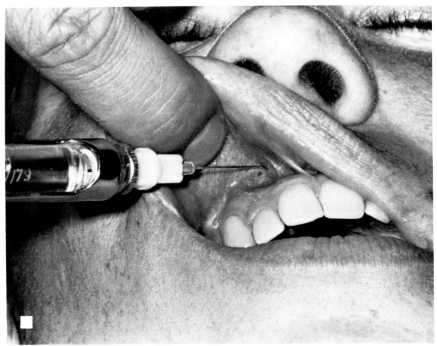

Figure 5.25. Maxillary anterior infiltration.

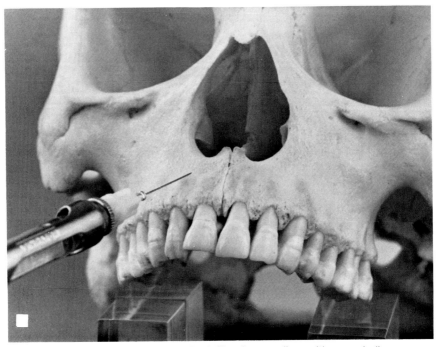

Figure 5.26. Maxillary anterior infiltration needle position on skull.

almost contacted. Aspirate and inject the solution at this point. Do not scrape the periosteum. The ideal deposition site is next to, but not touching, the periosteum (bone) as this is uncomfortable. If the needle can be stopped before contacting the periosteum, the injection will be just as effective as if the bone was contacted.

[Needle size: 25- or 27-gauge, long or short; volume: 0.9 ml (½ cartridge)]

The area of analgesia will be the selected tooth pulp, its associated buccal bone and periosteum and the associated buccal gingivae.

In adults, the maxillary 1st molar usually requires two infiltrations, one over the mesial buccal root and a second over the disal buccal root. The malar process of the zygomatic arch is low on the maxilla at this location, too dense for adequate diffusion of the agent, and is centered between the buccal roots of the maxillary 1st molar. This necessitates approaching the mesial root from the mesial and the distal root from the distal.

Technique for Multiple Tooth Analgesia by Infiltration

Because of the anatomy of the superior dental plexus and the schematic differentiation of the anterior, middle, and posterior superior alveolar nerve fibers, specific injections carry their names. These injections are done in the same manner as individual tooth infiltrations but because of diffusion of the anesthetic agent, multiple teeth will be anesthetized.

ANTERIOR SUPERIOR ALVEOLAR INFILTRATION (ASA) (FIGS. 5.27 and 5.28)

1. Retract the lip apically until the mucosa is taut to expose the buccal alveolus and the depth of the mucobuccal fold.

2. Identify the area and mentally visualize where the apex of the maxillary cuspid is located.

3. Insert the needle at the height of the mucobuccal fold and direct it to just above the apex of the maxillary cuspid.

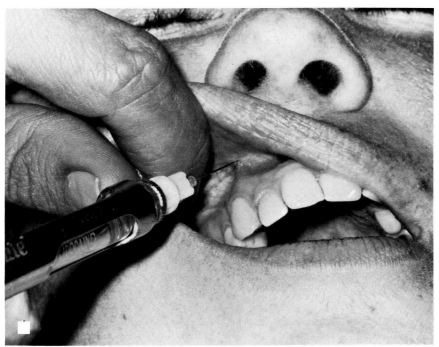

Figure 5.27. Anterior superior alveolar infiltration.

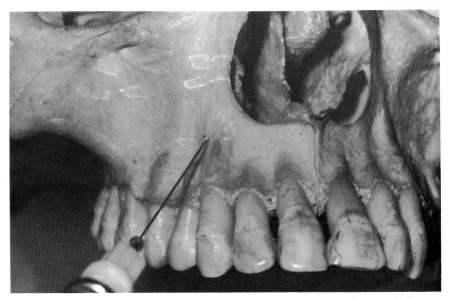

Figure 5.28.   Anterior superior alveolar infiltration needle position on skull.

4. Advance the needle until the bone is almost contacted but do not scrape the periosteum. Aspirate and inject at this point.

[Needle size: 25- or 27-gauge, long or short; volume: 0.9–1.8 ml (½–1 cartridge)]

The area of analgesia will be the maxillary cuspid, lateral and central incisor pulps, associated buccal bone and periosteum, associated buccal gingivae, and the ipsilateral upper lip (see Fig. 5.78).

MIDDLE SUPERIOR ALVEOLAR "INFILTRATION" (MSA) (FIGS. 5.29 and 5.30)

1. The injection technique is the same as the ASA except the needle is directed to just above the apex of the maxillary 2nd bicuspid. Aspirate and inject at this point.

[Needle size: 25- or 27-gauge, long or short; volume: 0.9–1.8 ml (½–1 cartridge)]

The area of analgesia will be the 1st and 2nd maxillary bicuspid pulps and the mesial buccal pulp of the maxillary 1st molar, the associated buccal bone and periosteum, and associated buccal gingivae (see Fig. 5.78).

POSTERIOR SUPERIOR ALVEOLAR "INFILTRATION" (PSA) (FIGS. 5.31 and 5.32)

1. The injection technique is the same as the ASA and MSA "infiltrations" except the needle is directed to just above the apices of the most posterior maxillary molar—either 2nd or 3rd. Aspirate and inject at this point.

[Needle size: 25- or 27-gauge, long or short; volume: 0.9–1.8 ml (½–1 cartridge)]

As the needle target area moves posteriorly, the line of insertion becomes more angled to the front of the mouth rather than following the long axis of the teeth. For the PSA "infiltration," the needle puncture point is at the greatest concavity of the mucobuccal fold and may be at the 2nd molar level with the tip of the needle being advanced to the apical bone of the maxillary 3rd molars. If the maxillary 3rd molar is missing, the deposition site is just above the apical area of the maxillary 2nd molar.

The area of analgesia will be the distal buccal and palatal pulp of the maxillary 1st molar, pulps of the maxillary 2nd and 3rd molars, the associated buccal bone

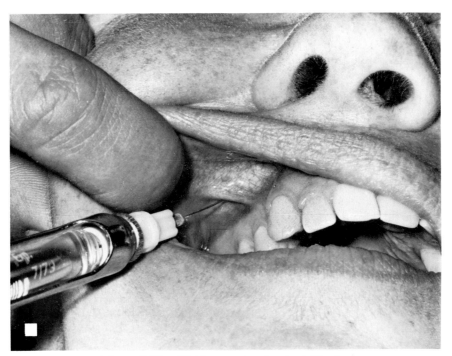

Figure 5.29.   Middle superior alveolar infiltration.

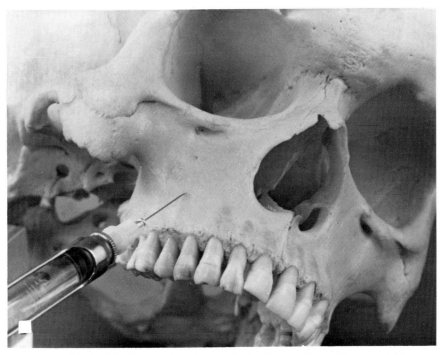

Figure 5.30.   Middle superior alveolar infiltration needle position on skull.

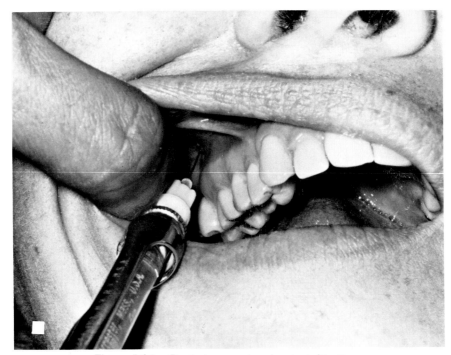

Figure 5.31.   Posterior superior alveolar infiltration.

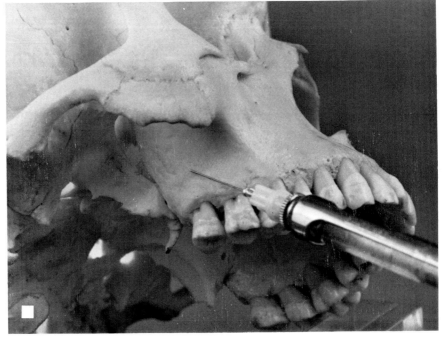

Figure 5.32.   Posterior superior alveolar infiltration needle position on skull.

and periosteum and associated buccal gingivae. The palatal bone associated with the maxillary molar palatal root is not anesthetized (see Fig. 5.78).

Techniques for Maxillary Block Injections

Block injections are more reliable than infiltrations if the needle placement is accurate, and the duration of analgesia is longer. Accuracy is very important as the efficiency of the injection is related to the distance over which the agent must diffuse to reach the nerve trunk.

POSTERIOR SUPERIOR ALVEOLAR NERVE BLOCK (FIGS. 5.33 and 5.34)

The posterior superior alveolar nerve fibers can be anesthetized before they enter the posterior aspect of the maxilla. This is differentiated from the PSA "infiltration," where diffusion of the agent through cortical bone is necessary. The block technique is a more predictable method of achieving analgesia of the PSA

area of innervation. The target fibers are located in soft tissue on the posterior superior maxilla and are blocked before they enter the maxilla through multiple foramina. The technique is as follows:

1. Palpate the most superior and posterior depth of the maxillary mucobuccal fold and the depression of the fold as it turns inward and upward.

2. Retract the buccal mucosa laterally to expose the greatest concavity of the fold and mentally visualize the posterior aspect of the maxilla. The patient's mouth should be only half open for this and the mandible shifted to the side of the injection. This moves the coronoid process and the ramus away from the tuberosity, allowing greater access and visibility. As the patient relaxes the mandibular muscles and moves the mandible laterally, the buccal mucosa can be retracted superiorly as well as laterally to tense the mucosa.

3. The needle is inserted on a line 45° to the maxillary occlusal plane and 45° to

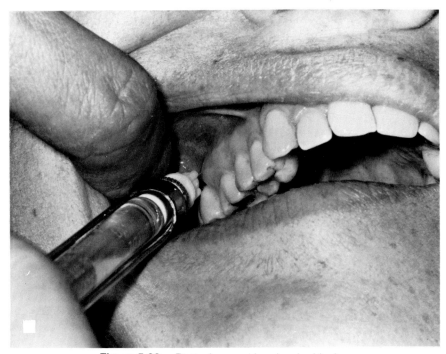

Figure 5.33.   Posterior superior alveolar block.

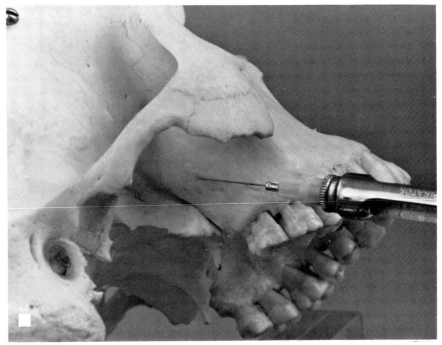

Figure 5.34.   Posterior superior alveolar block needle position on skull.

the sagittal plane of the head. It enters the tissue at the height of concavity of the mucobuccal fold and is advanced parallel to the posterior surface of the maxilla. The needle should be as close to the bone as possible, but without scraping the periosteum.

4. Depth of insertion is 2 cm or half the length of a long needle. Bone should not be contacted. Aspirate and inject at this point.

[Needle size: 25- or 27-gauge long. A short needle should not be used because it would be inserted over ¾ of its length. Volume: 0.9–1.8 ml (½–1 cartridge)]

The area of analgesia is the same as the PSA "infiltration" and will be the distal buccal and palatal pulp of the maxillary 1st molar, pulps of the maxillary 2nd and 3rd molars, the associated buccal bone and periosteum, and the associated buccal gingivae. The palatal bone associated with the maxillary 1st molar palatal root is not anesthesized (see Fig. 5.78). This injection technique is more efficient and reliable than the PSA infiltration but it has a

higher incidence of complication. this complication is hematoma formation because of needle-damaged vessels on the posterior of the maxilla.

INFRAORBITAL BLOCK (FIGS. 5.35 to 5.37)

The infraorbital nerve block is a method of securing analgesia of the ASA nerve plexus and in some cases portions of the MSA nerve plexus plus cutaneous structures. It is more efficient and reliable than the ASA "infiltration" and can be used routinely or when infection of the anterior teeth contraindicates needle placement in the apical area. The technique is as follows:

1. The patient must look straight forward. Locate the supraorbital notch and the infraorbital notch on roughness of the zygomaticomaxillary suture line.

2. Retract the upper lip upward and outward, exposing the convexity of the mucobuccal fold lateral to the maxillary second bicuspid. The infraorbital foramen

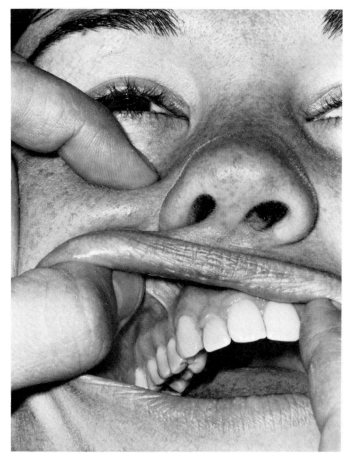

Figure 5.35.   Palpating infraorbital notch.

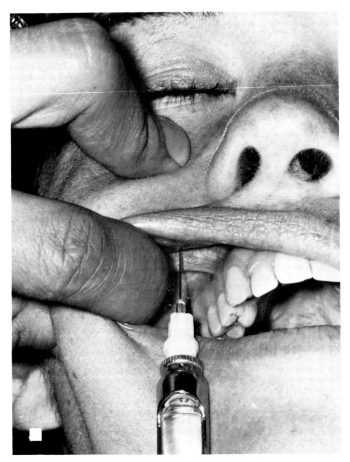

Figure 5.36.   Infraorbital block. Needle in line with pupil and infraorbital notch.

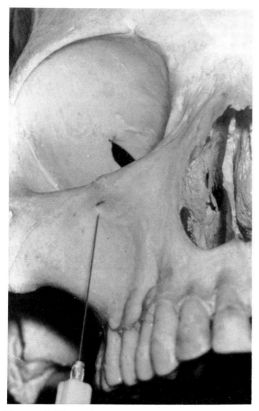

Figure 5.37. Infraorbital block needle position on skull.

lies on a line that traverses the supraorbital notch, pupil in forward state, and infraorbital notch (Fig. 5.35).

3. The palpating finger should be moved from the infraorbital notch to the depression on the inferior surface of the infraorbital rim. This is the infraorital foramen.

4. The needle enters the mucosa approximately 1 cm away from the alveolus in the mucobuccal fold lateral to the maxillary 2nd bicuspid and is directed to the area identified as the infraorbital foramen. The bone of the undersurface of the infraorbital rim should be gently contacted at this point (Figs. 5.36 and 5.37).

5. The needle tip does not have to enter the foramen to achieve analgesia but should be at the opening. The depth of needle penetration can be judged by estimating the distance from the palpating finger to the mucobuccal fold penetration point. It averages between 1 and 2 cm. Aspirate and inject at this point. Overinsertion is stopped by the undersurface of the infraorbital rim or is felt by the palpating finger.

6. As the agent is injected, the space occupied in the tissue by the solution will be felt to increase in size by the palpating finger and confirm proper needle position.

[Needle size; 25- or 27-gauge long; volume: 0.9–1.8 ml (½–1 cartridge)]

The area of analgesia will depend on how much of the anesthetic solution enters the infraorbital canal. The innervation of the ASA nerve fibers will definitely be anesthetized, as well as some or all of the MSA fibers. The variable MSA analgesia is related to anesthetic entering the foramen and the relative anterior or posterior point at which the MSA plexus fibers descend from the infraorbital nerve. The area of analgesia will include the ipsilateral lower eyelid, side of the nose, overlying cutaneous structures and the upper lip (see Fig. 5.78). The needle insertion path is through the levator angular oris muscle so some resistance may be encountered as the needle is advanced. Some advocate firm finger pressure over the foramen to physically force the anesthetic solution into the foramen. This may help to a limited degree but is not necessary for success.

NASOPALATINE NERVE BLOCK

Analgesia of the palatine nerves is not as commonly used as the buccal alveolar blocks and infiltrations. It is advisable to secure palatal anesthesia for placement of the rubber dam clamp for aggressive periodontal therapy or when accessory pulpal innervation is suspected in maxillary teeth. It is always necessary for surgical manipulation of maxillary teeth and palatal gingivae. The technique of the nasopalatine nerve block is as follows (Figs. 5.38 and 5.39):

1. Identify the incisive papillae.

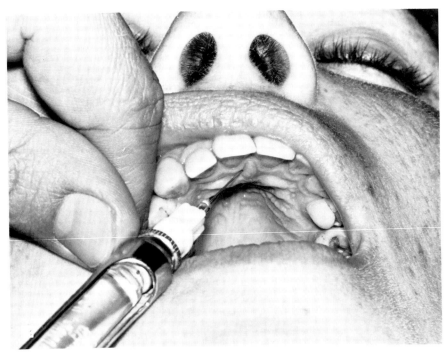

Figure 5.38.   Nasopalatine block.

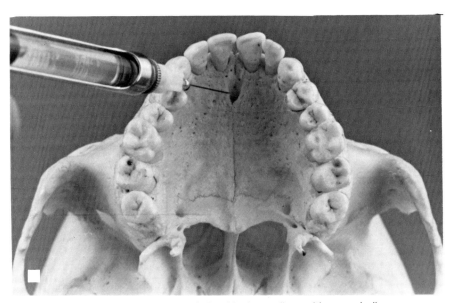

Figure 5.39.   Nasopalatine block needle position on skull.

2. Needle penetration is just to the side of the incisive papillae and directed to a point ½ cm deep and directly under the papillae or unti bone is reached (whichever occurs first). This will be at or above the nasopalatine canal. It is not necessary to enter the canal.

3. Aspirate and inject at this point.

[Needle size: 25- or 27-gauge, long or short. If a buccal injection has been previously administered, use the same needle. It is not necessary to change needles. Volume: 0.25–0.5 ml (⅛–¼ of a cartridge) or less if blanching of the tissue occurs.]

The area of analgesia will include the anterior palatal gingivae from cuspid to cuspid and the palatal bone and periosteum of the cuspids and incisors. Sensory innervation of the cuspid palatal periosteum and gingivae is shared with the anterior palatine nerve. This single injection anesthetized both the right and left nasopalatine nerves (see Fig. 5.78).

The nasopalatine injection is quite uncomfortable. This discomfort can be minimized by first giving a midline buccal infiltration, then infiltrating the interdental papilla between the central incisors and finally administering the nasopalatine. It is still uncomfortable but less so than if given first or alone. Another technique for minimizing the discomfort of this injection is to apply pressure to the area for 30 seconds with a topical anesthetic-soaked cotton-tipped applicator. While holding this pressure, insert the needle, aspirate, and inject.

ANTERIOR PALATINE BLOCK

The anterior palatine nerve block is used for the same purposes as the nasopalatine nerve block. The technique is as follows:

1. Identify the greatest concavity of the posterior hard palate in the 2nd and 3rd molar area. Palpate this site with a cotton tipped applicator and locate the depressable tissue found approximately halfway between the alveolar crest and the midline. The greater palatine foramen lies under this tissue. In some cases, a small depression will be seen next to the alveolus of the 2nd and 3rd molar area, identifying the canal opening (Fig. 5.40).

2. Needle insertion is from the opposite side of the mouth to the mentally visualized area of the foreamen (Figs. 5.41 and 5.42).

3. The needle is inserted to a depth of

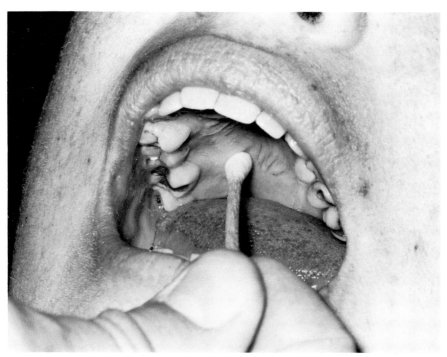

Figure 5.40. Cotton-tipped applicator over area of greater palatine foramen.

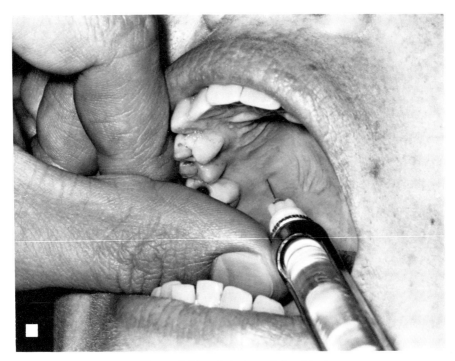

Figure 5.41. Anterior palatine block.

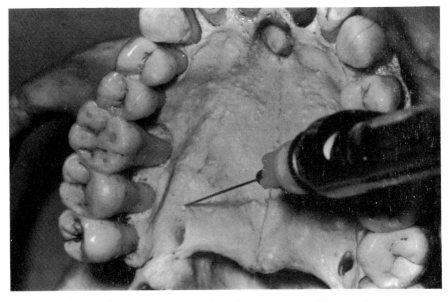

Figure 5.42. Anterior palatine block needle position on skull.

0.5 cm or until bone is reached. Aspirate and inject at this point.

[Needle size: 25- or 27-gauge short or long. Needle choice is on the basis of the previous buccal injection. Volume: 0.25–0.5 ml (⅛–¼ cartridge) or less if blanching of the tissue occurs.]

The area of analgesia will be the posterior palatal gingivae from the cuspid, to the 3rd molar, to the midline and associated palatal periosteum. Sensory innervation of the cuspid palatal bone, periosteum, and gingivae is shared with the nasopalatine nerve (see Fig. 5.78).

This injection is uncomfortable, just like the nasopalatine injection. Discomfort can be minimized if pressure anesthesia is applied to the area of the canal for 30 seconds prior to the injection. This is done with a cotton-tipped applicator as the topical anesthetic is applied. While the pressure is maintained, the needle is inserted and the injection made.

PARTIAL PALATINE BLOCK

A partial palatine injection can be given at any point along the forward course of the anterior palatine nerve. It is given in the greatest concavity of the hard palate midway between the alveolar crest and the midline and one tooth posterior to the desired area of analgesia (Figs. 5.43 and 5.44).

INFERIOR ALVEOLAR BLOCK (MANDIBULAR BLOCK)—STANDARD OR ROUTINE APPROACH

The inferior alveolar nerve block is probably the most frequently used dental injection as it is given for most restorative and surgical procedures on the mandibular teeth. It is also the most difficult to master because of the small target area located deep to the overlying mucosa. This target site has the most variability of the common injections and the efficiency of the standard mandibular block is the least of all injections. Precise technique will overcome many of the problems historically encountered.

The target site for anesthetic deposition is the anterior border of the inferior alveolar nerve, above the mandibular foramen. The mandibular foramen is located in the middle to posterior third of the ramus of the mandible, in an anterior posterior direction and at a variable distance above or below the mandibular occlusal plane. The anterior most portion of the inferior alveolar nerve, the target site,

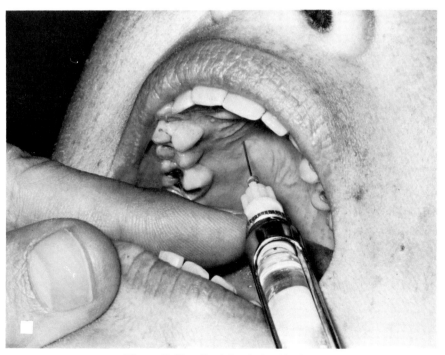

Figure 5.43. Partial palatine block.

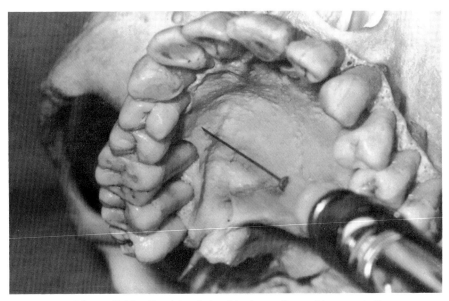

Figure 5.44. Partial palatine block needle position on skull.

is anatomically located in the middle of the ramus. This target area is in the mandibular sulcus and is a confined space bordered inferiorly by the attachment of the sphenomandibular ligament and insertion of the internal pterygoid muscle; laterally by the ascending ramus; medially by the internal pterygoid muscle; anteriorly by the fascia of the buccinator muscle and anterior attachment of the sphenomandibular ligament; and posteriorly by a lobe of the parotid gland. A loose connective tissue anatomical space exists for several centimeters above the target site. Any error in placement other than superiorly will result in solution deposition below the inferior limit of the mandibular sulcus and in an area too dense for diffusion of the agent to reach the nerve. All of the borders of the mandibular sulcus are dense connective tissue, muscle, or bone. Injection into this tissue will result in an anesthetic failure. The technique of the injection is as follows:

1. The patient's mouth must be opened as wide as possible. The *thumb* of the noninjecting hand is placed over the pter-ygomandibular triangle and then pulled laterally until the deepest depression in the anterior border of the ramus is felt. This depression is called the coronoid notch (Figs. 5.45 and 5.47).

2. As the thumb slides laterally onto the coronoid notch the loose tissue of the pterygomandibular triangle is pulled with it, creating a tense area for needle penetration.

3. The first or second finger of the noninjecting hand palpates and grasps the posterior portion of the ramus, finding a slight soft tissue depression. Force this finger as far superiorly as the ear will allow it to go (Figs. 5.46 and 5.47). The line established between the thumb and finger establishes the vertical height of the *target area* in the mandibular sulcus. The mandibular foramen will always be on or below this line. The mandibular foramen is in different relative locations, above and below the mandibular occlusal plane in children and adults. It is below the occlusal plane in children and at or above in adults. In edentulous individuals it cannot be compared to the occlusal plane. Regardless of the foramen's height,

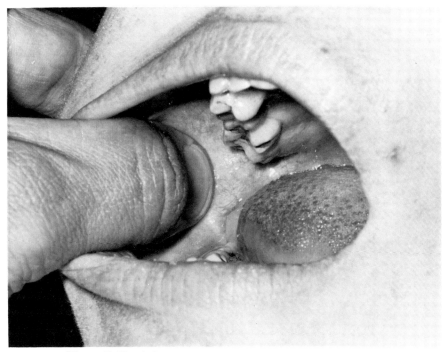

Figure 5.45. Inferior alveolar block intraoral thumb position.

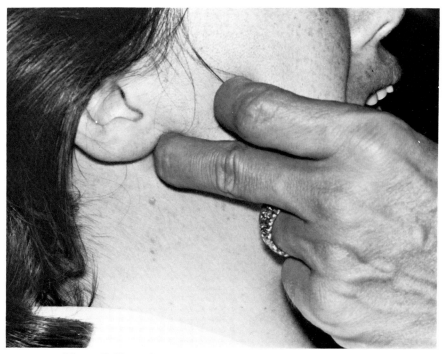

Figure 5.46. Inferior alveolar block extraoral finger position.

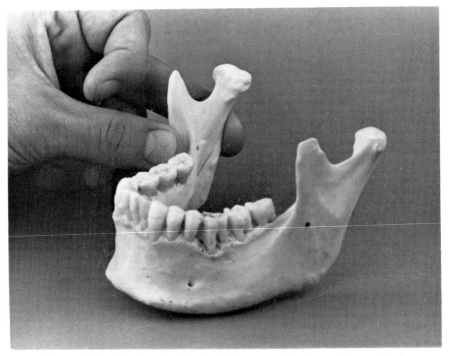

Figure 5.47. Inferior alveolar block finger and thumb position on skull.

in any age group, it will be on or below the line established by the thumb (anterior border) and finger (posterior border) location.

4. The anterior-posterior location of the anterior border of the inferior alveolar nerve, which is the *target site*, is located midway between the stabilizing thumb and finger and on the line of the thumb and finger. This point must be mentally visualized in the tissue, and the needle tip advanced to the site (Figs. 5.47 and 5.48). This thumb-finger grip also establishes the relative flare of the ramus and ensures control of the patient's mandible during the injection (Fig. 5.47).

5. The line of needle insertion is from the opposite mandibular bicuspids and directed to the mentally visualized anterior border of the inferior alveolar nerve in the mandibular sulcus.

6. The needle is inserted to the target site until bone is gently contacted. Depth of penetration is estimated by the thumb-finger position but it is rarely over 2 cm, or less than 1 cm. This depth may vary in

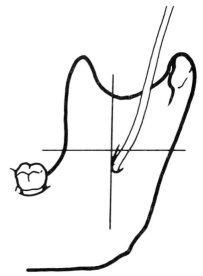

Figure 5.48. Schematic of mandibular foramen and average anatomical position of inferior alveolar nerve.

large individuals or in a child (Figs. 5.49 and 5.50). The *long* needle is always inserted at least ½ of its length but never over ¾ of its length. Aspirate and inject. If bone is contacted before ½ of the needle

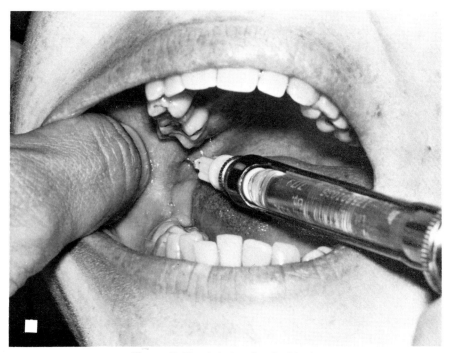

Figure 5.49. Inferior alveolar block.

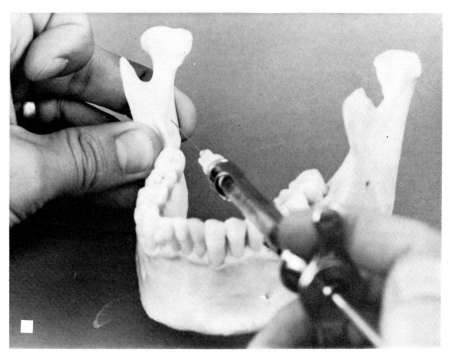

Figure 5.50. Inferior alveolar block needle position on skull.

is inserted, the mandible is either very small or most likely the internal oblique ridge has been contacted necessitating redirection.

[Needle size: 25- or 27-gauge long; volume: 0.9–1.5 ml (½–¾ cartridge). Save the unused portion of this cartridge for the lingual block and the long buccal block.]

The area of analgesia will be the pulps of the mandibular teeth, the buccal periosteum and the bone from the 1st bicuspid to the midline, the buccal gingivae from the 1st bicuspid to the midline, and the mucosa and cutaneous epithelium of the ipsilateral lower lip (see Fig. 5.79).

The mucosal penetration point varies, but lies within the pterygomandibular triangle. The line of insertion should penetrate the posterior aspect of the buccinator muscle and be just lateral or anterior to the pterygomandibular raphe. On some occasions, the needle will pass through the leading edge of the internal pterygoid muscle resulting in some resistance and discomfort. This cannot always be predicted or avoided (Fig. 5.51). The height of insertion is usually above the occlusal plane but always dictated by the palpating thumb and finger height.

The technique is the same for the left and right side with the technique previously described being for a right-handed operator for a right inferior alveolar nerve block. If the injection is to be for the left inferior alveolar nerve all positions and descriptions are exactly the same. The palpating-stabilizing hand is placed over the patients' head in a "head-lock" position so the thumb still palpates the coronoid notch and the finger, the depression on the posterior ramus.

This standard technique for inferior alveolar nerve analgesia is suitable for children, adults, dentulous, and edentulous individuals, without modification.

LINGUAL BLOCK

The lingual nerve block can be given as a specific injection or included as part of the inferior alveolar nerve block. An in-

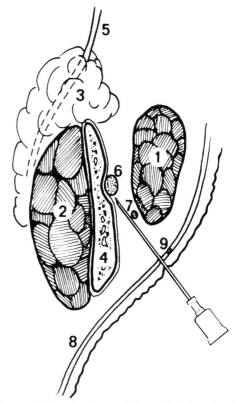

Figure 5.51. Anatomical view of inferior alveolar block anatomy. *1*, internal pterygoid muscle; *2*, masseter muscle; *3*, parotid gland; *4*, ramus; *5*, facial nerve; *6*, inferior alveolar nerve; *7*, lingual nerve; *8*, buccinator muscle; *9*, pterygomandibular raphe.

ferior alveolar nerve block will usually anesthetize the lingual nerve unintentionally because of diffusion. A specific lingual nerve block will anesthetize the lingual nerve but rarely or only partially anesthetize the inferior alveolar nerve. These two nerve blocks are routinely given together for restorative and/or surgical procedures. The technique is as follows:

1. After deposition of the anesthetic agent at the mandibular sulcus for the standard inferior alveolar nerve block, the needle is withdrawn *one-half* of its inserted depth on the same line as it was inserted.

2. This is the approximate location of the lingual nerve (Fig. 5.51). The injection of the lingual nerve is made at this location (Fig. 5.52), after aspiration.

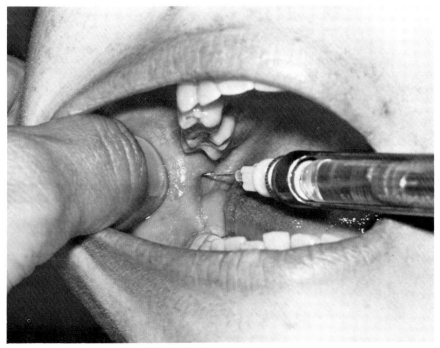

Figure 5.52. Lingual block.

[Needle size: 25- or 27-gauge long (same needle as the standard inferior alveolar block); volume: 0.5 ml (¼ cartridge)]

The area of analgesia will be the lingual periosteum of the mandibular teeth to the midline, the associated lingual gingivae, the floor of the mouth to the midline and the anterior two-thirds of the tongue to the midline (see Fig. 5.79). The chorda tympani (nerve) will also be anesthetized as it courses with the lingual nerve. This will result in loss of taste sensation in the anterior two-thirds of the tongue.

A partial lingual nerve block can also be made, where the lingual nerve enters the floor of the mouth, next to the lingual alveolar bone, one tooth posterior to the desired area of analgesia. Needle insertion is approximately 2 mm in depth and after aspiration 0.5 to 1.0 ml of solution is deposited (Figs. 5.53 and 5.54).

BUCCAL NERVE BLOCK (LONG BUCCAL NERVE BLOCK)

The buccal nerve block (long buccal nerve block) should be considered a routine part of mandibular anesthesia for re-storative procedures and is mandatory for surgical procedures of the mandibular posterior teeth. Analgesia of the buccal gingivae is helpful for application of rubber dam clamps, helpful for matrix and wedge placement, and the buccal nerve has been implicated in accessory innervation of the mandibular molars. Mandibular molar anesthesia will be more successful if the long buccal nerve block is routinely given along with the standard inferior alveolar and lingual nerve block. The technique is as follows (Figs. 5.55 and 5.56):

1. Identify the joint on the ascending ramus where the buccal nerve crosses from the medial to the external oblique ridge at the height of the occlusal plane.

2. The needle is inserted at the height of the occlusal plane, posterior to the mandibular 3rd molar into the soft tissue near the external oblique ridge. Depth of penetration is 1 to 2 mm.

[Needle size: 25- or 27-gauge long (same as the standard inferior alveolar nerve block and the lingual nerve block). Volume: 0.25–0.5 ml (¼ cartridge)]

The area of analgesia will be the buccal

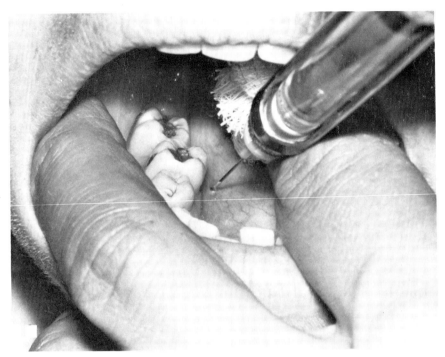

Figure 5.53. Partial lingual block.

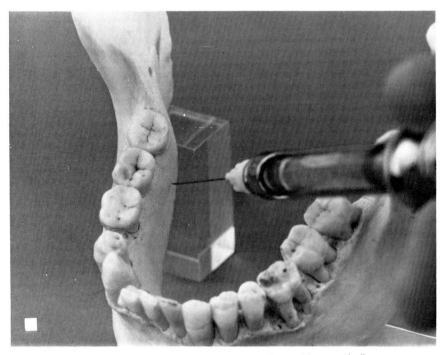

Figure 5.54. Partial lingual block needle position on skull.

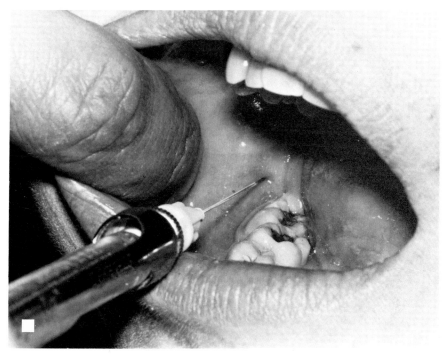

Figure 5.55.   Buccal block.

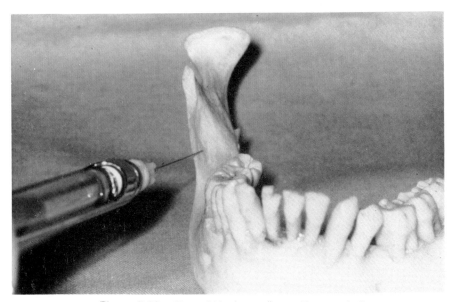

Figure 5.56.   Buccal block needle position on skull.

periosteum of the mandibular molars and 2nd bicuspid and their associated buccal gingivae (see Fig. 5.79).

The standard inferior alveolar, lingual, and buccal nerve blocks should all be considered part of routine posterior mandibular analgesia. These injections are given in a series with approximately ½ of the cartridge for the inferior alveolar, ¼ for the lingual, and the last ¼ for the buccal nerve.

Mental Nerve Block and Incisive Nerve Block

The mental nerve block achieves analgesia of the terminal branch of the inferior alveolar nerve at the mental foramen. The injection technique is as follows (Figs. 5.57 and 5.58):

1. Slide a palpating finger down the buccal alveolus between the mandibular bicuspids to the area between the apices of these teeth. A bump or in some cases a depression will be found between the apices, quite deep in the concavity of the mucobuccal fold. This represents the mental foramen and/or the mental neurovascular bundle.

2. The foramen opens in a posterior direction so it is difficult to advance a needle into the canal. When the foramen is identified, the needle is inserted into the mucobuccal fold to the identified target area. The line of insertion is perpendicular to the mandibular occlusal plane and 20 to 40° lateral to the long axis of the bicuspids.

3. The needle is advanced until bone is gently contacted. Aspirate and inject. Depending on whether the needle tip has entered the foramen, the anesthetic will be deposited at the entrance of the foramen resulting in a *mental block* or into the foramen where it anesthetizes the incisive branches of the inferior alveolar nerve resulting in the *incisive block* and a *mental block*.

[Needle size: 25- or 27-gauge, long or short; volume: 0.9 ml (½ cartridge)]

The area of analgesia of the mental and incisive nerve block are as follows.

A mental nerve block results in analgesia of the buccal gingivae and periosteum of the mandibular 1st bicuspid, cuspid, and incisors to the midline. It also provides analgesia of the mucosa and cutaneous epithelium of the ipsilateral lower lip (see Fig. 5.79).

An incisive and mental nerve block re-

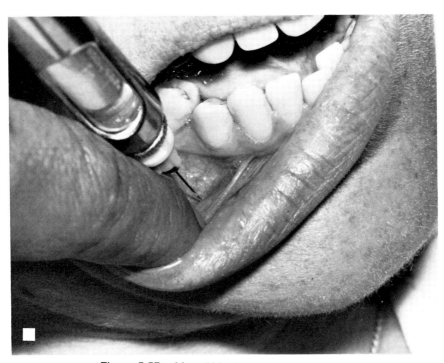

Figure 5.57.   Mental block and/or incisive block.

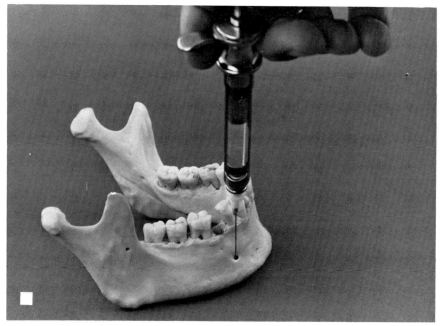

Figure 5.58. Mental and/or incisive block position on skull.

sults in analgesia of the mental nerve area plus pulpal analgesia of the mandibular 1st bicuspid, cuspid, and incisors to the midline and the associated buccal bone (see Fig. 5.79.)

"Gow-Gates" Inferior Alveolar Nerve Block

The Gow-Gates approach to analgesia of the inferior alveolar nerve is relatively new in the United States, although the technique has been used by its originator, George A. E. Gow-Gates, for many years in Australia. It has been demonstrated to be quite effective in achieving analgesia of the mandibular dental structures. With one injection, inferior alveolar and lingual nerves are anesthetized. The anesthetic solution is deposited *via* an intraoral approach at the neck of the translated condyle. The rational of this approach to the inferior alveolar nerve is to deposit the anesthetic solution at a site along the course of the nerve that is more proximally (centrally) located than the mandibular foramen. The inferior alveolar nerve is in close proximity to the trans-

lated condylar neck and therefore easily reached at this point. The injection technique is as follows:

1. The mandible must be in the translated position. This is done by having the patient open as *wide* as possible. The condyle will now be anterior to the condylar fossa. *Wide open* is critical as the condyle must be as far forward as possible.

2. The extraoral landmark of the intertragic notch is identified and can be marked by index finger position or with a disposable needle cover (Fig. 5.59).

3. The retracting (intraoral stabilizing) thumb identifies the coronoid notch on the anterior ramus of the mandible and retracts the cheek anteriorly and laterally (Fig. 5.60).

4. The intraoral puncture site is located just lateral to the pterygomandibular depression but medial to the tendon to the temporalis muscle and at the vertical height of the distal lingual cusp of a normal maxillary 2nd molar (Fig. 5.60).

5. The line of needle insertion is from the contralateral corner of the mouth to the ipsilateral intertragic notch, but parallel to the angulation of the ipsilateral

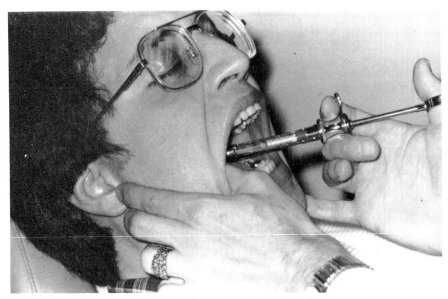

Figure 5.59. Extraoral "Gow-Gates" injection positioning. The index finger points to the intertragic notch.

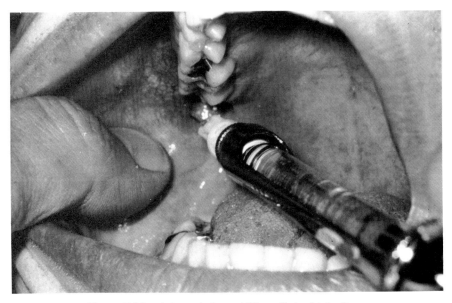

Figure 5.60. Intraoral view of "Gow-Gates" injection.

ear to the face. The flare of the ear is reported to indicate the relative flare of the mandibular ramus.

6. This line will intersect the neck of the translated condyle at a needle depth of approximately 25 mm (with variation). Bone *must* be contacted to confirm proper needle tip location (Figs. 5.61 and 5.62).

7. After osseous contact, withdraw the needle 1 mm, aspirate and inject.

[Needle size: 25- or 27-gauge long; volume: 1.8 ml (1 cartridge)]

Gow-Gates originally recommended 2.2 to 3.0 ml of anesthetic solution; however, in the United States, this would require using disposable parenteral injection

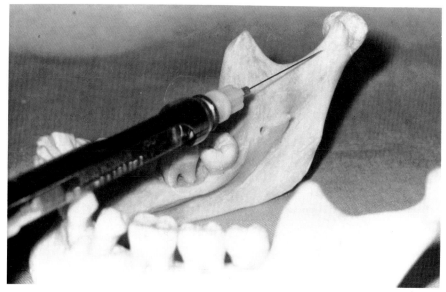

Figure 5.61. "Gow-Gates" needle position on skull.

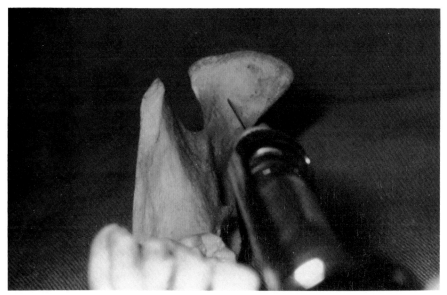

Figure 5.62. "Gow-Gates" needle position on skull.

equipment and multidose vials of anesthetic. Recent reports of clinical trials with the "Gow-Gates" injection indicate that the standard 1.8-ml cartridge of anesthetic is suitable. There is a small decrease in efficiency as the volume of fluid decreases but not enough to warrant using unfamiliar equipment.

The area of analgesia is the distribution of the inferior alveolar nerve and the lingual nerve. This includes the pulps of the mandibular teeth, the buccal periosteum and bone from the 1st bicuspid to the midline, the buccal gingivae from the 1st bicuspid to the midline, and the mucosa and cutaneous epithelium of the ipsilateral lower lip. It also includes the lingual periosteum of the mandibular teeth to the midline, the associated lingual gingivae, the floor of the mouth to the midline and the anterior two-thirds of the tongue to the midline (see Fig. 5.79).

Original reports indicated that the buccal nerve was consistently anesthetized by the "Gow-Gates" injection which would have made this an intraoral, 3rd division, trigeminal nerve block. It is now confirmed that buccal nerve anesthesia is variable and must be separately administered to insure analgesia.

"Akinosi" Inferior Alveolar Nerve Block

A third approach to the inferior alveolar nerve was recently reported. This involves depositing the anesthetic solution at a site midway between the mandibular foramen and the "Gow-Gates" site, with the *mouth closed.* This injection has specific advantage for the patient who cannot open because of trismus or pain or who has a limited opening making the standard inferior alveolar nerve block or the "Gow-Gates" injection difficult to administer. These are specific reasons to use the "Akinosi" injection but it can also be used as a routine approach. The technique is as follows:

1. The mouth is closed but the muscles should be relaxed so the cheek can be retracted (Fig. 5.63).

2. Intraorally, identify the coronoid process and retract the cheek.

3. Align the needle and syringe, parallel to and along the line of the maxillary 2nd and 3rd molar mucogingival junction. The marginal gingivae can also be used. This line of insertion is also parallel to the maxillary alveolus.

4. Insert the needle 2.5 to 3.0 cm into the soft tissue overlying the medial aspect of the mandibular ramus, between the ramus and the maxillary tuberosity. Aspirate and inject at this point (Figs. 5.63 and 5.64).

[Needle size: 25- or 27-gauge long; volume: 1.8 ml (1 cartridge)]

The area of analgesia will be the pulps of the mandibular teeth, the buccal periosteum and bone from the 1st bicuspid to the midline, the buccal gingivae from the 1st bicuspid to the midline, and the mucosa and cutaneous epithelium of the ipsilateral lower lip. Since the injection site is higher than the standard inferior alveolar nerve site, the lingual nerve is also anesthetized. This area of analgesia

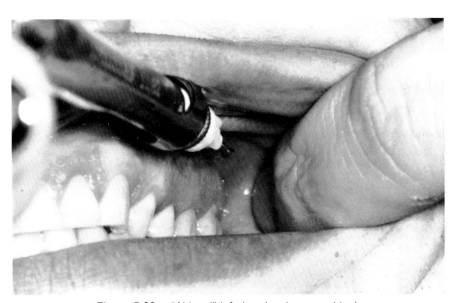

Figure 5.63. "Akinosi" inferior alveolar nerve block.

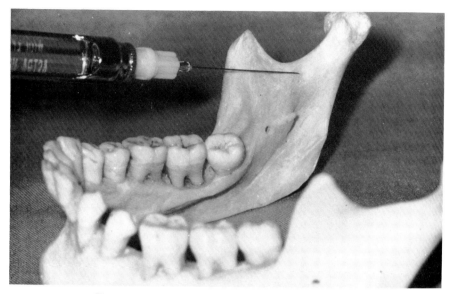

Figure 5.64. "Akinosi" needle position on skull.

will include the lingual periosteum of the mandibular teeth to the midline, the associated lingual of the tongue to the midline (see Fig. 5.79). The buccal nerve is variably blocked with this technique and a buccal nerve block must be separately administered to insure analgesia.

The term *tuberosity injection* has been applied to this technique of inferior alveolar anesthesia, presumably because it is given at a vertical height, even with the maxillary tuberosity. Tuberosity is a misnomer, however, so should not be used as a descriptive term since the technique is directed at the mandible.

Periodontal Ligament Infiltration (Intraligamentary Anesthesia)

The periodontal ligament (PDL) infiltration directs the anesthetic solution into the periodontal ligament, and under pressure forces the agent into this connective tissue to the apex of root. The agent then can block all nerve fibers entering the apex, whether from the primary innervation or from accessory or supplemental innervation. The solution would also block fibers entering lateral canals of the

root. The injection can be used as a primary method for *single tooth analgesia* or can be used as a supplemental injection to reinforce incomplete analgesia from the primary anesthetic technique.

Single tooth analgesia is a specific reason for using the PDL infiltration. A supraperiosteal technique can be employed in the maxilla but not in the adult mandible. A PDL infiltration will effect single tooth analgesia in either jaw. The technique is as follows:

1. The injection can be administered with the standard dental syringe or with the specially designed periodontal ligament syringes.

2. The needle is inserted, forcefully, but without buckling, along the long axis of the selected tooth, at an acute angle to the tooth, into the periodontal ligament (Figs. 5.65 and 5.66).

3. Create pressure in the cartridge by forcefully attempting to advance the piston on the regular dental syringe or by activating the level or trigger on a PDL syringe. This pressure must be maintained for 20 to 30 seconds.

4. Back pressure is critical to the technique and if the plunger in the cartridge

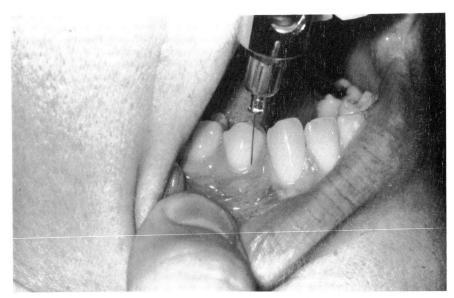

Figure 5.65. Periodontal ligament infiltration using a 30G, ultra-short needle on a periodontal ligament (PDL) syringe.

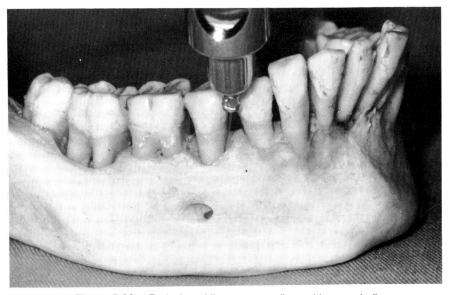

Figure 5.66. Periodontal ligament needle position on skull.

moves more than a few tenths of a millimeter during the 20 to 30 seconds, the needle is not in the PDL and the anesthetic solution will not enter the PDL. The feel of the injection can be experienced by injecting into a standard wood pencil.

5. The site of needle placement for any tooth is at the line angles, and is administered as one injection per root for multirooted teeth. For single rooted teeth, both mesial and distal line angle sites (two sites per tooth) should be used.

[Needle size: 25-, 27- or 30-gauge, short or long. The ultra-short 30-gauge needle is helpful in entering the PDL space and minimizing buckling, but 27- or 25-gauge long or short needles are also satisfactory (Fig. 5.67). The standard short or long needle lengths may require finger support to prevent needle buckling. For this injection, the needle can be bent at the hub to improve access and visability but this is not required. This is one of the two injections which can safely be administered with a bent needle. Volume: a few drops from a standard syringe or the metered volume of 0.1–0.2 ml from the PDL syringe. The gingival tissue will blanch.]

The area of analgesia will be the individual tooth pulp and the adjacent bone and gingiva at the injection site. If full gingival analgesia is required, the buccal, lingual, mesial and distal gingivae must be injected, using more PDL sites or with intrapapillary infiltrations (Fig. 5.68). It is not necessary to aspirate before a PDL infiltration as the only vessels present are capillaries, too small for the needle to enter.

The PDL infiltration had been used only sparingly until the early 1980s. It has not been subject to the same long term evaluations as other injection techniques; however, it appears to be safe and without

short or long term sequellae. Because of its newness, and until further use is monitored, some would consider it a supplemental rather than a primary injection. Its use to date has been safe and it has shown an efficiency rate equal to other techniques. Current literature should be monitored closely as with all new techniques.

(The American Dental Association Council on Dental Materials, Instruments, and Equipment issued a statement in February of 1983 recommending that the periodontal ligament injection be used only as an adjunct to conventional techniques).

Intrapapillary Infiltration

The intrapapillary injection is basically a submucosal-paraperiosteal infiltration. The technique is similar to other soft tissue infiltrations and is used for analgesia of the gingivae and the injection of vasoconstrictors in locals for control of hemorrhage from restrictive, periodontal, and surgical procedures. The technique is as follows (Fig. 5.68):

1. The needle is inserted approxi-

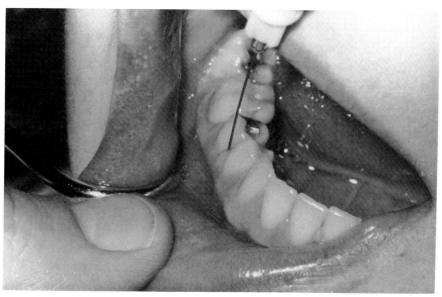

Figure 5.67. Periodontal ligament infiltration using a 27G short needle and a standard dental syringe.

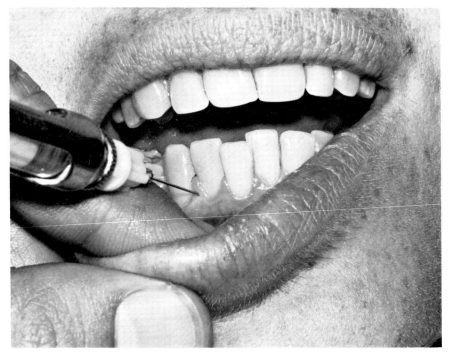

Figure 5.68.   Intrapapillary infiltration.

mately 1 mm into the desired papillae and the solution injection.

[Needle size: 25- 27- or 30-gauge long, short, or ultrashort. The size of the needle is of minimal concern in this injection because of the shallow penetration and absence of vessels that could be entered by the needle. The needle used for the primary injection of the area is usually used. Changing needles is not necessary. Volume: 0.2 ml or less. The solution is injected until the tissue blanches.]

Intrapulpal Infiltration

The intrapulpal injection is used only for pulp canal instrumentation after the chamber is opened. It is a supplement to other block or infiltration methods when complete analgesia is not achieved. The technique is as follows (Fig. 5.69):

1. A bend is placed in the needle (if necessary) to allow access of the needle tip into the pulp canal of the selected tooth. This is the second of the two injections that can safely use a bent needle. (The first was the PDL infiltration).

2. After gaining access to the pulp chamber, the needle tip is inserted as deeply into the canal as possible, and the anesthetic forced under pressure into the remaining pulpal tissue.

[Needle size: 25-, 27- or 30-gauge long or short; volume: $\frac{1}{2}$ ml]

The area of analgesia is the remaining pulpal contents. This analgesia may result from pressure anesthesia of the injection as much as the pharmacological action of the agent.

Intraseptal-Intraosseous Infiltration

The intraseptal and intraosseous infiltration injections involve infiltrating the cancellous bone at the desired site. They are used to achieve analgesia when other methods of infiltration or block fail to achieve adequate pain relief. *The injections are very effective but result in a blood level of the anesthetic agent and vasoconstrictor additives comparable to that of an intravascular injection. Therefore, are used only as a last resort and then only rarely.* The technique is as follows:

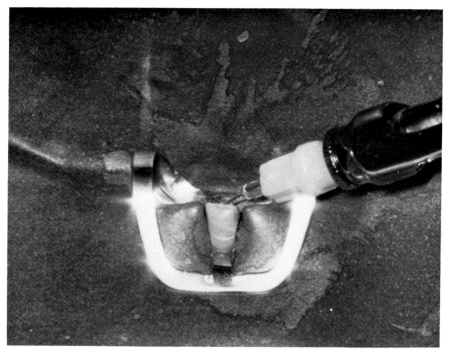

Figure 5.69. Intrapulpal infiltration.

1. Procure paraperiosteal analgesia of the proposed site.

2. If the intraseptal bone is chosen, an 18- to 22-gauge disposable parenteral needle is forced through the crestal bone and the injection made into the cancellous bone.

3. If the cortical bone near the apex is chosen, a hole in the cortical bone must first be made with a small bur (Fig. 5.70).

4. Through this hole, a 25-gauge dental needle is forced into the cancellous bone to the approximate area of the root apex (Fig. 5.71).

5. If the specially designed 30-gauge intraosseous dental needle is chosen it is forced through the cortical bone into the cancellous bone at the desired site (Fig. 5.72) without prior drilling of a cortical hole.

6. Aspirate and inject.

[Needle size: as listed in each technique; volume: 0.2–0.9 ml (¼–½ car-

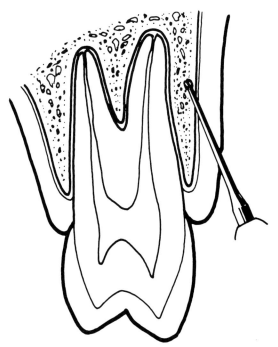

Figure 5.70. Schematic of bur penetrating cortical bone.

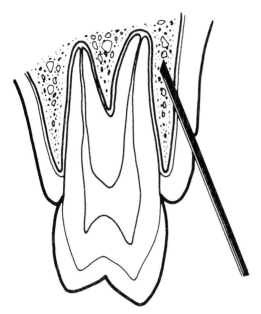

Figure 5.71. Schematic of intraosseous injection.

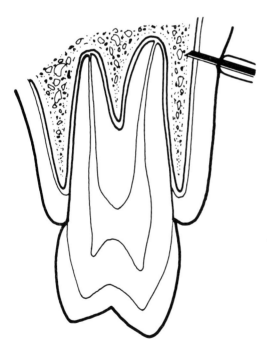

Figure 5.72. Schematic of intraosseous infiltration using an intraosseous needle.

tridge). The dose must be kept to a minimum.]

The area of analgesia is the immediate area of the injection and innervated areas of nerves in the injected area.

Trigeminal, 2nd, and 3rd Division Blocks

Second and third division blocks are injections infrequently used for common restorative and surgical dental procedures as the more peripheral injections previously discussed are adequate. They can be used, however, to great advantage to minimize anesthetic dose when a large area of the oral cavity must be anesthetized or when local infection is present and a more central injection site is desired. Main nerve trunk anesthesia is more desirable than numerous peripheral blocks or infiltrations as it keeps the total dose of the anesthetic agent low.

The 2nd or maxillary division of the trigeminal nerve can be reached by either an intraoral or extraoral approach. The 3rd division of the trigeminal nerve can only be completely blocked by an extraoral approach.

INTRAORAL MAXILLARY NERVE BLOCK (2nd DIVISION BLOCK)

A maxillary nerve block is used to achieve wide spread anesthesia of the maxilla when infection contraindicates routine injections, to reduce the dose of the agent, for extensive maxillary restorative or surgical procedures and for diagnostic analgesia. The injection technique is as follows (Figs. 5.73 to 5.75).

1. Identify the greater palatine foramen as in the anterior palatine block and secure analgesia of the anterior palatine nerve.

2. The line of needle insertion is parallel to the posterior maxillary alveolus on the side to be injected. The angle of insertion to the maxillary occlusal plane is dictated by the angulation of the greater palatine canal. This ranges from 45 to 85°. The greater palatine foramen is found by sounding until the needle enters the canal.

3. Advance the needle gently to a depth of 2.5 cm but never greater than 3.0 cm. After advancement to this depth, aspirate and inject.

[Needle size: 25-gauge long; volume: 1.8 ml (1 cartridge)]

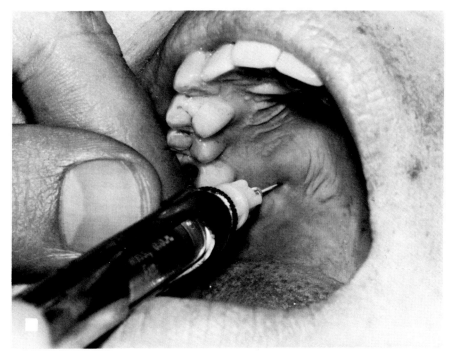

Figure 5.73. Intraoral 2nd division block.

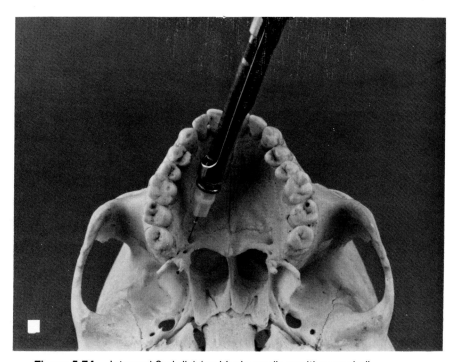

Figure 5.74. Intraoral 2nd division block needle position on skull.

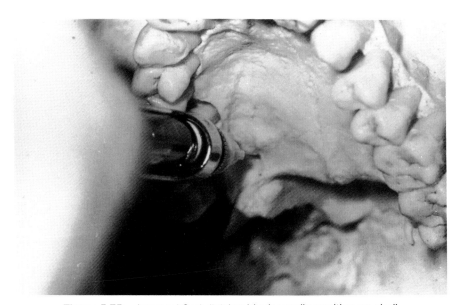

Figure 5.75.   Intraoral 2nd division block needle position on skull.

The area of analgesia will include the entire distribution of the maxillary nerve. This anesthetizes the hemimaxilla (see Fig. 5.78).

No bone is contacted after the needle is in the canal and at no point should the needle bend or be forced against resistance. If obstruction is encountered, the injection should be discontinued. Because of the needle tip proximity to the optic nerve and nerves of ocular motor control, temporary blindness and ocular deviation may occur. Temporary paralysis of the extrinsic eye muscles is not uncommon. These complications disappear as the action of the anesthetic agent dissipates. On aspiration, if air bubbles into the cartridge, the medial wall of the canal was penetrated and the needle tip is in the nasal cavity.

EXTRAORAL MAXILLARY NERVE BLOCK

The indications for an extraoral 2nd division block are the same as the intraoral except it can be used when opening of the mouth is not possible. The complications are also the same. The technique is summarized as follows but the exact technique is not given because it is not considered a routine injection for general dental practitioners.

The injection requires a surgical scrub preparation of the skin just below the zygomatic depression. After preparation of the skin, an intradermal anesthetic injection of the site is made. In this area of skin analgesia, a 4-inch 22-gauge needle is inserted through the zygomatic depression and the sigmoid notch until the tip contacts the lateral pterygoid plate. This depth is marked on the needle but cannot exceed 4.5 cm. The needle is then withdrawn and reinserted in an anterior superior direction into the pterygopalatine fossa to the previously marked depth. After aspiration an injection of 3 ml of anesthetic agent is made. The technique requires equipment not normally a part of intraoral injections and cannot be made with the dental syringe, needles, or cartridges (Fig. 5.76).

EXTRAORAL MANDIBULAR DIVISION BLOCK

The extraoral mandibular division block should be considered for the same purposes as the extraoral maxillary division block. It is done in a similar manner and requires similar equipment. It is not

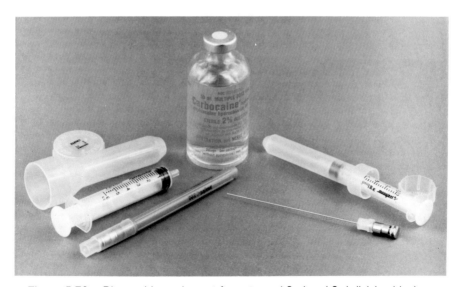

Figure 5.76. Disposable equipment for extraoral 2nd and 3rd division blocks.

Table 5.1.
Maxillary Arch Analgesia

Injection	Result
Single tooth	
Infiltration	Good success
PDL infiltration	Good success without lip anesthesia
Multiple teeth	
Multiple PDL infiltrations	Time consuming
ASA, MSA, PSA infiltrations	Good success
Infraorbital	Good success, wider spread facial anesthesia, some MSA innervation in addition to ASA innervation
PSA block	Higher positive aspiration rate than PSA infiltration, increased rate of hematoma formation, slightly greater efficiency than PSA infiltration
2nd division block	Increased complication rate, greater efficiency than individual area techniques

Abbreviations: PDL, periodontal ligament; ASA, anterior superior alveolar; MSA, middle superior alveolar; PSA, posterior superior alveolar.

Table 5.2.
Mandibular Arch Analgesia

Injection	Result
Single tooth	
PDL infiltration	Good success, alternative to inferior alveolar techniques
Incisor infiltration	Poor success, alternative to inferior alveolar techniques
Multiple teeth (anterior)	
Mental block	Poor success
Incisive branch block	Good success, but difficult to administer; alternative to inferior alveolar techniques
Inferior alveolar technique	Good success; see comparison in Table 5.3
Multiple teeth (posterior)	
Inferior alveolar technique	See Table 5.3

considered a routine injection for general dental practitioners.

The injection requires a surgical scrub of the skin just below the zygomatic depression. After preparation of the skin, an intradermal anesthetic injection of the site is made. In this area of skin analgesia, a 4-inch, 22-gauge needle is inserted through the zygomatic depression and the sigmoid notch until the tip contacts the lateral pterygoid plate. This depth is marked on the needle but cannot exceed 5 cm. The needle is then withdrawn and reinserted upward and posteriorly into the area of the foramen ovale to the previously marked depth.

After aspiration, an injection of 3 ml of anesthetic agent is made.

The technique requires the same extra equipment as the extraoral 2nd division block (Fig. 5.76).

CHOOSING THE APPROPRIATE INJECTION TECHNIQUE

After reviewing the many different injection techniques, it is apparent that more than one technique can be used to effect analgesia of any specific area. Tables 5.1 and 5.2 outline and review techniques used to produce analgesia of the maxillary and mandibular arches. Table 5.3 summarizes and compares the techniques that are used to effect analgesia of the inferior alveolar nerve. The standard, "Gow-Gates," and "Akinosi" techniques should all be considered suitable choices and any could be routinely administered.

Figure 5.77 illustrates the difference in

Table 5.3.
Inferior Alveolar Nerve Analgesia Techniques

Technique	Efficiency	Comment
Standard inferior alveolar block	65–85%; 10–15% positive aspiration Need separate lingual block Need separate long buccal block Variable mylohyoid block	Commonly used
Gow-Gates inferior alveolar block	91–100%; less than 2% positive aspiration Achieves lingual block Achieves mylohyoid block Variable long buccal block	Slower onset of analgesia
Akinosi inferior alveolar block	93%; aspiration rate not reported Achieves lingual block Achieves mylohyoid block Variable long buccal block	Can be given to a patient with trismus; difficult to visualize the path of needle insertion
3rd division block	Excellent; aspiration rate not reported Not routinely used	Increased complication rate

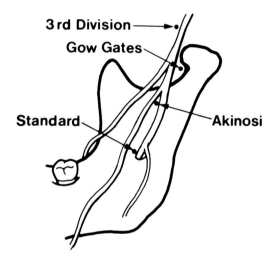

3 rd Division
Gow Gates
Standard
Akinosi

Figure 5.77. Inferior alveolar nerve injection sites.

anesthetic deposition sites among the different inferior alveolar nerve blocking techniques. As the injection site moves central (proximal) from the mandibular foramen, the efficiency of analgesia improves. This is reflected in the reported efficiencies of 65 to 85 per ccent with the standard inferior alveolar block to 91 to 100 per cent with the "Gow-Gates" technique.

Tables 5.4 and 5.5 outline the routinely used maxillary and mandibular injection techniques and the areas that are anesthetized by these injections. The num-

bered areas correspond to those in Figures 5.78 and 5.79.

Pulpal analgesia is the most difficult to achieve of all intraoral tissue. Surgical analgesia for manipulation of bone, periosteum, and gingivae is the easiest to achieve. Surgical procedures of the teeth and bone and traumatic manipulation of the gingivae do require additional anesthetic injections, but they are to anesthetize additional nerves which innervate the lingual and palatal gingivae, not to achieve a greater depth of pulpal analgesia.

Tables 5.6 and 5.7 outline the appropriate local anesthetic techniques to use when securing analgesia for restorative (pulpal analgesia) and/or surgical procedures (pulpal and gingival analgesia) of the maxillary and mandibular teeth.

EVALUATION OF DENTAL ANALGESIA

After completion of the selected injection technique, time is necessary for complete diffusion and absorption of the anesthetic agent into the target nerves. Subjective information which the patient relates to you concerning the feeling of anesthetic action should be apparent within 2 to 3 minutes of most injections. Up to 10 minutes may be necessary for complete operative analgesia to be present. Subjec-

Table 5.4.
Maxillary Injection Techniques

Anterior superior alveolar infiltration	3*
Middle superior alveolar infiltration	2
Posterior superior alveolar infiltration	1
Posterior superior alveolar nerve block	1
Nasopalatine nerve block (bilateral effect)	4
Anterior (greater) palatine nerve block	5
Middle and posterior palatine nerve block	6
Infraorbital nerve block	3, some of 2
2nd division nerve block	1, 2, 3, 4, 5, 6

* Area shown in Figure 5.78.

Table 5.5.
Mandibular Injection Techniques

Standard inferior alveolar nerve block	7, 8, 9*
Akinosi injection	7, 8, 9, 11
Gow-Gates injection	7, 8, 9, 11
Mental nerve block	9
Long buccal nerve block	10
Lingual nerve block	11
3rd division nerve block	7, 8, 9, 10, 11
Incisive nerve block	8, 9

* Area shown in Figure 5.79.

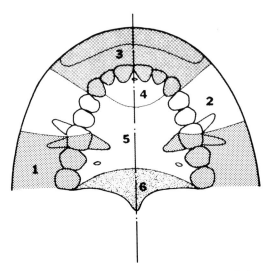

Figure 5.78. Schematic of innervation of the maxilla. *1*, posterior superior alveolar plexus innervation; *2*, middle superior alveolar plexus innervation; *3*, anterior superior alveolar plexus innervation; *4*, nasopalatine nerve innervation; *5*, greater or anterior palatine nerve innervation; *6*, middle and posterior palatine nerve innervation.

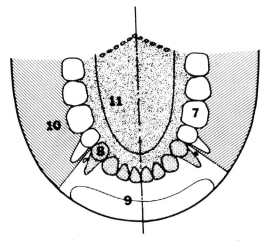

Figure 5.79. Schematic of innervation of the mandible. *7*, inferior alveolar nerve innervation; *8*, incisive nerve innervation; *9*, mental nerve innervation; *10*, buccal nerve innervation; *11*, lingual nerve innervation.

tive symptoms include a feeling of tingling and fullness in the innervated area. Objective signs of an adequate depth of operative analgesia can be determined by pricking the associated soft tissue with a sterile explorer or the needle tip. The patient must differentiate between pressure and pain as the sensation of pressure will remain as this is not affected by blocked sensory and pain fibers. The final determination of analgesia depth is made when instrumentation is initiated.

Apprehensive patients may emotionally be unable to differentiate pressure, vibration, and noise from pain and actually interpret these as painful stimulation. When this occurs, a form of conscious sedation behavior modification, or even general anesthesia may be necessary to accomplish the dental therapy. The operator must develop objective tests to evaluate and separate operative pain from apprehension. These can include activat-

Table 5.6.
Maxillary Injections for Specific Teeth

Tooth	Single Tooth Buccal Infiltration		Superior Plexus Infiltration		Infraorbital	Nasopalatine	Anterior Palatine
Maxillary incisor							
Restorative	Yes	or	ASA	or	Yes	plus	
Surgical	Yes	or	ASA	or	Yes	Yes	
Maxillary cuspid							
Restorative	Yes	or	ASA	or	Yes	plus	plus
Surgical	Yes	or	ASA	or	Yes	Yes	Yes
Maxillary bicuspid							
Restorative	Yes	or	MSA	or	?		plus
Surgical	Yes	or	MSA	or	?		Yes
Maxillary 1st molar							
Restorative			MSA and PSA				plus
Surgical			MSA and PSA				Yes
Maxillary 2nd and 3rd molars							
Restorative	Yes	or	PSA				plus
Surgical	Yes	or	PSA				Yes

Table 5.7.
Mandibular Injections for Specific Teeth

Tooth	Inferior Alveolar Nerve Block — Standard		Gow-Gates		Akinosi		Incisive Block		Single Tooth Buccal Infiltration	Lingual Block	Buccal Block
Mandibular incisor and cuspid											
Restorative	Yes	or	Yes	or	Yes	or	Yes	or	? value		
Surgical	Yes	or	Yes	or	Yes	or	Yes	or	? value	Yes	
Mandibular 1st bicuspid											
Restorative	Yes	or	Yes	or	Yes	or	Yes		plus	Yes	
Surgical	Yes	or	Yes	or	Yes	or	Yes		plus	Yes	
Mandibular 2nd bicuspid											
Restorative	Yes	or	Yes	or	Yes				plus	Yes	plus
Surgical	Yes	or	Yes	or	Yes				plus	Yes	plus
Mandibular molars											
Restorative	Yes	or	Yes	or	Yes				Child only	Yes	Yes
Surgical	Yes	or	Yes	or	Yes				Child only	Yes	Yes

ing a slow speed handpiece and placing its head on enamel rather than the bur on dentine to differentiate vibratory response from a pain response. The high speed handpiece can be activated with the cavity prep protected from air, water, and the bur to differentiate noise from sensory stimulation. Another tactic is "exploring enamel," an insensitive tissue, with an instrument point to differentiate pressure from discomfort.

If objective analgesia is lacking, the primary injection should be repeated *once*, as the usual cause of incomplete analgesia is lack of precise technique. If this fails, several possibilities exist. First, severe inflammation in the area of the nerve may prevent complete pharmacological action of the anesthetic agent. It is now known what biochemical changes take place along the course of a nerve, so in addition to anesthetic action being altered by pH at the site, even a block attempt away from the clinical site of the inflammation may still not result in adequate analgesia.

A second possibility is accessory and/or crossover innervation. Crossover innervation occurs at all locations where two or more nerves anastomose in an area such as the midline, palatal cuspid region, and buccal gingivae in the mental region. Accessory innervation is theorized in the maxilla as palatal nerves could reach the pulps of maxillary teeth. In the mandible, accessory innervation is theorized as lingual, buccal, cutaneous coli, high division fibers from the inferior alveolar, and mylohyoid fibers could reach the mandibular teeth pulps. These accessory and crossover innervation situations are overcome by administering supplemental injections. Since many of these accessory innervations cannot be anatomically proven, it is the success of supplemental injections that perpetuates the theory of their existence.

Theoretically, a PDL injection will circumvent all possible situations because the anesthetic solution reaches the entire root area, apical and lateral. This is why it is used frequently as a very successful supplemental injection. It can be used for individual tooth analgesia as well.

Palatal accessory innervation of maxillary teeth is treated by administering a *partial palatal* infiltration injection at, or one tooth posterior, to the tooth in question. It can also be treated by administering a *nasopalatine* or *greater palatine* nerve block. Examples of maxillary supplemental injection sites are illustrated in Figure 5.80.

Mandibular accessory innervation possibilities are greater but are treated in a similar manner. The PDL is an excellent first choice supplemental injection. In addition, because of possible buccal nerve

innervation of mandibular posterior pulps, it is always advisable to secure buccal nerve analgesia as a routine part of inferior alveolar analgesia regardless of the anticipated procedure. If pulpal analgesia is still not sufficient, as an alternative or in addition to the PDL injection, a series of mandibular supplemental injections are given.

Without regard to sequence, these are the buccal infiltration, lingual infiltration, and the retromolar triangle infiltration. The buccal infiltration (Figs. 5.81 and 5.82) is given at the depth of the mucobuccal fold, below the apex of the tooth in question. The lingual infiltration is given one tooth posterior to the tooth in question, in the floor of the mouth at the junction of the alveolar bone and the floor of the mouth. The retromolar pad (Figs. 5.83 and 5.84). It is directed at high division inferior alveolar fibers which could have branched above the level of usual anesthetic deposition. These fibers can theoretically course down the anterior border of the ramus before entering the mandible. The buccal infiltration is for cutaneous coli nerve branches which could theoretically enter the inferior border of the mandible. The lingual infiltration accomplishes the same plus anesthe-

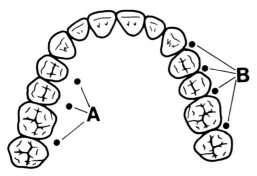

Figure 5.80. Maxillary supplemental injection sites. *A*, partial palatal infiltration sites; *B*, periodontal ligament injection sites.

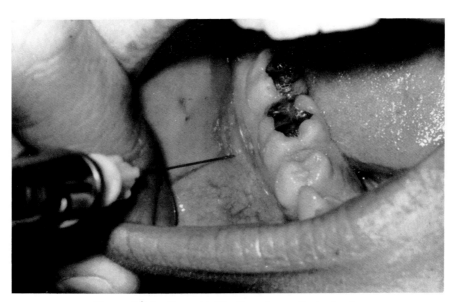

Figure 5.81. Buccal infiltration of mandibular teeth.

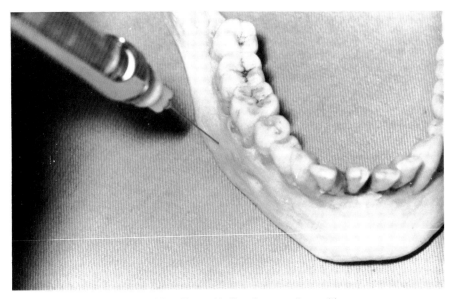

Figure 5.82.   Buccal infiltration needle position.

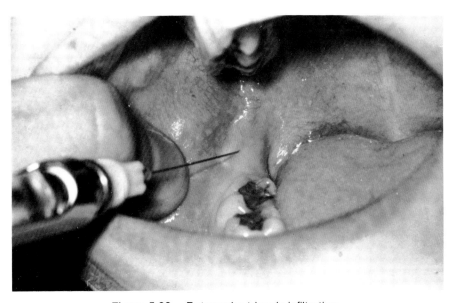

Figure 5.83.   Retromolar triangle infiltration.

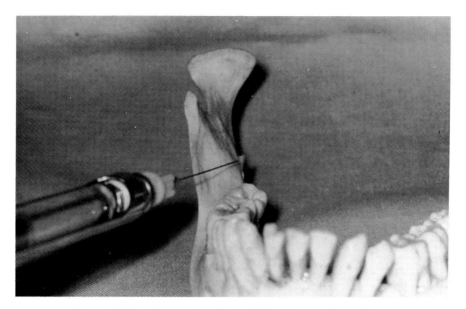

Figure 5.84. Retromolar triangle infiltration needle position.

tizes any mylohyoid branches which could enter the lingual of the body of the mandible. Each of these supplemental injections uses 1/3 of a cartridge (0.6 ml) of anesthetic. All three consume one full cartridge. Supplemental mandibular injection sites are schematically illustrated in Figure 5.85.

The chance of not achieving adequate analgesia because an agent has lost potency or "gone bad" is very remote, if not impossible, as long as the agent was stored and handled properly. Of course, expired solutions should not be used. Lack of technique is by far the biggest cause of "missed injections," followed closely by neural inflammation. Accessory innervation is a distant third. Apprehension and anxiety, if present, can be adequately controlled by proper patient handling and conscious sedation.

CONTROLLING THE PATIENT'S EMOTIONAL RESPONSE

The beginning student of local anesthesia should be totally engrossed with the anatomy of the injection site, needle placement, needle insertion and injection of the agent. After a short clinical expe-

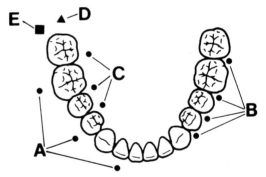

Figure 5.85. Mandibular supplemental injection sites. *A*, buccal infiltration sites; *B*, periodontal ligament infiltrations; *C*, partial lingual infiltration sites; *D*, retromolar triangle infiltration site; *E*, buccal nerve injection site.

rience, however, the technical aspects of the injection become automatic (not to say without thought) and more concentration can be directed to minimizing the patient's emotional reaction to the injection. the injection techniques presented earlier in this chapter are a safe method of administering local anesthesia. *They address physiology.* The patient's emotions are equally important and must also be addressed. The following are numerous tactics, some or all of which most dental practitioners use to divert the patient's attention away from the thought and sensation of the injection.

The most important aspect of minimizing the patient's emotional reaction is a rational explanation and then rhetoric *during* the injection. Each patient requires a different degree of explanation. A common error is to end statements such as "I am now going to anesthetize the area" with "OK?" Explain, but do not ask. This perpetuates procrastination. Rhetoric with the patient in this case does not mean requiring them to answer, as this is not possible during an injection, but may be statements like, "You'll feel my fingers squeeze your lip," "Please keep your eyes open," "Raise your hand when the area starts to become numb," and "Be sure to keep your mouth wide open." None of these actually have anything to do with the injection itself, but they do occupy the patient's mental processes with things other than the injection.

The person who is totally adverse to the injection may not be adequately controlled by this one-sided conversation but most individuals will accept this type of dental care with minimal complaint. Other forms of patient management such as conscious sedation, hypnosis, and acupuncture are available for the extremely difficult patient.

Two other tactics which deserve reiteration are *true rules* of administration. These are chair position and rate of injection. The reclined chair position should be used routinely. This virtually eliminates syncope. The rate of injection is also extremely important in controlling discomfort and is probably the one single most important facet of a comfortable injection. Administering an injection quickly so the patient can "get it over with" is not only painful, but potentially dangerous.

Anesthetic agents will diffuse through tissue, but not as fast as the liquid can be injected. Even at a rate of one cartridge per minute, the agent does not diffuse as quickly as it is injected. This rate does,

however, allow the tissue time to stretch with minimal discomfort as opposed to placing excess tension on connective tissue fibers and thus stimulating free nerve endings in the epithelium and periosteum. Connective tissue itself has minimal pain perception but the physical act of overstretching and tearing can result in operative and postoperative discomfort and edema.

The topical anesthetic should also be considered an aid in giving comfortable local injections. It most definitely will reduce or eliminate painful stimulation from the needle tip passing through the most superficial layers of the epithelium. However, it does not penetrate to sufficient depth to result in an injection that is imperceptible. Periosteum and muscle fibers are sensitive and when contacted will result in mild stimuli. Other tactics are necessary to complete the comfortable injection. The topical alone is not a panacea.

Some have recommended injecting a drop of anesthetic solution ahead of the advancing needle to minimize discomfort. This will anesthetize tissue, but anesthetics do not act immediately and if every millimeter of tissue were to be anesthetized, ahead of needle advancement, considerable time would be consumed. It must also be kept in mind that connective tissue is very insensitive and an inadvertent intravascular injection could occur. This technique of injection is not absolutely condemned but it does have only minimal value and even a small intravascular injection should be avoided.

A drop of anesthetic on the tissue before injection is another method used by some. This results only in the same effect as a topical anesthetic.

Physical manipulation of tissue will distract the patient's attention from epithelial penetration and minimize sensation of the advancing needle. This manipulation can take several forms, the most common being squeezing tissue with the hand that retracts and tenses the mucosa. Other physical distractors include pulling the lip and mucobuccal fold tissue over the needle tip rather than pushing the needle into the tissue. There appears to be no real difference between the two. Squeezing or pushing on tissue such as the palate, ascending ramus, and forehead also can act as excellent distractors. Any of these, especially when combined with a verbal narration of the "pinch" or "squeeze" or "mosquito bite" diverts the patient's attention to something other than the needle puncture.

Warming of the anesthetic solution has been advocated and apparently used by many, as commercial cartridge warmers are available. The validity of injecting a solution of near body temperature seems appropriate but with a slow injection technique the solution reaches body temperature very quickly as it courses through the needle. Even room temperature solutions do not cause discomfort or tissue damage. A cold solution, below room temperature, may be slightly uncomfortable but still not harmful. If the solution is at room temperature when injected, there is no need for supplemental warming. A procedure which must be avoided is storing cartridges in a warmer. Increased temperatures cause deterioration of the agent and those warmers that use an electric light to produce heat add to the problem, as light is another factor resulting in shortened shelf life.

A tactic that has virtually no substantiated benefit is to rub the site after completion of the injection. The rationale of this is to push or squeeze the solution through the tissue. There is no scientific evidence that this in any way hastens diffusion of the agent. If the anesthetic has been deposited in the correct anatomical location and at the recommended slow rate, subjective symptoms of numbness will already be apparent to the patient by the time the needle is withdrawn. The act has more emotional value, possibly to the practioner, than the physical value for the patient.

Rhetoric is always advocated as a means of distracting the patient and in rendering a rational explanation of the procedure, but certain words and phrases must be avoided. *Do not promise* what cannot be delivered, such as an injection the patient cannot feel. Modern techniques minimize discomfort but are not imperceptible. The words that should be avoided include: *pain*—use "discomfort"; *shot*—use "anesthetic administration"; *needle*—lead the conversation away from this as there are not always suitable substitutes.

Many other methods of emotional control may be encountered or taught by dental practitioners. Each should be thoroughly understood and proven safe before use and the full scope of psychological and physiological action must be considered. The foregoing discussion should provide a basis of comparison and insight as to how each new tactic or technique must be evaluated before use.

Bibliography

Adatia AK: Innervation of mandibular central incisors. *Oral Health* 69(10):53–56, 1979.

Akinosi JO: A new approach to the mandibular nerve block. *Br J Oral Surg* 15:83–87, 1977

Carter RB, Keen EN: The intramandibular course of the inferior alveolar nerve. *J Anat* 108:433–440, 1971.

Cook W: The cervical plexus and its probable role in the oral operator's field. *Dent Items* 73(4):356–361, 1951.

Council on Dental Materials, Instruments, and Equipment: Status Report: The Periodontal Ligament Injection. *J Am Dent Assoc* 106(2):222–224, 1983.

Dobbs EC, DeVier C: L-Arterenol as a vasoconstrictor in local anesthesia. *J Am Dent Assoc* 40:433–436, 1950.

Dover WR: The mandibular block injection—why it sometimes fails. *Oral Health* 61:12–14, 1971.

Evers H, Haegerstam G: *Handbook of Dental Local Anesthesia.* London, Schultz Medical Information, 1981.

Frommer J, Jele FA, Monroe CW: The possible role of the mylohyoid nerve in mandibular posterior tooth sensation. *J Am Dent Assoc* 85:113–117, 1972.

Gow-Gates GAE: Mandibular conduction anesthesia: a new technique using extraoral landmarks. *Oral Surg* 36(3):321–330, 1973.

Gow-Gates GAE, Watson JE: The Gow-Gates mandibular block: further understanding. *Anesth Prog* 24:183–189, 1977.

Gustainis JF, Peterson LJ: An alternative method of mandibular nerve block. *J Am Dent Assoc* 103:33–36, 1981.

Hayward J, Richard ER, Malhotra SK: The mandibular foramen: its anteroposterior position. *Oral Surg* 44:837–843, 1977.

Jorgensen NG, Hayden J: *Sedation, Local and General Anesthesia in Dentistry*, ed 3. Philadelphia, Lea and Febiger, 1980.

Levy TP: An assessment of the Gow-Gates mandibular block for third molar surgery. *J Am Dent Assoc* 103:37–41, 1981.

Malamed SF: The Gow-Gates mandibular block. *Oral Surg* 51(5):463–467, 1981.

Petersen JK: The mandibular foramen block. *Br J Oral Surg* 9:126–138, 1971.

Reitzik M: Inferior dental nerve block, a modified technique. *J Can Dent Assoc* 46(7):449–450, 1980.

Roberts DH, Sowray JH: *Local Anesthesia in Dentistry*, ed 2. Bristol, John Wright and Sons, 1970.

Robertson WD: Clinical evaluation of mandibular conduction anesthesia. *Gen Dent* 27(5):49–51, 1979.

Rood J: Some anatomical and physiological causes of failures to achieve mandibular analgesia. *Br J Oral Surg* 15(1):75–82, 1977.

Shields PW: Further observations on mandibular anaesthesia. *Aust Dent J* 22(5):334–337, 1977.

Sicher H: The anatomy of mandibular anesthesia. *J Am Dent Assoc* 33:1541–1557, 1946.

Stibbs GD, Korn JH: An evaluation of the local anesthetic, mepivacaine hydrochloride, in operative dentistry. *J Prosthet Dent* 14(2):355–364, 1964.

Sutton RN: The practical significance of mandibular accessory foramina. *Aust Dent J* 19(3):167–173, 1974.

Walton RE, Abbott BJ: Periodontal ligament injection: a clinical evaluation. *J Am Dent Assoc* 103:571–575, 1981.

Walton RE, Garnick JJ: The periodontal ligament injection: histologic effects on the periodontium in monkeys. *J Endocrinol* 8(1):22–26, 1982.

Walton R, Garnick J: Pulpal anesthesia with the PDL injection: clinical and histologic evaluation. *J Dent Res* 59(A):467, 1980.

Watson JE, Gow-Gates GAE: A clinical evaluation of the Gow-Gates mandibular block technique. *NZ Dent J* 72:220–223, 1976.

Weil C, Welham FS, Yacker RF: Clinical evaluation of mepivacaine hydrochloride by a new method. *J Am Dent Assoc* 63:26–32, 1961.

Yamada A, Jasstak JT: Clinical evaluation of the Gow-Gates block in children. *Anesth Prog* 28(4):106–109, 1981.

CHAPTER 6

Complications of Local Anesthesia

Problems, complications, and reactions to local anesthetics are rare when correct chair position and proper techniques are used. Certain problems such as anaphylaxis and allergy are presented in Chapter 7 in the section on management, although the specific aspects of these as they relate to dental local anesthesia will be included in the following discussion. Any deviation from normal could be considered a complication and should be avoided if at all possible. Most reactions can be avoided if the rules for proper drug administration are followed, as complacency and sloppy technique needlessly increase risk. Most problems, when they occur, are more annoying than dangerous, but even the mildest and simplest complication can become severe if not understood and treated. The following discussion is intended to acquaint the practitioner with all types of problems so that if they do occur, appropriate care can be rendered.

SYNCOPE

The most common untoward reaction to all dental therapy is syncope, and it will continue to be a common problem until all dental injections are done in a reclined position. The problem is almost entirely psychogenic and relates to how the patient reacts to discomfort and psychological stress. A complete discussion of the physiological mechanism can be found in basic physiology texts. In summary, the mechanism is one of neurogenic shock, also alled the vasovagal response. Peripheral vasodilatation occurs, allowing blood to pool in the lowest portion of the body. Normal vascular tone is in equilibrium with total blood volume, but when vessels in the extremities and abdomen dilate, blood pools. The most superior portion of the body is then depleted of an adequate blood supply because of gravity. This produces a corresponding loss of cerebral blood pressure and a relative lack of cerebral oxygenation from lack of blood flow. The lungs are oxygenating the blood adequately, but this blood does not reach the brain in sufficient volume to maintain consciousness.

Rarely is the problem hazardous, although without definitive therapy, it could be serious. Loss of consciousness from syncope does not usually occur without prodromal symptoms such as sweating, nausea, rolling eyes, pallor, and dizziness, which the patient will relate to the operator or should be noticed by the operator. If the initial signs of syncope are detected before loss of consciousness, the "faint" can usually be aborted by placing the patient in a reclined position and diverting their attention. Simple physical maneuvers such as having the patient breathe deeply and slowly, briskly tapping a foot, or any other mental function that keeps attention away from the syncopal reaction and/or dental procedure that is causing the neurogenic shock will accomplish the diversion. Chair position, however, is the most important aspect, since the patient is not lacking oxygen or the stimulus to breathe, only adequate blood volume to the brain. To treat syncope, the patient must be reclined with the legs level or slightly above the head. At no time should the trunk be higher than the head as this causes venous congestion in the upper body and the weight of the visceral organs can impair diaphragmatic function, making breathing more difficult. The operator must do this immediately, as the dental chair keeps the patient's head above the trunk and legs. Seizure activity may accompany syncope, but this does not change the diagnosis or treatment. Seizures from syncope cease when adequate blood flow returns to the brain. This confirms that the seizure is from syncope and not drug overdose.

The most unfortunate aspect of syncope is that the entire foregoing discussion should be superfluous as the occurrence can be virtually eliminated by practicing all aspects of dentistry in a reclined position.

ALLERGY

There is an unfortunate tendency to label many syncope-prone patients as being allergic to local anesthetics. Therefore, specific differentiation must be made between the two. Allergy to local anesthetic agents is a rarely encountered problem but is the reaction most feared. Since the introduction of amide anesthetics, the true incidence is extremely low. Procaine and other ester derivatives have a higher incidence of true allergic reactions. The most conclusive study in this area tested three amide agents—lidocaine, prilocaine, and mepivacaine—and three ester agents—procaine, tetracaine, and chloroprocaine. Patients were divided into two groups, those with a prior history of allergic reactions to anesthetic agents and those without. The results showed that regardless of history, no patients were allergic to the amide agents, while there were substantiated reactions to the ester agents. The allergen is *para*-aminobenzoic acid, the metabolite of ester hydrolysis.

The problem in clinical practice is that some amide commercial preparations previously contained methyl paraben as a preservative and antibacterial. This agent is chemically related to *para*-aminobenzoic acid and results in cross-sensitivity. A clinical situation then exists where allergic reactions can occur in response to the preservative in the local without allergy to the anesthetic agent itself. Anesthetic cartridges are commercially available without methyl paraben but the drug circular (package insert) must be consulted to ascertain which additives, if any, are present as this information is not normally advertised or displayed on the dental cartridge. All of the popular local anesthetic agents, as of 1982, no longer contained methyl paraben. Some agents, before that date, did. Local anesthetics in multi-dose vials still contain methyl paraben. Most topical anesthetics are ester derivatives and contain methyl paraben, so allergy is more likely than with amide injectables.

Allergic manifestations can take multiple forms, the least severe being cutaneous or mucosal eruptions such as vesicles, bulla, and urticaria, and the most severe being anaphalactoid with bronchospasm, dyspnea, cyanosis, hypotension and peripheral vascular collapse. Reactions can also be localized, widespread, immediate or delayed. Immediate widespread reactions are potentially more life-threatening than the delayed localized type, although all must be treated when present.

Mild manifestations are treated with an antihistamine such as diphenhydramine hydrochloride and the more severe with a combination of adrenaline, corticosteroids, and antihistamines. Specific treatment may be found in Chapter 7. It should be emphasized that most patients who feel they are allergic to local anesthetics ("caine" drugs or "all local anesthetics"), or have been told they are allergic to local agents, should be questioned very carefully to ascertain if the problem they report is truly an allergy. The majority of problems labeled "allergy" are not and can be explained on the basis of syncope, intravascular injections, or any of the other complications of local anesthesia discussed in the following. The alternatives to local anesthesia for dental therapy, although available, are few and not as convenient. The choice of general anesthesia is very expensive and of needless risk unless absolutely necessary.

Allergy testing is indicated if the patient's prior history is that of true sensitization. The procedure of testing is technically easy but somewhat risky. The possibility of precipitating mild and even severe reactions is possible and the practitioner must be ready to treat these reactions and provide complete life support for the patient if and when they occur. For these reasons, highly suspect patients should be evaluated by an allergist, medical center testing facility or other appropriate individuals to ascertain which agent or agents can be safely used. Testing to find the drug allergy source is unnecessarily dangerous. Routine in-office testing without appropriate informed consent and complete life support capabilities is not warranted.

BROKEN NEEDLE

The problem of broken needles is one that has been virtually eliminated by single use, disposable needles. Heat sterilizable needles lose strength and temper with time and, if overused, will break. Disposable needles rarely, if ever, break but when they do, it is because of excessive stress, bending induced by the operator, or sudden unexpected patient movement.

When a needle breaks it is almost always at the hub. Thus the absolute rule is that needles are never inserted more than $2/3$ to $3/4$ of their length. With this safety margin, if breakage occurs, the exposed end can be grasped with a hemostat and retrieved. If a needle is broken, great care should be exercised so that muscular action does not maneuver the needle into the tissue, thus obscuring its recovery. Several principles are involved to minimize and, in most cases, prevent needle

fracture. These are as follows:

1. Use single use, disposable needles.
2. Avoid using needles smaller than 25 or 27 gauge for deep tissue penetration.
3. Never insert a needle to the hub.
4. Avoid forcing the needle through resistant tissue (bone, cartilage) unless it is specifically designed for that purpose.
5. Avoid bending the needle before injection. Dental local anesthesia does not call for angled needles as all deep injections into oral tissue can be given with a straight needle. A bend can be placed before a periodontal ligament (PDL) or intrapulpal injection as these are not deep injections.
6. Never change needle directions while in the tissue—withdraw first.
7. Avoid sudden movements and do not alarm or surprise the patient. Any of these may cause the patient to make sudden unexpected movements.
8. Maintain finger rests and tissue support so that inadvertent patient movement can be controlled.

HEMATOMA FORMATION

Any time a needle is inserted through tissue, capillaries and, in some cases, larger vessels, may be punctured or torn. When this happens, extravasation of blood occurs. Clinical hematoma formation, however, is a rare occurrence. The posterior superior alveolar block is the injection where hematoma formation is most likely to occur. Needle penetration in the zygomatic area, behind the maxilla, courses near, through, or into the pterygoid venous plexus and on some occasions results in bleeding. Because the area is composed of loose connective tissue, the pterygomaxillary space can quickly fill with blood and result in almost immediate swelling (hematoma) of the area followed in several days by discoloration (ecchymosis) of the overlying skin and adjacent mucosal areas. Exacting technique will minimize intratissue bleeding but because of this risk, the posterior superior alveolar infiltration is usually chosen over the block.

The infraorbital nerve block is also susceptible to vessel penetration because it is one of the few areas where larger vessels are close to the skin. The inferior alveolar injection, "Gow-Gates" injection, and mental block injection may also result in vessel puncture and hemorrhage, but because the vessels are deeper in relation to overlying skin and mucosa, hemorrhage, when it occurs, may not be clinically evident.

Hematoma formation rarely requires specific treatment and will resolve in a few days without intervention. In fact, there are probably more deep, non-detected hematomas than there are those which are clinically evident. Symptoms, depending on the location and amount of bleeding, vary from minor soreness to considerable pain, swelling, discoloration, and temporary loss of function. Initial therapy, if deemed necessary, is the application of pressure to reduce intratissue bleeding. Cold pressure can be added to this. Pressure should be maintained for 5 minutes to control venous and arterial bleeding. By 24 hours, analgesics and rest for the affected area are the most appropriate care. Infection should not be a complication if aseptic techniques are followed. Patient reaction to hematoma formation relates to esthetics. Adequate explanation should put the patient at ease.

INFECTION

Infection can occur whenever non-sterile materials are introduced into the tissue and usually manifests within 24 hours of the injection. Fresh anesthetic solutions in single use cartridges and disposable needles have virtually eliminated infections from local anesthesia. However, errors in handling the needles and cartridges and improper mucosal preparation may result in infection. Topical disinfectants have been advocated for use at the puncture site and their use can be justified but they do not sterilize the mucosa,

as it is not yet possible to use agents strong enough to produce sterilization and yet not cause chemical injury. If the puncture site is dry and free of debris, the chance of infection is remote. Advancing a needle into or through infected tissue or through visible surface debris can carry microorganisms deeper into the tissue and must be avoided. Aseptic techniques which must be followed to prevent infection are as follows:

1. Autoclave or heat-sterilize syringes.
2. Dry and wipe mucosa before injection.
3. Use anesthetic cartridge on only one patient. Always discard unused portions even with techniques that use only a few drops of anesthetic. Aspiration and tissue fluid reflux contaminate solution.
4. Keep needle capped before use and recap after use. Inspect needle before use to insure the sterile seal is not broken.
5. Never resterilize single use needles.
6. Disinfect anesthetic cartridge diaphragm and inspect cartridge before use.
7. Do not store anesthetic cartridge in disinfectant solution.
8. Practice scrupulous personal hand hygiene and aseptic office techniques.

If infection should occur, it is treated with appropriate antibiotics.

PAIN ON INJECTION

Pain on injection or at least discomfort is not something that can absolutely be avoided. As discussed in the section on controlling the patient's emotional response, most discomfort can be minimized, but the discomfort of the needle tip passing through muscle, contacting periosteum, or contacting a nerve trunk is real and can only be partially eliminated. There are specific pain responses which may occur during the course of an injection that point to specific complications. The specific complaint of burning sensation is a symptom of contaminated anesthetic solution. This can happen if the dental cartridges are stored for extended periods in disinfectants or cold sterilization media. The diaphragm and/ or plunger may leak if left submerged. Ideal disinfection of the diaphragm is accomplished with 91 per cent isopropyl or 70 per cent ethyl alcohol just prior to use. No other disinfection is necessary. Do not store cartridges in any solution or media.

When the anesthetic agent is contaminated with alcohol or other disinfectants, severe local tissue toxicity results and chemical damage to the injected tissue and adjacent neural structures is possible. This can lead to prolonged anesthesia and/or paresthesia of tissues innervated by the damaged fibers. Nerve fibers are slow to regenerate so chemical damage to them can be permanent.

Most pain on injection is from injection pressure produced by a rapid injection rate. This can be minimized by injecting slowly, at least one minute per cartridge. Injecting faster is very uncomfortable. Discomfort on needle insertion through the mucosa has been proven to not vary among the 25-, 27-, and 30-gauge needles; however, there are still some who insist that the 30-gauge needle is more comfortable.This is probably due to the speed with which anesthetic can be forced through the lumen of this small needle in relation to a 25-gauge needle. The needle slows the injection rate and thus there is less discomfort.

Pain on injection can also occur if the operator has been so accurate in needle placement that the tip touches a nerve trunk. This problem is entirely *unavoidable*. When it happens, the patient will mention the feeling of an "electric shock" in a peripheral innervated area. In the standard inferior alveolar injection, if the lingual nerve is contacted, the sensation will be in the tongue and if the inferior alveolar nerve is contacted, the sensation will be in the lower lip. If this should happen, the needle should be withdrawn approximately 1 mm, reaspirated, and the injection continued. Rarely will this cause nerve damage; however, it is possible. Anesthesia is effected very quickly as the nerve is immediately bathed in the agent. It should be re-emphasized that the problem cannot be prevented and is the result of extremely accurate needle placement.

PARESTHESIA

Paresthesia is defined as an abnormal neural sensation. In the clinical situation, paresthesia is a *subjective complaint*. It does not specifically mean anesthesia, hypoalgesia, or hyperalgesia; however, on *objective evaluation* it could be any of these. The patient will complain of a feeling of "numbness," "coldness," or a "tingling" sensation in the affected area. It usually becomes apparent when the local anesthetic action wanes and a residual feeling of "numbness" remains.

Paresthesia is caused by damage to a nerve from physical, usually surgical, or chemical trauma. If a surgical procedure was not done in the area, the physical trauma could be from the needle tip contacting a nerve trunk. This may or may not have been noted during the injection. Chemical injury from contaminated anesthetic would probably be noted because of the severe burning sensation on injection. In either case, there is no treatment for paresthesia. The objective extent of the neural deficit should be ascertained by specific cranial nerve evaluation. This can be done by the practitioner or on referral. The patient should be *reassured* that neural healing occurs, but is slow. It can take weeks, months, or even years for complete healing or regeneration. Most paresthesias resolve in the first few months, but permanent paresthesia is possible. Since there is no specific therapy, the status and extent of the area involved must be monitored. Referral for monitoring, if resolution is not quick, is wise since the patient will undoubtedly have questions as to why it happened. A second, uninvolved party can answer these and reinforce the unavoidable nature of paresthesias from needle trauma. Only time will resolve the phenomenon.

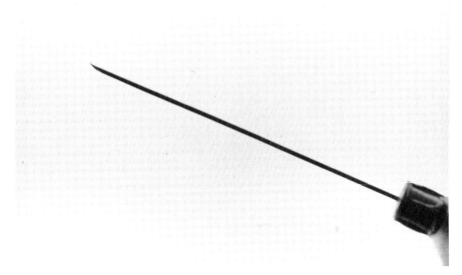

Figure 6.1.   Bur on tip of needle.

Other local "trauma" to the nerve that can result in temporary anesthesia or paresthesia include inflammation, hematoma around the nerve trunk, and burs on needle tips from heavy bone contact.

If bone is contacted forcefully, the tip of the bevel will bend and, on withdrawal, tear tissue (Fig. 6.1). The drag created is easily felt in the syringe. A needle that drags should be changed. Burs are difficult to see but can be found by pulling the needle over a sterile piece of gauze to see if it catches. Needles used for PDL injections should not be used for other areas of the mouth as the PDL technique frequently creates burs.

Sterilizable reusable needles historically posed this same needle trauma problem, as reuse and abuse dulled the points and created burs on the bevels. This, no doubt, increased the incidence of needle trauma.

TOXICITY ULCER (ISCHEMIC ULCER)

Every anesthetic has a specific local irritancy capacity. This phenomenon, however, is rarely encountered and happens only when the agent remains in a confined localized area for an extended period or is not dissipated or diluted by tissue fluids. This situation is compounded when a vasoconstrictor is used and the agent is injected into relatively avascular tissue such as the palate, gingival papillae, or mucobuccal fold. The clinical reaction manifests as an ulcer in the area of the injection which becomes apparent several days after the procedure (Figs. 6.2 and 6.3). The duration of the lesion is approximately 10 to 14 days and usually resolves without complication or treatment. These necrotic ulcers were once thought to be solely the result of inadequate blood supply to the area from intense vasoconstriction and consequent tissue death, hence the term ischemic ulcer. Evidence now exists which indicates that these ulcers are the result of the local tissue toxicity of the anesthetic agent which has been held at the injection site, undiluted, as a result of the vasoconstrictor. It appears that the incidence of these ulcers is low and is not related to differing concentrations of vasoconstrictors, only the presence or absence of a vasoconstric-

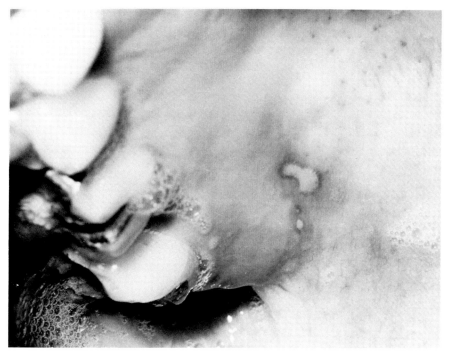

Figure 6.2. Local toxicity ulcer on hard palate (ischemic ulcer).

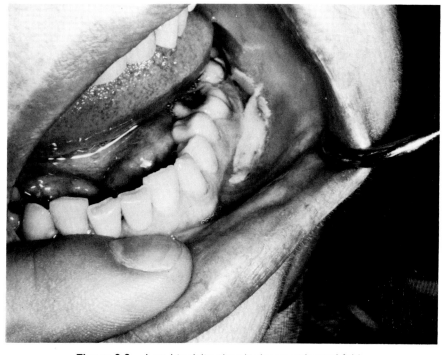

Figure 6.3. Local toxicity ulcer in the mucobuccal fold.

tor. Again, no specific treatment is indicated as the lesions are self-limiting. The patient does deserve an explanation.

TOPICAL CHEMICAL INJURY

All topical anesthetics possess differing degrees of local tissue toxicity. The mucosa of the oral cavity is susceptible to injury if these agents remain in contact with the tissues for too long. The time a topical anesthetic agent can remain safely in contact is in relation to its potency and chemical irritating capacity. All topicals are different and leaving them routinely in contact for 1 to 2 minutes may produce tissue sloughing. Follow each agent's specific manufacturer's directions. If the directions say 30 seconds, 2 minutes will produce injury. Figure 6.4 illustrates sloughing tissue from a topical anesthetic chemical injury. The lesion is self-limiting and requires no therapy.

SYSTEMIC TOXICITY

Toxicity of the central nervous system can occur in two ways after dental injection; first, through an overdose, and second, from a "temporary overdose" caused by an intravascular injection. The first, true overdose, should be absolutely avoided by being cognizant of the total dose of the drug given the patient. Definite guidelines based on body weight are given in Chapter 3. Errors are made when the practitioner is lulled into the relative safety of adult doses of locals. If adult doses are mistakenly given to children or debilitated patients, toxic symptoms result.

Temporary overdoses occur when normally safe subcutaneous doses of local anesthetics are injected into vascular channels. Aspiration should minimize this but it is not flawless. Certain injections have a higher incidence of positive aspiration (standard inferior alveolar, up to 12 per cent) but any soft tissue injection (maxillary infiltration less than 1 per cent) can be mistakenly given into a vessel. The flaws in aspiration are from either aspirating the side of a vessel onto the bevel of the needle or moving the needle tip during the injection, inadvertently, from an extravascular to intravascular site.

If the anesthetic injection is made into a vascular channel, the toxicity of the agent is much greater than if slowly absorbed into the blood stream from a subcutaneous site. The toxic effects of anesthetics and/or vasoconstrictors on the

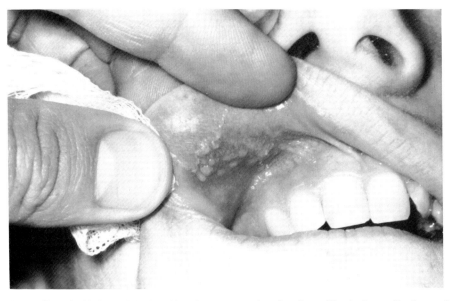

Figure 6.4. Chemical injury with sloughing from excessive duration of topical anesthetic application.

central nervous system and cardiovascular system are discussed in Chapters 2 and 3.

The speed with which the injection is made is critical in determining the severity of the toxic reaction which occurs from an intravascular injection. A slow venous injection allows time for the agent to be diluted in the general circulation, and only a minor, if any, effect will be noticed. The amount of local anesthetic introduced into the circulation by this method will probably be clinically undetectable. The vasoconstrictor, however, may produce clinical symptoms of dizziness, palpation, headache, and a sensation of "flying apart." the vasoconstrictor is quickly metabolized so the effects are short-lived. Hopefully the patient is healthy enough and has enough pulmonary and cardiovascular reserve to withstand the effect.

A fast (contraindicated) injection in a vein gives much less time for dilution as a bolus dose of the agent reaches target organs. This can result in more severe symptoms from either the local agent or the vasoconstrictor.

Injection into an artery has potentially more serious consequences. (Aspiration does not differentiate arterial from venous blood.) A slow arterial injection is no worse and possibly less hazardous than a slow venous injection because the agent is dispersed to small capillaries and then venous dilution before reaching either the heart or brain. A local consequence may be vascular constriction from the vasoconstrictor and this would manifest as blanching of the vascularized tissue. Permanent damage or serious sequelae do not result from the local effect.

A fast intra-arterial injection has potentially the most severe consequences. A rapid injection into an artery produces a reverse blood flow because of the pressure of the injected fluid. This reverse flow will allow a bolus of anesthetic and/or vasoconstrictor to enter the external carotid artery and in continued retrograde flow to reach the common carotid where it is dispersed to the internal carotid artery. A bolus of local anesthetic in this artery directly exposes the central nervous system to a transient but high dose of the agent. It can account for severe toxic reactions such as seizures and unconsciousness when only a small dose is administered. Reverse arterial flow can account for other bizarre symptoms of unwanted anesthesia, to be discussed later.

Treatment of toxic symptoms is dictated by the severity of the response. The effects of vasoconstrictor drugs on the central nervous system cause minor symptoms, for only a few seconds to minutes. The drugs are metabolized quickly and so lasting effects are not expected. Specific treatment, other than reassurance, is rarely necessary. Overdose and toxic symptoms from the local anesthetic agent require more specific supportive therapy. As discussed in the section on physiology and pharmacology of local anesthetic agents, the major clinical effect of a toxic reaction is central nervous system depression; however, the initial clinical symptom is likely to be excitation and/or seizures as inhibitory centers are initially depressed. This is followed by clinical CNS depression as the reaction worsens. (Review Chapter 2.)

Specific therapy for emergencies is discussed in Chapter 7, although for the general dental practitioner, the primary objective, regardless of diagnosis, as it may not initially be known, is basic life support. Overtreatment with drugs may make the situation worse. Simple syncope, vasoconstrictor venous injection, and true toxic overdose share some of the same symptoms such as excitation, seizures, and loss of consciousness. Therefore, in an emergency situation, specific "diseases are not treated," only the symptoms and maintenance of homeostatic mechanisms, with emphasis on the airway, breathing, and circulation (the ABC's of cardiopulmonary resuscitation).

IDIOSYNCRASY

Idiosyncratic responses are those complications that are individual to the patient. They rarely can be predicted and usually do not fit the pattern of other well defined reactions. Some define it as any reaction that is not allergic or toxic, but that definition is really too broad. Psychogenic factors undoubtedly play a very important role in these types of complications. Examples are symptoms of allergy when no allergy exists, toxic symptoms when the dose is well below the maximum allowable, and other unexplainable phenomena. Idiosyncrasy is a term used as a "catch-all" and should not be overused. Every effort should be made to diagnose the specific complication and explain its occurrence. Unfortunately the human biological system does not always react in the expected manner.

BLANCHING

Blanching of tissue can occur at the site of needle insertion or peripheral to the injected area. If it is at the puncture site, it is the result of an excessive volume of the agent or reduced blood flow through the tissue because of the vasoconstrictor. This degree of reduced blood flow does not result in tissue damage but may account for toxicity ulcers as discussed earlier. Figure 6.5 illustrates blanching after soft tissue injection of the buccal mucosa for a benign tumor removal.

If the blanching is peripheral to the area of the injection, two possible explanations are traumatic needle stimulation of sympathetic fibers or intra-arterial injection. Stimulation of sympathetic pathways will reduce blood flow to the innervated areas but is extremely rare and does not usually result in complications. Intra-arterial injections have been discussed under systemic toxicity. This also does not result in serious sequelae. Of course, if all of the anesthetic is injected intra-arterially, no analgesia will result.

UNWANTED ANESTHESIA

Occasionally anesthesia of nerves not selectively anesthetized occurs. This is quite common in anterior maxillary injections as the solution diffuses to fifth cranial nerve sensory fibers and to seventh cranial nerve motor fibers, affecting

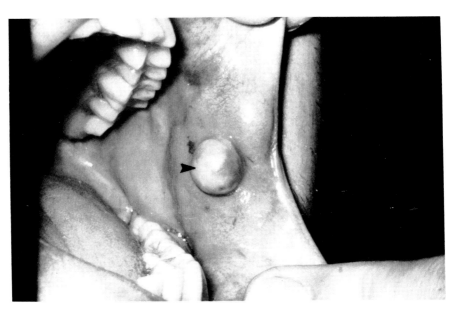

Figure 6.5. Blanching of soft tissue from vasoconstrictor in a local anesthetic, injected for surgical excision of inflammatory fibrous hyperplasia.

muscular function in the local area. Complete seventh nerve anesthesia may also result from deposition of the anesthetic solution into the parotid capsule during inferior alveolar injections. Once the anesthetic is in the parotid capsule it diffuses to the seventh nerve which courses through the gland. Symptoms are those of Bell's palsy and include ipsilateral loss of motor control of the buccinator muscle, inability to raise the corner of the mouth, and inability to voluntarily wink or close the eye (Fig. 6.6). If the needle tip is directed too deeply and posteriorly in carrying out an inferior alveolar block, it can enter the parotid capsule. This can be avoided by correct needle placement. Figure 6.7 illustrates how it can happen. If the full dose of the anesthetic is injected into the parotid gland, no mandibular anesthesia will occur. The paralysis of the facial nerve, of course, is temporary and will resolve as the agent is absorbed, redistributed, and metabolized. Specific therapy is necessary even though the problem is self-limiting. The affected eye *must* be protected from trauma, dust, and other flying debris since the lid will not close and the motor aspect of the lid reflex, conjunctival reflex, and corneal reflex is lost. The affected eye can be pro-

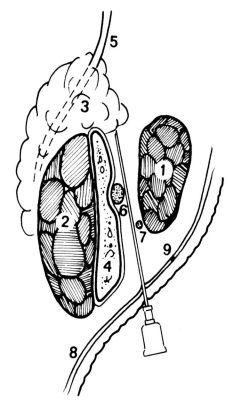

Figure 6.7.   Misdirected standard inferior alveolar nerve block into the parotid gland. *1*, internal pterygoid muscle; *2*, masseter muscle; *3*, parotid gland; *4*, ramus; *5*, facial nerve; *6*, inferior alveolar nerve; *7*, lingual nerve; *8*, buccinator muscle; *9*, pterygomandibular raphe.

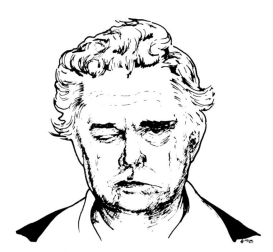

Figure 6.6.   *Left,* Seventh cranial nerve paraplysis from deep standard inferior alveolar nerve block attempt.

tected by manually closing the eye and taping it shut until motor function returns. Under no circumstances should the patient be allowed to leave the operatory without either motor function of the lid or mechanical protection for the eye. Anesthetic in the parotid capsule will not anesthetize the inferior alveolar nerve.

Other rare occurrences such as temporary blindness and loss of motor control of the eye may also occur. These are thought to be the result of retrograde blood flow from an intra-arterial injection allowing anesthetic to reach the internal maxillary artery. From this artery the agent is distributed across vascular anastomoses to the ophthalmic and lacrimal arteries, thus affecting the sixth cranial nerve and the orbital contents.

There is also a risk of ocular motor paralysis and optic nerve anesthesia if a needle is advanced far into the infraorbital foramen. The infraorbital fissure is sometimes a true canal with a thin roof and other times a fissure allowing easy needle penetration into the orbit and, in rare cases, even into the globe. This problem should never exist but it is easy to see that if the anesthetic solution is deposited in these locations, bizarre, temporary loss of function could occur.

Other major vessels and nerves are located throughout the vicinity of the course of the fifth cranial nerve and inadvertent needle placement could reach the vagus nerve, the carotid sheath, and the cervical sympathetic plexus. None of these are reached with normal needle insertion. All involve extremely deep and medial placement in attempting an inferior alveolar nerve block. Specific treatment of these is usually not necessary but the bizarre neurological symptoms are, at the least, startling.

SELF-INFLICTED INJURIES

Self-inflicted injuries result from trauma to an anesthetized tissue. The most common sites are lips, cheek, and tongue. Severe injury can be inflicted by chewing and biting on anesthetized soft tissue. The patient or the patient's guardian must be warned and advised to not allow this to happen. The most common problem is lip biting and occurs frequently in children and the mentally retarded. An example of the severity of this phenomenon can be seen in Figure 6.8. Another example of tongue biting is illustrated in Figure 6.9. The dentist is not legally liable for this type of complication *if* the individual or guardian is forewarned and advised.

Other major self-inflicted injuries include soft tissue burns from eating or drinking hot foods before return of normal sensation. The occurrence of these problems can be minimized by choosing an anesthetic solution of appropriate duration for the anticipated procedure. It is

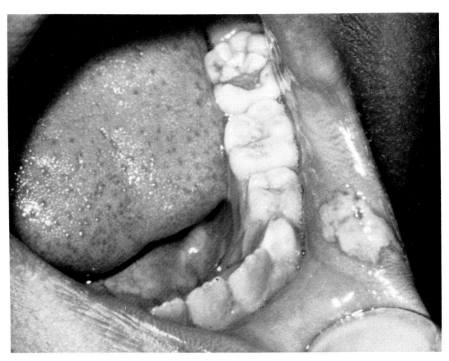

Figure 6.8.   Clinical result of self-inflicted injury from lip biting.

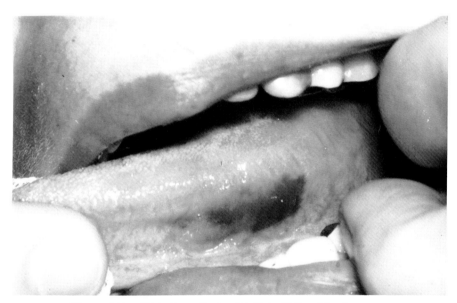

Figure 6.9. Clinical result of self-inflicted bite of the tongue.

inappropriate to produce mandibular soft tissue anesthesia of 3 to 4 hours' duration when the procedure requires only 15 minutes of operating anesthesia. The problem of self-inflicted injuries may become more common in the future because of the recent introduction of extended duration anesthetics. These agents provide not only long duration operating analgesia but also many hours of postoperative analgesia at surgical sites. For this reason extended duration anesthetics must be carefully used in children and the mentally retarded. Treatment of these injuries cannot be categorized as each must be handled as an individual traumatic soft tissue injury. Serious injuries may result, even to the extent of requiring primary closure. Most, however, require only an explanation of the occurrence.

GAGGING

Loss of sensation in the soft palate and pharyngeal area in some cases results in gagging. This occurs when an anterior palatine block also results in analgesia of the middle and lesser palatine nerves. When an anterior palatine block is given, the patient should be forewarned that loss of sensation in the soft palate causes an "odd" feeling which results from not being able to feel swallowing. This feels especially "odd" when a bilateral anterior palatine block is given. The patient should be reassured that they can swallow and there is no problem. If reassurance is not sufficient, a form of conscious sedation should be used to control this overt gagging.

PERIODONTAL LIGAMENT INJECTION COMPLICATIONS

All information to date indicates that the PDL injection is safe and without serious sequelae. The technique has not been widely used and must still stand up to the test of time. There has been one report of a tooth loosening 5 minutes after a PDL injection, and the patient removing it with finger pressure. One misadventure does not condemn a technique. The current literature should be monitored to confirm continued safety.

TRAUMATIC PREDISPOSITION OF SPECIFIC ULCERS

Recurrent intraoral herpes, recurrent herpes labiales, and recurrent aphthous ulcers are lesions which have trauma as a predisposing factor. The primary etiol-

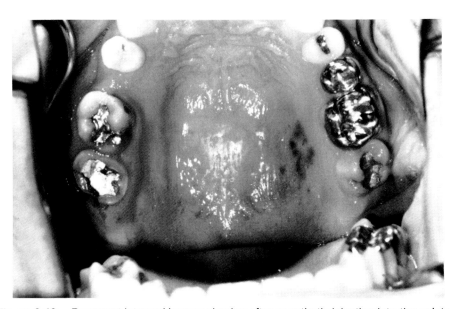

Figure 6.10.   Recurrent intraoral herpes simplex after anesthetic injection into the palate.

ogy of the diseases are latent herpes simplex infection for the first two and an autoimmune etiology for recurrent aphthous ulcers. Figure 6.10 illustrates recurrent intraoral herpes lesions on the palatal tissue in the vicinity of a recent palatal injection. This lesion will occur 2 to 3 days after the tissue trauma. Needle penetration is sufficient to induce such a lesion in susceptible individuals. Intraoral recurrent herpes must be differentiated from the singular toxicity ulcer (ischemic ulcer) in Figure 6.2. Both lesions heal in 10 to 14 days and do not require specific treatment.

Safe use of local anesthesia is assured by minimizing the dose and using exacting injection technique.

Bibliography

Aldrete JA, Johnson DA: Allergy to local anesthetics. *JAMA* 207:356–357, 1969.

Aldrete JA, Johnson DA: Evaluation of intracutaneous testing for investigation of allergy to local anesthetic agents. *Anesth Analg* 49:173–181, 1970.

Aldrete JA, Narang R, Sada T, et al: Reverse carotid blood flow—a possible explanation for some reactions to local anesthetics. *J Am Dent Assoc* 94(6):1142–1145, 1977.

Arora S, Aldrete JA: Investigation of possible allergy to local anesthetic drugs. *Anesthesiol Rev* 3:13–16, 1976.

Campbell RL, Gregg JM, Levin KJ, et al: Vasovagal response during oral surgery. *J Oral Surg* 34:690–700, 1976.

Campbell RL, Mercuri LG, Sickels JV: Cervical sympathetic block following intraoral local anesthesia. *Oral Surg* 47(3):223–226, 1979.

Cole JK: Ocular complication resulting from intraarterial injection during inferior alveolar nerve anesthesia. *Anesth Prog* 29(1):9–10, 1982.

Kramer SL, Milton VA: Complications of local anesthesia. *Dent Clin North Am* 17:443–460, 1973.

Malamed SF: *Handbook of Medical Emergencies in the Dental Office*, ed 2. C.V. Mosby, St. Louis, 1982.

Mitchell DF, Standish SM, Fast TB: *Oral Diagnosis/Oral Medicine*, ed 3. Philadelphia, Lea & Febiger, 1978.

Nelson PW: Injection system (letter to editor). *J Am Dent Assoc* 103(5):692, 1981.

Noble JR: The patient with syncope. *JAMA* 237:1372–1376, 1977.

Raymond LB: Angioneurotic edema with idiopathic pigmentation of the lip: a case report. *J Dent Child* 38:351–353, 1971.

Reidenberg MM, Lowenthal DT: Adverse nondrug reactions. *N Engl J Med* 279:678–679, 1968.

Management Problems of the Anesthetized and Sedated Patient

The use of monitors, the problems of airway management, evaluation of cardiovascular status and certain features of emergency care are directly applicable to the anesthetized and sedated patient. It is the duty of the dentist to ensure that no harm results from therapy, and for this reason the use of monitors assumes particular importance in patient care. Monitors give early warning of changes in physiological stauts.

MONITORING AND MONITORS

Continuous observations is the principal function of the doctor in charge of treatment. It involves use of all the senses—vision, hearing, touch, and smell—together with the application of judgment in determining which changes are significant. Other features such as the chart, stethoscope, blood pressure device and thermometer are all ancillary aids to judgment. Monitoring, albeit only observation, should always be indicated as being performed by the doctor during patient care. It is the principal reason that necessitates a doctor's presence during sedation and anesthesia. However, as the complexity of sedative practice, anesthesia, or surgery increases, the need for additional information increases. The information required to make adjustments is obtained more frequently if more major procedures are being performed. The more frequently the information is determined, the less the disturbances in physiology occur. Thus the simple monitor of patient observation devices used for local anesthesia, expands to monitoring of respiration by

the reservoir bag in inhalation analgesia, suggests the need of a respiratory monitor when intravenous sedation is being performed, and further progresses to the use of an intra-arterial monitor if hypotensive techniques are used for oral and maxillary facial surgery. The object is to achieve patient safety. The addition of equipment, especially electronic equipment, extends the central nervous system responses of the observer with the advantage of sensitivity, speed and recording. It is imperative that it work without neglecting the patient. Complex gadgetry may divert attention from danger signs that do not require measurement but only common-sense interpretation. Measurement is not an end in itself or a substitute for judgment, but rather an indispensable foundation for informed management of the patient. Of all the available devices, the chest stethoscope provides the most reliable ancillary aid for monitoring the patient.

Drugs induce changes in various tissues and organ systems by direct or indirect action. The changes induced are dependent on the pharmacological properties of the agents, methods of administration, their drug concentrations, biotransformation, and excretion. The various methods and parameters utilized to monitor patients are directed at detecting immediate direct or reflex changes. The information obtained will permit alteration of the agent as necessary to prevent or minimize any irreversible reaction which may be precipitated.

Acceptable practice dictates that all patients must be monitored when any drug is administered. The high incidence of cardiovascular disease alone, affecting 20 million people (13.2 per cent of the population) should alert us to the possible potential hazards associated with anesthesia and sedation. Thus, continuous monitoring of patients is mandatory to detect any abrupt change in the patient's status, in order to reduce the morbidity and mortality associated with sedation and anesthesia.

Monitoring of all patients, irrespective of the operative procedure, is only one adjuvant toward a rational and acceptable method of patient management. The accuracy and reliability of the data obtained from monitoring should facilitate early recognition and diagnosis of any change of the patient's physical status and eliminate all the available information to establish an accurate diagnosis prior to instituting treatment and be continually alert to observe the patient closely and make second to second adjustment and assessment of the patient's total condition.

Strict reliance on a single monitor measuring only one physiological parameter can be misleading and potentially hazardous. For example, in a clinical situation, the diagnosis of acute myocardial infarction by electrocardiographic alteration may be erroneous since these changes may be delayed 12 to 18 hours or may not even occur on the ECG; thus, enzyme studies, vital signs, and clinical assessment are also of paramount importance in establishing the diagnosis. No single sign or symptom or single monitor may be pathognomonic and diagnostic of a particular condition, for the total patient must be evaluated in respect to individual findings.

The ideal mechanical monitor should fulfill certain basic requirements of performance. It must be accurate in the measurement of the parameter monitored and, in addition, be able to reproduce the same performance in the same or other patients. It should have simplicity in design to obviate mechanical failure and to be applicable to all patients. Placement should be accomplished by auxiliary personnel and discomfort to the patient should be minimal. It should provide useful and meaningful information but yet not require great technical skill and knowledge for interpretation. It should not be prohibitive in cost, restricting its use and acceptance. It is obvious that to date no such ideal monitor exists.

Respiration

Observation of the respiratory movements provides an important assessment of one vital function. Verification of the fact that the patient is breathing spontaneously is of paramount importance both in anesthetized and in conscious patients. The loss of spontaneous respiration is an immediate signal of respiratory depression and if not corrected immediately will lead to severe tissue anoxia, circulatory arrest, and death. Of all the available devices for patient monitoring, the chest stethoscope provides the most reliable ancillary aid (Figs. 7.1 and 7.2).

RESPIRATORY RATE

Alteration of the respiratory rate and rhythm are usually "early" signs of physiological change in the patient. Tachypnea, an increase in the frequency of respiration, is frequently caused by apprehension and pain. During light anesthesia and early onset of hypotension an increase in respiratory rate is often observed. Thus, close monitoring of the respiratory rate is an excellent means for observing early changes. Tachypnea should be differentiated from hyperpnea, which is an increase in both the depth and rate of respiration. Tachypnea may reduce the tidal volume and, although increasing respiratory minute volume, may decrease the amount of alveolar ventilation. The alveolar ventilation is the amount of gas which participates in gaseous exchange in the pulmonary alveoli

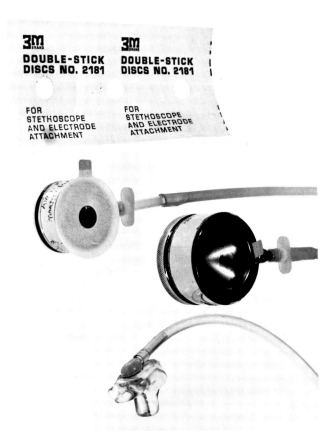

Figure 7.1.   The chest stethoscope can be simply placed using the 3M disc which is adhesive on both sides. The individually formed earpiece allows close, continuous monitoring of heart tones and respiration.

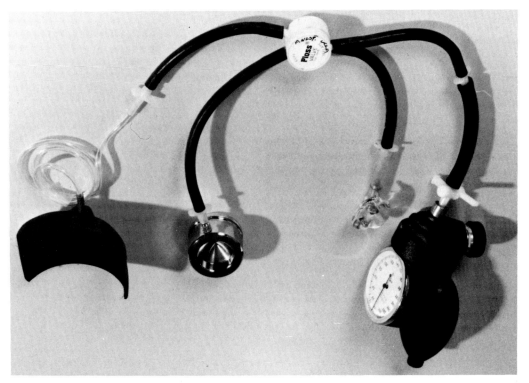

Figure 7.2. The Ploss valve allows automatic change from cardiac monitoring to measurement of blood pressure. It is activated by the pressure generated in the cuff.

and is a function of the respiratory rate and tidal volume less the dead space. Tachypnea may potentially reduce the volume of the alveolar ventilation with a decrease in available oxygen to tissue (hypoxemia).

Monitoring the respiratory rate is important since hyperventilation leads to hypocarbia, resulting in marked change in various organ systems. Hypocarbia induces cerebral vasoconstriction with a decrease in cerebral blood flow and possibly cerebral hypoxia. In addition, there is a reduction of the cardiac output with a decrease in arterial oxygenation.

RESPIRATORY RHYTHM

Principal factors affecting the rhythm of respiration are: 1) pain; 2) systemic conditions: electrolyte abnormalities, diabetic acidosis, central nervous system lesions, cardiovascular depression, myocardial infarction, hypotension; 3) level of anesthesia: premedication, induction, depth; 4) respiratory obstruction. The most frequent cause in alteration of respiratory rhythm is related to the depth of anesthesia.

The presence of respiratory obstruction or pain will alter respiratory rhythmicity as will certain systemic diseases and acute emergency situations. Cheyne-Stokes respiration is a manifestation of severe respiratory depression, which may indicate irreversible and late symptoms of respiratory depression of varied etiology.

RESPIRATORY OBSTRUCTION

Partial obstruction of the airway may occur without the usual stertorous sounds frequently associated with upper airway obstruction. An indirect yet very effective indicator of respiration is the central venous pressure. A catheter placed in the superior vena cava of right atrium will be affected by variations in the transpulmonary pressure. Thus, subtle changes in transpulmonary pressure which occur during respiratory obstruction will be no-

ticed immediately which would not be detected by observation of the patient. Apnea has been observed for short intervals of time during anesthetic induction with ultra-short acting barbiturates which are not clinically discernible yet can be demonstrated by continuous recording of the central venous pressure.

The clinical signs most frequently associated with upper airway obstruction are cyanosis, stertorous breathing, and tracheal or sternal retraction. Hypoxia and hypercarbia will result from airway obstruction with cyanosis as a late manifestation of partial or total respiratory obstruction.

PATIENT COLOR

Patient color is frequently used as a clinical sign of adequate oxygenation and perfusion of the peripheral tissue. Thus, abnormality affecting the arterial oxygen tension, decreased inspired oxygen concentration, decreased alveolar ventilation, insufficient hemoglobin, and the configuration of the oxyhemoglobin dissociation curve are but some factors which will reduce the amount of oxygen available to the skin tissue. In addition, adequate cardiac function is essential to maintain adequate perfusion. Thus, the rate of oxygen delivery and tissue utilization of oxygen will affect patient color. Skin color is also a subjective sign dependent on lighting, skin thickness, and the area viewed.

Cyanosis or blueness occurs as a result of hypoxemia with an abnormal increase in reduced hemoglobin as when 5 g of reduced hemoglobin per 100 ml blood are present. Because of the thinness and extensive vascularity of the oral mucosa and its accessibility during dental surgery, it is an ideal area for observing capillary blood behavior.

Observation of the patient's color is an easy and simple method of monitoring patients, although several pitfalls in diagnosis of arterial hypoxemia due to cyanosis should be mentioned. Pink lighting is suggested because cyanosis can go unrecognized or be attributed to the blueness of other shades of lighting. A minimum of 5 g of reduced Hb is necessary before cyanosis will occur; thus, with any reduction in the total red cell mass (hematocrit) whether by hemolysis, hemorrhage, or anemia, cyanosis may develop only when severe hypoxia is present. Alterations in hemoglobin, is sulf- or methemoglobin can be produced by sulfonamides or acetanilide.

Hypotension with severe to moderate peripheral vasoconstriction causes a marked reduction in capillary blood flow. The reduction in blood flow will increase the oxygen extracted; thus, a greater amount of reduced hemoglobin is present. Pallor may be more frequently associated with hypoxemia in the presence of hypotension and/or reduction in total red cell mass (hematocrit).

Variabilities in visual perception and experience of the observer are essential criteria when color is used as a method of monitoring. Comroe reports a study where subjects were given mixtures of high, normal, and low oxygen to breathe. The observers were to classify the subjects in three categories—pink, slight cyanosis, or definite cyanosis. In a group of patients breathing low concentrations of oxygen (arterial saturation 81 to 85 per cent), 49 per cent of the observers responded with a diagnosis of definite cyanosis, 37 per cent with slight cyanosis, and 14 per cent accurately classified the patient as "pink." Thus, strict adherence to available data and close observation of the patient are the essential criteria in assessing the significance of patient color.

OXYGENATION

The amount of oxygen in inspired gases can be determined with a Pauling oxygen meter, which uses the paramagnetic properties of oxygen for assessment of percentage. However, delivery of oxygen does not guarantee its uptake; thus assessment of arterial oxygen saturation or tension should be known.

The oxygen saturation of the arterial blood can be measured indirectly by the application of an oximeter to the vasodilated ear lobe. Vasodilatation is necessary so that capillary and arterial blood become approximated. It measures the ratio of reduced to oxygenated hemoglobin present by a photoelectric cell which absorbs light of differing wave lengths.

The partial pressure of oxygen in arterial blood can be measured by direct arterial sample and assessing the oxygen tension with an oxygen electrode. The electrode assesses electrical current in the blood which is linearly related to oxygen tension.

A recent development is the transcutaneous oxygen and carbon dioxide electrode which estimates the capillary tensions of these gases. In clinical practice it gives values that are below those obtained by direct measurement of arterial gas tensions, but the differences are constant. Response time for oxygen tension changes is rapid, and it provides a noninvasive monitor which, to date, has not caused the burns which have occasionally occurred with the ear oximeter.

Blood flow through the lung is not all arterialized since all the blood is not exposed to the inspired oxygen; this is known as a shunt. Anatomical shunt is always present and is that blood which flows through the bronchial, pleural, and Thebesian veins which is 2 per cent of the total cardiac output. Physiological shunt occurs when blood flows to collapsed areas of lung (atelectatic) or when blood flow/ventilation (Va/Q) imbalance exists. It is possible to evaluate the degree of shunt by knowing the alveolar and arterial oxygen tensions (see Table 1.3).

CARBON DIOXIDE

The carbon dioxide tension in blood can be measured directly or indirectly.

End-tidal air is representative of alveolar air and thus pulmonary capillary blood; end-tidal carbon dioxide tension is measured by absorption of infrared light which increases temperature and pressure in a chamber reflecting the partial pressure of carbon dioxide. The accuracy of the method can be improved by collecting a rebreathed gas sample which is more in equilibration with the alveolar air. If an arterial blood sample is obtained, the partial pressure can be determined with electrodes which measure either CO_2 tension or pH changes.

Cardiovascular

Next to direct visualization of the patient, monitoring of the cardiac cycle has been an effective and classic method of monitoring. The continuous auscultation of heart sounds serves as an index of cardiac dynamics. Cardiac rate, rhythmicity, and quality of the heart sounds are significant indicators of physical condition.

The *sine qua non* of monitoring is the "degree of change" from control or normal. It is imperative that baseline determination of the vital signs or physiological parameters to be monitored be determined at the time of consultation or preoperative examination and repeated prior to induction.

CARDIAC RATE

Alterations of the cardiac rate may occur during anesthesia. Bradycardia, a decrease in the cardiac rate below 60 beats per minute, or tachycardia, a rate greater than 100, may occur as a direct or reflex effect of the anesthetic agents. The prolonged duration of unrecognized bradycardia may lead to severe complications. The most frequent causes of bradycardia are: 1) anesthetic overdose: a) premedication, b) anesthetic induction, c) anesthetic maintenance; 2) reflex: a) pain, light anesthesia, b) hypertension, c) increased vagal tone, 3) direct cardiac depression.

Thus, continuous monitoring of the cardiac rate can provide valuable information regarding the status of the patient. The principal determinants of the myocardial oxygen consumption which best correlate with the degree of myocardial work or "strain on the heart" are determined by three factors: myocardial wall tension; level of myocardial contractility; and cardiac rate. Thus, continuous auscultation of the cardiac rate has important physiological significance. A useful index of cardiac oxygen consumption is the rate-pressure product, that is, the product of cardiac rate and systolic blood pressure. The normal peak range for adults is 7500 to 15,000. Increase of the rate beyond this range due to elevation of blood pressure or cardiac rate indicates excessive oxygen consumption. The use of this number has been developed in studies of cardiac anesthesia, where direct measurements of oxygen consumption have been readily obtained. It is a useful index of cardiac activity, that is, oxygen consumption.

Alteration in cardiac rhythm can be detected immediately during continuous monitoring. Cardiac arrhythmias occur frequently, even in normal man. Their identification and treatment (if necessary) are essential for the maintenance of normal cardiac dynamics. The first heart sound varies with the intensity of force of ventricular systole, and the loudness will vary with the magnitude of the diastolic pressure. The intensity of the second heart sound will vary with the height of the arterial pressure.

There are several advantages to cardiac auscultation. Principally, it is a continuous method where any abrupt alteration in rhythmicity, quality of heart sounds, and cardiac rate will be detected immediately. The use of the precordial and esophageal stethoscopes are the two most frequently used methods. The precordial stethoscope may present certain disadvantages. Markedly obese patients or patients with increased anterior posterior diameter of the thoracic cage (i.e., emphysema) have diminished heart sounds. Proper placement and securement of the stethoscope head to the chest, which may prove difficult in some patients, is of paramount importance. The esophageal type requires the patient to be asleep prior to insertion, a distinct disadvantage during the induction period of anesthesia.

BLOOD PRESSURE

Measurement of the blood pressure has been another of the classic methods of monitoring, yet the blood pressure does not indicate the adequacy of tissue perfusion. Various factors markedly influence the magnitude of the blood pressure: blood volume, myocardial function, cardiac output, peripheral vascular resistance, and the degree of atherosclerosis of the vascular system, among others. The blood pressure is the sum total of all these factors. Thus, marked alteration of the blood pressure may indicate alteration in these various physiological parameters with the possibility of impending danger. In addition, it is the main determinant of cerebral perfusion and is therefore a highly significant parameter which can be measured.

The systolic pressure is the highest pressure attained to overcome vascular resistance during ventricular systole. The diastolic pressure corresponds to the pressure at cardiac rest. The blood pressure may be measured by direct intra-arterial method or indirectly by the Riva-Rocca method. The direct method is the most accurate method for measuring the blood pressure. The necessity of intra-arterial catheterization renders this method impractical for use with every patient. Thus, the Riva-Rocca method is the most frequently used method. Comparison of the intra-arterial with the cuff method of blood pressure determination shows systolic and diastolic pressures correlate closely. The cuff method will show pressures lower than the intra-arterial determination; the discrepancy is attributed to cuff dynamics.

Certain sources of error may occur with the cuff method of blood pressure measurements. The diaphragm and blood pressure cuffs should not be so tight as to compress the brachial artery, as this will lead to a higher diastolic pressure reading secondary to venous stasis and a high systolic reading due to arterial wall compression. A diaphragm and cuff which are too loose will lead to lower systolic and diastolic readings.

The cuff diameters or length should cover at least two-thirds of the upper arm to give readings more closely related to true systolic and diastolic pressure. An excessively wide cuff will give higher readings; close attention must be given to cuff size in the pediatric patient as well as in the extremely thin or obese patient. Rapid deflation of the cuff is another common error in blood pressure measurement. Rate of deflation should approximate 10 mm Hg per second and will preclude error of the auscultatory gap which may occur with rapid deflation, when with reduction of the pulse pressure rapid cuff deflation leads to error. The Korotkoff sounds become inaudible with pressure reductions to 40 mm Hg or with severe vasospasm. In the poor risk patient or when extensive surgery is necessary, the intraarterial method may be indicated for continuous monitoring of the arterial blood pressure.

When patients are monitored by the use of blood pressure, a stable baseline should be obtained in which large fluctuations are avoided; this is most significant in the potential hypertensive patient. A blood pressure reduction from 170/110 mm Hg to 120/80 mm Hg will cause marked alteration in perfusion of vital areas and difficulties in prevention or treatment of severe hypotension with subsequent development of cerebral vascular neuropathies.

Although there is variability in the

blood pressure within the same individual and it is not a continuous method of monitoring, it remains an important and easy parameter to monitor.

Numerous electronic blood pressure measuring devices have been developed which will provide adequate evaluation of systolic and diastolic blood pressures throughout a dental procedure (Fig. 7.3). The availability of inexpensive equipment from catalog order films voids any excuse for not monitoring this parameter during patient care in dentistry.

PULSE AND PULSE MONITORING

Palpation of the peripheral vessels elicits information on cardiac cycle, cardiac rate, and cardiac rhythm. The quality or intensity of the pulse is a subjective finding. Continuous tactile monitoring of the peripheral pulse may be impractical; thus, various types of sensing devices are used to monitor the peripheral pulse. The plethysmograph type of monitors are of the volume pressure or optical density type. The photoelectric type of plethysmograph utilizes a crystal sensitive to various optical densities. The pulsatile nature of blood flow and the vascular tree creates differences in optical density. The difference can be detected by the optical crystal. The electronic energy developed may be represented graphically on paper or through the use of speaker and amplifier. The sound created is synchronized with cardiac rate.

The volume pressure type is used on the finger or peripheral limb. A narrow

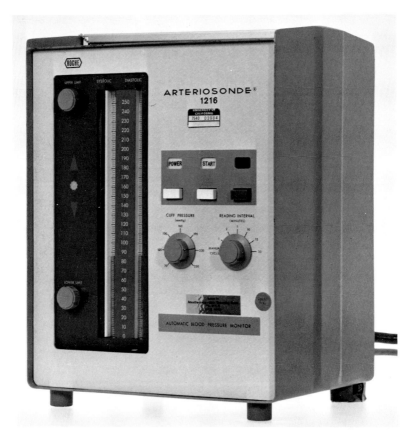

Figure 7.3. Systolic and diastolic blood pressure can be recorded automatically and displayed repeatedly up to 1-minute intervals by this type of apparatus. It is expensive, and adequate data can be provided by commercially available automatic devices, which range in price from $60 to $300.

column of mercury is placed on the finger or toe, dimensions of which will fluctuate in size corresponding to pulsation. Change in electrical resistance is measured, and energy may be transferred to activate either a visual or auditory modality.

The main disadvantages to plethysmography is the inherent complexity of the electric circuits. Improper placement and patient movement will give negative results, while in severe hypotension or intense vasoconstriction, the efficacy of pulse monitors is markedly reduced. They do not provide any information as to the intensity or quality of the pulse.

ELECTROCARDIOSCOPE AND ELECTROCARDIOGRAM

The electrocardiograph is not practical for continuous monitoring in the operating room. The electrocardioscope is an electrocardiographic monitoring device differing from ECG only in that there is no written record. The electrocardioscope is becoming a standard parameter in monitoring patients during anesthesia. It measures the electrical activity of depolarization and repolarization of the cardiac cycle, but it is unable to measure the integrity of myocardial contractility. The ECG may not show any abnormal tracing in the failing or compensated myocardium (Fig. 7.4).

The ECG will detect immediately conduction defects or alteration in rhythmicity. Identification of the abnormality may be done immediately. The ECG may detect myocardial ischemia by elevation in the S-T segment or T wave configuration. Its most important function is to differentiate the diagnosis of cardiac asystole from ventricular fibrillation, of paramount importance since the treatment of ventricular asystole and ventricular fibrillation is different. Thus an ECG unit should be available whenever anesthetic agents are to be used.

The standard leads are: lead I: right arm-left arm; lead II: right arm-left leg;

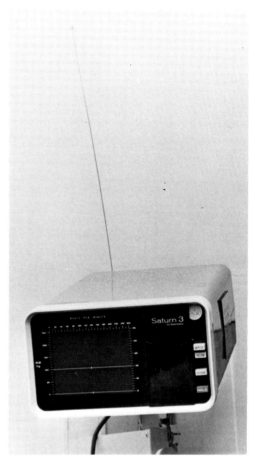

Figure 7.4. The electrocardioscope illustrated is activated by telemetry and obviates the need for connecting leads to the machine from the patient.

lead III: left arm-left leg. A wave complex is developed with the following characteristics: P wave: depolarization of auricle; P-R interval:transmission from S-A node to A-V node; QRS complex: depolarization of ventricle; S-T segment: excited state of ventricle; T wave: ventricular repolarization.

During routine monitoring, lead II is the most useful lead since the electrical axis measured will produce the best visualization and greatest deflection of the P wave. This facilitates the evaluation of conduction of the cardiac impulse from the S-A node to the terminal portion in the ventricle. Electrode paste is imperative with lead placement to reduce skin resistance and assure good patient contact for a diagnostic ECG trace.

Several manufacturers have electrocardioscopes available which are ideal monitors for anesthesia. They are small, compact, and portable and run at various speeds of 25, 50, 100 mm per second to examine configuration more closely. Some manufacturers have incorporated features to read the cardiac rate directly. During each cardiac cycle an auditory sound may be triggered and an alarm is immediately activated when no trace appears. Although the electrocardioscope does not fulfill all the requirements of an ideal monitor, it should always be available to differentiate the diagnosis of ventricular tachycardia and ventricular fibrillation or establish the diagnosis of cardiac asystole. A defibrillator is available, the paddles of which serve as electrodes for an ECG trace.

Central Nervous System

The integrity of the central nervous system is assured in local anesthesia and dental analgesia by continuous verbal contact with the patient. However, in general anesthesia only indirect observations can be made. The signs of general anesthesia reflect neuromuscular effort rather than central nervous system influences. Once consciousness is lost, then it is only possible to detect central nervous system depression in stage 4 of anesthesia, that is, when medullary depression occurs with respiratory and cardiovascular depression. The electroencephalogram is an attempt at central nervous system monitoring.

ELECTROENCEPHALOGRAPHY

The use of electroencephalography (EEG) is of limited usefulness for monitoring during clinical anesthesia, certainly in dental anesthesia. Changes in superior vena cava pressure exert greater influence on the EEG than does anesthetic depth, as do many other factors. Its use

has been relegated to indicate depth of anesthesia and the presence of life in open heart surgery or resuscitation.

NERVOUS CONDUCTION

Monitoring of this function is discussed in the section on muscle relaxants; a blockade monitor should always be available for use when muscle relaxants are used.

Temperature

Routine physical examination includes temperature recording. Hospital practice requires continuous monitoring of the temperature during operative procedures under general or regional anesthesia. Outpatient anesthesia does not preclude the necessity of monitoring of the temperature; a noninvasive technique with a skin probe is simple.

A 1-cm disc which adheres to the forehead and gives a changing readout of temperature is available. It is disposable and relatively inexpensive, but does not seem to be indicated for use in dental care.

Conclusion

No monitoring equipment can ever completely replace the human element necessary for effective monitoring. Monitoring equipment is only an adjuvant for obtaining additional data or information. It is the responsibility of the doctor to interpret and use the information in making the proper and necessary adjustment. No machine as yet is capable of making the appropriate and instantaneous adjustment necessary during anesthesia; thus, the ultimate efficiency of any monitor can only be as vigilant, as foolproof, as accurate, as the alertness and knowledge of the doctor.

EMERGENCY CARE

An emergency is a sudden or unexpected condition which, if unrecognized or inadequately treated, can cause significant morbidity or mortality.

Prevention is always easier than a cure. Therefore, since outpatient dental anesthesia or analgesia is always elective, it is incumbent upon the person or persons responsible for patient management to adequately screen all patients for pre-existing systemic disease preoperatively and select only healthy patients for outpatient procedures, particularly for anesthesia. Recognition of pre-existing conditions and careful monitoring will facilitate early diagnosis of impending complications and prompt institution of appropriate treatment.

All personnel involved in patient management should be adequately trained in resuscitation. Periodic attendance at and certification in cardiopulmonary resuscitation should be the expected standard of care. Office drills involving all personnel should be performed at frequent intervals to keep skills current. The office anesthesia evaluation periodically required of all members of the American Association of Oral and Maxillofacial Surgeons is an excellent example of self-regulation of performance standards in office practice and could be implemented throughout the dental profession.

A portable emergency cart containing all necessary resuscitation equipment and drugs should be immediately available where patients are treated. Printed cards should list indications and proper dosages of each drug to facilitate rapid and appropriate administration in emergency conditions. Drugs should be immediately replaced after each use and reviewed at frequent intervals to replace out-of-date preparations. Equipment should be checked at the start of the day to ensure proper function. A source of oxygen and suction should be available in each operatory and recovery area.

Planning for emergency care should include establishment of a relationship with a nearby physician qualified in resuscitation who will respond immediately to a call for assistance. The office emergency plan should include listing of telephone numbers for the physician, ambulance, and nearest hospital emergency room so that the appropriate telephone calls can be made without delay if assistance is needed in the office or the patient requires transportation to the hospital for definitive therapy.

The Certificate in Basic Life Support in Cardiopulmonary Resuscitation provided by the American Heart Association is a requirement for many state licensures; in addition, many dentists have also become certified in advanced life support. The various courses approved by the American Heart Association provide all the necessary information for the practitioner.

Circulatory Arrest

The final common pathway of hypoxia and hypercarbia, if not corrected, is cessation of effective heart action, or circulatory arrest. This is a critical emergency demanding immediate expert attention, as failure to perfuse the brain with oxygenated blood causes irreversible neurological damage within 4 minutes or less. Early diagnosis and effective cardiopulmonary resuscitation provide adequate perfusion of oxygenated blood to other vital organs as well, such as heart, liver, and kidneys, and determines the degree of tissue necrosis or reversibility. In fact, when hypoxia has preceded circulatory arrest, irreversible neurological damage occurs earlier than 4 minutes.

Circulatory arrest is usually not a sudden phenomenon, but rather it is often preceded by cardiac arrhythmias, hypotension, respiratory obstruction, or cessation of breathing. Careful monitoring frequently demonstrates the prodromal situation in time to correct the underlying etiology and prevent significant morbidity or death.

Various studies have documented the incidence of circulatory arrest in the medical/surgical hospitalized patient under general anesthesia as between 1:2340 and 1:3000. The incidence is greater among pediatric and geriatric patients and in patients with pre-existing systemic disease. In 1972 a survey by the American Society of Oral Surgeons reported only 11 fatalities among 5,250,000 outpatient anesthetics administered by qualified oral surgeons. Selection of healthy patients for dental procedures is undoubtedly a contributing factor to the lower mortality rate in comparison to hospitalized patients. However, there is also the difficulty of gathering accurate data on office practice where all cases of mortality may not have been reported.

Circulatory arrest is a general term for failure to perfuse vital organs with oxygenated blood. The basic conditions in which this can occur are cardiac asystole, ventricular fibrillation, and electromechanical dissociation. Regardless of which of these events has occurred, prompt recognition of circulatory arrest and immediate institution of resuscitation efforts are mandatory.

DIAGNOSIS

Prodromal signs usually appear before circulatory arrest and indicate hypoxia and/or cardiac failure. In the awake patient cerebral hypoxia causes restlessness, anxiety, and disorientation. Respiratory signs and symptoms include dyspnea, tachypnea, gasping, laryngeal stridor, pallor, and cyanosis. Cardiovascular signs are venous distention, irregular pulse, hypotension, and profuse diaphoresis. Appropriate action at this time may avert circulatory arrest.

When circulatory arrest has occurred the carotid and femoral pulses are absent; the radial pulse is not a dependable guideline. Blood pressure is unobtainable. The heart sounds are not audible by auscultation. There may be gasping respirations or complete cessation of respiratory effort. Pupillary dilatation occurs within 1 to 2 minutes of arrest and indicates brain anoxia. There is absence of bleeding and dark colored blood in the surgical field. The patient becomes flaccid. There may be convulsions. If a cardiac monitor is present it may show cardiac asystole or ventricular fibrillation. On the other hand, electromechanical dissociation may be associated with a relatively normal tracing. Once the diagnosis of circulatory arrest is suspected, basic life support must be initiated immediately. The earlier resuscitation is begun, the better the patient's chance for survival.

PERSONNEL

Basic to successful resuscitation of the patient who has sustained circulatory arrest is a well-trained staff who undergo frequent periodic emergency drills to keep their skills current. An organized effort in which each member of the team knows his job is the result of careful planning and training.

The American Heart Association, the American Red Cross, and other organizations offer comprehensive courses in cardiopulmonary resuscitation (CPR).

In the office or clinic, organization of the resuscitation team is the responsibility of the doctor in charge. Although CPR can be carried out by one person, at least for a short time, the availability of three trained persons is highly desirable. The ideal team for resuscitation in the office probably includes five members. One person ventilates the patient, one person performs external cardiac massage, one person administers drugs, one person acts as an in-the-room circulator and keeps a written record of time of arrest, treatment, and drugs given, and one person is available to call for assistance according to a prearranged plan.

EQUIPMENT AND DRUGS

Oxygen and the means for delivery should be available in all patient care areas. A resuscitation bag (Fig. 7.5) or a positive pressure resuscitator should be available which will allow positive pressure ventilation and also deliver oxygen when the patient is breathing spontaneously. There are reports that a patient has been successfully resuscitated and ventilated utilizing the nasal mask of an

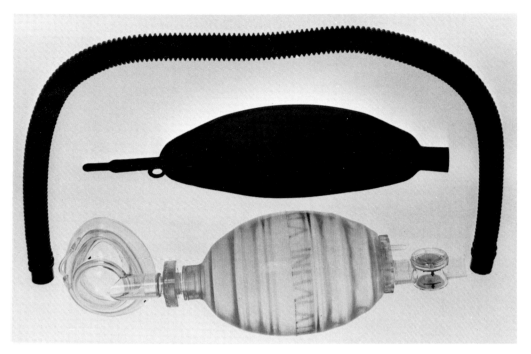

Figure 7.5.   If a resuscitation bag is used, then to achieve good oxygen levels in the inspired gases, a tail must be placed on the bag.

analgesia machine. It requires more skill than is usually possessed by the general dentist.

A complex drug inventory may result in inappropriate treatment. It is better to have a few well-understood medications available and accessible. A series of pre-loaded syringes may be of value, particularly if color-coded and of different shapes. They should be covered with cellophane to allow checking and an expiratory date of all medications noted. A suggested basic list and suggested adult dosage follows:

Epinephrine 1:1,000	0.5 mg/ml	0.2 ml
Epinephrine 1:10,000	0.5 mg/ml	1 ml
Isoproterenol inhaler (Isuprel)		
Atropine 0.4 mg/ml		1 ml
Diphenhydramine (Benadryl)	50 mg/ml	1 ml
Diazepam (Valium) 5 mg/ml		1 ml
Hydrocortisone (Solucortef) Mix-O-Vial	100 mg	1 ml
Nitroglycerine tablet	0.32 mg	1 tab
Naloxone (Narcan)	0.4 mg/ml	0.5 ml
Ephedrine 50 mg/ml		0.5 ml
Lidocaine 50 mg/ml		50 mg
Mephentermine (Wyamine)	30 mg/ml	1 ml

Esophageal Airway

This (Fig. 7.6) is frequently used by paramedical personnel and will allow adequate ventilation if the operator is unable to achieve adequate ventilation with a resuscitator or bag and mask. It can be used for prolonged periods, and studies show oxygen levels to parallel those obtained with an endoctracheal tube. There are some hazards in that perforation of pharyngeal and laryngeal tissues can occur, but these are a small penalty to pay for adequate resuscitation with prevention of regurgitation.

Death in the Dental Office

Loss of a patient's life during treatment in the dental office is an unexpected and catastrophic event for all concerned. Grief of the patient's immediate family may lead to unpleasant or irrational behavior in the presence of others. Dismay of office personnel may lead to errors in handling a delicate matter. Such eventualities, although difficult to contemplate, should always be planned for. Selection of

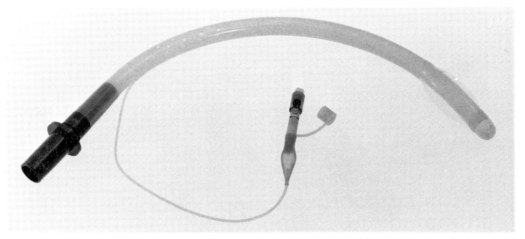

Figure 7.6. The esophageal airway illustrated is an extremely useful device for ventilation of the apneic patient and is advocated for use by those unskilled in intubation. The cuff is inflated in the esophagus, which prevents regurgitation and on blowing down the tube, air is forced into the oropharynx, inflating the patient.

healthy patients for office procedures, adherence to accepted techniques, use of safe and workable equipment, and the presence of a well-trained staff do much to prevent significant morbidity or mortality.

In the event that a death occurs in the dental office the following procedures are suggested to make the situation easier on all concerned. Have the receptionist excuse all other patients from the waiting room, explaining that an emergency has occurred requiring immediate attention by the doctor. No further details should be given. Inform the relatives what has happened in the privacy of your office. Tell them that the patient collapsed, everything possible was done, but that resuscitation was unsuccessful. Express grief and sympathy, but do not admit liability or errors in judgment. If no family members are in the office, contact the closest relative, state that a serious emergency has occurred, everything possible is being done, and request that they come promptly. Try to avoid stating over the telephone that the patient is dead. Notify the coroner and your insurance carrier immediately. Prepare a complete and accurate record of the event, its treatment,

and the probable cause of death. Make no other statements without legal representation.

Ventilation

It is the function of anesthesia and analgesia to provide pain relief with minimal physiological impairment. To achieve this requires satisfactory ventilation, that is, adequate oxygenation and elimination of carbon dioxide. It is fundamental to all sedation and anesthesia practice. Probably the majority of problems that arise during sedation are respiratory.

Conditions which interfere with adequate ventilation of the patient produce a decrease in blood oxygenation (hypoxia) and accumulation of carbon dioxide (hypercarbia). Complete lack of tissue oxygenation, anoxia, can produce irreversible brain death within $3\frac{1}{2}$ minutes or sooner. Hypoxia and hypercarbia both produce myocardial irritability and increase the likelihood of serious cardiac arrhythmias, predecessors to ventricular fibrillation or cardiac standstill.

Adequate perfusion of the tissues with well-oxygenated blood is essential for the maintenance of normal metabolic functions. When tissue cells are forced to function under hypoxic conditions, cellular metabolism is abnormally altered. A shift from aerobic to anaerobic glycolysis causes increase in lactic acid production. This tissue acidosis reduces cellular efficiency, particularly in areas readily susceptible to hypoxia, such as the myocardium and brain.

The partial pressure of carbon dioxide in arterial blood is the principal factor controlling spontaneous respiration in normal subjects. Carbon dioxide appears to affect respiration by a central action on the medullary centers, as denervation of the aortic and carotid chemoreceptors has little effect on the ventilatory response to changes in blood carbon dioxide tension. Small increases in the partial pressure of carbon dioxide in arterial blood have a stimulating effect on the medulla, causing increase in rate and depth of respiration (hyperpnea). Larger increases, however, depress the medullary respiratory center. Decrease in arterial blood oxygen tension elicits reflexes mediated by the aortic and carotid chemoreceptors which stimulate respiration. However, such hypoxic stimulation does not occur until the arterial oxygen tension falls to 30 mm Hg, a dangerously low level. Since the combination of hypoxia and hypercarbia exerts serious depression on respiration, establishing a vicious cycle of ventilatory deterioration, prompt recognition and treatment of ventilation problems are of prime importance.

HYPOXIA

The term hypoxia refers to oxygen lack from any source. The signs and symptoms of hypoxia depend on the severity and rate of onset. In the conscious patient there may be loss of consciousness or a more gradual dulling of intellect. The subject is usually unaware of the change as judgment is impaired. A primary sign is tachycardia with a slight rise in blood pressure. Tachypnea tends at first to be shallow and periodic. Sweating and cyanosis develop concomitantly.

Anoxia refers to complete lack of oxygen but is often used synonymously with hypoxia.

The margin of safety in the healthy individual is slight because of the characteristics of the oxygen-hemoglobin dissociation curve. With an inspired oxygen level of 8 per cent the patient may be all right; between 6 and 7 per cent the status is variable; and at 5 per cent death ensues. The changes noted may be irrevocable. Brain damage at autopsy may be minimal, as it requires survival for at least 3 days following a hypoxic episode for detectable microscopic damage to develop, and this accounts for the many negative autopsies following anesthetic accidents.

The causes of hypoxia during analgesia and anesthesia are: 1) inadequate concentration of oxygen; 2) mechanical problems in the machine, such as a) flow meter defect or b) empty oxygen cylinders; 3) ventilation defects due to inadequate ventilation, respiratory obstruction or abnormal ventilation/perfusion ratios; 4) depressed cardiac function; 5) overdose of drugs; and 6) effects of surgery.

EXCESS OXYGEN

No problem is presented with the administration of 100 per cent oxygen in anesthesia and analgesia. It can, however, if administered for prolonged periods, lead to pulmonary problems. In man, when oxygen is inhaled for periods of more than 24 hours, there is carinal irritation which produces substernal distress and cough. It can lead to pulmonary congestion, pulmonary edema, and tracheobronchitis. Paresthesia can occur in the extremities, together with muscular pains. Some of the changes of oxygen toxicity are related to CO_2 retention. If oxygen is given at 3 atm pressure, then enough is dissolved in the plasma to provide the oxygen requirement of the tissue. As CO_2 removal is dependent upon reduced hemoglobin, none is available for its rapid removal from the tissues. CO_2 is retained within the tissue, and convulsions occur owing to retention of the CO_2. Excess oxygen does not depress respiration because the carbon dioxide level is unaltered. Oxygen lack plays a part in the control of respiration only when severe and PaO_2 has fallen to 30 mm Hg.

The cardiovascular effects of breathing 100 per cent oxygen include a reduction in heart rate and cardiac output and increased peripheral resistance and systemic blood pressure; 100 per cent oxygen indeed acts as a vasopressor.

The patient with severe chronic obstructive pulmonary disease (COPD) presents problems for dental treatment. A high inspired oxygen concentration (FIO_2) given in conjunction with a depressant drug such as a narcotic or barbiturate could produce apnea, as CO_2 narcosis can develop. In the normal patient, respiratory drive is predominantly due to carbon dioxide and oxygen is not a factor in respiratory stimulation. However, for a patient with COPD, hypoxemic drive is of significance, and elevation of the oxygen tension may eliminate this hypoxic drive. Thus, although oxygen tension is adequate, carbon dioxide can rise to levels which will produce narcosis and apnea. Pulmonary function tests and hospitalization are necessary for such patients prior to sedation or general anesthesia. In such patients consciousness must first be affected and the respiratory center depressed by other agents before these conditions can arise. The administration of nitrous oxide-oxygen sedation alone will not produce apnea in such patients.

CARBON DIOXIDE

Carbon dioxide is the waste product of tissue metabolism. Normal ventilation maintains the arterial carbon dioxide tension within narrow limits. The balance between production and elimination is affected by anesthesia and analgesia. Elevation of the normal arterial carbon dioxide level is a normal concomitant of the agents used for anesthesia and analgesia. Anesthetic and analgesic agents depress the respiratory center and consequently elevate the respiratory threshold to carbon dioxide levels; therefore, higher levels of carbon dioxide are required to drive ventilation. Equipment can readily increase the tendency to elevations of $PaCO_2$ because of increases in equipment dead space.

Respiration is one of the principal methods of short term maintenance of pH. Acid-base balance over the long term, in excess of 24 hours, can be achieved by renal excretions of ions or cations. The maintenance of pH within limits of 7 to 7.70 is that compatible with life.

Carbon Dioxide Excess

The factors in production of CO_2 excess are respiratory depression, anesthetics, and narcotics; respiratory obstruction; faulty equipment, stuck valves, and increased resistance; inadequate carbon dioxide absorption; and severe bilateral lung disease.

Mild hypercapnia, PCO_2 50 mm Hg, is a frequent concomitant of anesthesia with spontaneous respiration, and it may be unrecognized. Severe degrees of hypercapnia are associated with progressive narcosis and coma; it may indeed resemble curarization with tracheal tug, and eventual respiratory failure. The clinical effects of hypercapnia are increased cerebral blood flow and rise of cerebral spinal fluid pressure, which leads to postoperative headache; a rise in circulating catecholamines, with the development of potential cardiac arrhythmias and sweating; tachycardia and rise in blood pressure. Although there is a central vasomotor effect of vasoconstriction, the peripheral action of CO_2 produces vasodilatation which will result in increased bleeding, and increased rate and depth of respiration.

These changes, if not corrected, will

lead to eventual cardiovascular collapse and respiratory arrest. An additional problem arises with hypercarbia in that changes in pH affect the desired concentrations of the active fractions of drugs and relaxants. Occasionally, sudden lowering of a chronic elevated CO_2 tension can result in severe hypotension and arrhythmias.

Carbon Dioxide Lack

Hypocarbia is due to voluntary hyperventilation, which occurs with anxiety or artificial ventilation under anesthesia. It is probably the commonest cause of fainting in the dental chair.

The effects of carbon dioxide lack are reduction of cerebral blood flow and cerebral oxygen tension with subsequent clouding of consciousness and analgesia. Hypocarbia protects against cardiac arrhythmias, and falls in blood pressure develop if positive pressure ventilation raises mean intrathoracic pressure.

Tetany is seen only with spontaneous hyperventilation of prolonged nature.

An advantage of hyperventilation under general anesthesia is that the amount of anesthetic required can be reduced. It is possible to perform major operations with nitrous oxide-oxygen and curare only, provided that adequate hyperventilation is maintained throughout the operation. The advantages in this reduction of anesthesia probably outweigh the disadvantages of decreased cerebral circulation and cerebral oxygenation. In the dental patient who is in good health, this type of anesthesia is satisfactory and can be considered a safe and satisfactory practice, reducing the amount of anesthetic required for the procedure.

Airway Management

Airway problems account for the majority of incidents that occur in sedative and anesthetic practice. Care of the airway in all patients is a priority often relegated to an unlicensed person.

PREOPERATIVE

Many aspects of the medical history (allergies, asthma, tracheal abnormalities) will predict many problems and a review of previous records or consultation with the patient's previous anesthetist is indicated. Clinical features to note at the preoperative physical examination include nasal configuration, presence of defective, loose teeth or heavy calculus, and general shape of the mandible.

SITES OF OBSTRUCTION

Obstruction can occur anywhere in the airway. Upper airway obstruction often can be corrected simply by correct positioning of the mandible, tongue, or oral packing. Lower airway obstruction may require special expertise, equipment, or procedures for successful management.

Mouth

Complete closure of the mouth occurs with the edentulous patient, and the normal anatomical configuration of the jaw is lost. An oral airway cut short may be helpful. It is not wise to attempt to overcome the problem of the edentulous mouth in the early phases of anesthetic induction with a full-sized oropharyngeal airway. Extension of this airway into the pharynx of the patient who is not fully anesthetized may cause coughing, struggling, or laryngospasm. Sometimes the airway problem in an edentulous patient is best overcome by leaving both dentures, if available, in the patient's mouth until induction is complete.

Removable partial dentures can become dislodged and obstruct the airway. Therefore, partial dentures should always be removed prior to induction of anesthesia.

Tongue

When the musculature of the tongue loses tone it will fall back against the posterior wall of the pharynx. The tongue is the principal cause of upper airway obstruction. The tongue problem can be overcome by exerting pressure against the angle of the mandible to bring it forward.

Nose

The majority of patients have one nostril through which they breathe better than the other. This should be ascertained in the preoperative evaluation. At least one patent nasal passage is essential for inhalation to prevent mouth-breathing and air dilution of inspired gases.

Larynx

In laryngospasm, coughing, or swallowing there is glottic closure as the intrinsic muscles of the larynx adduct the vocal cords (Fig. 7.7). Closure of the false cords by action of the aryepiglottic muscles occurs, the larynx ascends, reducing the distance between the thyroid cartilage and hyoid bone, and the epiglottis rotates posteriorly to cover the entrance to the larynx.

Tracheobronchial

Lower airway obstruction presents greater problems to the anesthetist as the area is not directly visible nor amenable to simple external manipulations. Tracheal narrowing (tracheomalacia) from

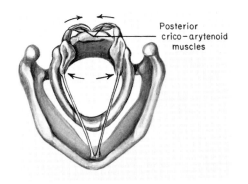

Figure 7.7. The only muscle of the larynx which abducts the vocal cords is the posterior cricoarytenoid.

Posterior crico-arytenoid muscles

the effects of long term endotracheal intubation or tracheostomy, direct tracheal injuries, or a congenital web should be ascertained at the preoperative evaluation. The trachea or mainstem bronchi may be partially obstructed by adjacent masses such as tumor or enlarged lymph nodes. Hoarseness of the voice secondary to tumor invasion of the recurrent laryngeal nerve may alert the anesthetist to such a problem. The degree of airway obstruction generally becomes much worse under sedation or anesthesia, and such patients are poor risks for office anesthesia. The trachea and large bronchi may be obstructed by foreign material from the operative site in the oral cavity (blood, tooth fragments) or by regurgitated and aspirated liquid or solid stomach contents. An adequate oropharyngeal pack and an appropriate period of preanesthetic fasting are standard preventive measures. Narrowing of the smaller bronchial airways may occur during an acute asthmatic attack, after aspiration of liquid vomitus or during an anaphylactic reaction.

MANAGEMENT OF RESPIRATORY OBSTRUCTION

The upper airway is readily observable and easily accessible to manipulations. Therefore, diligent attention to the upper airway is paramount in preventing or promptly correcting any obstruction. Upper airway obstruction is essentially recognized by noisy respirations, retraction of suprasternal neck muscles, and cyanosis. Four common causes of upper respiratory obstruction to consider are improper patient position, inadequate support of the upper airway, mechanical factors, and anatomical considerations (Figs. 7.8 and 7.9).

Improper Patient Position

The majority of dental procedures are done in a sitting or semi-reclining position. Proper positioning of the patient is

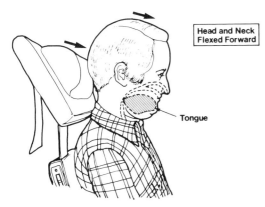

Figure 7.8. When the head is flexed, the soft tissues, particularly the tongue, close the airway.

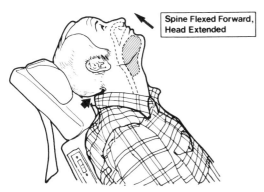

Figure 7.9. If the neck is flexed at the cervical spine and extended at the occiput, the soft tissues open and a good airway can be established.

the first essential in assuring a patent airway during anesthesia.

The contour type of dental chair with adjustable backrest and headrest is recommended. The backrest is placed in an upright position 90° to the contour seat. The patient is instructed to sit erect in the chair, and the level of the backrest is fitted to be directly below the superior border of the scapula. The midportion of the headrest should be in the area of the occipital protuberance and superior nuchal line. The head should be positioned slightly anterior by flexion of the neck so that when the mouth prop is inserted, the mandibular symphysis almost touches the sternum. The head is then extended by bilateral anteriorly applied force at the angles of the mandible. Extension of the

cervical spine causes the tongue and epiglottis to fall backward and places undue strain on cervical muscles.

Adequate stabilization of the patient must be maintained even when an endotracheal tube is in place. During manipulation or instrumentation for dental or oral procedures counter-force is necessary to immobilize the head and jaw, prevent trauma to the temporomandibular joint or cervical spine, and avoid movement or displacement of the endotracheal tube.

MANAGEMENT DURING ANESTHESIA

Head Position

The head should be placed so that there is flexion at the cervical spine and extension at the occiput, as though "sniffing the morning air." This is done by placing a small pillow under the head or pushing the headrest of the dental chair forward. This position provides maximal opening of the airway. Hyperextension of the head without flexion of the cervical vertebrae reduces the airway by diminishing the diameter of the oropharynx. Excessive rotation of the head to one side or the other should be avoided as circulation to the brain or cervical spinal cord may be significantly decreased in some patients.

Jaw Position

The tongue is controlled by positional changes of the mandible. Maximum forward position of the tongue and opening of the airway is achieved by bringing the mandible forward. This is done by exerting forward pressure against the angle of the mandible and forward and upward pressure beneath the chin.

Proper head and jaw position are the most important techniques in maintenance of the airway.

Support of the Upper Airway

With the onset of surgical anesthesia or deep sedation muscular relaxation occurs, and the tongue falls backward against the posterior pharyngeal wall, causing upper airway obstruction. Control of the airway must commence promptly at this time. Support of the mandible must be continued throughout and it can be fatiguing even during a short procedure of 5 to 10 minutes' duration. To open an airway obstructed by the tongue, lifting of the bony chin is superior to neck lift or jaw thrust. The flexed fingers of one hand are placed beneath the mandibular symphysis in the submental region and anterosuperior traction is steadily applied. The opposite hand may be used to bring the mandibular angle forward or stabilize the mandible and head for operative manipulations. Forearms of the anesthetist are rested on the patient's shoulders to lessen fatigue. Pressure should never be applied to the neck in the proximity of the bifurcation of the common carotid artery. Unilateral or bilateral carotid compression with direct or reflex decrease in cerebral blood flow could be disastrous.

Mechanical Factors

An oropharyngeal pack during surgical procedures or a rubber dam during restorative procedures should always be placed before beginning instrumentation in any patient whose protective pharyngeal and laryngeal reflexes are obtunded. Blood, mucus, and other foreign material is then excluded from the oropharynx, and aspiration into the tracheobronchial tree is avoided. Oropharyngeal packs should not be allowed to slip posteriorly into the airway. Long, heavy suture or cord should be attached to packs to facilitate their easy removal. Loose placement of the pack may allow mouth-breathing and air dilution of inhalation agents.

Endotracheal and nasopharyngeal tubes should be moderately flexible. Some tubes are susceptible to kinking, increasing air flow resistance and the work of respiration, or causing complete obstruction. Blood, mucus, or lymphoid tissue can partially or totally obstruct the tip or lumen of a tube.

For induction of inhalation analgesia and anesthesia or for oxygen administration it is essential that the mask fit well to prevent dilution of the administered gases with room air. If the patient breathes room air, induction time will be prolonged. Prolonged induction increases the risk of vomiting.

Presence of a nasal mask is not stimulating to the patient, so lighter anesthesia is required than for placement of a nasopharyngeal tube. A broad nose may not allow adequate placement or seal of the mask. Access to operative procedures in the anterior maxilla may be compromised by the presence of the nasal mask on the upper lip.

Excess mucus production by the struggling patient may cause laryngeal stridor or spasm during the second stage of anesthesia. Selection of a type of mask is a matter of personal preference as long as the requirement for a tight fit is met. A leak as small as a 15-gauge needle may allow air dilution of up to 60 per cent. The fit of the mask is more a function of manual skill than the manufacturer's design.

An oral airway keeps the tongue forward and assists airway maintenance during anesthesia. They are available in various sizes (pediatric to adult) and extend from the lips to the posterior pharynx. In this position the airway will hold the tongue forward, preventing contact with the posterior pharyngeal wall and occlusion of the airway. Airways are made of plastic, rubber, and metal; the metal airway can be a traumatic instrument if not inserted with extreme care and is best avoided. The airway should be well lubricated, and care should be taken not to damage the teeth. The oropharyngeal airway does not guarantee a patent airway. Proper head and jaw position must be maintained. If the oropharyngeal airway is not inserted properly, it can displace the tongue posteriorly and occlude the airway. If an airway is inserted when the anesthesia is too light, contact of the airway with the epiglottis or pharynx can initiate the gag reflex, vomiting, or laryngospasm.

There is a variety of nasopharyngeal tubes; however, the soft plastic or soft rubber tube is preferred because it does not traumatize the nasopharynx during its passage. The average length for a nasopharyngeal tube for a given patient is the distance from the ala of the nose to the tragus of the ear. If there is no flange on the tube, or if it is not used with a connector, a safety pin should be placed through it to prevent its inhalation. Although passage of a nasopharyngeal tube is stimulating to the patient, lighter anesthesia is required for tube passage than for placement of an oropharyngeal airway. The bevel on the nasopharyngeal tube is cut for insertion into the right nostril; if it is inserted into the left nostril, the position of the tube should be checked to ensure that the end of the tube is not occluded against the tonsil or pharyngeal wall. The largest possible nasopharyngeal tube should be passed to allow laminar flow of gases; the opposite nostril should be occluded to prevent air dilution during inspiration. Binasal pharyngeal tubes are also available; the two small tubes provide an adequate diameter for air flow and reduce the likelihood of nasal trauma. An advantage of the nasopharyngeal tube in dental anesthesia is that the oral pack can be placed snugly against the tube to reduce mouth-breathing, limit air dilution of the anesthetic gases, and prevent laryngeal contamination. Disadvantages include deeper anesthesia required for their passage than for the nasal mask, production of cardiac arrhythmias during passage, and possible trauma to nasal or pharyngeal tissues.

Anatomical Considerations

The obese patient and the patient with a short, thick neck ("bullneck") are poor candidates for ambulatory anesthesia and care must be exercised with intravenous sedation. Endotracheal intubation is often indicated. In nonintubated patients control of the airway is difficult or impossible, and the level of anesthesia is often erratic. Injection of an induction dose of intravenous barbiturate into such a patient may cause immediate total airway obstruction, a frightening experience for attending personnel. Even in the intubated grossly obese patient the excessive weight of adipose tissue on the thorax and abdomen has a depressing effect on the depth of respiration, allowing hypercarbia and hypoxia to occur if continual support of ventilation is not given.

The patient with a severely retruded mandible is at great risk for airway obstruction during anesthesia. It is difficult to adequately elevate the mandible forward to open the airway. The anterior position of the larynx in such patients makes direct laryngoscopy for placement of an endotracheal tube a difficult task requiring skill and experience.

Limited mouth opening or cervical spine immobility secondary to infection, trauma, congenital, or arthritic conditions poses special problems. Large infectious swellings around the mandible and neck can produce rapid obstruction of the airway during anesthetic induction. Anesthesia should not be started in such patients unless access to the airway is guaranteed beforehand, usually by awake nasoendotracheal intubation or tracheotomy.

Massive salivary gland enlargement has been reported during induction of general anesthesia. If it occurs, bilaterally, severe respiratory embarrassment develops, similar to airway obstruction seen in Ludwig's angina. Etiology may be excessive coughing and straining with increased saliva production and obstruction of salivary outflow.

Extreme hyperextension or rotation of the cervical spine during attempts at airway control must be avoided. Strain of cervical musculature or cervical spine or spinal cord injury can occur. Prolonged extreme hyperextension of the cervical spine during total muscular paralysis for repeated attempts at endotracheal intubation has caused spinal cord infarction. Excessive rotation of the cervical spine compromises cerebral circulation in some patients.

Decrease in thoracic wall or lung compliance interferes with adequate ventilation because the chest and lungs cannot expand fully. The patient with kyphoscoliosis often has a fixed thoracic cage, while the patient with pulmonary fibrosis cannot fully expand his lungs because of loss of elasticity in pulmonary interstitial tissue.

Laryngeal Stridor and Spasm

It is important to distinguish between laryngeal stridor and laryngospasm. Laryngeal stridor may be either inspiratory or expiratory. Inspiratory stridor occurs during deep anesthesia. The reduction of skeletal muscle tone results in adduction of the vocal cords. As the anesthetic gases flow through the narrowed glottic opening during inspiration, the vocal cords partially impede the flow of the gases into the trachea, producing the characteristic stridulous sound. Lightening the anesthesia usually corrects this problem. Expiratory stridor most often occurs in response to stimulation under too light a plane of anesthesia. It is frequently accompanied by tachypnea or hyperpnea, and it may progress to laryngospasm.

Laryngospasm is a rare occurrence with inhalation anesthesia and is not a feature of conscious sedation but a frequent accompaniment of intravenous anesthesia. The usual initiating stimulating factor is blood or mucus in the airway. The spasm is usually made worse by the accompanying hypoxia and hypercarbia. Suctioning of the airway and administration of 100 per cent oxygen following suctioning of the pharynx to remove blood or mucus usually relieves the spasm. Laryngospasm

is made worse by the accompanying hypoxia and hypercarbia. If laryngospasm has developed during the administration of a volatile anesthetic agent, then this agent should be turned off. If suctioning and oxygen are not effective, the administration of a 10- to 20-mg dose of succinylcholine intravenously will be adequate to relieve most cases of laryngospasm and allow positive pressure ventilation with oxygen. Prior to the administration of succinylcholine to relieve laryngospasm foreign material should be aspirated from the pharynx; otherwise, foreign material could be forced into the tracheobronchial tree. Injection of succinylcholine into the tongue will produce rapid relaxation of the cords when an intravenous line is not present. It may relieve those who are anxious about their ability to handle laryngospasm to know that the authors have rarely had to use succinylcholine.

Laryngospasm

Complete or partial closure of the laryngeal airway can be sudden, and immediate treatment is required. Both the true and false vocal cords are in adduction (closure) during laryngospasm. Minimal or complete absence of respiratory exchange causes rapid onset of hypoxia and hypercarbia with their associated hazards.

Upper airway obstruction above the level of the cords is characterized by low pitched inspiratory sounds and is corrected by proper positioning of the head and mandible. Initially laryngospasm is recognized by the characteristic high pitched crowing sounds during inspiration which occur with partial closure of the rima glottidis. Once complete closure of the laryngeal aperture has occurred, active attempts at spontaneous respiration are continued by the patient, and inspiratory movements of the thorax and abdomen can be seen until anoxia and hypercarbia cause respiratory arrest.

Laryngospasm can be directly correlated with anesthetic technique. During stage II of inhalation anesthetic induction the pharyngeal and laryngeal reflexes are hyperactive and closure of the cords is stimulated by pain, excessive secretions, premature surgical manipulations, or rapid increase in concentration of inhalation anesthetic agents. Once stage III, plane 2 of surgical anesthesia is achieved, laryngospasm should be a rare occurrence, especially if anesthesia is maintained solely with inhalation agents. Induction and maintenance of light anesthesia with barbiturates such as thiopental or methohexital are associated with an increased incidence of laryngospasm. The ultra-short acting barbiturates have a parasympathomimetic action which increases vagal influence on the vocal cords. During light barbiturate anesthesia, with or without nitrous oxide-oxygen, stage III, plane 2 is usually achieved, and pharyngeal and laryngeal reflexes are easily stimulated by surgical manipulations, blood, secretions, or misplaced oropharyngeal packing.

Laryngospasm may be induced directly or by reflex activity. Direct induction of vocal cord closure is caused by stimulation of foreign material, such as blood, mucus, tooth fragments, or misplaced gauze packing, on the pharynx or epiglottis. Pain is the most common cause of reflex laryngospasm. Periosteal stripping during a light plane of general anesthesia is a frequent initiating factor. Rapid increase in concentration of inhaled anesthetic vapors, parasympathomimetic activity of ultra-short acting barbiturates, and increase in vagal tone are other examples of stimuli which evoke reflex laryngospasm.

It has been stated that before death occurs the vocal cords will relax, and the patient will make one last inspiratory effort ("penultimate breath"). Waiting for such an event to occur in order to begin ventilating a moribund patient may prove disastrous. The rapid oxygen desaturation of arterial blood and accumulation of carbon dioxide may have already initiated irreversible changes in brain cells or extreme hyperirritability of the myocardium with onset of ventricular arrhythmias or fibrillation. Even following total denitrogenation of arterial blood by breathing 100 per cent oxygen for several minutes, arterial oxygen tension will fall dangerously low after breathing an anoxic mixture of gases for 90 seconds or less. Therefore, active treatment of laryngospasm must be initiated immediately as it is recognized.

Treatment of laryngospasm involves immediate termination of anesthetic induction or surgery, clearing of the oral cavity and pharynx, administration of 100 per cent oxygen, and, if necessary, a muscle relaxant. The bite block, if present, should be kept in place for access while the oropharyngeal pack is removed and the mouth and pharynx are gently cleared of blood, mucus, tooth fragments, and other foreign material. The pharynx and paralaryngeal and epiglottic areas are best avoided unless gross contamination exists. Strong anterior traction should not be placed on the tongue. The soft palate, pharynx, base of tongue, and epiglottis send sensory impulses via the glossopharyngeal (IX) nerve and receive motor nerve supply from the vagus (X) nerve. Stimulation of these areas, especially in the presence of hypoxia and hypercarbia which increases vagal tone, can increase laryngospasm and precipitate cardiac arrest (Figs. 7.10 and 7.11).

When vocal cord closure is incomplete, as indicated by high pitched stridor, 100 per cent oxygen is administered by controlled ventilation with gentle pressure by full-face mask. If no respiratory exchange takes place, the cords have completely closed, and a short acting muscle relaxant must be given immediately. Succinylcholine (10 to 20 mg intravenously or by sublingual injection) produces relaxation of the cords in most cases in a matter of seconds and allows ventilation of the patient by full-face mask. Occasionally a second dose of succinylcholine is necessary to procure adequate vocal cord relax-

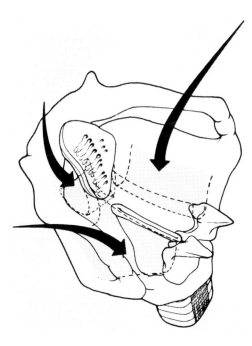

Figure 7.10. If positive pressure ventilation is given during laryngeal spasm, air is forced into the piriform fossae and vallecula. There is then soft tissue closure of the airway which compounds the spasm.

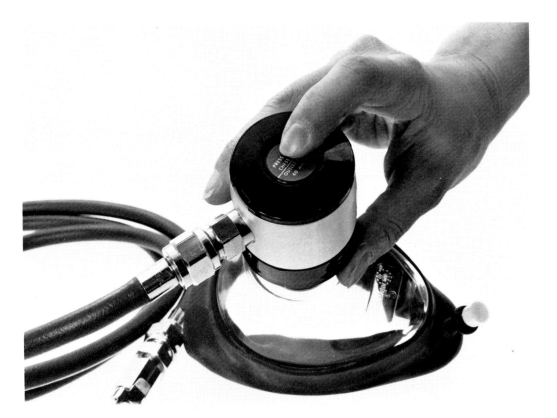

Figure 7.11. A Robershaw resuscitator is preferable to a bag and mask for the inexperienced. The oxygen flow is activated by the valve which inflates the patient. In addition, if the patient breathes spontaneously, high flows of oxygen are delivered at inspiration.

ation, but the risk of cardiac arrest following multiple doses of succinylcholine needs to be considered. Following administration of succinylcholine, controlled ventilation is maintained until return of adequate spontaneous respiratory effort.

Cricothyroid Puncture. If laryngospasm is not relieved by the above methods or the administrator is anxious about the use of succinylcholine or inability to perform laryngoscopy, then cricothyroid ligament puncture (coniotomy) is a lifesaving procedure (Fig. 7.12). The cricothyroid ligament which lies between the cricoid and thyroid cartilages in a relatively bloodless area. The cricothyroid airway is only temporary; its objective is to provide oxygen for a short period while the patient overcomes the laryngospasm. To and fro ventilation will not occur, but the anatomical configuration of the vocal cords is such that gas can exit but not enter. A 13-gauge needle produces an adequate temporary airway and is less traumatic than the commercially available cricothyroid trocar. The 13-gauge needle or trocar is directed inferiorly in the trachea to prevent perforation of the posterior wall of the trachea and injury to the esophagus.

Bronchospasm

Bronchospasm is neither transitory nor prone to spontaneous remission. Life-

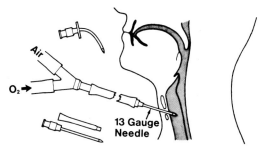

Figure 7.12. A tracheal plastic catheter is a useful instrument for puncture of the cricothyroid membrane. A 12- to 14-gauge needle may be used. Both are probably preferable to the commercially available cricothyroid trochar. A T-connector is needed for attachment of oxygen to the needle.

threatening interference with adequate ventilation requires termination of bronchospasm by the use of drugs and ventilatory support.

The incidence of bronchospasm associated with general anesthesia is low, although patients with pre-existing pulmonary disease are at increased risk. Etiology of bronchospasm includes respiratory infection (especially bronchitis from chronic cigarette smoking), inhaled foreign bodies or toxic pollutants, bronchial asthma, reflex activity secondary to release of vasoactive amines (kinins, serotonin), during pulmonary embolism, and reflex smooth muscle spasm due to increased vagal tone during painful procedures under light anesthesia or traction on viscera. In the known asthmatic patient drugs such as thiopental and morphine may initiate bronchospasm and should be avoided.

The pathophysiology of bronchospasm simulates an acute asthmatic attack with spasm of bronchiolar smooth muscle, edema of peribronchiolar tissues, narrowing of the smaller air passages with air trapping and increased pulmonary secretions. The development of bronchospasm initiates a marked decrease in total ventilatory exchange. The thoracic cage is fixed in an expanded inspiratory position due to trapping of air distal to the narrowed bronchioles and the lungs rapidly lose compliance and become more difficult to ventilate. Diffuse wheezes, especially during expiration, are heard on auscultation throughout the chest. Other causes of increased airway resistance, such as upper airway obstruction, kinked and misplaced nasopharyngeal or endotracheal tubes, or plugging of the tube with foreign material, should be ruled out before making the diagnosis of bronchospasm.

Treatment of bronchospasm requires immediate control of the upper airway with positive pressure ventilation to prevent hypoxia and hypercarbia. Adequate ventilation of the patient is dependent upon drug therapy to reverse bronchial smooth muscle spasm. Drug therapy is more effective and less likely to produce severe cardiac arrhythmias if hypoxia, hypercarbia, and respiratory acidosis are not present. An adrenergic substance, such as adrenalin (0.1 to 0.3 mg intravenously) or isoproterenol (1 mg in 250 ml of 5 per cent dextrose and water at a rate of 40 to 60 drops per minute intravenously) is recommended for an immediate relaxing effect on bronchiolar smooth muscle. Isoproterenol may also be given by inhaler via the anesthetic circuit. Sustained effect is produced with aminophylline, 6 to 9 mg/kg in 100 ml 5 per cent dextrose and water, given by intravenous drip over 20 minutes to reduce the incidence of hypotension, gastric upset, and cardiac arrhythmias. Corticosteroid therapy is not helpful during immediate treatment as it takes approximately 2 hours after a dose to reach maximal anti-inflammatory effect. For prolonged effect, especially when bronchodilating drugs are not producing optimal effects or the patient will require extended therapy, large doses of steroid hydrocortisone, 200 mg, or dexamethasone, 20 mg, can be given intravenously.

Pulmonary Aspiration

Entrance of foreign material into the tracheobronchial tree is an acute emergency which can rapidly terminate fatally if not prevented or properly managed. During dental procedures under sedation or general anesthesia foreign material may be aspirated into the lungs from either the oral cavity or the stomach at any time when the patient's protective pharyngeal and laryngeal reflexes are obtunded. Hence this problem is not a feature of conscious sedation, where by definition protective reflexes are active.

Secretions, blood, tooth, or bone fragments may be aspirated if adequate suction is not available to clear this debris. A well-placed oropharyngeal pack also prevents such material from passing into the pharynx where it can gain access to the laryngeal aperture. The presence of a cuffed endotracheal tube is another preventive measure.

An appropriate period of fasting prior to anesthesia or analgesia, usually 4 hours, should render the patient's stomach empty at the time of anesthetic induction. Unfortunately, multiple factors, including anxiety, pain, narcotics, trauma, and shock, delay gastric emptying time, and the stomach may not be empty as expected. Gastric contents may gain access to the lungs by either vomiting or regurgitation. The incidence of pulmonary aspiration of gastric contents has been reported to vary between 0.03 and 26.3 per cent. The highest incidence occurs in obstetric patients, followed by upper abdominal surgery. Fifteen to 25 per cent of all maternal mortality and 11 per cent of all anesthetic mortality are due to pulmonary aspiration.

Aspiration of material into the tracheobronchial tree is usually easily recognized. Rapid, deep swallowing movements may precede active vomiting, which usually occurs during induction of or recovery from anesthesia. Regurgitation is a passive, and often silent, process. However, once foreign material gains entrance into the lungs, there is immediate onset of coughing, severe wheezing, difficulty in ventilating the patient, tachypnea, tachycardia, and cyanosis.

The pathophysiology of pulmonary aspiration differs depending on the type of material which enters the lungs. Solid material, debris from the oral cavity or solid food from the stomach produces mechanical blockage of larger airways and causes sudden total obstruction. Liquid gastric contents with a pH below 2.5 are highly irritating and produce an intense chemical inflammatory response (the so-called aspiration pneumonitis or Mendelson's syndrome) rapidly causing severe edema, secretions, bronchospasm, hypoxia, and hypercarbia, progressing to consolidation.

Management must be instituted immediately. Lower the patient's head and turn it to the right. Clear the mouth and pharynx of all liquid and solid debris manually and with a large bore suction. Access to the lower airway should be gained with endotracheal intubation or bronchoscopy and all visible material rapidly removed. Ventilate the patient with 100 per cent oxygen. If liquid gastric contents were aspirated, pass a nasogastric tube into the stomach and check the pH of the gastric aspirate. If the pH is above 2.5, a chemical pneumonitis will probably not develop. Continue to clear the tracheobronchial tree of all debris by suctioning alternating with oxygenation. If the gastric pH is below 2.5, full treatment of aspiration pneumonitis must be given. Clear all visible liquid material from the lungs by suctioning. Irrigation with saline or bicarbonate solutions is controversial; while it may neutralize some of the acidic aspirate, it also tends to spread it to other parts of the lungs. The patient will probably require bronchodilators and mechanical ventilation. Aminophylline in a loading dose of 6 to 9 mg/kg given intravenously over a 20-minute period helps reverse bronchospasm, but the patient should be monitored for hypotension and cardiac arrhythmias. Although their effect is delayed, steroids in large doses, hydrocortisone, 200 mg, or dexamethasone, 20 mg, should be given intravenously to help reduce the massive inflammatory response. Transfer of the patient to a respiratory intensive care unit is required for further definitive care. Antibiotics may be needed for treatment of documented pulmonary infection, but they are not an essential part of emergency management of aspiration pneumonitis. Despite treatment the mortality rate may exceed 60 per cent.

Apnea

Apnea may be attributable to a number of medical emergencies. Prolonged apnea due to anesthetic agents or muscle relaxants has occurred in dental anesthetic practice, with fatal results.

The often inadequate facilities for providing artificial or controlled ventilation which may be present in the dental office would seem to contraindicate the routine use of muscle relaxants in outpatient dental practice. When prolonged apnea occurs, treatment with intermittent positive pressure ventilation is indicated until the situation has been evaluated. If prolonged apnea develops in the dental office and continues for 20 to 30 minutes, that is, within the usual maximum period of time allowed for outpatient anesthesia, it would be preferable to transfer the patient to a hospital to allow more efficient artificial ventilation until apnea is reversed.

FACTORS COMMON TO EITHER TYPE OF RELAXANT

1. Central depression due to the action of either opiates, intravenous barbiturates, or other anesthetic agents. Clinical awareness of the method of administering anesthesia will make this apparent.

2. Hypocarbia. Vigorous artificial ventilation following the administration of a relaxant drug will result in the lowering of carbon dioxide tension. Respiration will not restart until the respiratory threshold to carbon dioxide tension is reached. If the patient is allowed to remain apneic, the carbon dioxide tension will be restored. Administration of 100 per cent oxygen during the period of apnea allows apneic oxygenation to maintain adequate levels of oxygen tension.

3. Hypercarbia. Because of hypoventilation or inadequate elimination of carbon dioxide from the anesthetic circuit, hypercarbia can develop. Hypercarbia can be a respiratory depressant. Vigorous artificial ventilation will decrease carbon dioxide tension.

4. Metabolic acidosis. Metabolic acidosis will rarely be encountered in dental anesthesia other than inpatient hospital practice. Metabolic acidosis can produce prolonged apnea.

5. Reflex. Reflex overstimulation of the Hering-Breuer reflex by vigorous expan-

sion of the lungs with artificial ventilation can produce apnea; a decreased effort of artificial ventilation will decrease this reflex activity. The presence of the endotracheal tube can reflexly inhibit respiration; removal of the endotracheal tube will often be the initiating factor in resumption of spontaneous ventilation.

d-TUBOCURARINE OR GALLAMINE

Many disorders of potassium metabolism will produce a central and peripheral action that will produce prolonged apnea. The electrolyte imbalance which this implies is not generally seen in dental practice.

SUCCINYLCHOLINE

Succinylcholine as classically administered in the dental office can often produce prolonged apnea due to several factors.

1. Atypical pseudocholinesterase which will not metabolize succinylcholine adequately may be present.

2. Electrolyte imbalance possibly related to drug therapy allows abnormal reactions at the motor end plate, with consequent prolonged depolarization.

3. A low pseudocholinesterase can be an acquired condition, with resultant delay in metabolism of succinylcholine. Overdosage of succinylcholine will produce manifestations of prolonged apnea, and it is recommended that 1 g of succinylcholine be not exceeded. It is the duration of depolarization which is significant, however, rather than the amount. One gram in 10 minutes is less of a problem than 200 mg in 1 hour. In addition, in large doses, metabolism of succinylcholine to succinylmonocholine can result in the accumulation of the metabolite at the muscle end plate with consequent prolonged apnea.

4. Dual block. The initial depolarizing action of succinylcholine can be followed by a neuromuscular blockade which is non-depolarizing. It is usually produced if intermittent repeated injections of succinylcholine are given and is reversed by neostigmine.

DIAGNOSIS OF PROLONGED APNEA

1. A clinical checklist of the possible causes should be gone over by the anesthetist.

2. The nerve stimulator can be used. In this the electrodes are placed over the ulnar nerve, and an electrical twitch stimulus is given which produces contraction of the little finger. It can then be followed by a tetanic stimulation; a subsequent twitch stimulus will produce a maximal response in the patient with a non-depolarizing block, but in the patient with a depolarizing block there will be no improvement in response.

3. A test dose of edrophonium can be given which will improve the block produced by a non-depolarizing agent.

Cardiovascular Problems

Most emergency situations involving the cardiovascular system are precipitated by hypoxia or hypercarbia. However, patients with pre-existing heart disease are at greater risk than healthy patients. A thorough preoperative history and physical examination will identify most patients with existing cardiovascular problems and those with significant risk factors. Warning signs and symptoms are usually present prior to an emergency. Patients with significant cardiovascular disease are generally not good candidates for outpatient general anesthesia or intravenous sedation, which will cause respiratory depression.

Twenty-eight million people in the United States have some form of heart ailment, and 650,000 of these die each year from heart disease. One million persons experience a heart attack (myocardial infarction) in the United States annually, of which 350,000 die outside of a hospital within the first 2 hours after the onset of symptoms.

Risk factors which help identify those patients most likely to experience myocardial infarction include: hypertension—blood pressure above 140/90 mm Hg; high serum levels of cholesterol and triglycerides; obesity; lack of physical exercise; chronic cigarette smoking; diabetes mellitus; family history of heart disease, especially premature (under 40 years of age) myocardial infarction; stress; male sex.

Symptoms which usually indicate cardiovascular disease can be elicited during the medical history and include: angina pectoris (chest pain on exertion, exposure to cold, excitement, or after a heavy meal, and relieved by rest or nitroglycerine); dyspnea on mild exertion; orthopnea; paroxysmal nocturnal dyspnea; ankle edema; intermittent claudication; heart palpitations (especially if accompanied by dizziness, dyspnea, or chest pain); history of previous myocardial infarction, hypertension, cerebrovascular accident (stroke), rheumatic or syphilitic valvular heart disease, or congestive heart failure.

SYNCOPE

Some patients react during a period of stress with a strong vasovagal response. The reflex bradycardia and peripheral vasodilatation produce a profound fall in cardiac output and cerebral perfusion. If the patient is not supine, cerebral blood flow is reduced and the patient may lose consciousness (syncope). A convulsion may occur secondary to cerebral hypoxia. The entire episode can be quite frightening to bystanders. In the dental office syncope most frequently occurs during placement of an intravenous needle or injection of local anesthetic. Young, healthy, muscular males seem unusually susceptible.

Initial signs and symptoms of vasovagal syncope include nausea, pallor, diaphoresis, and slowing of the pulse. If it is untreated at this point, cyanosis, profound hypotension, loss of consciousness, and convulsions occur.

Treatment is indicated without delay as soon as the syndrome is suspected. Place the patient supine and elevate the legs above heart level, administer 100 per cent oxygen by mask, monitor blood pressure and heart rate. If the heart rate is above 60 per minute the systolic blood pressure above 90 mm Hg, no drug therapy is indicated and the event will be corrected by the maneuvers described above. If systolic blood pressure is below 90 mm Hg and heart rate is below 60 per minute, give atropine, 0.6 mg intravenously, to reduce vagal activity and increase heart rate. If heart rate improves but blood pressure remains low, a vasopressor may also be required.

Most patients respond rapidly to proper positioning and administration of oxygen. They appear clinically normal with acceptable blood pressure and heart rate within a few minutes. However, severe depression of stroke volume and cardiac output persists for over 1 hour after recovery from syncope. Sedation or general anesthesia should, therefore, be deferred for at least 2 hours or until the next day.

HYPOTENSION

Significant drop in blood pressure (defined as decrease in excess of 15 per cent) can occur before, during, or after the administration of sedation or anesthesia. When mean arterial pressure drops below approximately 60 mm Hg, adequate perfusion of the heart, brain, and kidneys no longer occurs. Metabolic acidosis develops, causing intense arteriolar vasodilatation and spasm of capillary sphincters. Pooling of blood in precapillary areas removes it from the effective circulating blood volume with decrease in venous return and cardiac output. If severe hypotension is left uncorrected, myocardial infarction, stroke, acute renal failure, or irreversible shock can develop. Frequent blood measurements are imperative during the administration of sedative or anesthetic drugs which can cause peripheral vasodilatation or myocardial depression.

Some of the anesthetic-related causes of arterial hypotension are listed in Table 7.1. Knowledge of the etiology of hypotension is critical to its rational treatment.

When hypotension is related to inadequate circulating blood volume (various types of shock), treatment must include replacement of adequate amounts of the appropriate fluids (blood, plasma, electrolyte solutions). Vasopressors are no longer considered rational in most cases of shock because they intensify the vasoconstriction which is already compromising circulation to vital organs.

A patient with a diseased myocardium who becomes hypotensive may be affected adversely by vasopressors. The increase in peripheral resistance caused by vasoconstriction may increase the work load and oxygen consumption of the diseased (decompensated) heart beyond its reserve and precipitate acute congestive heart failure or myocardial infarction.

The hemodynamic effects of the various sympathomimetic drugs used as vasopressors have been attributed to their differential actions on two types of adrenergic receptors, the α and β receptors. This classification of adrenergic receptors is based on their response to the sympathomimetic amine isoproterenol (Isuprel). Beta receptors are those most responsive to isoproterenol (peripheral vasodilatation, increase in rate and strength of myocardial contraction), while those least responsive are α receptors. α receptors are responsible for peripheral vasoconstriction (skin, mucosa, intestine, and kidney) and are stimulated most by norepinephrine. Epinephrine has mixed effects. At low concentrations β receptors are predominantly stimulated, while both α and β receptors are stimulated by larger doses (0.3 to 0.5 mg in adults).

The aim of vasopressors in treating hypotension is to restore adequate perfusion to vital organs, including the heart, without increasing cardiac work and oxygen consumption past the tolerance of available myocardial reserve. The β-adrenergic agents, such as epinephrine and isoproterenol, have both a chronotropic (increase in rate) and an ionotropic (increase in strength of contraction) effect on the myocardium. Stroke volume and cardiac output are increased, but so are cardiac work and oxygen consumption. Increased cardiac rate shortens the period of diastole when perfusion of the coronary arteries occurs. Thus, the increased oxygen demand of the myocardium which is stimulated to contract with greater strength is supplied with less oxygen when increased cardiac rate interferes with coronary artery perfusion. This is a dangerous situation in the heart with little or no reserve.

α-Adrenergic agents, such as methoxamine and phenylephrine, have their main effect on peripheral blood vessels producing vasoconstriction. However, since the heart must pump against increased peripheral resistance, cardiac work is indirectly increased. Increased vagal activity is stimulated by increased blood pressure, and the heart rate slows by reflex action. When selecting a vasopressor for treatment of hypotension, the choice depends upon the cause of lowered blood pressure and whether α- or β-adrenergic effects will best return blood pressure to acceptable levels. In many cases of hypotension, as mentioned above, a vasopressor is not the drug of choice.

A number of vasopressors used in treatment of hypotension have been evaluated

Table 7.1.
Drug Related Causes of Hypotension

Therapeutic drugs used prior to anesthesia
Excessive premedication
Overdose of general anesthetics
Vascular absorption of local anesthetics
Raised airway pressure
Hemorrhage
Reflex activity to surgical maneuvers
Change in position of the patient
Cardiovascular disease
Septic shock
Incompatible blood transfusion
Anaphylactic reaction

for their α and β effects. Their effects and appropriate doses are listed in Table 7.2.

Examples of hypotension in which use of a vasopressor is indicated are excessive premedication and overdose of general anesthetic agents. Both have a depressant effect on the myocardium and a relaxing effect on peripheral blood vessels. A vasopressor with both α and β effects most appropriately corrects this type of hypotension.

Vasopressor therapy for hypotension occurring during acute congestive heart failure or acute myocardial infarction is seldom indicated. The underlying cause of lowered blood pressure is usually failure of the decompensated myocardium to pump effectively, cardiogenic shock. Agents which directly (β) or indirectly (α) increase the work load of the heart only intensify the decompensation of the already overloaded myocardium. Generally, an agent which improves the efficiency of the myocardium, less oxygen consumption per unit of output, such as a digitalis preparation (digoxin, ouabain) is the agent of choice for cardiac decompensation.

HYPERTENSION

Hypertension can be dangerous in that rupture of a cerebral aneurysm can occur in an otherwise healthy patient. It can lead to increased work for the heart and will frequently cause cardiac arrhyth-

mias. Diagnosis of the cause can usually lead to prompt treatment of the problem and rapid reversal of the increased blood pressure. Causes are usually hypoxia, hypercarbia, light anesthesia with excess stimulation, or overdose of epinephrine.

If a careful preoperative evaluation is made then hypertension can be anticipated if the patient has been treated with tricyclic antidepressant drugs, and subsequently given exogenous catecholamines.

The urgent treatment of hypertension of unknown origin is diazoxide (Hyperstat) in a dose of 300 mg. The other alternative is hydralazine (Apresoline) in a dose of 20 mg. These medications will produce an increased pulse rate and thus cardiac output, and therefore should be avoided in cardiac failure. If it is possible, nitroprusside (Nipride) is indicated as it does not cause an increase in rate.

CARDIAC ARRHYTHMIAS

The significance of irregularities in cardiac rhythm lies in their interference with normal ventricular filling, myocardial contractility, coronary artery perfusion, stroke volume, and potential for progression to circulatory arrest. Pre-existing cardiac arrhythmias should be recognized and adequately treated before surgery. The recognition of complex arrhythmias is not a necessary part of the education of the dentist performing local anesthesia or

Table 7.2.
Mode of Action of Selected Vasopressors

	Activity		IV Dose		
	α	β	Single	Infusion (in 500 ml D$_5$W)	Tachyphylaxis
Ephedrine	Yes	Yes	10–25 mg		Yes
Dopamine (Intropin)	Yes	Yes		200 mg (2–20 μg/kg/min)	
Norepinephrine (Levophed)	Yes	Yes		2–4 mg	
Mephentermine (Wyamine)	Yes	Yes	10–30 mg	500 mg	
Metaraminol (Aramine)	Yes	Slight	0.5–2.0 mg	100 mg	Yes
Methoxamine (Vasoxyl)	Yes		3–5 mg	40 mg	
Phenylephrine (Neosynephrine)	Yes		0.2–0.5 mg	10–20 mg	

conscious sedation. Some basic arrhythmias can be recognized without the use of the electrocardiogram.

Alterations in cardiac rhythm may be rapid (tachycardia, greater than 100 beats per minute or slow (bradycardia), fewer than 60 beats per minute, and atrial or ventricular in origin. Bradycardia may cause significant decrease in cardiac output and drop in mean arterial pressure because even though each heart beat may produce an adequate stroke volume, not enough beats occur each minute to sustain adequate perfusion. By critically shortening the time between each heart beat, tachycardia reduces ventricular filling and coronary artery perfusion, both of which occur during diastole. Some rapid atrial irregularities, such as atrial fibrillation or atrial flutter, require medical treatment for adequate control of cardiac rate. However, atrial arrhythmias are not usually immediately life threatening. They seldom occur de novo during anesthesia; they should be recognized and treated preoperatively. Ventricular arrhythmias are generally more ominous. They may appear for the first time suddenly during anesthesia, and they have the potential to progress to ventricular fibrillation.

The causes of cardiac arrhythmias associated with anesthesia include pre-existing cardiac disease, hypoxia, hypercarbia, hypertension, patient anxiety, type of anesthetic induction, reflexly due to light anesthesia, anesthetic overdose, and electrolyte imbalance. Patients with pre-existing heart disease should be identified by careful preanesthetic evaluation. Agents and techniques should be selected which expose such patients to a minimum of risk. The method of anesthetic induction influences the incidence of cardiac arrhythmias. During induction with inhalation agents ventricular arrhythmias are frequent, probably secondary to increased secretion of endogenous catecholamines. The incidence of arrhythmias was significantly reduced during inhalation induction of general anesthesia by administering propranolol (children, 5 mg; adults, 10 mg), a β-adrenergic blocker, orally prior to induction. Anesthetic induction with the ultra-short acting barbiturates is associated with a low incidence of cardiac arrhythmias.

Imbalance of electrolytes, especially potassium, can cause myocardial irritability. Patients on diuretic therapy lose excessive potassium in their urine, which if not replaced by daily supplementation, causes hypokalemia. Chronic hypercarbia is often present in patients with chronic pulmonary disease. If excessive carbon dioxide is removed by vigorous controlled ventilation in such patients there is a rapid shift of potassium ions from the extracellular to the intracellular space with resultant hypokalemia and frequent cardiac arrhythmias. The other causes of cardiac irregularities are best avoided by careful adherence to proper anesthetic technique.

Treatment of cardiac arrhythmias during anesthesia begins with appropriate monitoring for early recognition. An oscilloscope allows visualization of the electrical activity of the heart so that recognition of various irregularities is possible, and rational treatment can be provided. Immediately as a significant arrhythmia is observed, the initial course of action is to stop surgical manipulations, check the patency of the airway, turn off the anesthetic agents, and administer 100 per cent oxygen. Further treatment depends upon the type of arrhythmia and whether it persists or reverts to normal sinus rhythm.

Sinus Tachycardia

The rate is greater than 100 beats per minute. The rhythm is regular, and each QRS complex is preceded by a P wave. It occurs in apprehensive patients (Fig. 7.13).

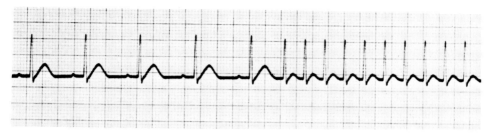

Figure 7.13. Paroxysmal tachycardia is evidenced by sudden increases in rate from an ectopic pacemaker. Numerous causes and therapies have been advocated. It is not a serious arrhythmia unless prolonged.

Supraventricular Tachycardia

If supraventricular tachycardia does not respond to the normal treatment modalities, such as carotid massage, phenylephrine, edrophonium and propranolol, then verapamil, a calcium-blocking agent, can be given in an initial dose of 5 to 10 mg and repeated in 30 minutes if the response is inadequate. Overdose will result in hypotension, atrioventricular block, or cardiac asystole.

Sinus Bradycardia

The rate is less than 60 beats per minute. The rhythm is regular, and a normal P wave precedes each QRS complex. This rhythm is normal when seen preoperatively in well-conditioned athletes, especially long distance runners. It may also be a prodromal sign of vasovagal syncope. During general anesthesia bradycardia is generally a sign of anesthetic overdose. Slow cardiac rhythm makes it easier for ectopic foci in the ventricular myocardium to initiate irregular beats; atropine may prevent such a tendency by increasing the rate of discharge of the SA node.

Premature Ventricular Contractions (PVCs)

An extra heart beat may occur when an ectopic focus in one of the ventricles initiates a contraction. Most premature ventricular contractions are followed by a compensatory pause. Isolated PVCs may occur during anesthesia in healthy patients. However, patients subjected to hypoxia and hypercarbia or who have preexisting heart disease frequently develop significant ventricular arrhythmias. The danger of such arrhythmias is their potential to progress to ventricular fibrillation if not recognized and treated. Treatment is lidocaine (100-mg intravenous bolus), followed by an intravenous lidocaine infusion of 1 to 4 mg per minute (1 g in 500 ml of 5 per cent dextrose in water) to maintain suppression of ventricular irritability.

Ventricular Tachycardia

This arrhythmia presents a grave, life-threatening situation, since inadequate ventricular filling and decreased coronary artery perfusion lead to loss of myocardial efficiency and reduced cardiac output. It may also be a precursor to ventricular fibrillation. The rate is 100 to 250 beats per minute, and the rhythm is usually regular.

Treatment includes intravenous lidocaine. If the clinical situation is critical (circulatory collapse, loss of consciousness), then cardioversion, synchronized with the QRS complex to prevent "R-on-T phenomenon," should be performed immediately.

ACUTE CONGESTIVE HEART FAILURE

The diseased myocardium is susceptible to failure of adequate pumping action if the cardiac work load is excessive (increased peripheral vascular resistance, excessive fluid replacement), if the myocardium is depressed (excessive premedication, overdose of general anesthetic agents), or if inadequate oxygen is supplied to the myocardium (hypoxia, decreased coronary artery perfusion by hypotension, or cardiac arrhythmias). While the patient with a normal heart usually tolerates such conditions for a reasonable period of time, the patient with heart disease may rapidly develop acute congestive heart failure and pulmonary edema. Patients with ischemic or hypertensive heart disease are especially susceptible.

Symptoms are progressive and include dyspnea, orthopnea, and paroxysmal nocturnal dyspnea. Signs include tachycardia, tachypnea, and cardiac enlargement. Progression causes right-sided heart failure. Failure of the right ventricle to empty adequately during systole causes pitting edema (particularly of the lower extremities), passive congestion of the liver, distended neck veins, and decreased renal perfusion with lowered urine output and fluid retention. Such patients should be recognized preoperatively and prepared with digitalization and diuretic therapy.

ACUTE MYOCARDIAL INFARCTION

Acute myocardial infarction (ML, coronary occlusion, heart attack) may occur during, prior to, or in the postoperative period. The classic signs and symptoms of severe crushing chest pain with radiation to the left upper extremity, nausea, pallor, and feeling of impending doom may not be recognizable in a sedated or anesthetized patient. A high index of suspicion should be maintained, especially among those patients with high risk factors or positive medical history.

Myocardial infarction should be suspected during or after operation when severe hypotension, cardiac arrhythmias, congestive heart failure, or pulmonary edema appear suddenly and without apparent reason. Anoxia, hypotension, overdose of general anesthetics or analgesics, and excessive blood loss are frequent precipitating factors. Diagnosis of acute MI generally is made on the basis of history, physical examination, electrocardiographic changes and increase in serum enzymes. An adequate history is often impossible in an obtunded patient, and pain is not present early in 5 to 10 per cent of cases, especially diabetics. The ECG is positive in only 85 per cent of patients. It may take several hours or even days for the ECG and serum enzyme changes to become apparent.

Myocardial infarction is a potential complication during or after surgery. In patients with no history of previous myocardial infarction the incidence is approximately 0.13 per cent. However, the risk is greatly increased in patients who have suffered previous infarcts. In several studies results varied, but the risk decreases to 10 per cent 6 months postinfarction and to normal after 2 years. Risk factors associated with significnatly increased infarction rates include preoperative hypertension, intraoperative hypotension, and operations of more than 3 hours' duration. Mortality rate for reinfarction after operation is approximately 50 per cent. The complications most frequently associated with mortality in myocardial infarction include shock, acute congestive heart failure, and cardiac arrhythmias.

Immediate treatment of a suspected or confirmed myocardial infarction includes administration of oxygen, loosening of clothing, and elevation of the head to ease breathing, morphine (2-mg increments intravenously) for relief of pain, calm reassurance of the patient by attending personnel, and transfer to a coronary care unit as soon as possible. Prophylactic use of lidocaine (100 to 300 mg intramuscularly) has been advocated to reduce incidence of fatal arrhythmias during transport of the patient to hospital facilities.

CEREBROVASCULAR ACCIDENT

Cerebrovascular accident (CVA, stroke, cerebral apoplexy) is a general term for a spectrum of syndromes occurring secondary to occlusion of the blood supply to specific areas of the brain. Vascular occlusion may arise from thrombosis (85 per cent of cases), intracranial hemorrhage (12 per cent), or embolization from distant sites (3 per cent). Contributing factors include decreased cerebral blood flow associated with hypotension, myocardial infarction, or acute congestive heart failure. Patients with valvular heart disease, cardiac arrhythmia, or infective endocarditis may release emboli which travel to the cerebral circulation. Hypertensive patients are particularly at risk to develop a cerebrovascular accident.

The early signs and symptoms of cerebrovascular accident may mimic those seen in the early postanesthetic period. Nausea, vomiting, headache, vertigo, and dyspnea are early symptoms. A stroke generally progresses, however, to produce a neurological motor and sensory deficit representing a specific area of brain damage. Suspicion of a stroke should initiate supportive care and immediate consultation with a neurologist for definitive diagnosis and treatment.

FLUID MANAGEMENT IN DENTAL ANESTHESIA

Fluid management begins during the preoperative visit. Fluid and electrolyte deficits should be recognized and corrected before operation. While this is primarily the surgeon's responsibility, the anesthetist may be involved as a consultant.

An intravenous drip should be started on every patient before the induction of intravenous anesthesia in all but the briefest cases. In addition to the administration of fluids, the intravenous route can be used to inject anesthetic drugs as required or as a rapid route of administration of emergency drugs.

During anesthesia and surgery deficits in fluid and electrolytes and maintenance requirements should be provided. Following operation adequate fluids must be provided to supply maintenance requirements and continuing blood losses. Studies have emphasized the inability of dental patients to take adequate oral nourishment and fluids following oral surgical procedures. Since the anesthetist often shares responsibility for postoperative, as well as intraoperative fluid management, the following suggestions are helpful in managing the overall fluid requirements of the dental anesthesia patient.

1. Replace fluid deficit caused by preoperative fasting. This deficit, usually 5 per cent of blood volume or 250 to 500 ml in adults, is generally a water loss with superimposed metabolic acidosis. A solution of 5 per cent dextrose in water or lactated Ringer's solution is suitable.

2. Replace fluid losses during operation due to ventilation through an endotracheal tube, sweating, and formation of edema fluid. These losses average 5 to 10 ml per kg body weight per hour with highest value for small children. Replacement with a balanced electrolyte solution (e.g., lactated Ringer's) is recommended.

3. Blood losses, additionally, should be replaced as they occur with normal saline, lactated Ringer's solution, or other balanced electrolyte solution. In the presence of persistent cardiovascular instability or blood loss in excess of 1 liter in adults, whole blood should be given. Gravimetrically measured blood loss should be increased by one-third to equal actual blood loss.

4. The minimal fluids given intravenously during a dental anesthesia case of 30 minutes or less should be 500 ml to replace fasting deficits and the usual fluid losses incident to anesthesia. Lactated Ringer's solution is recommended. Thereafter, fluid maintenance requirements

should be given at the rate suggested in paragraph 2 above.

5. Postoperative fluid requirements should include the following: a) replacement of continuing blood loss (with whole blood or balanced electrolyte solution); b) provision of minimal daily fluid requirements (2000 to 3000 ml per day or 1300 to 3000 ml per sq m of body surface area per day; see above); c) replacement of abnormal fluid losses: vomiting, diarrhea (water and electrolytes according to loss); elevated body temperature (500 ml per day, for every degree of temperature elevation, replace with hypotonic saline, e.g., 5 per cent dextrose in 0.11 per cent NaCl).

6. Recording of all intake and output aids in detecting the nature and amounts of fluid deficits or excesses.

7. If long term provision of intravenous fluids is necessary after dental anesthesia, consultation with a fluid balance specialist may be indicated.

During the operation the anesthetist should constantly monitor the patient for signs of over-replacement. Auscultation of the lungs for the onset of rales is helpful. Vigorous fluid replacement may cause urinary bladder distention which can interfere with respiration or cause neurogenic reflex depression of blood pressure. In lengthy cases, insertion of a urinary catheter and measurement of urine output is advisable. Normal urine output is at least 50 ml per hour. Values less than this in a patient with normally functioning kidneys usually indicated under-replacement of fluids. At the opposite end of this spectrum, the clinician should consider oliguria or anuria secondary to acute tubular necrosis and renal shutdown, which usually results from prolonged shock or other situations in which poor perfusion of the kidneys occurs.

If available, the values obtained from monitoring central venous pressure or doing serial blood volume determinations can be helpful in assessing fluid replacement if they are correlated with clinical findings and good judgment. These more complicated methods of monitoring are generally used only in major surgical procedures.

Allergic Reactions

True allergic reactions develop as a result of immunological sensitzation. Prior exposure to the offending drug or antigen is necessary in order for production of antibodies to occur. Subsequent exposure to the drug causes formation of antigen-antibody complexes, which is the basis for the clinical manifestations of the allergic reaction. Drug allergy may appear clinically as any one of a number of symptom complexes whose onset may be acute or delayed and whose clinical course may be mild or severe. Clinical manifestations include skin reactions (urticaria, rash, pruritis, eczema), drug fever, organ-specific reactions, serum sickness, and anaphylaxis.

Anaphylactic shock represents an acute, life-threatening emergency characterized by hypotension, bronchospasm, urticaria, diffuse erythema, pruritis, laryngeal edema, cardiac arrhythmias, and hyperperistalsis. This allergic reaction is most frequently associated with intravenous or intramusclar drug administration. Therefore, it can occur during administration of intravenous sedatives or anesthetic agents. Atopic patients (persons with asthma, allergic rhinitis, or atopic dermatitis) have an increased likelihood of anaphylactic reactions.

It has been estimated that 5 per cent of hospital admissions are due to drug reactions, and a minimum of 15 per cent of hospitalized patients have at least one adverse reaction to a drug. Unfortunately, in the minds of many patients any untoward drug reaction is an allergic reaction. A careful history will usually disclose whether the patient has a true allergy or has experienced a toxic, idiosyncratic or neurogenic reaction (syncope) or a known side effect of the drug. Skin testing is sometimes used to disclose sensitivity to certain drugs, especially penicillin. However, a small amount of drug injected intradermally may itself provoke an anaphylactic reaction. If the test dose is not given in a proper intradermal wheal, a reaction may not occur in an allergic patient. Therefore, it is recommended that skin testing for allergy be done only by practitioners with specialty training in this field of medicine.

In dental anesthesia, acute anaphylactic reactions have been reported to local anesthetics, preservatives used in local anesthetics, methohexital, and thiopental. True allergic reactions probably account for less than 1 per cent of all systemic complications associated with local anesthetics. These reactions have occurred more often in the past with procaine than with the local anesthetic agents (lidocaine, mepivacaine) now more commonly used. Methylparaben (methyl-p-hydroxybenzoate), an alkyl ester of p-hydroxybenzoic acid and, therefore, similar to benzoic acid ester local anesthetics (procaine, tetracaine), is used as a preservative in anesthetic carpules of procaine and lidocaine. It has been implicated as the offending agent in allergic reactions when one of these two local anesthetics has been given. Mepivacaine (Carbocaine) is supplied in carpules without methylparaben. Six cases of acute allergic reaction to the ultra-short acting barbiturate, methohexital, have been reported. The first sign of this reaction was sudden onset of hypotension, followed shortly by skin rash, wheezing, cyanosis, sneezing, rhinorrhea, periorbital edema, abdominal cramps, urticaria, and pruritis. The series of events occurred in patients anesthetized with methohexital, nitrous oxide-oxygen, with or without 2 per cent lidocaine with 1:100,000 epinephrine.

The life-threatening aspects of acute anaphylaxis include the effects of massive release of vasoactive substances on pulmonary and vascular smooth muscle, and edema of airway soft tissues, epiglottis, larynx, trachea, bronchi, and bronchioles. Vasodilatation with peripheral pooling, impaired venous return, and reduced cardiac output cause hypotension and inadequate organ perfusion. Bronchospasm and edema of the airway produce hypoxia or anoxia. Termination in cardiac arrest occurs rapidly if treatment is not instituted immediately. Epinephrine (0.3 to 0.5 ml of 1:1000 solution) is given subcutaneously unless full-blown shock is present, in which case it is diluted and given intravenously. Epinephrine acts in at least two ways, by interfering with further mediator release, histamine, kinins, and other vasoactive amines, and by antagonizing the effects of these mediators on end-organ receptors. One hundred per cent oxygen is administered. Additional treatment may be required for hypotension, cardiac arrhythmias, laryngeal edema, or bronchospasm. Observation over several hours and repeated doses of medications may be required. Persistent hives, rash, pruritis, and allergic manifestations may require a several-day course of antihistamines (diphenhydramine 25 to 50 mg 3 to 4 times daily) and steroids (prednisone 5 mg twice daily). Following recovery the patient should be informed of the reaction and the name of the offending drug so that this information can be given to any physician or dentist who provides future treatment.

Malignant Hyperthermia

Recently, a number of cases of rapid rise in body temperature under general anesthesia, often terminating fatally, have been reported in the literature. Identification of patients at risk, prompt recognition of the condition if it occurs, and appropriate treatment of malignant hyperthermia are essential in the modern practice of anesthesia and analgesia.

It has been estimated to occur in 1 in 10,000 anesthetic exposures. Malignant hyperthermia is more common in males, children, teenagers and young adults. It usually occurs during anesthesia with halothane and succinylcholine, but has been reported with nitrous oxide alone. The patient or his family may have a history of localized or diffuse muscle disease, strabismus, ptosis, kyphoscoliosis, spontaneous hernia, generalized muscle weakness, or skeletal muscle atrophy. Susceptible patients and relatives may have an increased serum level of the enzyme creatine phosphokinase (CPK).

Initially, the clinical syndrome of malignant hyperthermia presents as violent fasciculations after administration of succinylcholine, followed by skeletal muscle rigidity including isolated masseter spasm. At this time an initial rise in rectal temperature may be seen, with subsequent rises as fast as 1°F every 5 minutes to as high as 112°F. Decreased pulmonary compliance or chest wall rigidity, tachypnea, mottled cyanosis, and ventricular arrhythmias occur in rapid succession. Arterial blood gas measurements reveal decreased oxygen tension and pH and increased carbon dioxide.

The pathophysiology of malignant hyperthermia is the result of a defect in muscle cell membranes. After exposure to a triggering agent, either uncontrolled release or blocked uptake of calcium ions by the sarcoplasmic reticulum of the muscle cell occurs. Increased free intracellular calcium ions produce massive accelerated muscle cell metabolism with sustained muscular contractions and excessive heat production. The rapid metabolic rate consumes excessive oxygen, produces large amounts of carbon dioxide and hydrogen ions, and causes hypoxia, hypercarbia, and acidosis. Adenosine triphosphate (ATP) is used so rapidly that very little remains to supply energy to transport systems to the cell membrane. As a result, myoglobin, potassium, and phosphate leak out of the cell. Such a process of muscle cell derangement may occur at a low rate in susceptible patients before administration of general anesthesia and could account for the increased serum level of CPK preoperatively in these patients.

Prompt treatment of malignant hyperthermia is required to prevent mortality. Administration of anesthesia is terminated and 100% oxygen given. Dantrolene, 1 to 10 mg per kg, is specific therapy. Rapid cooling of the patient is achieved by use of a cooling blanket, rectal or gastric lavage with iced saline, administration of chilled intravenous fluids, and small doses of chlorpromazine to produce peripheral vasodilatation and prevent shivering. Respiratory exchange is managed by intubation and use of a volume-controlled ventilator to overcome decreased pulmonary compliance. Procainamide or procaine is given (1 g in 500 ml 5 per cent D/W intravenous drip) to promote uptake of free ionic, calcium by the sarcoplasmic reticulum. Lidocaine or other amide type local anesthetics cause release of free calcium and are contraindicated in the treatment of malignant hyperthermia. Metabolic acidosis is corrected by intravenous sodium bicarbonate. Hyperkalemia, caused by excessive release of cellular potassium, may require treatment by infusion of dextrose, insulin, and bicarbonate. Myoglobinuria may lead to acute renal failure. Brain damage may occur secondary to hypoxia. Transfer of the patient to an intensive care unit is indicated as soon as possible.

The mortality rate among reported cases of malignant hyperthermia is up to 70 per cent, but with dantrolene therapy it is substantially reduced.

Bibliography

Aarons EF: What if a patient dies in your office? *Med Econ* 49:195, 1970.

Allen DG, Morris LE: Central nervous system effects of hyperventilation during anaesthesia. *Br J Anaesth* 34:296, 1962.

American Heart Association and National Academy of Sciences—National Research Council: Standards for cardiopulmonary resuscitation (CPR) and emergency cardiac care (ECC). *JAMA* 227 (Suppl.):837, 1974.

American Society of Oral Surgeons Committee on Anesthesia: A.S.O.S. anesthesia morbidity and mortality survey. *J Oral Surg* 32:733, 1974.

Cameron JM, Goldman V, Paul DM: Deaths with dental anesthetics. (Corr.) *Anaesthesia* 26:252, 1971.

Campbell RL, Gregg, JM, Levin KJ: Vasovagal response during oral surgery. J Oral Surg 34:698, 1976.

Comroe JH, Jr, Botelho S: The unreliability of cyanosis in the recognition of arterial anomexia. Am J Med Sci 214:1, 1947.

Courville CB: Asphyxia as a consequence of nitrous oxide anesthesia. Medicine 15:129, 1936.

Driggs RL, O'Day RA: Acute allergic reaction associated with methohexital anesthesia: report of six cases. J Oral Surg 30:906, 1972.

Everett GB, Allen GD: Cardiac asystole following repeated administration of succinylcholine chloride: a case report. J Oral Surg 30:209–211, 1972.

Goldman L, Caldera DL, Nussbaum SR, et al: Multifactorial index of cardiac risk in noncardiac surgical procedures. N Engl J Med 297:845, 1977.

Guildner CW: A comparative study of techniques for opening an airway obstructed by the tongue. J Am Coll Emerg Phys 5:588, 1976.

Guntheroth WG, Abel FL, Mullins GL: The effect of Trendelenburg's position on blood pressure and carotid flow. Surg Gynecol Obstet 119:345, 1964.

Heller ML, Watson TR: The role of preliminary oxygenation prior to induction with high nitrous oxide mixtures: polygraphic PaO_2 study. Anesthesiology 23:219, 1962.

Hickler RB, Vandam LD: Hypertension. Anesthesiology 33:214, 1970.

Katz RL, Bigger JT, Jr: Cardiac arrhythmias during anesthesia and operations. Anesthesiology 33:193, 1970.

Kelman GR, Nunn JF: Clinical recognition of hypoxaemia under fluorescent lamps. Lancet 1:1400, 1966.

Kennedy WF, Bonica JJ, Ward RJ, et al: Cardiorespiratory effects of epinephrine when used in regional anesthesia. Acta Anaesth Scand (Suppl.) 23:320, 1966.

Levine HD, Phillips E: An appraisal of the newer electrocardiographic: correlations in one hundred and fifty consecutive autopsied cases. N Engl J Med 245:833, 1961.

Malach M: Lidocaine for ventricular arrhythmias in acute myocardial infarction. Am J Med Sci 257:52, 1969.

Mendelson CL: Aspiration of stomach contents into the lungs during obstetric anesthesia. Am J Obstet Gynecol 52:191, 1946.

Merin RG: Slow channel inhibitors, anesthetics and cardiovascular function. Anesthesiology 55:198, 1981.

Meyer RA, Allen GD: Blood volume studies in oral surgery: II. Postoperative complications and the state of hydration. J Oral Surg 26:800, 1969.

Michenfelder JD, Fowler WS, Theye RA: CO_2 levels and pulmonary shunting in anesthetized man. J Appl Physiol 21:1471, 1966.

Parker CW: Drug allergy. N Engl J Med 292:511, 732, and 457, 1975.

Parks CR: Operative fluid shifts: a review of the literature. Anesth Analg 45:495, 1966.

Saidman LJ, Eger EI, II: Effects of nitrous oxide and of narcotic premedication on the alveolar concentration of halothane required for anesthesia. Anesthesiology 25:302, 1964.

Shires T, Jackson DE: Postoperative salt tolerance. Arch Surg 84:703, 1962.

Steen PA: Myocardial reinfarction after anesthesia and surgery. JAMA 239:2566, 1978.

Tolas AG, Allen GD: Propranolol in prevention of cardiac arrhythmia. J Oral Surg 28:181, 1970.

Tolas AG, Allen GD, Ward RJ, et al: Monitoring during anesthesia. Oral Surg 19:317, 1965.

Verne D: Water and electrolyte balance: a review. J Oral Surg 23:609, 1965.

CHAPTER 8

Gases

Physical laws govern the behavior of gases. An understanding of this behavior is helpful in the proper use and administration of gaseous agents for analgesia and anesthesia.

The terms *vapor* and *gas* are not readily distinguishable from each other. However, vapor generally refers to the gaseous state of a substance which at room temperature and atmospheric pressure is a liquid. Ether or halothane vapors are examples. A gas is a substance which at room temperature and pressure exists only in the gaseous state. Liquefaction is impossible since the temperature of the room is above the *critical temperature* of the gas. The critical temperature is that degree to which a gas must be cooled before it can be liquified by pressure. A gas such as nitrous oxide is stored as a liquid under high pressure in cylinders. For oxygen it is −116°C at 2000 psi and for nitrous oxide, 36.5°C at 750 psi.

Critical pressure of a gas is that pressure to which the gas must be compressed before it liquifies.

A gas always occupies its entire container and has an inherent tendency to expand. The volume of a gas varies inversely with the pressure to which it is subjected, the temperature remaining constant (*Boyle's law*).

When a gas is heated, molecular movement increases and the gas tends to expand. *Charles' Law* states that at a constant pressure, the volume of a gas is directly proportional to its temperature. If this expansion is prevented, the number of molecular impacts on the walls of the container increases and the pressure rises.

At the same temperature and pressure the same number of molecules of any gas occupies the same volume (*Avogadro's law*). The pressure of a gas is a measure of the molecular bombardment on each unit area of the wall of its container in unit time. In a mixture of gases each gas exerts the same pressure which it would if it alone occupied the container (*Dalton's law*). The pressure each gas exerts is called its *partial pressure*, and the total pressure of the mixture is the sum of the partial pressures of the constituent gases. Each constituent gas in a mixture exerts the same proportion of the total pressure as its volume is of the total volume. The principles of the effects of temperature and pressure are of concern in preparing anesthetic gases for storage in tanks and their administration from these tanks (Fig. 8.1).

Gases dissolve in liquids. The amount of a gas which dissolves in a given liquid is directly proportional to the pressure of the gas (*Henry's law*). The higher the temperature of the liquid, the less the amount of gas that goes into solution. At any given temperature and pressure a gas dissolves in a given liquid only to the extent that when no further gas dissolves in the liquid a state of equilibrium exists between the gas and liquid. The liquid is then a *saturated solution* with respect to the gas dissolved. The gas in solution exerts the same *tension* as the partial pressure of the gas over the liquid with which it is in equilibrium.

Diffusion or intermolecular mingling can take place through a permeable membrane. Diffusion is a molecular movement and should not be confused with movement in bulk, for which some external

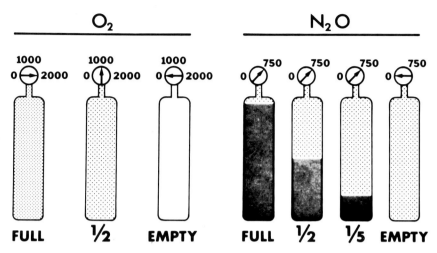

O_2

N_2O

FULL   ½   EMPTY   FULL   ½   ⅕   EMPTY

Figure 8.1. The nitrous oxide cylinder registers full until more than four-fifths empty because it is stored mainly in liquid form.

force such as gravity must be applied. Diffusion is aided by differences in pressure or tension. If a gas exists on either side of a membrane, the direction of its diffusion is determined not by any difference in amount but by any difference in the partial pressures which it exerts on either side of that membrane. The same consideration applies to a gas diffusing into or through a liquid. Diffusion also depends on molecular weight, and the rates of diffusion of gases at identical partial pressures are inversely proportional to the square roots of their molecular weights (*Graham's law*). Thus, oxygen (mol. wt. 32) diffuses more rapidly than carbon dioxide (mol. wt. 44), and, despite the greater solubility of carbon dioxide, the pressure gradient of CO_2 is less; inadequate ventilation may maintain an adequate PaO_2 but not eliminate carbon dioxide.

Under the same conditions of temperature and pressure, gases dissolve to different extents in any liquid. The volume of gas which dissolves in a unit volume of solvent, measured under the conditions of temperature and pressure at which solution occurs, is termed Ostwald's *solubility coefficient*. For example, when the blood solubility of an inhalation anesthetic agent is high (e.g., methoxyflu-

rane), alveolar concentration does not equilibrate rapidly with inhaled concentration. As so much of the agent is taken up from the alveolar air and dissolved in the blood, the agent takes a long time to reach equilibration. Once equilibration is achieved, alveolar tension rises rapidly. Induction of anesthesia is therefore slow. The reverse is true for gases of low blood solubility (e.g., nitrous oxide).

A clinical application of gas solubility is seen in nitrous oxide uptake and elimination during anesthesia and analgesia. Nitrous oxide is 15 times as soluble as nitrogen and 100 times as soluble as oxygen in blood.

At the conclusion of nitrous oxide administration, excretion occurs so rapidly that the percentage of nitrous oxide in the alveolus is increased, and consequently there is a fall in the alveolar oxygen percentage. The partial pressures of oxygen and nitrogen are thus lowered, and hypoxia can develop. It is the phenomenon of *diffusion anoxia*. This accounts for the routine of administering 100 per cent oxygen at the conclusion of nitrous oxide-oxygen anesthesia.

The uptake of nitrous oxide can be hastened by preoxygenation. If oxygen is given for 120 seconds, the nitrogen in the lung is eliminated. The greater solubility

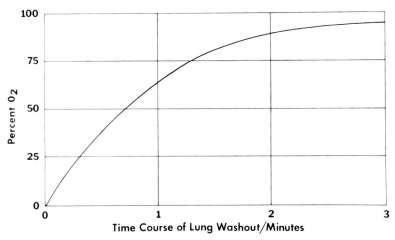

Figure 8.2. The graph shows the rapid washout of nitrogen from the lung when 100 per cent oxygen is inhaled.

factor of nitrous oxide over oxygen as opposed to nitrogen results in a more rapid uptake of nitrous oxide by the blood and in consequence increases the speed of induction (Fig. 8.2).

UPTAKE OF ANESTHETIC GASES AND VAPORS

The general laws governing diffusion, solubility, and the relations of volume, pressure, and temperature apply to the uptake of anesthetic gases and volatile anesthetic agents (vapors). Uptake of inhalation agents is dependent on function of four factors: apparatus and system, the lungs, the circulation, and the tissues. The uptake follows the following pattern:

Essentially, the apparatus delivers the concentrations selected. The higher the concentration and flow rate, the more rapidly alveolar equilibrium is reached. In a nonrebreathing system the patient breathes the same concentration delivered by the machine. In a circle system, there is some rebreathing which tends to dilute the concentrations during the induction.

The alveolar concentration in the lungs is directly related to the concentration delivered and the ventilation of the lungs, and inversely related to the rate at which the agent leaves the alveoli to enter the circulation. The molecules of inhalation agent diffuse across the alveolar membrane into the pulmonary circulation almost instantaneously.

The difference in tension of a gas in the alveolus and in the venous blood returning to the lungs determines the actual tension gradient. The speed at which equilibrium between alveolar and blood tension is achieved depends not only on how much gas the tissues extract during the circulation time, but also on the solubility of the particular agent in blood. The blood/gas *partition coefficient* is a term used to describe how a gas or vapor is distributed at equilibrium between these two media. For example, if the concentration of an anesthetic in blood was 2 volumes per cent and was in equilibrium with a concentration in the alveolus of 1 volume per cent, the blood/gas partition coefficient would be 2. The higher the partition coefficient, the greater the agent's solubility in blood.

The greater the agent's solubility in blood, the longer it takes to reach equilibrium between alveolar tension and arterial tension. This increases induction and recovery times, as maximal effect of an inhalation agent is related to the establishment of equilibrium between arterial and alveolar tension of the agent.

The rate of blood flow through pulmonary capillaries depends on cardiac output. An increase in cardiac output means that a greater amount of vapor or gas is removed from the alveolus, a fall in alveolar concentration occurs causing blood and tissue tensions to fall, and the plane of anesthesia lightens.

Uptake of inhalation agents by the tissue depends on the tissue tension gradient, tissue/blood partition coefficient, and tissue blood supply. Once equilibrium is reached between the tissue and blood tensions, saturation has occurred and no further uptake occurs in that particular tissue. The tissue/blood partition coefficient determines the rapidity with which inhalation agents saturate tissues, the least soluble reaching equilibrium and maximum effect earliest. Most inhalation agents have similar blood and tissue solubility. An exception is halothane, which has a solubility in muscle and brain three times that in blood. Adipose tissue, which has a special affinity for inhalation agents as they are all lipid-soluble, continues uptake throughout an anesthetic and significantly slows recovery.

Uptake by tissues is dependent on their vascular supply. The brain and other vital organs (heart, liver, kidneys) with rich vascular supply initially receive a high proportion of inhalation agent. Later there is a redistribution of the agent as it comes into equilibrium with the other body tissues. Relatively large amounts must be given during induction because of the recirculation of the agent to tissues other than the vital organs. As these depots (muscle, fat) become saturated (*secondary saturation*), smaller amounts are required to maintain the effect. Thus in administering nitrous oxide-oxygen inhalation sedation it is of value to give quantity as well as a high percentage during induction so that a steady state can be rapidly reached.

Emergence from inhalation anesthesia or analgesia involves all the factors mentioned in uptake operating in reverse. Recovery is in fact a re-equilibration of the body with atmospheric air, and it is more rapid when secondary saturation of body tissues has not had time to occur.

TECHNICAL ASPECTS: GAS PREPARATION AND STORAGE

Oxygen and nitrous oxide are prepared, purified, and stored under pressure in metal cylinders. Oxygen is stored in the gaseous state, while nitrous oxide is stored in the liquid state. Various sizes of cylinders are available for use, depending on whether they are attached to a portable apparatus or kept in a central gas supply. The large G cylinders contain 5,300 liters of oxygen, and 13,830 liters of nitrous oxide when converted to gaseous form. In the manufacture of nitrous oxide great care is taken to remove all water vapor before the gas is compressed into cylinders. The cooling which inevitably takes place when the cylinder valve is opened is sufficient to freeze any residual water vapor in the nitrous oxide and block the exit valve.

The control of the flow of gas under high pressure from cylinders presents problems. A very small movement of the tap produces a large alteration in gas flow. For any given setting of the tap the gas flow falls with the drop in pressure inside the cylinder. If a constant flow rate is to occur with variation in cylinder pressure, the cylinder tap requires frequent adjustment, a bothersome task. Placing a reducing valve between the cylinder and flowmeter overcomes these difficulties (Fig. 8.3). In addition, adjustment of flow is more accurate, and the valve prevents excess wear in the flow meters. A reducing valve is conventionally placed on the cylinder itself, eliminating the need for cumbersome high pressure tubing between cylinder and valve. Cylinder pressure is no longer a problem until the tank is empty, as the gases leave the reducing valve at the constant set low pressure (usually about 45 psi).

Flow meters are incorporated to deliver

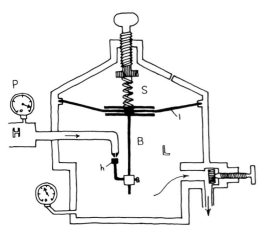

Figure 8.3. A two-stage reducing valve rather than the simple reducing valve illustrated is used to limit the gas pressure to the flow meter to about 50 psi.

accurately the desired flow rates of gases from the cylinders to the patient. Flow rate settings in liters per minute are provided on the face of the flow meter. The interdependence of flow rate, size of orifice, and pressure difference on either side of the orifice is useful in the construction of the main types of flow meters.

The dry flow meter has three main variations:

1. Rod. Found on older Heidbrink machines mounted vertically with upper end of rod indicating flow. Accuracy range is approximately ±7 per cent.

2. Rotameter. Drawn glass tubes, increasing in diameter from bottom to top, with frictionless, freely rotating aluminum bobbin indicating flow. Tubes are vertically positioned and are the most accurate of the flow meters (±2 per cent). Should be used only for the gas indicated, as at low flows the annular space is equivalent to a tube and viscosity of the gas determines flow, while at high flows the annular space is equivalent to an orifice and density of the gas determines flow. This is the type of flow meter found on most quality anesthesia machines.

3. Ball and tube. Pressure of gas pushes the ball up an inclined plane. Turbulence about ball and friction of ball against tube are factors in movement. Tube is ground

with the desired taper. The usual accuracy is ±5 per cent. This type of flow meter is generally utilized for quality analgesia machines.

Conventionally, all gas cylinders, tubing, wall outlets, and flow meters conform to a *standard color code* to minimize confusion or errors in administering the proper gases.

Standard color coding of gas cylinders is as follows:

Oxygen—green
Nitrous oxide—blue
Compressed air—pink
Carbon dioxide—gray
Cyclopropane—orange

Each wall outlet is constructed to allow plug-in by only one type gas line for safety (Figs. 8.4 to 8.6).

OXYGEN

Physical Properties

Oxygen is a tasteless, colorless, odorless gas, occurring in 20.9 per cent concentration in air. Its specific gravity is 1.105 (air: 1.000) and its molecular weight is 32. Oxygen is prepared commercially by fractional distillation of liquid air and stored in gaseous form in green-colored cylinders at a pressure of about 2000 psi.

Oxygen cannot be ignited, but its presence aids combustion. Oxygen under pressure may cause an explosion in the presence of oil or grease, so these substances are not used on reducing valves, cylinder outlets, or wall outlets.

Clinical Use of Oxygen

There are three principal factors responsible for carrying sufficient oxygen to the tissues. These are: (1) the blood flow (indirectly related to cardiac output), (2) the hemoglobin concentration of the blood, and (3) the oxygen saturation of the blood (oxygen dissociation curve). Any one of these factors may be reduced by as much as one-third without causing significant problems in a healthy patient.

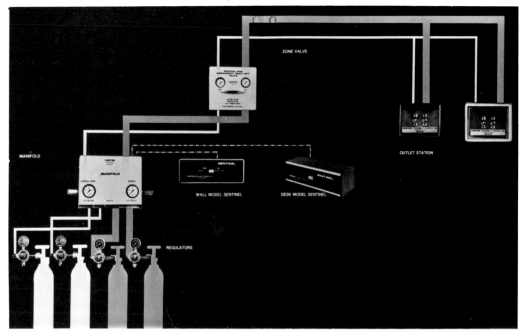

Figure 8.4. The diameter index safety system (DISS) will not allow connection of the wrong gases to the machine. This does not preclude connection of the wrong pipes to the outlet, but the use of ½-inch and 1-inch pipes prevents this error. (Courtesy Porter Instrument Company.)

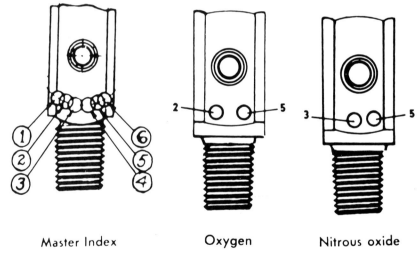

Master Index   Oxygen   Nitrous oxide

Figure 8.5. The pin index safety system (PISS) prevents connection of the wrong cylinder to the yoke for any particular gas.

However, if each of them is reduced by this amount the effect may be lethal.

It is often erroneously assumed that an anesthetized patient will be adequately oxygenated if he breathes a concentration of oxygen similar to that present in room air (20 to 21 per cent). However, recent work has shown that for a variety of reasons the anesthetized patient requires more oxygen than the conscious patient breathing room air. Following administration of an analgesic or anesthetic agent the available oxygen in the inspired air should be increased to at least 30 per cent

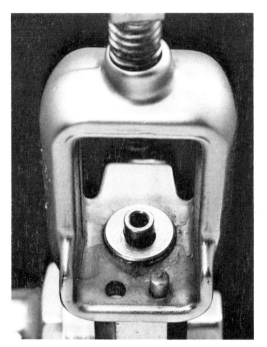

Figure 8.6. The pins can be broken on the yoke which allows connection of the wrong cylinder.

to compensate for the inadequate ventilation, a normal concomitant of anesthesia and analgesia.

One factor tending to lower arterial oxygen tension in anesthetized patients is hypoventilation caused by depressant effect of the anesthetic agents. The deficient tidal exchange causes dead space gases to be moved to and fro with inadequate amounts of these fresh gases reaching the lung alveoli. Hypoventilation leads not only to lowered arterial oxygen tension, but to increased carbon dioxide tension with its potential hazards.

Oxygenation of venous blood is one of the main functions of the lungs. The commonest failure of oxygenation is that inspired air and pulmonary blood flow do not meet together in the correct proportions. The *ventilation-perfusion ratio* is the relationship between the amount of inspired air and the amount of blood reaching a single lung alveolus. In the normal lungs of a conscious patient, the overall effect, although far from precise, is to maintain a fairly constant oxygen

saturation of arterial blood. During anesthesia the phenomenon of *venous admixture* becomes important in lowering the arterial oxygen tension. Venous admixture refers to that portion of blood leaving the right side of the heart that fails to become oxygenated. Venous admixture includes both an *anatomical shunt* and *maldistribution* or physiological shunt. Anatomical shunt is that portion of the blood which passes through the Thebesian and bronchial vascular systems to nourish the heart and lungs. The blood is not oxygenated, but it arrives at the left side of the heart to dilute the oxygenated blood returning from the lung alveoli. In a conscious normal patient, the anatomical shunt represents 2 per cent of the total cardiac output. Maldistribution or physiological shunt (V_A/Q abnormality, where V_A = alveolar ventilation and Q = cardiac output) is that portion of pulmonary blood flow which passes through *relatively* underventilated lung, or may be present if blood does not flow through ventilated lung. If atelectasis is present, that portion of the lung will be *totally* underventilated. Under general anesthesia the total venous admixture (or shunt) may rise to 10 to 15 per cent. It is greater during controlled ventilation than when spontaneous respiration is used. Further, inspired oxygen requirements tend to rise proportionally with the length of the anesthetic, corresponding to progressive development of small miliary atelectatic areas in the lungs (see Table 1.3).

General anesthesia does have a role in raising the arterial oxygen tension. Unconsciousness lowers the metabolic rate, and total body oxygen consumption may decrease by 15 to 20 per cent. If the patient breathes a mixture of nitrous oxide and oxygen, the concentration effect increases the oxygen tension of the blood during the period of uptake. If hyperventilation is used during anesthesia, the alveolar oxygen tension can be increased.

Unless hyperventilation is used, however, the effects of the usual hypoventilation caused by anesthetic agents and the effect of pulmonary shunt raise the administered oxygen requirements of the anesthetized patient above 20 per cent. In otherwise healthy patients, without hypoventilation, severe anemia, or reduced cardiac output, 30 per cent oxygen is usually sufficient to maintain arterial oxygen tension above 80 mm Hg, in which case hemoglobin saturation is above 93 per cent.

In conscious inhalation sedation, the oxygen percentage will always be above that of room air. It is given before and after the administration of conscious sedation, as the uptake and elimination of nitrous oxide can be increased due to the relative solubilities in the blood of oxygen and nitrous oxide. Adjustment of nitrous oxide levels following the administration of oxygen is much more rapidly accomplished. Preoxygenation of the patient is also a useful technique to reduce atmospheric pollution with nitrous oxide.

At the conclusion of the operation, the administration of 100% oxygen will prevent diffusion anoxia and also aid in the more rapid removal of nitrous oxide. Diffusion anoxia is a condition that theoretically occurs in general anesthesia. The rapid elimination of nitrous oxide from the blood into alveolus at the conclusion of the operation results in a high partial pressure of nitrous oxide in the alveolus; thus the oxygen percentage in the alveolus falls.

All local or general anesthetics and sedative and narcotic drugs have potential for causing severe respiratory depression or respiratory arrest. Since the dentist is using one or more of these drugs in his daily practice, oxygen must be readily available in his operating and recovery rooms. The administration of oxygen is universal treatment for nearly all medical and anesthetic emergencies. Facilities are required for administration of oxygen under positive pressure to the patient who has severely depressed respiration or has stopped breathing.

An anesthetic or analgesic machine is an ideal apparatus for oxygen administration as it generally has flush valves to provide large amounts of oxygen rapidly and a reservoir bag to provide artificial ventilation as required. Portable oxygen tanks and masks are satisfactory providing the patient is breathing spontaneously. Administration of oxygen through a Robertshaw resuscitator or other similar resuscitative device allows the dentist to provide artificial ventilation as needed and should be available in the absence of an anesthetic or analgesic machine.

NITROUS OXIDE

Physical Properties

Nitrous oxide is a sweet-smelling, colorless, nonirritating gas. It is heavier (specific gravity 1.5) than air. This has practical significance for the anesthetist as nitrous oxide can be allowed to flow over the face of a resistant child with the mask held out of sight above the patient's head until consciousness is lost.

Commercial nitrous oxide is prepared by gently heating ammonium nitrate to 240°C. The gas is then compressed in stages to remove impurities such as ammonia, water, and nitric oxide. Nitric oxide is the major impurity and has caused some fatalities due to pneumonitis and pulmonary edema. As it is lighter than nitrous oxide, it is evolved first from a gas cylinder, and it is an irritating and pungent gas. Thus the simple precaution of smelling the gas before delivery to the patient avoids a potential hazard.

Nitrous oxide diffuses through rubber in small quantities, which can be compensated for during anesthesia by using high flow rates. In addition nitrous oxide will pass through the wall of the cuff on an endotracheal tube. Pressure in the cuff rises and can cause damage to the tracheal mucous membrane.

The blood/gas solubility coefficient of nitrous oxide is 0.47. Since it is only slightly soluble in blood relative to other anesthetic agents it very rapidly reaches equilibrium between alveolar and arterial tensions, accounting for rapidity of induction and short recovery time in anesthesia. Nitrous oxide must be given continuously to counteract this evanescent effect. Nitrous oxide is 15 times as soluble in blood as is nitrogen, but has 100 times the solubility of oxygen in blood.

The clinical application of this physical feature is seen in the use of preoxygenation to speed induction of anesthesia into nitrous oxide and oxygen. The converse is noted when 100 per cent oxygen is given at the conclusion of an operation with nitrous oxide-oxygen, to avoid diffusion hypoxia.

Nitrous oxide is neither inflammable nor explosive, unless exposed to oil or grease under pressure as warned on all reducing valves and wall outlets. However, it will support combustion of other agents even in the absence of oxygen, since its decomposition products are nitrogen and oxygen (Fig. 8.7).

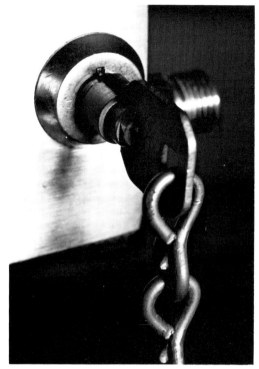

Figure 8.7.   Nitrous oxide-oxygen conscious sedation machines may be locked to prevent use by unauthorized personnel or the gases may be stored in a locked cupboard.

Uptake and Distribution

The uptake of nitrous oxide is rapid and may equal 1 to 2 liters per minute initially before the vascular organs (brain, heart, kidneys, liver) become saturated. After 10 to 15 minutes these organs reach equilibrium with arterial tension and uptake decreases to 300 to 500 ml per minute, mostly in muscle. After an hour of anesthesia, uptake is about 100 to 200 ml per minute, partly being absorbed into fat and partly to replace loss by diffusion through skin.

Uptake of nitrous oxide is facilitated initially by using high flow rates and high concentrations. Flow rates of at least 8 to 10 liters per minute are necessary in order to flush out the anesthetic system, particularly when a circle system is used, to reduce dilution by residual air in the lungs, and to replace alveolar gases lost by uptake (Fig. 8.8). Prior denitrogenation by breathing 100 per cent oxygen for 2 to

3 minutes also facilitates uptake of nitrous oxide by removing nitrogen from alveolar air and arterial blood. Further, the higher the concentration of the inspired gas, the more rapid the rise of the alveolar concentration toward that inspired. For example, it takes 4 to 5 minutes to reach 80 per cent of the inspired concentration in the alveoli when 1 per cent nitrous oxide is breathed, but only 1 minute when 100 per cent nitrous oxide is inspired (Fig. 8.9).

One hundred per cent concentration of nitrous oxide can be given for 1 to 1½ minutes following denitrogenation before hypoxia occurs. Since normal ventilation removes 85 per cent of the original gases within the lung in less than 1½ minutes, it is obvious that inspiration of 100 per cent nitrous oxide for longer than this results in hypoxia. The clinical practice of administering 100 per cent nitrous oxide for speedy induction of anesthesia has been condemned as unnecessary and dan-

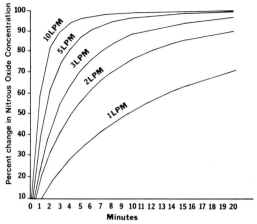

Figure 8.8. The rate of change in nitrous oxide-oxygen concentration in a circle system with increasing flow rates is well demonstrated in a study which was performed by Eger, E. I., II in 1960. It demonstrated the need for high flows at induction.

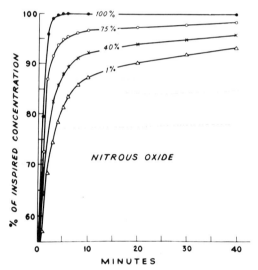

Figure 8.9. The graphs indicate the approach of alveolar nitrous oxide concentration to that in the inspired gases. The higher the concentrations of nitrous oxide breathed, the more rapidly alveolar arterial nitrous oxide reaches equilibrium with that inspired. The inspired concentrations are indicated on the respective curves. (Reprinted with permission from Eger, E. I., II.: Factors affecting the rapidity of alteration of nitrous oxide concentration in a circle system. *Anesthesiology* 21:348, 1960.)

gerous (Fig. 8.10). A double blind study compared 100 per cent nitrous oxide with oxygenated mixtures of nitrous oxide in

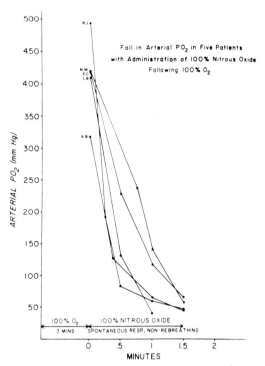

Figure 8.10. The graph shows the rapid fall in arterial oxygen tension which occurs when 100 per cent nitrous oxide is breathed following 100 per cent oxygen inhalation. (Reprinted with permission from Heller, M. L., and Watson, T. R.: The role of preliminary oxygenation prior to induction with high nitrous oxide mixtures. *Anesthesiology* 23:219, 1962.)

their rapidity of induction. Expert clinicians could not determine differences in speed of induction. As high percentages of nitrous oxide can be given, and it has a high solubility relative to nitrogen, large amounts of nitrous oxide are taken up during induction. Thus, a minute volume of 5 liters per minute can be increased by as much as 1 liter per minute, to give an effective minute volume of 6 liters per minute. This is known as the "concentration effect" and is another feature which accounts for the rapid induction of anesthesia or analgesia with nitrous oxide (Figs. 8.11 and 8.12).

In combination with this effect during induction is the "second gas effect." If an adjuvant gas vapor is given with nitrous oxide, the increase of effective ventilation results in increased uptake of the adju-

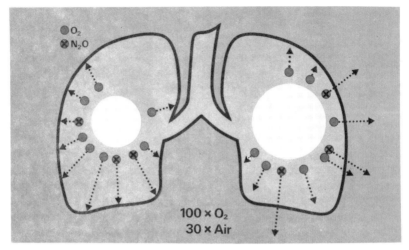

Figure 8.11. The representative lungs show the concentration effect in nitrous oxide uptake due to its higher solubility in blood, as compared to oxygen.

vant. Thus, induction of anesthesia with other agents is aided by concomitant administration of nitrous oxide.

The elimination of nitrous oxide from the body is a mirror image of its uptake, with output high during the first few minutes and continually decreasing amounts lost thereafter. During the first few minutes of output, diffusion anoxia may occur as large amounts of nitrous oxide leave the blood and dilute the oxygen concentration in inspired air reaching the alveoli. Adequate oxygenation is assured by administering 100 per cent oxygen for a few minutes following termination of nitrous oxide.

Pharmacology

Many of the effects previously attributed to nitrous oxide are the result of its use in hypoxic or anoxic concentrations. During anesthesia the oxygen in nitrous oxide is not available for metabolic needs. Cyanosis, jactitations, convulsions, respiratory arrest, decreased mental acuity, idiocy, cerebral edema and death have all been observed during or following a nitrous oxide anesthetic.

Studies in hyperbaric chambers have confirmed that nitrous oxide is an anesthetic agent. The development of anesthe-sia with a mean minimum anesthetic concentration of 104 per cent at sea level pressure accords well with the theoretical concentration calculated from the minimum anesthetic concentration (MAC) and the oil/gas coefficient (OG). Thus, MAC $\times$ OG = K(143). MAC = 143/1.4 $\times$ atmospheric pressure, and approximates to 100 per cent.

Because of its lack of potency nitrous oxide is a relatively safe agent when administered with adequate oxygen. Supplementation with other agents to preclude the need for hypoxic techniques has become established in modern anesthetic practice.

The most significant effects of nitrous oxide administered with adequate oxygen are on the central nervous system. The analgesic effects of nitrous oxide on painful stimuli and other modalities of sensation have been objectively shown and are of major importance in inhalation analgesia in dentistry. Short term memory is affected, given an amnesic effect. Euphoria is frequent. During induction with nitrous oxide, as the other sensory functions are reduced, the patient's hearing predominates, with even minor sounds greatly amplified. Extraneous noise is obviously detrimental during induction of anesthesia.

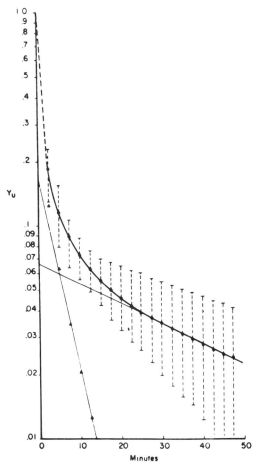

Figure 8.12. The graph is a composite of results for five subjects, and the range is indicated by the bars. Alveolar concentration of nitrous oxide rapidly approaches that of the inspired concentration. At $Y_u = 1$, the alveolar concentration is 0, at $Y_u = 0.1$, the alveolar concentration is already 90 per cent of that inspired. (Reprinted with permission from Salanitre, E., Rackow, H., Greene, L. T., Klonymus, D., and Epstein, R. M.: Uptake and excretion of subanesthetic concentrations of nitrous oxide in man. *Anesthesiology* 23:814, 1962.)

Nitrous oxide used in 70 per cent concentration is more effective than narcotics in reducing the minimum anesthetic concentration (MAC) of other principal anesthetic agents (e.g., halothane). There, 70 per cent nitrous oxide is usually administered in general anesthesia to reduce the amount of the more potent agents required and reduce cardiovascular and respiratory depression from these agents.

Nitrous oxide itself has little effect on the cardiovascular system of an adequately ventilated patient, though it has a vasopressor effect when used with oxygen; but, if it is added to halothane-oxygen anesthesia, nitrous oxide produces cardiorespiratory depression (Fig. 8.13).

Respiration is not significantly altered by nitrous oxide. Secretions in the oral cavity, pharynx, or lungs are not stimulated and the sense of smell is depressed.

Profound muscle relaxation does not occur with nitrous oxide. Muscular rigidity or muscle spasm is seldom seen except during hypoxia.

Toxicity

Repeated exposure to nitrous oxide-oxygen sedation when used for recreational purposes will cause neurological deficits. Several dentists who presented with distal numbness of limbs and hypoactive reflexes and who felt something like an electric shock when the neck was flexed were found to have used nitrous oxide-oxygen daily for pleasure. The damaging effect of nitrous oxide on nervous tissue is related to subacute combined degeneration of the cord, a sequel of pernicious anemia. Nitrous oxide will oxidize cobalt. Vitamin B_{12} formation requires cobalt as

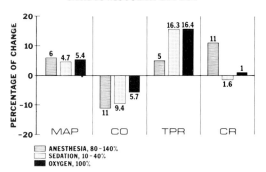

Figure 8.13. Comparative cardiovascular effects of nitrous oxide anesthesia, nitrous oxide-oxygen conscious sedation, and 100 per cent oxygen developed from several studies illustrates the minimal cardiovascular effects developed by conscious sedation with nitrous oxide-oxygen.

a co-factor of the enzyme methionine synthase. Six hours of exposure to nitrous oxide results in 3 days' suppression of vitamin B_{12} production. This toxic effect of nitrous oxide in man has been shown to be reversible. In rats nitrous oxide will significantly inactivate methionine synthase at 2500 ppm but not at 500 ppm. Thus a dose-response relationship has been developed which may indicate levels to which rooms should be scavenged for nitrous oxide; 400 ppm would be a safe mean level, with 200 ppm in the operating zone. Staff in unscavenged operating rooms have normal serum methionine levels, indicating that either inhibition is not occurring or diet will compensate. The toxic effect of nitrous oxide in man has been found to be reversible.

There have been isolated reports of malignant hyperpyrexia occurring in dental patients who only received nitrous oxide-oxygen. It is not a toxic effect of the gas, however.

Prolonged administration (over 48 hours) of nitrous oxide depresses bone marrow. Originally, this occurred during its use as a sedative for anterior poliomyelitis victims. Treatment of leukemia patients with prolonged nitrous oxide inhalation has caused reduction in white cell counts and sedation but no increase in longevity. During the relatively short term use of nitrous oxide for anesthesia or analgesia, none of these effects has been reported.

Chronic Exposure to Trace Contaminants in the Operatory

Over the past decade, there have been repeated reports that chronic exposure to trace contaminants of anesthetic gases in the atmosphere of the dental operatory or operating room is harmful. The original reports noted an increased morbidity in Russian anesthesiologists. Subsequent studies were performed elsewhere and implied a teratogenetic effect of anesthetic agents. Abortions were noted to be more common in personnel exposed to operating room gases. Naturally, the gases suspected were nitrous oxide and the volatile anesthetic agents. Note should be made, however, that other agents in the operating room atmosphere are more toxic than any of the routine anesthetic agents. Review of the studies on increased sterility and abortion in operating room personnel would suggest that statistically there is no significant difference between personnel subjected to stress and those who are exposed to anesthetic agents in trace amounts.

Several animal studies, both with nitrous oxide and volatile anesthetic agents, would indicate that exposure of a unique strain of rats to massive doses of anesthetic agent can result in teratogenetic effects and changes in the cerebral cortex.

It is extremely difficult to extrapolate such data from animals to humans. The level of exposure is massive in relation to the size of the animal, duration of exposure, and degree of exposure. The unique species involved in the studies could be a major factor in the development of the problems.

The original retrospective study of anesthesiologists indicated a greater incidence of specific diseases in anesthesiologists. The later prospective study failed to confirm these data. Indeed it was found that anesthesiologists exposed to anesthetic gases had a greater life expectancy than other physicians, except in regard to an increased incidence of suicide. The early studies showing changes in psychomotor performance in volunteers exposed to trace contaminants of nitrous oxide-oxygen, halothane, or enflurane indicated an impairment of performance. Two subsequent studies have failed to confirm these data.

The recent study conducted for the American Dental Association and reported in 1980 would indicate many more problems occurring in dentists and dental assistants than have been previously reported among anesthesiologists. The study has been subject to criticism, as epidemiologists consider the study to have been badly structured. In the study there was an attempt to determine a dose-response relationship. Dentists should exhibit more problems than the assistants; however, the assistants with probably much less exposure report a much greater incidence of problems. The percentage increase of neurological deficit in male dentists was 70%, while the assistants reported a 163% increase. The male dentist shows no increase in cancer, whereas the assistants report a 90% increase in cancer. The male dentist shows a 22% increase in kidney disease, whereas the assistant shows a 73% increase. These figures suggest either an astounding male-female difference to the response to nitrous oxide trace contamination or a more enthusiastic reporting of problems by the assistants, who may well be exposed for a briefer period.

Epidemiological criticisms of the methodology are: reliance on memory; the fact that some dentists have retired; and the possible financial advantages to complainants of problems. The response rates of personnel indicate that those with less exposure are less likely to respond, especially when the majority of the questions are considered to be loaded. The end points of the study are gross, abortion and malformation, and there is a lack of specificity. As regards mortality, there is no correlation with age, sex, the accuracy of the cause of death, comparative grouping, and the cooperation of those reporting. For cancer, there is no selectivity of comparisons and there is lack of specificity in reporting the type of cancer.

At present, it would seem to indicate that there is little evidence that real danger exists to the operator from chronic exposure to trace amounts of anesthetic agents. There is, however, technology available to reduce the level of contamination, and it would be perhaps of value for the dentist to consider at this time use of such equipment. The regulations posed by the regulating government agency call for more stringent regulation of the dentist than of the operating room. The facts currently available do not warrant such stringency. The current concept is that the dentist should consider the problem and decide if his circumstances warrant an improvement in nitrous oxide and anesthetic hygiene, and whether to use specific equipment to reduce contamination. A consideration in this regard may well be the attitude of the female assistants in the office. Their partial awareness of the problem and the general prevailing attitude of the public to pollution are factors to be considered in the use of antipollutant devices, even before legislation is enacted.

Clinical Applications in General Anesthesia

Nitrous oxide occupies an important role in general anesthesia. Because of its analgesic properties and lack of major cardiovascular or respiratory depression, it is usually included in inhalation anesthetic mixtures to reduce the requirements (MAC) of other, more potent agents. Nitrous oxide is not a potent anesthetic agent and can produce analgesia and amnesia in most patients. Stage III, plane 1 of general anesthesia may be reached in some patients using adequate oxygen. In many others, however, it is impossible to attain adequate surgical anesthesia, even for single tooth extractions, without introducing hypoxic mixtures or supplementing with a more potent agent. Because of appreciation of the hazards of hypoxia, the latter method is the one used in modern dental anesthesia.

Bibliography

ADA Ad Hoc Committee on Trace Anesthetic: A potential health hazard in dentistry. *J Am Dent Assoc* 95:750, 1977.

Bruce DL, Bach MH, Arbitt J: Trace anesthetic effects on perceptual cognitive and motor skills. *Anesthesiology* 40:45, 1974.

Campbell EJM, Nunn JF, Peckett BW: A comparison of artificial ventilation and spontaneous respiration with particular reference to ventilation-blood flow relationships. *Br J Anaesth* 30:166, 1958.

Cohen EN, Bellville JW, Brown BW: Anesthesia, pregnancy and miscarriage. *Anesthesiology* 35:343, 1971.

Cohen EN, Brown BL, Wu ML, et al: Occupational disease in dentistry and chronic exposure to trace anesthetic gases. *J Am Dent Assoc* 101:21, 1980.

Courville CB: Narcosis and cerebral anoxia. *Anesth Analg* 34:61, 1955.

Eisele JH, Smith NT: Cardiovascular effects of 40% nitrous oxide in man. *Anesth Analg* 51:956, 1972.

Fink BR: Diffusion anoxia. *Anesthesiology* 16:511, 1955.

Hayden J Jr, Allen GD, Butler LA, et al: An evaluation of prolonged nitrous oxide-oxygen sedation in rats. *J Am Dent Assoc* 89:1374, 1974.

Heller ML, Watson TR: The role of preliminary oxygenation prior to induction with high nitrous oxide mixtures: polygraphic PaO_2 study. *Anesthesiology* 23:219, 1962.

Hornbein TF, Eger EI, Winter PM, et al: The minimal alveolar concentration of nitrous oxide in man. *Anesth Analg* 61:553, 1982.

Lassen HCA, Henriksen E, Neukirch F, et al: Treatment of tetanus. *Lancet* 1:527, 1956.

Layzer RB, Fishman RA, Shafer JA: Neuropathy following abuse of nitrous oxide. *Neurology* 28:504, 1978.

Millard RI, Corbett TH: Nitrous oxide concentrations in the dental operatory. *J Oral Surg* 32:593, 1974.

Severinghaus JW: The rate of uptake of nitrous oxide in man. *J Clin Invest* 33:1183, 1954.

Smith G, Shirley AW: Failure to demonstrate effects of low concentrations of nitrous oxide and halothane on psychomotor performance. *Br J Anaesth* 48:274, 1976.

Thornton JA, Fleming JS, Goldberg AD, et al: Cardiovascular effects of 50% nitrous oxide and 50% oxygen. *Anaesthesia* 28:484, 1973.

Trieger N, Loskota WJ, Jacobs AW, et al: Nitrous oxide—a study of physiological and psychomotor effects. *J Am Dent Assoc* 82:142, 1971.

Vessey MC: Epidemiological studies of the occupational hazards of anesthesia. A review. *Anaesthesia* 33:430, 1978.

Wedley JR, Jaffe EC: Malignant hyperpyrexia and the dental outpatient. *Anaesthesia* 28:146, 1975.

CHAPTER 9

Equipment for Inhalation Analgesia and Anesthesia

It is important that any equipment brought into contact with the patient is such that experimental evaluation has demonstrated that it will not materially influence the normal physiological parameters of the patient. The various anesthetic circuits are detailed, and their principles should be understood before alterations are made in equipment. Most equipment, as supplied by the manufacturer, has been tested and evaluated by many investigators and anesthetists. The practice of modifying anesthetic machines for individual requirements should be done only with care and after consideration is given to the alterations in the basic physics of the equipment.

The problems of sterization of equipment are discussed, and the desirability of standardization is also noted.

The foregoing remarks apply with equal vigor to analgesia machines. Indeed, as many practitioners of analgesia have had less recent exposure to basic physics than anesthetists, they should approach modifications with even greater care.

ANALGESIA MACHINES

The machines used in dental analgesia are of the continuous flow type. Their function is to provide sufficient gases for the patient to breathe instead of the room air from which he has been removed.

Continuous Flow Machines

The basic parts of an analgesia machine with continuous flow are: 1) a source of gases at appropriate line pressure with two reducing valves; 2) flow meters to measure gas flow and which incorporate fail-safe mechanisms (Fig. 9.1); 3) a reservoir bag; 4) conducting tubes and face masks; 5) expiratory valves.

Flow meters are used to measure the liters per minute flow of gases. The most widely used variety of flow meter is the variable orifice dry flow meter, in which the gases flow from below upward through a tapered tube. As the gas flows, it elevates a bobbin, ball, or in some a rod. The annular space between the walls of the tapered tube and the bobbin, ball, or rod, through which the gas flows, varies according to the height of the bobbin or ball and may aproximate orifice or tubular flow. In the case of the rotameter, flow is read at the top of the bobbin and in the case of the ball, at the midpoint of the ball.

Older types of flow meter were the fixed orifice flow meters utilizing a Bourdon pressure gauge. The pressure was transmitted across a small orifice, which straightened a flexible metal Bourdon tube. Flow was related to pressure. The position of the needle indicator varied with the pressure, and gas flow was indicated in gallons per hour. The small orifice required to cause a pressure differential resulted in rapid blockage of the orifice, with resultant inaccuracies. At low flows even with a patent tube, accuracy was sacrificed.

Simple machines with a dial appeal to the dentist who does not wish to alarm the patient with complex apparatus. Dial types using a diaphragm regulator have been developed but they still do not show

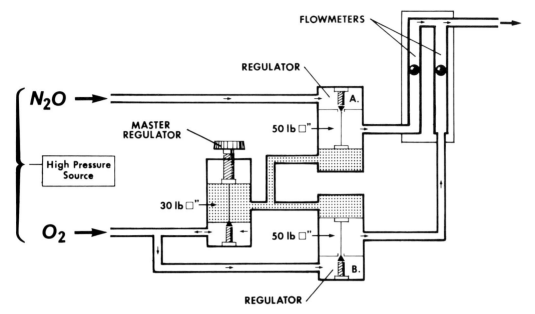

Figure 9.1. The safety systems built into the nitrous oxide-oxygen machine are based on the principle of a master regulator. If the pressure in the regulator falls below 30 psi, then the supply of nitrous oxide ceases. It can be set so there is minimal flow of oxygen at all times.

visual flow, and thus are open to criticism.

Another application of gas flow, through a fixed orifice with resultant pressure difference, is utilized in the water depression meter which had the same disadvantages. A more accurate water depression meter was that made by Foregger with a larger bore than the Bourdon gauge type.

The water sight-feed meter is no longer utilized. The gases bubbled through graduated holes in a tube below water level; gas flow was dependent upon the number of orifices through which gas was flowing. The method was highly inaccurate, as the turbulence of the water at high gas flows made visibility impossible. It did, however, provide a positive index of gas flow, and only the spinning of the rotameter provides such similar positive evidence of gas flow.

The principal types of flow meter used now are the variable orifice dry flow meters, rotameter, ball and rod. Their performance is based on the characteristics of the individual gas. Rate of flow varies with density and viscosity. Through an orifice the density of the gas determines the rate of flow which varies inversely as the square root of the density of the gas if the pressure difference is kept constant.

If the constriction is tubular, as at low flows, then viscosity determines the rate of flow of the gas. Gases of similar density cannot be used with any degree of accuracy through any of the variable orifice flow meters, as their viscosity may not be the same. And the reverse is true; gases with similar viscosities may have different densities.

The effect of altitude upon density and subsequent flow mesurement has little effect in normal practice, there being a 1 per cent error for every 1000-foot rise in altitude.

Changes in density occur with all gases administered, and if nitrous oxide-oxygen is given, the inaccuracies usually nullify each other. The influence of temperature change is minimal; increased density at lower temperatures will not affect the performance of the flow meter.

ROTAMETER

The gas passes up the tube, and the area of the annular space varies as the bobbin rises up the tube. Flow is directly proportional to the annular space; consequently, a linear scale can be used. The stream of gas impinges on the bobbin and causes rotation. As the bobbin does not touch the side of the glass, friction is eliminated. Accuracy of ±2 per cent can be expected. The only inaccuracy is from the weight of the bobbin, which is usually aluminum. As only weight is a feature, the inaccuracy is constant for all positions in the tube. The tube must be held vertically (Fig. 9.2).

BALL FLOW METER

The ball is forced up the tube by the gas. For greatest accuracy an inclined plane and two balls are used. Gas flow pushes the ball up the tube. The gas streaming around the balls produces local turbulence and viscosity effects causing differential loss of pressure, and the ball rises until the differences in pressure above and below the tube are equal. Two balls decrease the tendency to oscillate. Accuracy of ±5 per cent is expected and is least at lower flow rates. There is compound increase in diameter of the tube, and the changes over the lower part of the tube are too great for accuracy (Fig. 9.3).

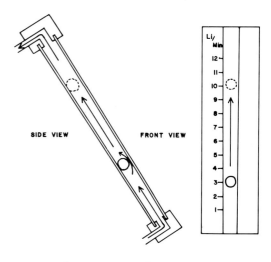

"BALL AND TUBE" FLOWMETER

Figure 9.3. Ball type flow meter showing inclined plane for greater accuracy.

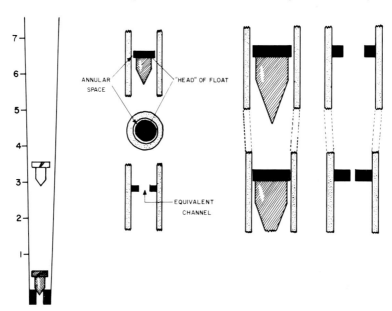

Figure 9.2. Diagrammatic representation of rotameter illustrating the change in orifice size with the compound increase in tube diameter.

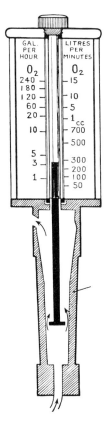

Figure 9.4. Rod type flow meter as used on the Heidbrink Kinet-o-Meter. (Reprinted with permission from McIntosh, R., Mushin, W., and Epstein, H. G.: *Flow meters: Physics for the anesthetist*, 2nd ed. Oxford and Edinburgh, Blackwell Scientific Publications, 1963.)

ROD FLOW METER

The gas flows through a lower conical tube, and a metal rod rides on the gas. It is pushed up into the glass tube where the scale is read. Accuracy is not as great as with the rotameter, because the scale is small for great variations in flow and the metal tube does not taper uniformly, changes from orifice to tube occur over a limited range; accuracy, therefore, is limited, ±7 per cent (Fig. 9.4).

INHALATION CIRCUITS

The basic circuits described are used with all continuous flow machines.

Principles in Circuits

As the administrator of analgesia inhalation agents is removing the patient from his natural environment, it is necessary to avoid any hazardous change in the respired atmosphere. Thus, it is essential that there be no fall in oxygen tension in the inspired gas, and that carbon dioxide not build up in the inspired atmosphere (Fig. 9.5).

RESISTANCE

The circuit should be such that there is no resistance to respiration. Thus, wide

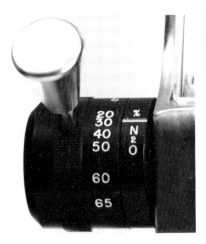
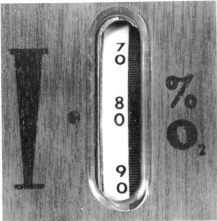

Figure 9.5. The contrasting concepts of a mixing dial are illustrated. Either the change in percentage of nitrous oxide or change in percentage of oxygen is chosen. The flow meter remains the final determinant of percentage.

bore tubes are essential, and the internal diameter of a breathing tube should not be less than 1 cm.

The valves in a analgesia circuit should not cause resistance to expiration. Expiratory valves should always be set at their minimal tension unless positive pressure ventilation is being used. The valves should be observed carefully as sometimes water vapor causes them to stick and thus increases resistance to expiration.

VOLUME FLOW RATE, LAMINA AND TURBULENT FLOWS

Poiseuille's Law

The volume of fluid flowing through a tube varies as to the fourth power of the diameter of the tube. Thus, the wider the tube, the less resistance there is to gas flow. The pressure drop or resistance is directly proportional to the flow rate. When the flow is rapid, it may become turbulent, and pressure loss rises with the square of the flow rate. The pressure loss or the development of turbulent flow can be varied by volume of flow or irregularities in the circuit. It is important that pressure loss not be allowed to develop as resistance to respiration results. Abrupt changes in tubes and connections, particularly constrictions, cause a change from turbulent to lamina flow with loss of energy. A smooth flow of gas offers less resistance than turbulent flow. The effort of respiration is minimal with smooth, wide bore tubes.

DEAD SPACE

It is important that the minimal amount of equipment dead space, additional respiratory gases which are not in contact with respiratory epithelium, be attached to the patient. Large masks, with expiratory valves not adjacent to the mask, result in increases in dead space. It is particularly important in children to avoid accumulation of dead space; otherwise carbon dioxide accumulates under the mask. In some of the older adult full face masks there is up to 150 ml of mask dead space. The Rendall-Baker-Soucek masks, developed conjointly by an anesthetist and dentist, are specifically for children and avoid instrumental dead space (Fig. 9.6).

RESERVOIR BAG

The purpose of the reservoir bag is to provide peak inspiratory flow and to allow intermittent positive pressure ventilation. During respiration, inspiration usually only occupies one-third of the respiratory cycle. The average adult minute volume is 7 liters. Thus, to inspire 7 liters in 1 minute, an inspiratory rate of 21 liters per minute is required if the average tidal volume is assumed to be 500 ml. Either a continuous flow of gases at 21 liters per minute can be provided or a reservoir can be used with a flow rate of 7 liters per minute and yet provide peak inspiratory flow rate of gases. It is important that a minimal volume of fresh gas be provided in the circuit. It is also important to remember that a reservoir bag is not a rebreathing bag (Fig. 9.7).

REBREATHING

A function of all modern equipment is to avoid rebreathing. This can be achieved with either a large flow rate, or by using carbon dioxide absorption. Unless carbon dioxide is removed, the expired gases should not be rebreathed. Artificial ventilation by means of intermittent squeezing on the reservoir bag is useful in anesthetic practice, but CO_2 must be eliminated before the gases are inspired.

Nonrebreathing Circuits

The disadvantage of a nonrebreathing circuit is economy. However, in relation to the other expenditures, the use of large amounts of gases cannot be considered an important factor.

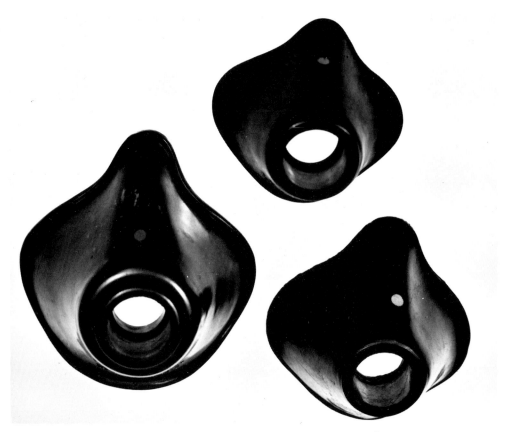

Figure 9.6.   Three sizes of Rendall-Baker-Soucek full face masks devised for children, which reduce mask dead space to a minimum.

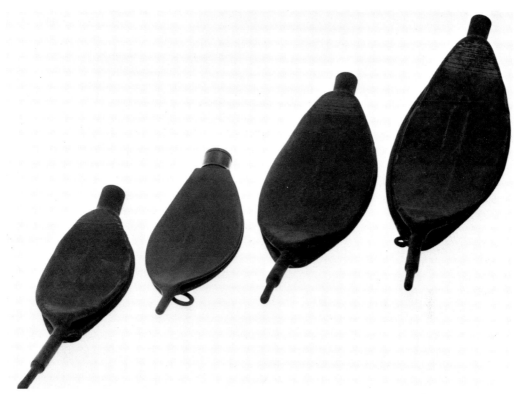

Figure 9.7. Reservoir bags range in size from 500 mm to 5 liters. As it provides the volume for peak inspiratory flow, the bag should be sufficiently large to prevent collapse of the bag with the large minute volumes generated in dental practice.

Attempts have been made to introduce humidifiers into dental practice to eliminate the potential hazards of dry gases. In procedures under general anesthesia lasting on the average 5 hours, no deleterious effects of dry gases in a nonrebreathing circuit were demonstrated. The additional complication of a humidifier may make for unnecessary hazards in the administration of analgesia.

MAGILL CIRCUIT

The setup of the Magill circuit can be seen in Figure 9.8. The principal features are adequate gas flow, a wide bore tube delivering gas to the patient, a reservoir bag, and an expiratory valve adjacent to the mask.

The minimal gas flow required is that which approximates the alveolar ventilation in the patient. The alveolar ventilation in the majority of people is usually 1 liter per minute less than the calculated minute volume. However, for convenience and a margin of safety, the usually required flow rate is that of the patient's minute volume, thus avoiding rebreathing (Fig. 9.9).

The hose delivering the gases to the patient must be of wide bore; the usual corrugated hose provides an adequate diameter. A corrugated hose dose not kink and allows distortion without narrowing of the tubing with subsequent increase in resistance. For inhalation analgesia the twin hoses can be replaced by a longer length of corrugated hose and a nasal

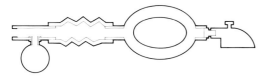

Figure 9.8. The Magill or Mapleson A circuit configuration is routinely used in dentistry for delivery of nitrous oxide-oxygen. The length of corrugated tubing is not critical, but increase in the length of the small bore tubing (1 cm diameter) beyond 45 cm length increases resistance beyond a recommended 0.5 cm H_2O.

mask with a single port. The hose is applied over the patient's head, a disadvantage for some hairstyles.

The expiratory valves are one-way spring-loaded of varying types. The standard types are: 1) the Heidbrink spring-loaded; 2) the McKesson with varying pressure settings; and 3) the Salt valve without spring, with pressure exerted by weight, which is useful for controlled respiration. The spring tension with spontaneous respiration should be the least possible while still remaining in excess of the collapsing pressure of the reservoir bag, which is approximately 0.5 cm H_2O.

The pressure graduations on the expiratory valves of nasal masks are of no significance and are only indications of antiquated anesthetic practice.

The introduction of a flap converts the expiratory valve into a one-way valve. Many one-way valves were developed in response to a requirement for artificial ventilation. They are used commonly in pediatric practice to ensure nonrebreathing. Their inherent disadvantage is that they require care in cleaning and disassembly; otherwise they soon lose their reliability (Fig. 9.10).

Many of the anesthetic nasal masks have valves fitted, and there is no need for an additional valve within the circuit. This type of circuit is classically used in outpatient dental anesthesia and analgesia. It can be altered to suit the individual requirement, provided the basic principles of the Magill circuit together with the basic principles of anesthetic circuits themselves are understood and appreciated (Fig. 9.11).

A disadvantage of the Magill circuit is that the expiratory valve should be as close to the patient as practical. In consequence, the expired gases often blow into the operator's face. Over a short time this is of little consequence, but during prolonged restorative operations the expiratory vapors are a nuisance to the operator. To overcome this problem, collecting devices have been made which attach to the

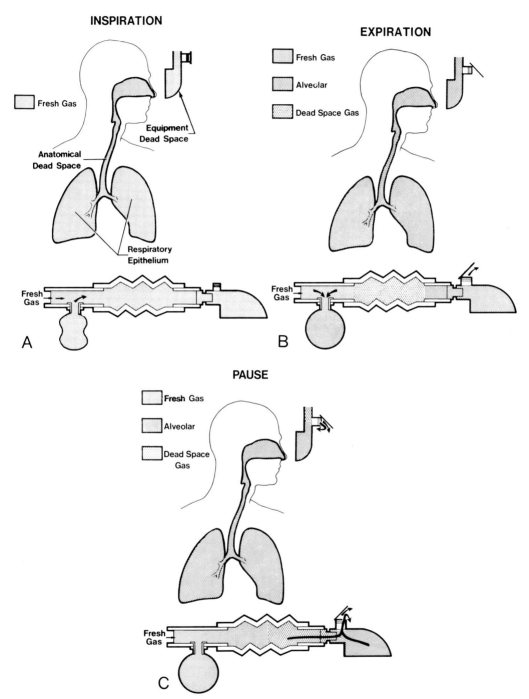

Figure 9.9. The respiratory patterns and gas flows in the Magill (Mapleson A) circuit illustrate the absence of rebreathing with spontaneous respiration.

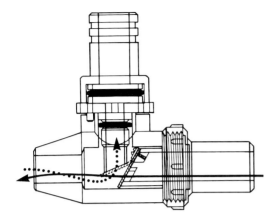

Figure 9.10. The one-way valve illustrated shows the pattern of gas flow. A similar valve may be fitted in circuit on conscious sedation machines.

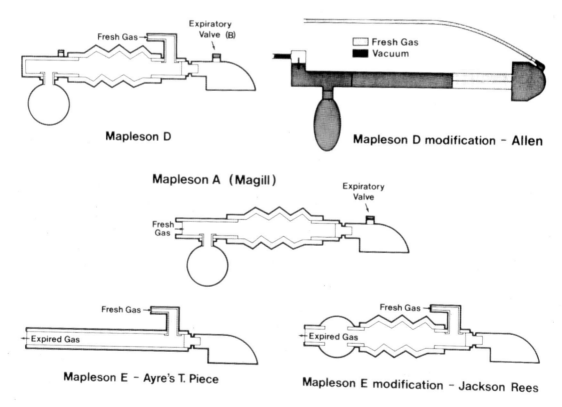

Figure 9.11. Various semi-closed systems can be used for nitrous oxide-oxygen sedation. Flow rates in excess of the minute volume are suggested to avoid rebreathing. The Mapleson D is useful as a scavenging circuit.

suction and thus evacuate the expired vapor (Fig. 9.12).

THE T-PIECE CIRCUIT

The basic circuit is that of a T-piece upon which various modifications have been imposed. Fresh gas flows into the right angle of the "T," one cross-limb of which is attached to a mask while to the other is attached wide bore tube open to atmosphere. Ayre's T-piece has the ad-

vantages that resistance to expiration is minimal and there is no rebreathing. In consequence, it is the method of choice of anesthesia for children, where resistance and rebreathing can be critical factors. The minimal flow rate required is 1½ to 2½ times the minute volume, in which case rebreathing does not occur. The expiratory limb of the T-piece should be equal to one-third of the patient's tidal volume, in order that air dilution of the

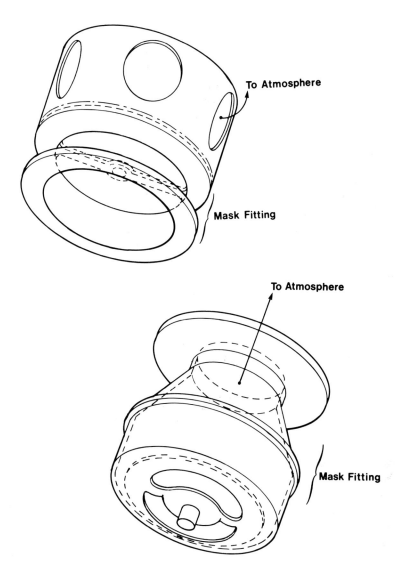

Figure 9.12.   Two simple expiratory valves are shown. Both have no adjustment which is ideal for conscious inhalation and sedation equipment. The lower valve can be used with a simple suction catheter to reduce nitrous oxide pollution in the dental operatory.

inspired gases does not occur. Expiration occupies one-third of the respiratory cycle; thus, the expired gases flow into the expiratory limb in this time interval. During the rest pause, again one-third of the cycle, fresh gas drives the expired gases out into the atmosphere. On inspiration only fresh gas remains for inspiration and is adequate in volume to prevent air dilution. Ayre's T-piece is simple, and in consequence few problems arise provided the basic principles are not violated. However, it is expensive in gas flow, and in basic form it is not recommended for routine use, as the interposition of a simple pop-off valve will accomplish much that is necessary. The important principles followed in the Ayre's T-piece are that 1) an adequate gas flow is provided; 2) the expiratory limb has a noncorrugated tube; and 3) the expiratory limb is left open to atmosphere.

The modifications which have been developed in this type of equipment are the placement of a bag with an open-ended tail on the expiratory limb. The intermittent closure of the open tail allows intermittent positive pressure ventilation. It should be emphasized that this expiratory tail should not be closed in any other way than intermittent closure with the ventilating hand.

DENTAL ANESTHESIA SETUP FOR ORAL SURGERY

In this section consideration is given to the use of anesthetic circuits related uniquely to outpatient general anesthesia for oral surgery. The use of a nasal mask or nasopharyngeal tube as an alternative is the method of patient administration.

The features of a nasal mask are that 1) the expiratory valve is the mask; 2) the pressure setting of the valve is set to minimal tension and the pressure markings are ignored; 3) the air diluent feature is closed, preferably eliminated; 4) the unique selection of nasal mask is left to the discretion of the administrator. There are many nasal masks available. The most critical feature is to achieve an adequate seal of the nasal mask without trauma to the patient and without obliteration of the airway. The fresh gas supply can be delivered in several ways: by narrow tubes on either side of the head; in a T-piece fashion over the top of the head; or through the tail of the reservoir bag over the back of the head. As long as the basic principles of minimal resistance, adequate diameter of tubing, and adequate gas flow are followed, then any method which suits the operator is satisfactory.

Nasopharyngeal tube features should be evident: 1) the tube should be soft; 2) the bevel should be cut adequately to provide minimal trauma to the nose, a 30° angle being preferable; 3) the tube should be patent before being introduced; 4) the expiratory valve should be attached close to the patient; and 5) nasal endotracheal connectors with a 45° angle should be used. The last requirement is essential when using nasopharyngeal tubes; otherwise there are problems of kinking and distortion. In children their proper length should be sought; the usual distance is that from the angle of the mouth to the tragus. A special selection of tubes for children is indicated; otherwise inadvertent endotracheal intubation can occur (Fig. 9.13).

Binasal tubes are a recent introduction in dental practice. It is possible to use smaller nasopharyngeal tubes with adequate gas flow. In an investigation comparing nasal mask and nasopharyngeal tubes, it was found necessary to use the widest possible bore nasopharyngeal tube to avoid respiratory resistance. The binasal tube will allow minimally sized nasopharyngeal tubes to be used with consequent reduction in trauma.

Carbon Dioxide Absorption

The technique of carbon dioxide absorption is not widely used in dental anesthesia or analgesia, probably because of

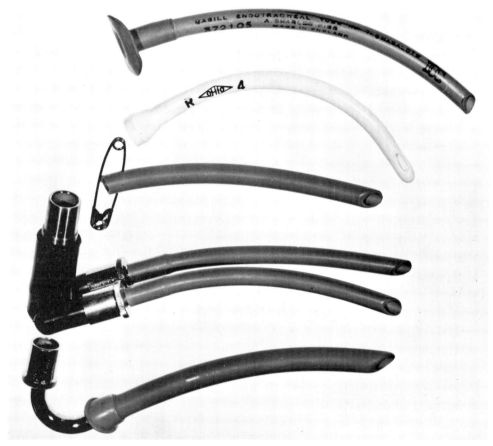

Figure 9.13. Various nasopharyngeal tubes used in dental anesthesia. The white plastic tube is hard and causes unnecessary trauma. The use of a flange, connector, or safety pin to prevent the tube entering too far into the nostril is a useful additional feature. The binasal tube allows placement of smaller tubes in each nostril.

the bulkiness of the equipment involved. There are, however, certain inherent advantages of carbon dioxide absorption: economy of gases, retention of heat, and maintenance of humidity. As these factors are significant only in prolonged cases, it may account for the unenthusiastic reception of the technique in dental anesthesias and analgesia.

Major disadvantages are clumsiness of equipment and lime dust in the system which can irritate the patient. Classically, the equipment was developed for the closed system where there was absence of leaks. As in outpatient dental anesthesia and analgesia this cannot be assured,

there was little advantage in applying the technique.

CIRCLE SYSTEM

The circle system has many advantages, not the least of which are that the bulky soda lime canister is removed from the patient and lime dust does not reach the patient. The disadvantages are that the valves in the circuit tend to stick and the very size of the canisters occupies much space in the operatory. The requirements for a circle system are that the unidirectional valve be situated such that gas can only flow in one direction in the circle, and further that an absorber of at least 2,000 g be used. The canister components are usually a double setup. Their average size is 1,000 ml containing 1,000 g of soda lime. Their efficiency rating is about 9 hours for an individual compartment. As the absorbent becomes utilized, the effective air space in the canister increases. The advantage of a two-compartment soda lime canister is that the compartments can be reversed, thus decreasing the air space. Moisture condenses in the reserve lime chamber, which becomes hydrated and is therefore more efficient when used. A clear-walled canister is important as color change can be visualized. A pH color indicator is included in the soda lime so that a color change occurs when the soda lime is exhausted (Fig. 9.14).

CHEMISTRY

The two types of carbon dioxide absorption are either soda lime or baralime. The mixture in soda lime consists of sodium or potassium hydroxide, 5 per cent, and calcium hydroxide, 95 per cent. In baralime it is 20 per cent barium hydroxide and 80 per cent calcium hydroxide. With soda lime a silicate should be included for hardness to reduce dust, and a certain amount of moisture should be available. The granular size should be four to eight mesh, allowing adequate surface area for carbon dioxide absorption with minimal intergranular space and consequent minimal dead space. Carbon dioxide dissolves in water, forming carbonic acid. In soda lime, the highly active sodium hydroxide reacts first, with H_2CO_3 forming NaOH, Na_2CO_3, and water vapor. Then the so-

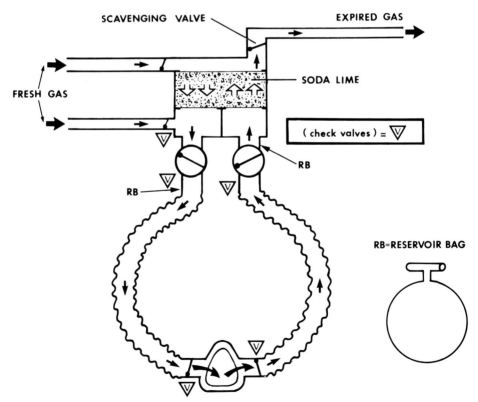

Figure 9.14. In a circle absorber system, the one-way valves and reservoir bag may be placed in various situations. Fresh gas is usually directed through the canister to ensure humidification. A major concern is not to use two valves in opposite directions. A major advantage is that scavenging of expired gases is simplified.

dium carbonate is reactivated by the calcium hydroxide.

$$2\,NaOH + H_2CO_3 \rightarrow$$
$$Na_2CO_3 + 2\,H_2O + heat$$
$$Na_2CO_3 + 2\,CaOH \rightarrow$$
$$Ca_2CO_3 + NaOH$$

Similarly for baralime, the barium hydroxide reacts with carbonic acid to form water and barium carbonate, which is then reactivated by the calcium hydroxide.

USE OF THE CARBON DIOXIDE ABSORPTION SYSTEM

A totally closed system with total rebreathing and carbon dioxide absorption requires a minimal flow rate of 300 ml of oxygen per minute, which represents the basal oxygen requirement of the average adult. It is now rarely used, and the majority of circle systems use flow rates somewhat comparable to the Magill system. It has become routine practice not to have a totally closed system, but to have a semiclosed system where the excess gases are vented to the outside, with total flow rates of between 3 and 5 liters. An inherent disadvantage of the system is increasing resistance, which makes it less than suitable for children.

Another disadvantage of the system is the large amount of dead space, which can be minimized if the unidirectional valves and the expiratory valves are placed adjacent to the patient; this then obviates the system's advantage of venting gases away from the operator.

The low flow rate used with circle absorber systems are an attractive feature. There are, however, two problems. Initially a large flow is required to give quantity of nitrous oxide for rapid uptake, but more important at low flow rate there is difficulty in achieving a satisfactory meter which determines the quantity of oxygen administered. Short of utilizing an oxygen analyzer, then it is difficult to ensure the concentration of nitrous oxide administered.

Other Classifications of Anesthetic + Analgesia Circuits

Circuits can also be classified according to the communication which they establish with the atmosphere and the degree of rebreathing in conjunction with carbon dioxide absorption.

CLOSED CIRCUIT

In a closed circuit all leaks must be eliminated from the system. A minimal flow rate of 300 ml of oxygen is given, and it is perhaps the most economical form of anesthesia. It is used in conjunction with a circle or to and fro soda lime system, and artificial ventilation is practical throughout the procedure. The patient is totally excluded from the atmosphere in both inspiration and expiration.

SEMICLOSED CIRCUIT

A semiclosed circuit is used with either the Magill circuit or an absorber system and is the most frequently used technique. The patient is excluded from the atmosphere at inspiration but the expiratory valve is partially opened to allow leak of gas excess on expiration. It is safer than the closed system, allowing a greater margin of safety.

OPEN CIRCUIT

In an open circuit no reservoir bag is used. The patient has complete access to the atmosphere as in the open drop method with gauze mask. For safety, 300 ml of oxygen are flowed under the mask throughout the period of anesthesia as the vaporized volatile agent will reduce the partial pressure of inspired oxygen. The patient is exposed to atmosphere on both inspiration and expiration.

SEMI-OPEN CIRCUIT

The semi-open circuit is the Ayre's T-piece where the patient has access to atmosphere at inspiration and expiration but no reservoir bag is used. The total gas flow is provided without utilizing room air.

INSUFFLATION

With the insufflation technique, gases are blown into the pharynx, and at inspiration and expiration the patient is able to breathe through the atmosphere. It requires no valve or reservoir bag, but there is no knowledge of inspired gas tensions. It is an older method which has fallen into disrepute and is not utilized.

STANDARDIZATION

Since 1946, attempts have been made to have simplicity and standardization of connections in all anesthetic equipment. The multiplicity of connections is worse in dental anesthesia. The 15-mm connections are used in both male and female patient breathing circuits, and the 22-mm connections in both male and female anesthesia machines. A committee of the American Society of Anesthesiologists has been formed to develop standardization in order to reduce hazards.

A connector attaches directly into the endotracheal tube; all other fittings are called adapters. The component nearest the patient is the patient end, and, at the machine, the machine end. There are straight endotracheal tube connectors, nominal 15 mm; right-angle curved endotracheal tube connectors, nominal 15 mm; and acute-angle curved endotracheal tube connectors, nominal 15 mm. The internal diameter has been accepted as the method for designating and identifying the connector (Fig. 9.15).

Certain basic concepts should be followed. The largest possible diameter straight connector should always be used so that resistance will be minimal, and there should be few variations in size between connectors so that turbulence will not develop. There are many adapters; a swivel, a Y, a canister, a nonrebreathing valve or other component, and a universal adapter. Prior to use of a strange anesthetic machine it is imperative that the connectors and adapters be mated to ensure fit.

DEVICES TO REDUCE OPERATING ROOM POLLUTION

Even though there have been no proven harmful effects of chronic exposure to anesthetic trace contaminant gases, the technology to reduce these contaminants is available. The suggestion that teratogenetic effects of these trace contaminants are possible makes it prudent to institute scavenging devices.

There are several factors which can re-

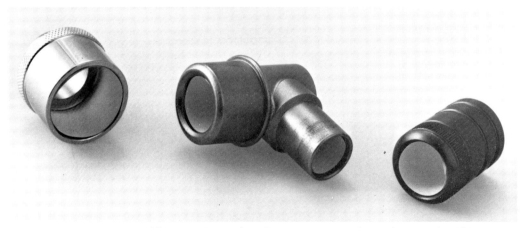

Figure 9.15. Fifteen- and 22-mm male and female connectors are becoming standard features on all equipment in order to simplify connections.

duce the contamination in the dental office, before the installation of scavenging equipment. Thus if the equipment is maintained and serviced regularly, leaks that occur in the gas conducting system from the tank to the nosepiece can be eliminated. The leaks will occur mainly at joints, in fittings on flexible hoses, or defective rubber goods. The technique of scavenging will vary with the type of office building and the suction or air conditioning in the operatory. It is imperative then that these factors be considered before a scavenging device is installed. Thus if suction is used to remove the gases, the suction apparatus must be built to NFPA code for removing flammable gases. If a passive system is used, then a means of evacuating the gas is necessary without recirculating the air within the building.

The requirements of scavenging equipment are that it be adaptable to the sedation or anesthesia machine and exhaust systems available. It must be constructed so that it does not interfere with the normal function of the breathing system, in that delivery of the gases is unaffected. Problems in this regard are the introduction of increased resistance and changes in dead space, gas concentrations, and pressure. In particular suction must not be allowed to be applied directly to the airway. Although this is not a major feature in dental practice where a semi-open circuit is usual, nonetheless suction applied directly to the airway would affect the function of gas delivery. In addition the equipment must be effective regardless of the heating and air conditioning system in use, and allow adequate disposal of the gases. The major problem is in the disposal of oxidizing agents. Finally the equipment must be capable of attaining a reasonable level of nitrous oxide and other agents within the breathing zone of the dentist.

Currently three major systems for the removal or scavenging of trace pollutants in the dental operatory are available.

1. *Suction.* In these circuits, an attempt is made to remove the expired gases around the nosepiece by suction. This can be accomplished as in the Brown mask by having a second mask outside the expiratory valve. Suction from 35 to 45 liters a minute is then applied to the double mask, and gases are effectively removed from the area of the anesthetist. A similar device can be constructed by the application of suction to the expiratory valve, taking care that adequate leakage around the edge of the nosepiece does not occur. The major disadvantage of the Brown mask is that the expiratory valve is lifted by suction, at inspiration, and air entrainment occurs. It is more efficient in preventing air entrainment at higher flow rates (Fig. 9.16).

2. *Passive evacuation.* This system involves evacuation of the gases from the expiratory valve by conducting the gases to an exit port or to an exit air conditioning vent. These circuits have been in use since the early 1970s, when the problem of removal of trace contaminants became most obvious. Several devices have been devised to evacuate the gas from the regular Magill nosepiece. Other modifications have been introduced which place the expiratory valve at the base of the anesthetic or conscious sedation unit, and thus reduce the bulk at the nosepiece. The modifications of the Mapleson D circuit are many, and provide adequate control of pollution levels. It must be emphasized that in this circuit great care must be taken to prevent leakage around the nosepiece, a sometimes difficult maneuver in conscious sedation, though readily achieved in general anesthetic practice (Fig. 9.17).

3. *Circle system.* The use of the circle system has not been common in outpatient dental anesthesia or analgesia. In dental practice it introduces other problems and for the dentist may prove less than satisfactory. However, as the expiratory valve is placed on the base of the

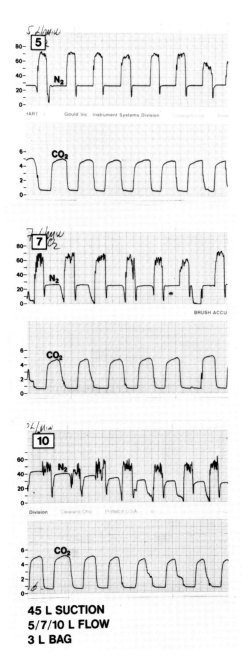

45 L SUCTION
5/7/10 L FLOW
3 L BAG

Figure 9.16. The Brown mask used to decrease nitrous oxide pollution in the dental operatory effectively removes most traces of nitrous oxide. However, at all flow rates, air dilution of the inspired mixture occurs. Nitrogen (*upper*) and carbon dioxide (*lower*) were measured under the double mask during respiration of 100 per cent oxygen. At inspiration as seen by the fall in CO_2 level, air entrainment occurs as noted by the peak in nitrogen levels. High flows and a larger reservoir bag decreased air dilution of inspired gas.

machine away from the operator, the apparatus for gas evacuation is less cumbersome. In the use of a closed system, care must be taken to ensure that the apparatus does not allow leakage around the nosepiece.

The use of an oropharangeal sponge pack will reduce the levels of nitrous oxide pollution and prevent leakage of nitrous oxide from the mouth. However, coughing, straining, and talking in procedure will always increase pollutant levels, and make difficult the maintenance of low levels of pollution in conscious sedation.

Other mechanisms have been suggested to reduce pollutant levels in the region of the operator and assistants. For example, the use of suction in the area of the mouth and around the nose will reduce the levels of nitrous oxide pollution during operative procedures. In addition, the use of an air sweep fan has been proposed which would reduce pollutant levels adjacent to the operator. A critical study of the numerous mechanisms to reduce operating room pollution have been performed by Donaldson. The systems studied were the Brown, the Dupaco, the Porter, and the Frazer-Harlake. All performed adequately, lowering the pollution level in the operative area to below recommended levels.

In summary, then, many pieces of equipment are available for the reduction of nitrous oxide pollution in the dental office, and many will continue to be devised. The critical feature is that these circuits do not alter the function of the apparatus in delivery of the agent to the patient, and further that they do not affect respiratory patterns during anesthesia.

It should be noted that currently there have been no attempts by OSHA to challenge the non-use of anti-pollutant devices in operating rooms. Legal action against hospitals which have not conformed have been dropped. It suggests that the anxiety level in the profession about this problem has been exaggerated.

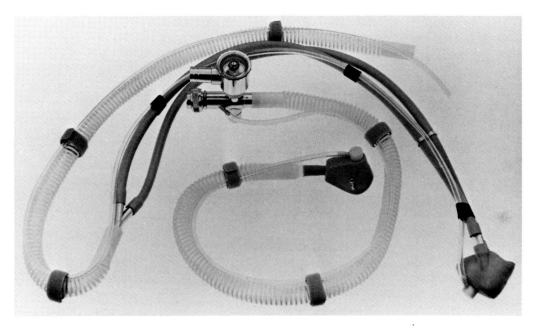

Figure 9.17. The modified Mapleson D circuit will reduce nitrous oxide pollution in dental operatory to acceptable levels. It can be used either as an overhead or twin hose circuit. A good mask fit is essential.

CLEANING AND STERILIZATION OF EQUIPMENT

Cleaning of Equipment

The removal of foreign matter from equipment is significant, in that mechanical cleanliness is in itself a factor in reducing bacterial infection. The items should be soaked, prerinsed, and the soil removed with ordinary scrubbing brushes. Test tube brushes are of value in cleaning, and the use of regular soap solutions with a detergent are adequate for such cleaning. The brushes themselves should be sterilized weekly. It is possible to use equipment which will not only wash but sterilize the anesthetic equipment and ultrasonic cleaning is available. Apart from the latter, however, this is an unnecessary expense in the dental operatory. The significant factor is that rinsing should remove soil and residual detergent. Drying of the equipment following rinsing is important both for equipment which will not undergo subsequent disinfection, and also for equipment which will be sterilized by soaking in the liquid chemicals or in ethylene oxide.

Sterilization

In regard to sterilization there is much controversy, and historically the safety of the transfer of infection by such equipment in dental patients has not posed a problem.

The presence or absence of infection allows the placement of equipment into three categories which can be decided by the operator.

CATEGORIES

1) Routine: patients in whom no infection is present. 2) Nonrespiratory contamination; the general range of localized and systemic infections, including *Staphylococcus*, *Streptococcus* (except A, B hemolytic), viral hepatitis, *Pseudomonas* etc. 3) Respiratory contamination: patients with pneumonia, bronchitis, and upper respiratory infections.

Contamination of soda lime is not a feature, and major contamination is not discussed, as it is rarely applicable to dental anesthesia.

PROCEDURES

Routine

1. Top surface of gas machine is stripped of all equipment and washed with Staphene.

2. Breathing circuit, *i.e.*, corrugated rubber tubing, reservoir bag, connectors, masks, and endotracheal tubes, are removed from machine and processed as described below.

3. All other equipment which has been in contact with the patient's airway—laryngoscope blades, oral airways, esophageal stethoscopes, etc.—removed and processed as below.

4. Metal equipment from above is washed in the ultrasound washer, dried, and autoclaved.

5. Rubber and plastic equipment is washed with Septisol, rinsed in water, soaked for 10 minutes in Cidex (glutaraldehyde), rinsed thoroughly in water, and air dried. Cuffs on endotracheal tubes which are not "built in" are removed prior to washing, washed and dried separately, and replaced after drying. Endotracheal tubes, when dry, are packaged in cellophane wrappers.

6. All other equipment which has been in contact with the patient but not the airway (e.g., ECG cables, blood pressure cuff, and stethoscopes) is wiped with alcohol and returned to service as soon as dry.

Nonrespiratory Contamination

1. All procedures listed for routine cases are followed, in addition to special procedures for this category.

2. Special care is taken to avoid accumulation of moisture on equipment surfaces (and particularly dextrose- or other nutrient-containing solutions).

3. Clean equipment is kept covered insofar as possible to avoid "fallout" of particulate material and droplets. Drawers in machines and carts are opened only as necessary.

4. At the conclusion of the case the anesthetist washes hands thoroughly with either pHisoHex or Septisol. The technical personnel do likewise after cleanup.

5. All equipment which has been in direct contact with patient but which is usually not considered contaminated (e.g., blood pressure cuff tubing) is wiped off with Staphene or alcohol, whichever is most appropriate.

6. All external surfaces of gas machine and anesthesia cart are wiped off with Staphene.

Respiratory Contamination

1. All procedures listed for minor contamination are followed in addition to special procedures for this category.

2. Several options for breathing circuits are acceptable and are processed as follows.

T-piece and Magill circuits, routine processing.

Nonrebreathing systems involving nonrebreathing valves, disinfection procedures are routine; the nonrebreathing valve is disassembled as necessary, washed with Septisol, rinsed, soaked in Cidex (glutaraldehyde), rinsed, and air dried.

A completely disposable circle system consisting of Dryden canister and valves with Ohio disposable tubing, Y-connector, and bag may be used. The entire breathing circuit is then discarded with contaminated material at the conclusion of the case.

The regular nondisposable canister and valves already on the machines may be used with a bacterial filter between patient and reservoir on the exhalation limb.

The regular circle system can be used

without a bacterial filter, but this is discouraged because of difficulty of disinfection. Should this system be used, tubing, bag, and connectors are processed routinely. The canister is emptied and soda lime is discarded. The entire canister and valve unit is completely disassembled, washed with Septisol, rinsed, soaked in Cidex (glutaraldehyde), rinsed, and air-dried.

GAS STERILIZATION

A useful sterilization technique for heat- or moisture-sensitive materials is ethylene oxide. The equipment will kill all microorganisms. The problem is that the gas can be toxic, particularly when inhaled, and in contact with the skin will cause dermatitis and blistering. It is necessary to stress that equipment which comes into the airway following ethylene oxide sterilization can produce skin reactions and laryngotracheal inflammation. For this reason the equipment must be used according to instructions. It has wide applicability and produces minimal damage to the equipment. A major disadvantage is the need for a large inventory of equipment to allow long periods of time for aeration of the sterilized equipment. Its application then probably is confined to large volume conscious sedation or anesthesia operations.

INSTALLATION OF NITROUS OXIDE-OXYGEN IN THE OFFICE

It is important to locate the nitrous oxide-oxygen storage within a minimal distance of outlets. The operatories in which it is installed should have easy access to the outside, and the lines for nitrous oxide-oxygen should be carried either overhead or in the floor. The installation should be in conformance with the local NFPA code, together with any local requirements. It is important that the system conforms to such regulations and is approved by the local fire prevention bureau or the State fire marshal. The contractor should be a licensed plumber who has had previous experience, and contact with another dentist who has had such an installation is suggested. The estimate should contain details of outlets, storage rooms, alarms, check valves, safeties and outlets.

It is important that local and state officials be present during the period when the system is purged, and that a high, pure dry nitrogen testing of the system is performed. In addition, a check is made for oxygen and nitrous oxide coming out of the respective outlets.

Bibliography

Adams D, Allen GD, Scaramella J: Modifying nitrous oxide analgesia circuits to reduce pollution in the dental operatory. *Anesth Prog* 23:176, 1976.

Allen GD: Nitrous oxide oxygen sedation machines and devices. *J Am Dent Assoc* 88:611, 1974.

Ayre P: The T-piece technique. *Br J Anaesth* 28:520, 1956.

Brown ES, Seniff AM, Elam JO: Carbon dioxide elimination in semiclosed systems. *Anesthesiology* 25:31, 1964.

Dorsch JA, Dorsch SE: *Understanding Anesthesia Equipment.* Baltimore, Williams & Wilkins, 1975.

Knudsen J, Lomholt N, Wisborg K: Postoperative pulmonary complications using dry and humidified anaesthetic gases. *Br J Anaesth* 45:363, 1973.

Mapleson WW: The elimination of rebreathing in various semi-closed anaesthetic systems. *Br J Anaesth* 26:323, 1954.

McCarthy FM, Shuken RA: Appraisal of the demand flow anesthetic machine and review of the literature. *J Oral Surg* 27:624, 1969.

Scaramella J, Allen GD, Adams D: Nitrous oxide pollution levels in oral surgery offices. *J Oral Surg* 36:441, 1978.

Swenson RD: Scavenging of dental anesthetic cases. *J Oral Surg* 34:207, 1976.

Whitcher CE, Zimmerman DC, Tonn FM, et al: Control of occupational exposure to nitrous oxide in the dental operatory. *J Am Dent Assoc* 95:763, 1977.

CHAPTER 10

Inhalation Analgesia (Sedation)

Inhalation analgesia is in the main confined to nitrous oxide-oxygen inhalation as other methods of inhalation analgesia have neither gained such popularity nor been so thoroughly investigated.

Inhalation analgesia is a safe practice which can be performed by any general dentist with adequate training. the basic principles of gas flow and physiology are the same in analgesia as in anesthesia. An understanding of the basics presented in the other chapters will aid the dentist in his understanding of inhalation analgesia. It must, however, be distinguished from anesthesia in that the patient does not lose consciousness and can always be roused. Verbal response is the best monitor of the level of analgesia. In addition, as the patient can consciously breathe room air, he may himself regulate the level of analgesia. This does not absolve the dentist from his responsibility in monitoring the patient and determining the depth of analgesia, but it is an additional safeguard. Patient regulation of level of analgesia also distinguishes anesthesia from analgesia. The use of inhalation analgesia is a successful and widespread technique of which the patient should not be deprived because of the dentist's inability to understand the basic principles upon which it is founded. As oxygen delivery equipment is essential in all dental offices, it is a small step to expand that equipment to provide inhalation analgesia.

DEVELOPMENT

The euphoria of nitrous oxide-oxygen has been known since described by Humphrey Davy in 1797 and the analgesia which paralleled this development also was noted. Thus, nitrous oxide has been available as a useful tool for relief of pain and anxiety during dentistry for two centuries. The vogue for nitrous oxide-oxygen analgesia has been periodic, achieving peaks of popularity and then declining. The decline in popularity can be related to the inaccuracy of machines available for the delivery of nitrous oxide-oxygen. The Heidbrink Simplex, which we have evaluated in the past, is representative of such inaccuracies, as indeed are the other commonly used dental analgesia and anesthesia machines, the McKesson Nargraff or Narmatic. The machines were used to deliver nitrous oxide in an intermittent fashion. Consideration of the basic physical properties of nitrous oxide indicates that this is not the way to administer an inhalation agent which has a relatively low blood/gas solubility coefficient, 0.46 (methoxyflurane 13.0). The alveolar concentration of nitrous oxide-oxygen mirrors the blood gas levels, and thus the inhaled concentration soon affects the tissue levels of the gas. The results of intermittent administration of nitrous oxide-oxygen can be seen in Figure 10.1. The calculated uptake demonstrates the evanescent effect of nitrous oxide-oxygen as opposed to the continuous activity of methoxyflurane. On delivery the majority of these machines are accurate, and thus the dentist using them could achieve satisfactory analgesia if administration were continuous. The machines become inaccurate after use, and the manufacturers recommend that they be checked at regular intervals. The absence of representatives capable of handling the technical aspects of the machines resulted

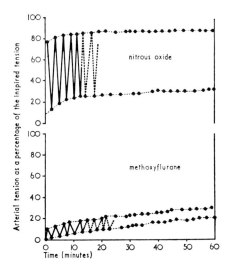

Figure 10.1. A comparative, computed uptake of nitrous oxide-oxygen and methoxyflurane by intermittent administration. The differences in the uptake of nitrous oxide as opposed to methoxyflurane are evident by the graph. (From Jones, P. L., Rosen, M., Mushin, W. W., and Jones, E. V.: Methoxyflurane and nitrous oxide as obstetrical analgesics. II. A comparison by self-administered intermittent inhalation. *Br Med J* 3:259, 1969.)

in this policy of maintenance not being followed. Consequently, the analgesia machine became inaccurate and analgesia was no longer obtained. It thus fell into disrepute. However, the current analgesia machines have flow meters which should obviate this problem, and analgesia should retain its rightful place in the pain control program for dentistry.

The general requirements of an analgesia machine are as follows. 1) It should be reasonably accurate (within 5 per cent of the indicated concentration). The rotameter is accurate to 2 per cent, and the ball flow meters to 5 per cent. 2) It is necessary that the analgesia machine be serviced within the local area by a salesman who is efficient, competent, and interested. 3) An oxygen flush should be available to deliver 100 per cent oxygen as required. 4) A central supply system of nitrous oxide and oxygen should be available, together with spare tanks for emergency use. 5) Many recommend that the analgesia machine should deliver a basic

2½ liters of oxygen so that a hypoxic mixture cannot be given by the dentist. 6) A fail-safe device should be incorporated so that if the line pressure of oxygen fails, then the supply of nitrous oxide is cut off.

OBJECT

The object of nitrous oxide-oxygen analgesia is primarily to relieve anxiety, and in addition it reduces the time span of awareness of the dental experience. Analgesia is an incidental extra possibly related to the development of self-hypnosis; 30 per cent of patients are placebo reactors. However, with nitrous oxide-oxygen definite periosteal analgesia can be produced, which parallels the increase in concentration. There is, however, no analgesia in the teeth. A good sound regional anesthetic is necessary for relief of tooth pain. Nitrous oxide analgesia is an approved and proven way of relief of anxiety in the conscious patient. The patient is conscious, and thus analgesia is 100 per cent safe. Mental impairment is significantly present, and this is the only object of modern day nitrous oxide-oxygen analgesia. The gag reflex is not depressed, but the technique of analgesia produces enough sedation to relax the patient who always gags when manipulations are made in the area innervated by the glossopharyngeal nerve.

METHODOLOGY

As a prerequisite for delivery of nitrous oxide-oxygen analgesia, it is essential that the dentist understand the basic physical principle of the gases and fundamentals of the gas machine in combination with the physiology of respiration, all discussed in other sections of this book. Without this basic understanding, the past absurdities which have developed in analgesia will recur, to the detriment of the patient.

EQUIPMENT

Equipment setups for either the Magill, T-piece, or circle systems can be used for administration of analgesia.

Machines

Continuous flow machines are used mainly for analgesia, the ball type flow meters with 5 per cent inaccuracy being the cheapest. Continuous flow machines are more accurate at high flow rates, and consequently, the higher flow rates which we choose to use may be best. The accuracy of the machine can be readily tested in all offices by the simple expedient of water displacement. If the success of analgesia begins to fail, then a check of the accuracy of the equipment is indicated. Magill circuit with a reservoir bag and minimal resistance tubing is the standard circuit for administration of nitrous oxide-oxygen analgesia.

Two misconceptions should be clarified: 1) that the gas delivered to the patient should be warmed—nasal breathing adequately warms the coldest air. The specific heat of air is only 0.35 cal per g, and thus any gases can be readily heated by the ambient atmosphere. 2) that the gas should be humidified. Again, the nasal mucosa readily humidifies the driest gases in desert climates. The brief period of inhalation analgesia poses no problem.

Nasal Masks

The minimal tension should be set on all expiratory valves, and in contradistinction to the nasal masks used for inhalation dental outpatient anesthesia, these masks should be soft. A soft mask allows a close approximation to the patient without marking the face. The sizes vary and should be chosen to fit each patient, and an adequate gas flow should be provided to prevent a dilution occurring through the side of the mask. The bore of the delivery tubes should be adequate for respiration without resistance.

Metal connectors from the mask to hoses are best avoided for analgesia as they tend to mark the face. The use of gravity will allow the heavier nitrous oxide to sink over the patient, and the semi-supine position for the administration of the gas will aid in administration.

The use of air dilution valves on nasal masks is a ridiculous attempt to provide a safety factor which is unnecessary, provided analgesia is understood by the dentist. The other purpose of the air dilution valve is to prevent the patient from feeling stifled. Understanding of the purpose of a reservoir bag in the provision of peak inspiratory flow and an adequate minute volume avoids the necessity for provision of such a feature. Air dilution introduces a high degree of inaccuracy in the volume of delivered gases; thus, the administration of analgesia becomes a mystic art rather than a science. Air dilution valves should be completely eliminated from analgesia equipment. The calculation of the degree of dilution is impossible. Each patient ceases to become a learning experience for the dentist, as relative responses cannot be compared.

Nasal Catheters or Cannulae

Studies with the administration of 100 per cent oxygen through nasal cannulae indicate that it is extremely difficult to elevate the arterial oxygen tension above 200 mm Hg. It is impossible to deliver accurate nitrous oxide-oxygen percentages to the patient by this method. It does provide easy access to the mouth, but it eliminates any scientific assessment of delivered concentrations. If nasal cannulae are used, high flows of gases are required to partially overcome the air dilution which occurs. It can be calculated that if 80 per cent nitrous oxide with 20 per cent oxygen is delivered at a total flow rate of 10 liters per minute, the inspired nitrous oxide percentage will be about 25 per cent. Unless concentrations of oxygen below 20 per cent are administered, it will not be possible to raise the concentration of nitrous oxide above the 25 per cent level.

Dental Aids

The use of a rubber dam, pharangeal sponge, or a moistened McKesson oropharyngeal pack aids in producing a dry field and protecting the airway. The use of continuous suction helps keep the airway clear and, in combination with a conscious patient, protects the airway.

APPROACH

It is valuable for the administrator of analgesia to have experienced the sensations of analgesia, in order that he may approach the patient with confidence. It is useful to spend some time with the patient describing the subjective sensations he will feel, such as the tingling and warmth, the ability to breathe through the mouth if he feels that he is slipping away, and the explanation that the dentist will still be there caring for the patient. Each dentist should develop his own technique and approach to the patient dependent upon his unique circumstances.

Food

It is best that the patient avoid large meals prior to operation because analgesia can produce nausea and vomiting. Although the airway is protected, the occurrence of such a situation in the office is not pleasant. It is suggested that a 3-hour interval be allowed following a large meal; fasting should be avoided. In our studies, patients complaining of nausea all had fasted prior to the administration of nitrous oxide analgesia.

Age

Patients under 3 years of age pose technical problems in approach, but there is no hazard to analgesia. As the patient approaches 5 years of age, he becomes more amenable to acceptance of the nasal mask. Children accept greater percentages of nitrous oxide for analgesia than do adults. The practice of combining an oral

or intramuscular premedication with nitrous oxide poses the potential problem of inducing general anesthesia.

Sex

The young teen-age female presents major problems in nitrous oxide-oxygen analgesia as she often exhibits hysterical symptoms. A female chaperone is essential in an office where nitrous-oxide oxygen is administered owing to the propensity of females under nitrous oxide-oxygen to have sexual abreactions.

Staff or Personnel

All the people on the staff should experience nitrous oxide-oxygen in order that they may exhibit confidence to the patient regarding administration. They should be familiar with recording data, monitoring the blood pressure and pulse, and changing concentrations if the dentist is involved in the dentistry.

Application

It is important for the operator to smell the mask each time prior to administration. This ensures that no impurities are present in the nitrous oxide, that leftover smells from the mask (as from the cleansing fluid) have been eliminated. The use of perfume on the mask may be indicated. The color of the equipment is important; black masks are psychologically negative and a lighter colored mask is a useful adjunct. The patient can be preoxygenated, which will aid in the uptake of nitrous oxide, but this is not essential. Nitrous oxide has a sweet smell, and the patient should be reassured that it is only the equipment that has an odor. Leaks around the mask must be avoided and gravity should be enlisted to allow flooding of nitrous oxide-oxygen over the patient. Once initiated, the application should continue. Nitrous oxide has a relatively poor solubility in comparison with other more potent anesthetic agents. Although it is given in high concentrations, it is rapidly eliminated. Nitrous oxide-oxygen is an evenescent analgesic and *must be given continuously.*

Delivered Volumes and Concentrations

The majority of patients (80 per cent) react to average concentrations of nitrous oxide in the manner illustrated in Figures 10.2 and 10.3). However, 10 per cent are underreactors. Thus, individual concentrations must be varied for each patient. It is useful to begin with a total 10-liter flow, as calculations of percentage changes are easier and flow meters are more accurate in this area. Changes in 5 per cent concentration produce changes in the patient's response. The onset of analgesia will develop in 1 to 2 minutes,

and concentration of nitrous oxide should never exceed 40 per cent unless the risk of induction of general anesthesia is accepted. It is useful to begin the initial concentration at 30 per cent and increase or decrease from the level depending upon the response of the patient. The duration of administration should be up to 4 hours, and, although excretion is rapid and recovery appears rapid, it should be realized that the excretion of nitrous oxide is dependent upon the total amount administered. Mental recovery occurs in 1 to 2 minutes. Cardiovascular stability returns to normal immediately.

Altitude will affect the activity of nitrous oxide-oxygen during conscious sedation. Thus, at an altitude of 5000 feet, the atmospheric pressure is only 630 mm Hg; this is 0.83 per cent of sea level atmospheric pressure. Thus, the partial

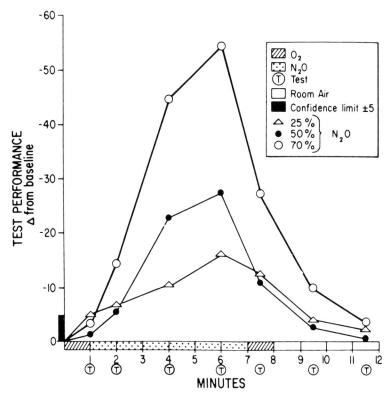

Figure 10.2. This study demonstrates a dose-response relationship between increasing nitrous oxide concentrations and increasing psychomotor effects. (Reprinted by permission from Trieger, N., Loskota, W. J., Jacoby, A. W., and Newman, M. G.: Nitrous oxide—a study of physiological and psychomotor effects. *J Am Dent Assoc* 82:146, 1971. Copyright, American Dental Association.)

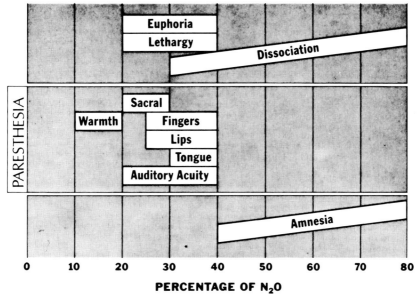

Figure 10.3. The majority of patients respond at the concentrations indicated. Tingling is often felt only in a single area. It does indicate analgesia in that area. Dissociation and amnesia increase with increasing concentrations of nitrous oxide.

pressure of administered nitrous oxide is reduced and the activity of nitrous oxide reduced by one fifth.

The use of the Bender Gestalt test by Trieger indicates that psychomotor function is normal 2 to 3 minutes after nitrous oxide analgesia. However, excretion of nitrous oxide continues long after administration. Detectable amounts have been collected in the expired air 4 hours after a 5-minute exposure to 10 per cent nitrous oxide. It is useful practice to administer 100 per cent oxygen at the conclusion of the procedure to allow a period of readjustment for the operator and aid in the excretion of the nitrous oxide-oxygen.

Dose Response

A definitive dose-response relationship to nitrous oxide oxygen has been demonstrated by Trieger. There is a progressive increase in psychosedation levels which will parallel the analgesic effects.

Signs and Symptoms of Analgesia

The subjective symptoms of nitrous oxide-oxygen analgesia related to the con-

Table 10.1
Other Symptoms of Nitrous Oxide-Oxygen Analgesia Which May Develop

	%
Warmth	10–20
Amnesia	40–55
Euphoria*	20–40
Loss of consciousness	60 →
Anesthesia†	80–140

* Most important adjunct—this is what is sought.
† As indicated by MAC.

centration of administered nitrous oxide are indicated in Figure 10.3. If the operator has himself experienced analgesia, he will appreciate that there is a considerable range of patient response. Table 10.1 shows additional subjective signs and symptoms which can occur. They are useful adjuncts in observing the patient. Figure 10.4 illustrates the objective signs and relates them to the concentration of nitrous oxide. It is essential that the operator understand the implications of each sign and symptom. The nausea and vomiting which occur are related mainly to the individual rather than the concentra-

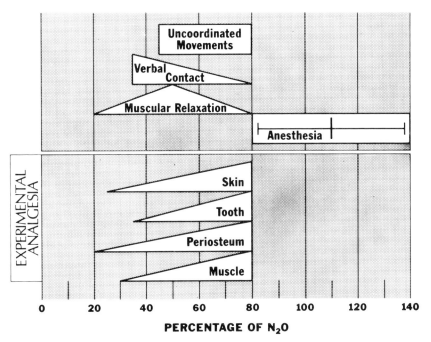

Figure 10.4. True analgesia develops in some areas with minimal concentrations of nitrous oxide. Uncoordinated movement is a signal to decrease the concentration of nitrous oxide.

tion of nitrous oxide-oxygen. But vomiting usually occurs when concentrations between 40 and 50 per cent nitrous oxide are administered. Nausea is an indication to decrease the administered concentration.

The subjective responses shown in Figure 10.3 indicate the range of concentrations over which responses are obtained. Not all features are exhibited by an individual patient.

Somnolence increases to anesthesia as the concentration of nitrous oxide rises, whereas dissociation reaches a peak with concentrations in the analgesia range. The dissociation is an unpleasant experience to pateints who do not like to surrender their personal control. Dreams are evident of overdose and early anesthesia. Sexual overtones indicate again the need for a chaperone (Fig. 10.5).

The objective responses are in the ranges we have elicited in the experimental situation and in demonstrations. It is desirable to maintain verbal contact for monitoring purposes, the basis of con-

scious analgesia. Uncoordinated movements occur with anesthetic induction, and increasing the concentration of nitrous oxide at this time is a common mistake. The concentration should be decreased; a response to surgical stimulation is not uncoordinated.

Sweating may be due to a vasovagal effect from which it should be distinguished.

Tooth sensitivity is unaffected until 50 per cent nitrous oxide concentration is reached. It then is in the area of anesthesia. The experimental pain in skin and mucous membrane can be relieved by nitrous oxide oxygen and is evident with low concentrations. Pain relief for muscle ischemia is profound and develops early. Thus, while conscious sedation with nitrous oxide-oxygen produces little analgesia in the tooth, true analgesia, pain relief without loss of consciousness, is produced for other pain modalities as in obstetrics and for tourniquet pain. The differing response to experimental pain with nitrous oxide-oxygen has been used

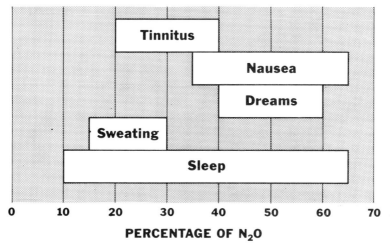

PERCENTAGE OF N₂O

Figure 10.5.   Dreams are associated with sleep and may be directed by positive suggestion prior to induction of conscious sedation.

experimentally to differentiate types of pain.

Periosteal analgesia at 40 per cent is profound. The other symptoms noted are more variable than those previously noted. Warmth may be localized to face and hands or a total body flush may be felt.

Amnesia is of great value as it allows long appointments with minimal patient recall.

The signs of early N_2O anesthesia should be noted and studied. If overdose occurs, it is important to reverse the effects before the excitement peak is reached. If respiration becomes slow and irregular and is associated with muscle movements, check the eyes for eyelids resisting opening and the eyeballs rolling.

Limits for Anesthesia

Table 10.2 shows the early signs of nitrous oxide-oxygen anesthesia. It has been demonstrated that the lower limit of nitrous oxide concentration which will produce anesthesia is 80 per cent. Thus, limitation of the nitrous oxide-oxygen delivered concentration to 40 per cent in analgesia provides an additional safeguard. There are some who may respond at a lower limit, and there should never

Table 10.2.
Signs of Early N_2O-O_2 Anesthesia

Slow breathing, becoming irregular
Breath holding
Grunting
Muscle movement
Large pupils that contract to light
Rolling eyeballs
Eyelids resist opening
Conjugate deviation of eyes
Increased pulse rate
Increased blood pressure

be any hesitation on the part of the operator to reduce the concentration of delivered nitrous oxide.

A major hazard is the attempt to increase the potency of nitrous oxide-oxygen analgesia, increasing the concentration of nitrous oxide above the usual limits. It must be appreciated that anesthesia then becomes a reality. The other hazard is the combination of analgesia methods such as intravenous techniques with nitrous oxide-oxygen in order to expand the analgesia field. This technique should only be followed if the operator feels confident that he can handle the problems of general anesthesia, and if he has the equipment available for meeting such problems.

SIDE EFFECTS
Exaggerated Sounds

With the decrease in other sensory input, the normal sounds become exaggerted. It is essential for ancillary personnel to appreciate this feature and in particular not drop instruments in an analgesia setting.

Sweating

Sweating can occur at any concentration immediately after induction. It is related to the individual's reponse. A common side effect of nitrous oxide-oxygen sedation which begins soon after administration, it is, in part, related to the release of catecholamines and peripheral vasodilatation. Although total peripheral resistance rises, a distinction must be made between this and vasodilatation of skin vessels. The peripheral resistance consists of the blood vessels in muscles, bowel, and gut. The skin is only one small area of peripheral resistance and nitrous oxide causes dilatation of skin vessels.

Peripheral Vasodilatation

Possibly peripheral vasodilatation can cause the sweating and is responsible for the feelings of warmth.

Nausea

Nausea is related to excess concentrations and is usually preceded by sweating. It will occur following prolonged administration of high concentrations, particularly in the 40 to 60% range, or those patients who are nauseated prior to beginning treatment.

Encapsulated Pockets

If the eustachian tube is blocked, the middle ear becomes a closed pocket of air. Nitrous oxide can accumulate and concentrate with consequent increase in total pressure which will cause ringing in the ear. It may be cleared by either a Valsalva maneuver or yawning.

Nitrous oxide will pass into pockets of gas in the bowel. If they are confined, they can cause distension.

Oxygen Toxicity

The problem of oxygen toxicity is often raised in regard to nitrous oxide-oxygen sedation. At normal atmospheric pressure administration of 100% oxygen for an excess of 24 hours results in tightness in the chest, dry cough, and sometimes hemoptysis. It is not a problem with nitrous oxide-oxygen sedation.

USES OF NITROUS OXIDE ANALGESIA

The safety of nitrous oxide is demonstrated by the numerous uses for nitrous oxide-oxygen. Thus, control of pain in coronary thrombosis and angina have been treated with nitrous oxide-oxygen. A fixed mixture of 50/50 nitrous oxide-oxygen Entonox is administered safely by trained personnel such as paramedics. It has been used in all forms of injury, particular safety being evident in head injury. Postoperative pain has been treated by nitrous oxide-oxygen, and 25 per cent nitrous oxide is equivalent in pain relief to 10 mg of morphine. Other uses have been for tension headaches, migraine, Raynaud's disease, bronchial asthma, leukemia, and it is the standard analgesic used during childbirth. Three million patient hours given in a controlled situation in Denmark have indicated no problems.

CONTRAINDICATIONS AND HAZARDS

Nitrous oxide-oxygen analgesia is contraindicated in any patient in whom any operative procedure would be contraindicated. Thus, nitrous oxide-oxygen analgesia will not expand the field of the operator into realms in which he should not proceed. If an elective procedure is not indicated, then nitrous oxide analgesia will not make it possible. Table 10.3 indicates the contraindications to nitrous oxide-oxygen analgesia. In addition, it is

Table 10.3.
Contraindications to Nitrous Oxide-Oxygen Analgesia*

Nasal obstruction
Pregnancy—first trimester
Asthma
Epilepsy
Psychiatric patients
Medications affecting patient's
  physiological reactions

* Problems which militate against any elective procedure.

important to realize that nasal blockage can be produced by crying; thus, if there is crying before analgesia, the nose will be blocked and it may not be possible to deliver the nitrous oxide-oxygen. Common sense dictates that coryza is an absolute contraindication to nitrous oxide-oxygen analgesia as well as a hazard of exposure to the operator. Pregnancy in the first 3 months is a contraindication, as it has been shown that nitrous oxide-oxygen can be teratogenic in the rat embryo. In addition, administration of prolonged nitrous oxide-oxygen has been shown to be toxic to white blood cells. Although there is no human indication of teratogenic effects of nitrous oxide, the cautious administrator will avoid known administration of nitrous oxide in the first trimester for the medical-legal problems which may develop. Epilepsy is a contraindication, as hyperventilation may occur during nitrous oxide-oxygen analgesia. Hyperventilation, it should be noted, is a technique for inducing epileptic focal responses in the EEG.

The patient who has bronchial asthma may respond poorly to nitrous oxide-oxygen analgesia in that application of the nasal mask may produce a confined feeling and production of an asthmatic spasm.

The psychotic patient is not a candidate for analgesia, as he may show posthypnotic responses. Care must be taken in administering inhalation analgesia to these patients in that they may respond to unthinking remarks with a postoperative trance. Finally, the patient who is on

mood-altering drugs should be viewed with great caution just as in general anesthesia. With proper patient selection problems should not occur.

CARDIORESPIRATORY EFFECTS OF ANALGESIC CONCENTRATIONS OF NITROUS OXIDE-OXYGEN

The cardiorespiratory effects of nitrous oxide-oxygen in concentrations up to 40 per cent nitrous oxide parallel those of inhalation of 100 per cent oxygen. There is a slight rise in mean arterial pressure related to an increase in total peripheral resistance. Cardiac output falls, as does the work of the heart. The results of studies which show changes in cardiac output and total peripheral resistance with nitrous oxide-oxygen are shown in Figure 10.6. The results are compared with the effects of 100 per cent oxygen inhalation (Table 10.4).

There have been numerous studies which indicate release of endogenous catecholamines during the administration of nitrous oxide-oxygen. In addition, studies performed with other drugs in combination with nitrous oxide-oxygen indicate differing cardiovascular effects. The

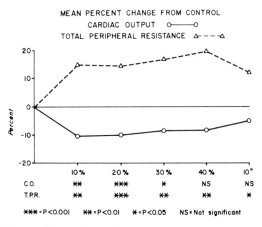

Figure 10.6. The effects on cardiac output and total peripheral resistance are explicable as due to the high concentrations of oxygen given. (From Everett, G. B., and Allen, G. D.: Simultaneous evaluation of cardiorespiratory and analgesic effects of nitrous oxide-oxygen inhalation analgesia. *J Am Dent Assoc* 83:129, 1971.)

Table 10.4.
Results of Inhalation of Various Concentrations of Nitrous Oxide-Oxygen Compared with Effects of Inhalation of 100 Per Cent Oxygen

	MAP	CO	CR	SV	TPR	PaCO$_2$
100% O$_2$	5.4 ± 1.7	−5.7 ± 3.3	−1.0 ± 2.2	−4.1 ± 2.7	16.4 ± 4.2	33.3 ± 1.4
10% N$_2$O	2.1 ± 2.2	−10.6 ± 2.2	−1.0 ± 1.9	−9.7 ± 1.8	14.7 ± 3.1	34.1 ± 1.2
20% N$_2$O	2.8 ± 2.4	−10.0 ± 1.2	−1.2 ± 1.8	−8.7 ± 1.8	14.2 ± 2.0	34.4 ± 0.9
30% N$_2$O	5.8 ± 2.4	−8.6 ± 2.9	−3.3 ± 2.1	−5.9 ± 2.7	16.6 ± 3.9	33.4 ± 1.2
40% N$_2$O	8.2 ± 2.1	−8.4 ± 4.1	−0.8 ± 4.2	−7.3 ± 2.0	19.7 ± 4.7	34.4 ± 0.7

No statistically significant difference was seen in any of the cardiovascular parameters measured at any concentration.

(From Everett, G. B., and Allen, G. D.: Simultaneous evaluation of cardiorespiratory and analgesic effects of nitrous oxide-oxygen inhalation analgesia. *J Am Dent Assoc* 83:129, 1971.)

Table 10.5.
Differing Cardiovascular Effects Noted with Positional Change and When Other Drugs are Combined with Nitrous Oxide-Oxygen

Drugs	CO	Rate	TPR	BP
N$_2$O 40% dental (Everett, G.B., and Allen, G.D., 1971)	−9	0	+20	+9
N$_2$O 40% supine (Eisele, J.H., and Smith, N.T., 1972)	−19	−15	+27	−3
N$_2$O + halothane (Smith, N.T., *et al.*, 1970)	−3	2	15	11
N$_2$O + morphine (Martin, W.E., *et al.*, 1970)	−21	−8	20	0
N$_2$O + morphine, coronary (Stoelting, R.K., 1972)	−34	−17	21	−13

influence of position is significant and is noted with nitrous oxide-oxygen and with diazepam. In mixing analgesic techniques, careful attention must be paid to prior and subsequently administered agents when using nitrous oxide-oxygen. Table 10.5 clearly demonstrates the influence of such drugs in combination with nitrous oxide-oxygen.

OTHER INHALATION AGENTS

It is of interest to note that diethyl ether is a potent analgesic agent. Used in concentrations of between 2 per cent in oxygen and 4 per cent in air, it is nonexplosive and thus has been used with cautery in cases of open heart surgery as the best supplement for maintenance of analgesia in the triad of balanced anesthesia. However, for routine practice, it is advisable to use nonexplosive agents, as the floors in dental offices are not conductive. Inadvertent increments in concentration could result in an explosion or fire hazard. Other agents available for inhalation analgesia are enflurane and methoxyflurane.

ADVANTAGES OF VOLATILE INHALATION AGENTS

The advantages of volatile inhalation agents for analgesia are 1) economy, 2) simple method of delivery, 3) potent, 4) oxygen can be added, 5) analgesia of the

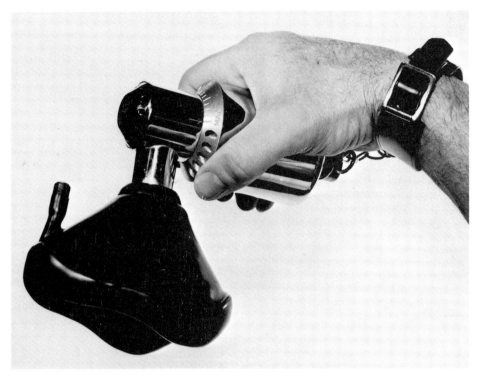

Figure 10.7. The Cyprane inhaler for methoxyflurane analgesia.

tooth and periosteum occurs, 6) vaporizers are available which will allow wide variations in concentration to be administered accurately.

DISADVANTAGES OF VOLATILE INHALATION AGENTS

Disadvantages are 1) odor, 2) potency results in ready change to anesthesia from analgesia, 3) vaporizers are easily modified and require frequent checking, 4) cardiac arrhythmias can easily develop and combinations with local anesthetics may be hazardous, 5) there is a potential upset of metabolism, as the agents are in part metabolized, 6) vaporization can be difficult, 7) oxygen is not a necessary accompaniment of the technique.

VAPORIZERS AVAILABLE FOR USE WITH VOLATILE ANALGESIC AGENTS

The vaporizers which are available for analgesia are the Duke inhaler or Cyprane

Table 10.6.
Percentage of Methoxyflurane Delivered by Cyprane Inhaler Determined by Sonic Analyzer

Maximal Intermittent Flow, 16–20 Min	Methoxyflurane Delivered	
	5 min	10 min
liters/min	%	%
2.25	0.73	0.7
5.1	0.63	0.53
7.5	0.51	0.45
9.6	0.35	0.4
10.1	0.35	0.4
11.8	0.35	0.33

inhaler (Fig. 10.7), which is held in the patient's hand and allows concentrations to be varied. It can be used with methoxyflurane. The delivered concentrations of methoxyflurane by the Cyprane inhaler are shown in Table 10.6. It is a stable inhaler though not temperature-compensated.

Temperature- and volume-compensated vaporizers are available which will deliver concentrations of methoxyflurane or enflurane in either air or oxygen.

AGENTS

Methoxyflurane

Methoxyflurane is used extensively in obstetrics. Its high potency and high solubility result in rapid uptake. It is not readily vaporized and, in combination with the low concentration, develops a stable analgesia pattern even though the drug is given intermittently. Once analgesia is established, intermittent administration of methoxyflurane will maintain analgesia. It is thus possible to use a vaporizer such as the Cyprane inhaler, in which the route of administration of the drug is the mouth, for dentistry where the operator and the administration of analgesia both require the same route. It can be administered in concentrations of 0.25 to 0.35 per cent, which will give satisfactory analgesia. The uptake of methoxyflurane compared to nitrous oxide as calculated by Mapleson and quoted by Jones *et al.* shows why satisfactory levels of methoxyflurane can be achieved when the drug is given intermittently. The greatest hazard of methoxyflurane would appear to be the potential to produce addiction. Of all the analgesic agents, methoxyflurane appears to give the greatest feeling of postoperative euphoria. It is an agent with minimal production of cardiac arrhythmias or even sensitization of the myocardium to injected epinephrine. It is metabolized by the body, and up to 45 per cent is excreted *via* the kidney. There is no indication of nephrotoxicity when the drug is given to the normal patient in small dosage.

Enflurane

Enflurane has been used for both obstetric analgesia and dental sedation. Early reports indicate it is a useful agent for dentistry.

Bibliography

Allen GD: The enigma of air dilution. Anesth Progr 17:52, 1970.

Chapman CR, Murphy TM, Butler SH: Analgesic strength of 33 percent nitrous oxide. Science 179:1246, 1973.

Cleaton-Jones P, Moyes DG, Whittaker AM: Clinical effects of nitrous oxide and oxygen mixtures at sea level and at 1700 metres altitude. Anaesthesia 34:859, 1979.

Freedman GL, Allen GD: Comparison of differing modalities of experimental pain in man. J Dent Res 49:378, 1970.

Hamilton WK, Eastwood DW: A study of denitrogenation with some inhalation anesthetic system. Anesthesiology 16:861, 1955.

Haugen FP, Coppock WJ, Berquist HC: Nitrous oxide hypalgesia in trained subjects. Anesthesiology 20:321, 1959.

Hornbein TF, Martin WE, Bonica JJ, et al: Nitrous oxide effects on the circulatory and ventilatory responses to halothane. Anesthesiology 31:250, 1969.

Jastak JT, Paravecchio R: An analysis of 1331 sedations using inhalation, intravenous or other techniques. J Am Dent Assoc 91:1242, 1975.

Jastak JT, Malamed SF: Nitrous oxide sedation and sexual phenomena. J Am Dent Assoc 101:38, 1980.

Jones PL, Rosen M, Mushin WW, Jones EV: Methoxyflurane and nitrous oxide as obstetric analgesics. II. A comparison by self-administered intermittent inhalation. Br Med J 3:259, 1969.

Kerr F, Ewing DJ, Irving JB, et al: Nitrous-oxide analgesia in myocardial infarction. Lancet i:63, 1972.

Persson PA: Nitrous oxide hypalgesia in man. Acta Odont Scand Suppl 7:1–98, 1951.

Pleasants JE: The case against relative analgesia. Dent Clin North Am 15:839, 1971.

Shulman M, Schmidt G, Sadove MS: Evaluation of oxygen therapy devices by arterial oxygen tensions. Dis Chest 56:356, 1969.

Smith WDA: Experiments demonstrating the uptake, distribution and elimination of nitrous oxide in the context of outpatient anaesthesia. Br J Anaesth 39:464, 1967.

Smith WDA: Uptake and elimination of inhalation anaesthetics during outpatient anaesthesia. Br J Anaesth 36:180, 1964.

CHAPTER 11

Intravenous, Intradermal, Subcutaneous, and Intramuscular Injection

The teaching of venipuncture must not be confined to dentists who intend to practice intravenous sedation or anesthesia. Should an emergency arise in the dental office which requires the use of intravenous drugs, the dentist must have the ability to administer these drugs competently. The requirements for safe venipuncture are a knowledge of the anatomy of the site of injection, a reliable, safe technique, and the ability to recognize and treat any problems that may arise.

ARTERIAL BLOOD SUPPLY AND THE VENOUS DRAINAGE OF THE UPPER LIMB

The upper limb is supplied by the brachial artery, which is an extension of the axillary artery. The brachial artery lies superficially throughout its course and passes deep to the bicipital aponeurosis where it can be palpated on the medial aspect of the cubital fossa. It normally divides into the radial and ulnar arteries 1 cm distal to the bend of the elbow and supplies the forearm and hand.

The venous return from the hand begins as small veins passing between the metacarpals and from the side of the fingers to form a dorsal venous network on the back of the hand (Fig. 11.1). Some of the venous return follows the major arteries; but of more clinical significance in venipuncture is the superficial venous drainage *via* the forearm (Fig. 11.2). This is composed of two major veins formed at the wrist, the basilic on the medial or ulnar aspect and the cephalic on the lateral or radial aspect. The basilic vein passes along the ulnar side of the forearm eventually penetrating the deep fascia, midway between the cubital fossa and the axilla. The cephalic vein traverses along the radial border of the forearm and cubital fossa and lateral to the biceps before penetrating the clavipectoral fascia to join the axillary vein just below the clavicle. A median vein draining the palmar surface of the hand can normally be found beginning at the wrist or mid-forearm. Its position is variable and it may not even be present. As it approaches the cubital fossa it divides into two more constant branches, one supplying the cephalic vein and one supplying the basilic vein. These branches are the median cephalic and median basilic veins, respectively. The latter is normally more prominent partly due to its receiving a contributory vein, the deep vein, which emerges from the investing fascia of the cubital fossa and partly due to its loose attachment to the enveloping fascia.

It should be noted that the above is a description of the standard formation of the superficial veins of the upper limb. There is great variation in the formation and position of these veins which has led to differences in the nomenclature used by anatomy texts.

Since the greatest fear in venipuncture is intra-arterial injection, it is important

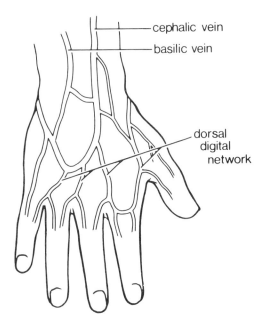

Figure 11.1. Dorsal digital venous plexus of hand. (From Everett, G. B., and Allen, G. D.: Intravenous therapy: a review of site selection and techniques. *Anesth Prog* 9:280, 1969.)

These anatomical situations must be kept in mind when inspecting the cubital fossa for a suitable vein. Often the most tempting choice of vein to be used is the

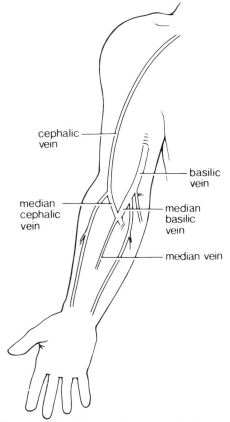

Figure 11.2.   Venous drainage of the forearm.

to remember that within the cubital fossa the median basilic vein is separated from the brachial artery and its accompanying median nerve only by the bicipital aponeurosis, a medial extension of the biceps brachial tendon which passes distally and medially (Fig. 11.3). In addition, the brachial artery may divide into the radial and ulnar arteries above the aponeurosis and either of the divisions may pass superficially within the cubital fossa. Approximately 18 per cent of the population have superficial arteries in this region, and this is bilateral in one-fifth of the cases. When this occurs, the radial artery usually passes under the bicipital aponeurosis to become superficial in the upper forearm and continue subfascially to the wrist. The ulnar artery, arising from a premature brachial bifurcation, is more likely to be found in a superficial location in the cubital fossa, either traversing the bicipital aponeurosis or piercing the aponeurosis at a variable location in the fossa or forearm.

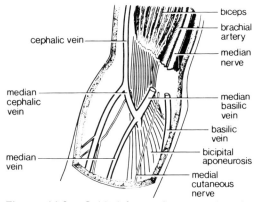

Figure 11.3. Cubital fossa demonstrating the close relationship of the brachial artery and median nerve to the median basilic vein. They are separated only by the bicipital aponeurosis.

median basilic. Should venipuncture be attempted here, however, there is the possibility of missing or passing through the vein, penetrating the bicipital aponeurosis and entering the brachial artery or injuring the median nerve. For this reason, the median basilic vein should not be used. It is safer to choose a vein on the lateral aspect of the fossa, such as the median cephalic or the cephalic.

Since veins on the forearm, distal to the cubital fossa, are loosely held by the investing fascia, they appear to be quite prominent but their mobility renders them difficult to enter when venipuncture is attempted.

No matter which vessel is chosen for the injection, the cardinal rule is that it must always be palpated before embarking on venipuncture. The presence of a pulse suggests an artery and an alternate vein should be sought.

CHOICE OF SITE OF INJECTION

There are two schools of thought regarding the site of intravenous injection, one favoring the dorsum of the hand and the other the cubital fossa or forearm. In general, minor complications using the back of the hand are frequent, while major complications occur only if the cubital fossa is used.

The greatest advantage of using the dorsum of the hand is the reduced possibility of intra-arterial injection as the arteries in this area are quite small, relatively deep, and have fewer abnormalities than those of the arm. Occasionally, pain in the hand is experienced during injection due to a rapid transfer of the injection solution to the arterial side *via* an arteriovenous fistula initiating transient vasospasm. Should an intraarterial injection be inadvertently given, the area supplied by the arteries in the hand is much smaller than that supplied by the major arteries of the arm and the consequences would, therefore, be less serious.

Although the veins on the back of the hand are often more prominent, they are only loosely bound by the superficial fascia and tend to move away from the needle point when attempting venipuncture. The veins are also small and more tortuous than those in the arm, again making entry more difficult. In addition, many intravenous agents are irritants and injecting them into such small veins increases the incidence of venous thrombosis and thrombophlebitis. Finally, from the patient's point of view, should a hematoma occur following venipuncture, it is noticeable on the dorsum of the hand whereas in the cubital fossa it can be hidden by long-sleeved clothing.

When the veins of the cubital fossa or forearm are used, the veins, being much larger, will allow rapid dilution of the drug and, therefore, lead to less venous irritation. Venipuncture is also facilitated there by the size of the veins and by the underlying aponeurosis holding them firmly in position in the cubital fossa. The major drawback of this site of injection is the presence of major arteries and nerves, increasing the possibility of penetrating these structures to cause intra-arterial injection or neuropathies. The proponents of this area claim that these risks are eliminated by the correct choice of veins and a safe venipuncture technique.

VENIPUNCTURE IN THE CUBITAL FOSSA

Venipuncture can be divided into distinct stages: 1) identification of the vein to be used; 2) "sterilization" of the area; 3) alignment of the needle; 4) penetration of the vein; 5) aspiration of the blood; 6) injection of the drug; 7) removal of the needle.

1. The patient is placed in the dental chair in the semi-supine position with the dentist sitting by his side facing the patient. The chair is then raised sufficiently to allow the patient's arm to slope downward, facilitating the pooling of the blood in the arm. Arterial pulsations should

now be palpated and arterial routes accurately identified with the patient's arm in a relaxed position (Fig. 11.4). This is accomplished with the arm not extended on an armboard and prior to tourniquet placement. The vein chosen for the venipuncture should also be palpated to ensure that indeed it is not an aberrant artery. The tourniquet is placed proximal to the proposed site of injection. Tourniquet pressure need provide only moderate venous obstruction as, even with this moderate pressure, arterial pulsations in small superficial arteries may be obliterated, a prime example being the superficial ulnar artery. The dental operating light should be directed transversely across the area, thus throwing the vessels into relief. Light aimed directly over the operating site may make the vessels more difficult to see.

2. The site of injection should be swabbed with alcohol for at least 30 seconds. Although this does not "sterilize" the epidermis, it does remove any obvious surface contamination and is expected by most patients as part of an acceptable procedure.

3. The operator's left hand is used to support the arm with his left thumb placed distal to the proposed point of penetration and lateral to the path of the vein

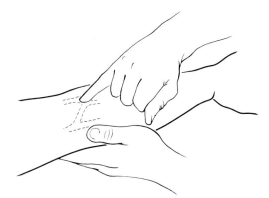

Figure 11.4. The first stage of venipuncture. Palpation to ensure that there is no pulsation to define the position of the brachial artery, which must be avoided.

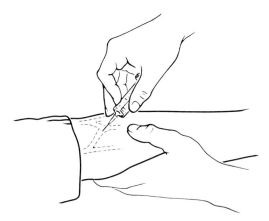

Figure 11.5. Alignment of the needle at 30° to the vein of choice with the left hand stabilizing the vein and the arm.

(Fig. 11.5). The thumb applies tension to the skin, pulling in the same direction as the vein runs. If tension is applied laterally, the vein will be compressed and also pulled to one side, making penetration difficult. Sometimes, the clinician or his assistant applies one or two drops of ethyl chloride on the area of penetration to achieve some surface anesthesia. With the advent of sharp disposable needles of small gauge, venipuncture can be accomplished painlessly without this embellishment.

The syringe is held in the right hand between forefinger and thumb with the remaining three fingers acting as stabilizers. The gradations on the syringe should be uppermost visible to the operator on injecting. The needle point is placed 1 cm behind the section of the vein to be entered, at an angle of 30° to the skin and, most important of all, in line with the vein.

4. The act of inserting the needle into the vein should be one smooth continuous motion. Once the lumen of the vein has been entered, the direction of the needle is altered to run parallel to the skin surface so that the needle is threaded into the vein for at least 1 cm.

It is claimed that if an artery has been entered, it will be evident at this stage by the appearance of blood pulsating back into the barrel of the syringe and by the bright red color of the blood. This should not be relied upon, since a small gauge needle may reduce the arterial force sufficiently to prevent this backflow and the color of venous blood varies from dark blue to bright red.

5. To confirm that the needle is now within the vein, aspiration is carried out (Fig. 11.6). The thumb of the left hand is transferred to the hub of the syringe to stabilize it while the right hand draws back the plunger. The left thumb should hold the syringe firmly but gently as too much pressure by the left thumb can force the needle through the vein wall. The amount of blood aspirated should only be sufficient to ensure that a vein has been entered. Aspiration should be completed before every injection and an incremental technique may require several aspirations. Should excessive blood be withdrawn each time, the operator will find that he eventually has a syringe full of blood, making aspiration difficult to assess.

6. Finally, the drug is injected (Fig. 11.7). Only a small increment of the drug should be given initially and the patient's reaction assessed. If there is complaint of pain at the site of injection, it suggests extravascular injection and may be accompanied by a slight swelling at the site

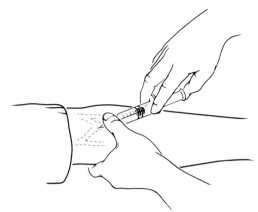

Figure 11.7. Injection of drug, having released the pressure in the tourniquet.

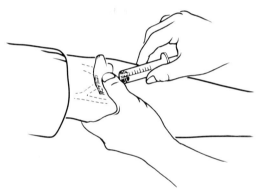

Figure 11.8. Removal of the needle and application of pressure over the area to prevent hematoma formation.

of injection. Pain or a burning sensation running up the arm is common with irritant drugs such as diazepam and is indicative of the drug irritating the vein wall. However, the most serious complaint is severe, acute pain running down the arm accompanied by blanching of the extremities. This is indicative intra-arterial injection and, hence, the reason for limiting the initial increment. In addition, if any immediate adverse reaction to the drug is seen, then the less drug given the better.

7. On completion of injection, a sterile gauze swab is held firmly over the venipuncture site, both while the needle is removed and for the following 2 minutes (Fig. 11.8). This will decrease the chances of hematoma formation.

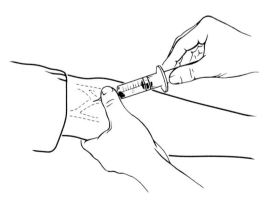

Figure 11.6. Following venipuncture, aspiration is carried out with the thumb of the left hand stabilizing the syringe.

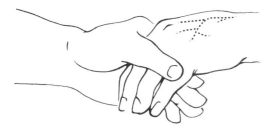

Figure 11.9. Hand position for intravenous injection in the dorsal of the hand.

VENIPUNCTURE IN THE DORSUM OF THE HAND

If the dorsum of the hand is to be used, the patient's hand should be clasped gently with the operator's left hand, his free thumb fixing the veins by applying tension of the skin distal to the site of venipuncture (Fig. 11.9). The thumb must be placed on the phalanges rather than the metacarpals to prevent obscuring the field and making the inclination of the needle too steep. The tourniquet is placed on the wrist and the stages of venipuncture carried out as already described.

DIFFICULT VEINS

Before a patient is offered intravenous sedation, he should be examined for suitable veins. It takes only a few embarrassing venipuncture failures on a nervous patient to reinforce this point. Generally, children are poor candidates for intravenous techniques as their veins are small and very often masked by subdermal fatty tissue. Obesity is also a problem in adults where even large veins may be difficult to see, although they can be palpated. Nervous patients may display poor veins because their fear leads to stimulation of the sympathetic system and subsequent vasoconstriction. This also occurs when the patient is cold, either due to the weather or to a cool operatory; therefore, try to relax the patient and have a warm environment in the dental office.

After a tourniquet is applied with the patient's arm positioned sloping down to enhance venous pooling in the arm, the chair light is shined across the arm, throwing the veins into relief. Venous pressure can be increased by the patient opening and closing his fist and veins will become more extended if the overlying skin is flicked with the finger. If the vein is not yet obvious, hot packs may be applied. Often a vein which cannot be seen can be found on palpation to be quite large and obvious. To confirm the vein's position, the forefinger is placed along the path of the vein and rolled back and forth. This should indicate the direction the needle must take and the depth at which the vein lies. Nitrous oxide-oxygen is sometimes used to bring up veins, since it both relaxes the patient and causes peripheral vasodilation. Upon successfully entering the vein, the nitrous oxide-oxygen may be terminated.

Whatever technique is used to find the difficult vein, it is important to wait until the veins are well extended before attempting venipuncture. The trauma of a failed venipuncture can cause collapse of the vein in addition to extravasation of blood.

COMPLICATIONS IN VENIPUNCTURE AND THEIR TREATMENT

The administration of drugs intravenously is a safe technique if the preceding instructions are followed, but where complications do arise, the operator should be able to recognize and treat them, and to analyze the problem.

The most common complication is hematoma. This is the result of extravasation of blood into the surrounding tissues and may be as mild as a small yellow blemish or may, in extreme cases, be an angry blue/red area several centimeters in diameter accompanied by mild edema and tenderness. It is caused by trauma to the vein either by inadequate venipuncture, by penetration through both walls of a vein, or by tearing of the vein wall by a blunt needle. The cause of hematoma is often lack of pressure over the venipuncture site after withdrawal of the needle. A sterile gauze swab should be held firmly over the venipuncture site for at least 2 minutes after withdrawal of the needle. Normally, a hematoma requires no treatment, although its breakdown and resolution will be enhanced by the application of hot packs.

Venous thrombosis also varies from a small painless nodule which can barely be palpated to a tender hard cord which runs the length of the vein. Often, like the hematoma, it is not noticed until several days after the venipuncture. The thrombosis is usually the result of injecting irritant solutions into small veins. The possibility of thrombosis can be avoided by the following: diluting irritant solutions beforehand; administering the drug via an intravenous drip of a carrier solution such as dextrose; injecting the drug slowly, thereby allowing it to be diluted by the blood; using only large veins; or by flushing the veins with a solution such as dextrose or saline after injection. Dissolution of the thrombus again will be enhanced by application of hot packs over the affected area. Recent studies indicate that venous thrombosis of some degree always occurs following injection of diazepam.

Phlebitis, or inflammation of the vein, may be seen as a red wheal following the course of the vein and is tender to palpation. The causes are similar to that of thrombosis and it is often accompanied by thrombosis, producing a thrombophlebitis. Thrombophlebitis may be accompanied by fever, malaise, and leukocytosis. Following the acute stage, which may last several days, the vein may remain tender for several weeks. The treatment for this condition when severe is 100 mg of phenylbutazone t.i.d. for 3 days. Not only will this provide analgesia, but its anti-inflammatory properties will also be beneficial. Since it may cause gastric irritation, it must be taken at meal times and prescribed only to patients with no history of gastric problems. Antibiotic coverage is also advisable due to the pos-

sibility of infection being present and application of hot packs will again facilitate the breakdown of the clot. Where the thrombus or thrombophlebitis is extensive, it is advisable to rest the affected arm by means of a sling to prevent further irritation and propagation of the clot.

Should a thrombus become infected, then suppuration with septicemia is a possible, but rare, complication, and is more likely to occur with an indwelling catheter than with a single intravenous injection. In addition to the treatment prescribed for thrombophlebitis, the patient would require hospitalization for observation.

Air emboli during injection is often a fear of both the patient and the novice operator. It can be avoided by ensuring that the system used is completely air-free and air-tight, whether it be a needle and syringe or a continuous drip system. Should a small air bubble enter the venous system, there is little cause for alarm as it will dissolve in the blood.

Intra-arterial injection of a drug may result in severe pain distal to the site of venipuncture, blanching of the hand, and loss of a radial pulse. The drug will not be diluted in the artery as it would in the veins which increase in volume as they follow their course. On the contrary, the drug will pass into ever-decreasing vessels, causing tissue damage, arteriospasm, and inflammation leading to thrombosis. The amount of thrombus formation will depend on the irritant properties and the volume of the solution injected. This, in turn, will determine the area involved, the degree of gangrene which may follow, and, therefore, the loss of tissue. Treatment must be immediate. Five to 10 cc of 1 percent procaine should be injected through the "indwelling" needle. This is important as once the needle is removed, the artery will be in spasm and impossible to find. The procaine will serve to dilute the injected drug, providing vasodilation of the peripheral vessels and giving some relief from the pain. This should suffice

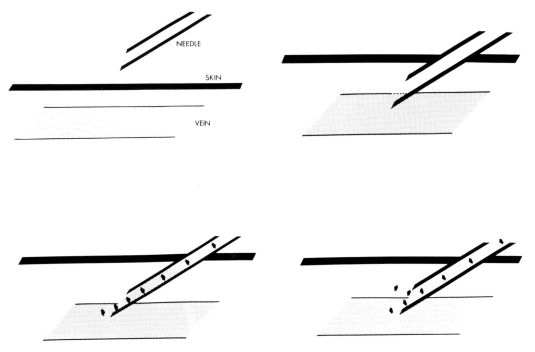

Figure 11.10. With the bevel of the needle up, blood may be aspirated but perivascular injection can still occur.

in the majority of cases to circumvent further problems. Additional treatment requires hospitalization and includes elevation of the extremity to heart level with immediate heparinization with 10,000 units intravenously followed by 5,000 units intravenously every 6 hours for 4 to 5 days. Dilatation of the arteries can be produced by sympathetic nerve block of the stellate ganglion or the brachial plexus. This, together with the use of narcotics, will alleviate the pain. Arteriography may be used to find the extent of damage, followed by thrombectomy to establish pulses in the major vessels. Resultant gangrenous areas are then treated surgically. The importance of recognizing vessels, injecting drugs slowly in increments, and diluting the drug where possible will now be recognized.

Perivascular injection should be suspected when the patient complains of pain at the site of injection accompanied by swelling of the tissues around this area. A positive aspiration test does not dis-

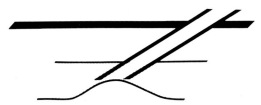

Figure 11.11. With the bevel of the needle pointing down, suction of the vein wall may cause blockage of the lumen on a negative aspiration test.

count possible perivascular injection. Especially with large bore needles inserted with the bevel up, it is possible to only partially penetrate a vein, thus allowing aspiration of blood but also extravascular injection (Fig. 11.10). For this reason, many advocate that the bevel of a needle should face downward during venipuncture. This, in turn, however, may produce the opposite phenomenon. The bevel of the needle may lie parallel to the vein wall and, on aspiration, draw up the vein wall to produce a negative aspiration test (Fig. 11.11). Injection could still be carried out painlessly, but by slight rotation of the needle will regain a reassuring positive aspiration.

EQUIPMENT FOR VENIPUNCTURE

Intravenous sedation technique has the advantage that very little equipment is required in addition to that used in a properly equipped dental office. Expensive, sophisticated equipment is available, however, and the denist must tailor his needs according to the techniques he will be using.

Tourniquets

A tourniquet in its simplest form is a length of rubber tubing tied in a slip knot proximal to the site of injection. Many other simple tourniquets are also available, all of which have the same problem—poor control of the pressure applied. A tight tourniquet will prevent arterial blood supply to the area, whereas a loose one will allow venous outflow. A sphygmomanometer taken just above the diastolic pressure point will overcome both these problems. In addition, once the sphygmomanometer is in place, it is an added incentive for the dentist to record the patient's blood pressure before each treatment.

Armboards

The purpose of an armboard is to keep the patient's arm immobilized during venipuncture and the subsequent injection of drugs. In its simplest form, it is a flat board supporting the arm with straps at both ends which transfix the wrist and upper arm. More complex types are bolted to the dental chair and have a wide range of position. These are a worthwhile investment where extensive sedation or general anesthesia techniques are used that require drugs to be given intermittently throughout the procedure. The simpler armboards can become quite uncomfortable if left in place for any time

and in some cases as the arm relaxes and flexes, the proximal restraining strap acts as tourniquet.

Instead of an armboard, the dental assistant can hold the patient's arm by the wrist with one hand, and support it under the elbow with the other during venipuncture. While standing at the side of the patient, she will act as a screen to the working area while conversing with and reassuring the patient. Where there is a continuous drip or intermittent injection, the needle can be taped in position and the arm then placed on the armrest of the chair. Fortunately, most dental chairs have armrests which are designed to cradle the arm comfortably for long periods of time. Those not so well designed can be adapted with a square of foam sponge placed in the region of the elbow. The arm will be sufficiently immobilized throughout the procedure if the wrist is lightly taped to the chair.

Needles

The first hypodermic needle in the form of a quill attached to a syringe is attributed to the combined efforts of the artist, Christopher Wren, and the chemist, Robert Boyle, in the 17th century. It was necessary at that time to use a lancet to cut down into the vein. Today's needles are so designed and manufactured that the skin is smoothly pierced, the vein entered, and fluids subsequently administered.

Modern disposable needles are made of stainless steel or aluminum, both of which are noncorrosive and inert. In addition to the bevels placed at the tips of the needles, some are coated with silicone to enhance penetration. The silicone also has the advantage of being hemorepellent, which minimizes clot formation.

Needles are classified according to their length and the gauge, the latter originally referring to the outside diameter of the needle, but now associated with the lumen size. The common range of needle gauge is from 14 to 25; the larger the gauge number, the smaller the lumen size. Large lumen needles need only be used where viscous fluids are involved.

Winged Needles

Winged infusion needles are originally called scalp vein needles. These were designed for venipuncture of the scalp vein of infants where the other superificial veins were inaccessible. Conventional needles were too long for this purpose and could easily penetrate the opposite wall of the vein. This was overcome by the shorter needle with wings that are taped to the scalp to secure the needle in place. The winged infusion set is now preferred by many for venipuncture in patients of all ages because of its versatility and re-

liability in maintaining a vein once inserted. It consists of a short stainless steel needle with normally two flexible wings mounted on the shank, and variable length of tubing attached to a female Luer adapter (Fig. 11.12). This can be fitted to various intravenous setups such as a single syringe or a continuous drip. The needle is held by the wings, which are folded together during venipuncture. The wings are laid flat and taped securely to the skin, assuring that the needle will remain in the lumen of the vein while allowing a degree of movement by the patient. A variation of the above is a single winged needle. Its main advantage is that should the lumen of the needle lie too close to the vein wall and thus prevent aspiration, it can be rotated 180°, which will free it from the vein wall (Figs. 11.13 to 11.16).

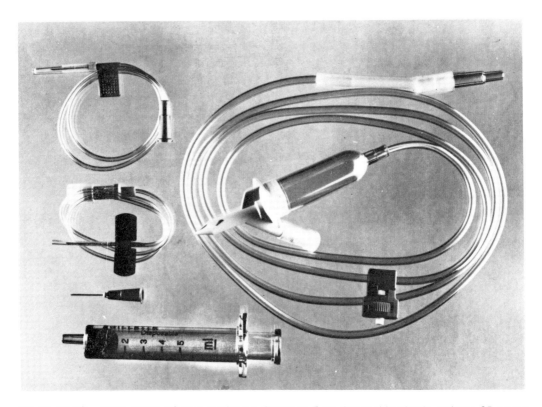

Figure 11.12. From *lower left* in a clockwise direction: 5-ml disposable plastic syringe; 25-gauge ⅝-inch needle; butterfly needle; "minicath" with single wing; veniset with bayonet connection and drip changer, wheel valve, and male Luer connection.

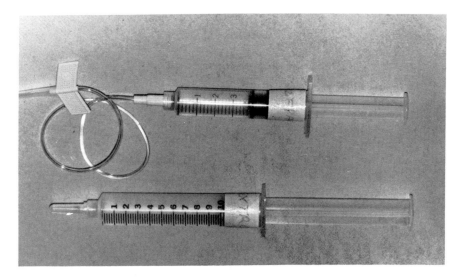

Figure 11.13. The two-syringe technique. The diazepam is placed in a 5-ml syringe with dextrose or saline in the 10-ml syringe. The contents of each syringe are clearly labeled but do not obscure the gradations. A 25-gauge needle may be used here.

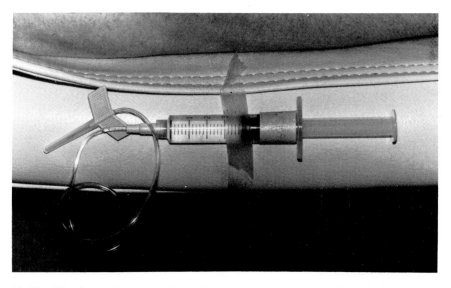

Figure 11.14. The two-syringe technique. Prior to venipuncture the 5-ml syringe is taped to the chair to free the operator's hands.

Continuous Drip Systems

Intravenous sedation or general anesthetic technique requires a continuous drip throughout to ensure that there is always a patent vein which can be used in an emergency. The individual dentist must assess whether the modality he is using necessitates such a procedure.

There are several solutions available for a continuous drip, the most common being dextrose, saline, and Ringer's solution. A veniset connecting the bottle fluid to the infusion device consists of several feet of clear flexible plastic tubing with a bayonet connection for the fluid at one end and a male Luer connection at the

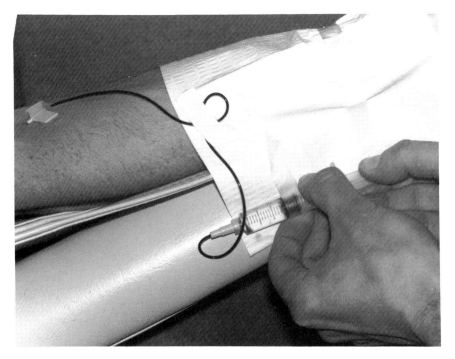

Figure 11.15.   The two-syringe technique. Following titration of the drug, blood is withdrawn to clear the excess diazepam from the extension tubing.

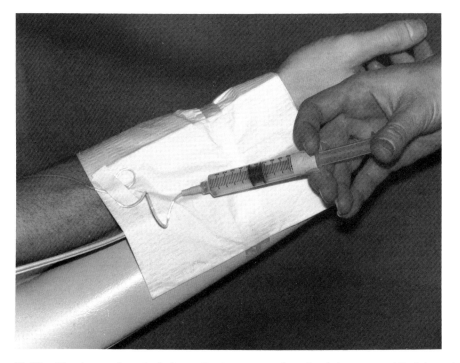

Figure 11.16.   The two-syringe technique. Dextrose or saline, 5 ml, is now rapidly injected. The remaining 5 ml can be given in increments over the next hour to maintain a patent vein.

other. Below the bayonet connection lies a clear plastic chamber through which the solution drips indicating the rate of flow. Further down the tubing, a valve is situated which regulates the rate of flow.

Once the veniset is attached to the suspended bottle of fluid and to the infusion kit, the valve is opened to allow the system to be completely filled with solution and cleared of all air bubbles. The valve is then closed, venipuncture and securing of the winged needle completed, and the patient's wrist taped to the arm rest. The valve is then opened to allow a flow of one drop every 1 or 2 seconds.

Close to the male Luer attachment of the veniset is a thicker portion of rubber tubing. When the drip is allowed to flow, this tubing may be pinched and quickly released to draw blood back momentarily into the system, thus indicating a patent vein. If the rate of flow is too rapid, this sign may be disguised (Fig. 11.17).

Intravenous drugs are then administered *via* this system by injecting the drug through the rubber tubing. Before doing so, however, it should be confirmed that the drug is compatible with the parenteral solution (Fig. 11.18).

The preceding information is basic for a dentist to safely administer an intravenous drug. The further requirements before embarking on intravenous sedation are clinical experience under supervision and the ability to choose a safe drug.

INTRADERMAL AND SUBCUTANEOUS INJECTION

Intradermal and subcutaneous injections are seldom used in dentistry. The intradermal or intracutaneous injection may be used mainly for diagnostic purposes, such as a tuberculin test, or a test for sensitivity to various substances. The solutions are injected in the corium of the skin from which they are absorbed slowly

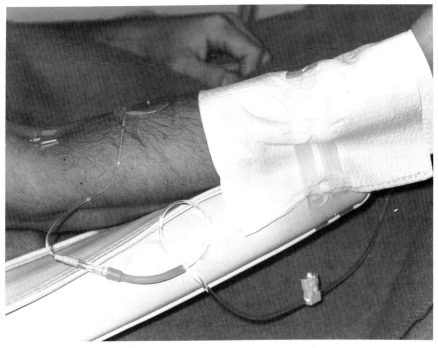

Figure 11.17. Intravenous drip technique. The gauge of the needle must be at least 23 to allow the flow of fluid. Note that the tubing is taped to the dental chair arm as a reminder to the patient that there is an intravenous needle in his arm. The wheel valve is brought close to area of operation to allow easy change of the flow rate.

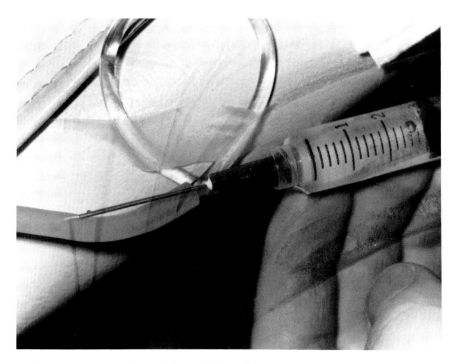

Figure 11.18. Intravenous drip technique. With a fairly rapid drip rate the diazepam is titrated through the tubing to the patient at the normal rate of titration. Excess tubing is taped to the chair to prevent the needle being accidently removed.

by the capillaries. Only small amounts of solution are injected—normally only a few drops. This method of sensitivity testing has the advantage of displaying the body's reaction to the substance clearly at a superficial level and, since so little agent is used, the reaction is normally localized with no systemic reaction.

A fine 26-gauge needle is inserted into the dermis at a 10° angle (Fig. 11.19) with the bevel up. Once the lumen is obscured the fluid is injected forming a slight weal. The needle is removed rapidly but the site is *not* massaged, since this may disguise any reaction to the substance. A subcutaneous injection of local anesthetic is advocated by some as a precursor to intramuscular injections to reduce the discomfort of this injection. However, the subcutaneous plexus of sensory nerves cause the subcutaneous injections to be even more painful than the intramuscular injection itself.

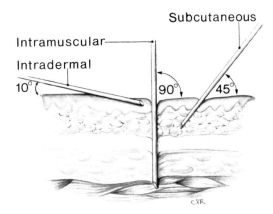

Figure 11.19. Angle of entry for intradermal, subcutaneous, and intramuscular injections.

Where a subcutaneous injection is deemed appropriate a ⅝-inch needle would normally be inserted at a 45° angle (Fig. 11.13). In an obese patient a ⅝-inch needle may not reach the subcutaneous tissues. This can be overcome by increasing the angle to entry to 90° and using a 1-inch needle.

The most common site for subcutaneous injections is the upper arm. The area of injection is swabbed with a gauze moistened with antiseptic and then the tissue is grasped between the forefinger and thumb. The needle is inserted rapidly to the required depth and the plunger of the syringe than retracted gently to determine whether the needle is in a blood vessel. Should the aspiration be positive and blood drawn back into the syringe the needle should be partially withdrawn and reinserted at a different angle. Only when a negative aspiration is obtained may the drug be slowly injected. Finally the needle is withdrawn quickly while applying pressure with a gauze swab at the site of injection and the area massaged with the swab.

INTRAMUSCULAR INJECTION

Since there are few nociceptors in deep muscle tissue intramuscular injections are often given for irritant solutions. This is also a route of administration which is seldom used for outpatient dentistry but is popular by some for administering preoperative sedatives to inpatients.

Absorption of the drug from the muscle tissues is relatively rapid due to the great vascularity of these areas. Peak blood levels are therefore reached more rapidly than if the drug was administered orally, although the intravenous route obtains the swiftest peak blood levels.

A dose of 2 to 5 ml of solution may be given intramuscularly with no notable tissue damage. Where larger amounts are necessary the drug should be given in divided dosages.

While the intramuscular route is therefore more rapidly effective than oral administration, it suffers from similar drawbacks. It is difficult to titrate the exact dosage required for each patient because of the delay in maximum effect of the drug and therefore empirical formulas

must be used, taking into consideration such factors as the patient's age, weight, and physical condition.

Sites of Intramuscular Injection

It is important that the muscle chosen for the injection be sufficiently large to absorb the volume of drug being used. It should also be situated in an area free of major nerves and blood vessels.

The *dorsogluteal* has for long been a popular site of injection. The area injected is on the upper, outer quadrant of the buttock, 5 to 7.5 cm below the iliac crest of the pelvic. A common error, however, is injecting too low because of erroneous determination of the iliac crest. To overcome this the iliac crest should be palpated rather than being identified visually. One hand is then placed on the gluteal muscle so that the forefinger and thumb outline the area of injection. Where the injection is too low the sciatic nerve may become involved (Fig. 11.20).

The anatomical landmarks of this site can be observed in obese patients because of the excessive adipose tissue being mistaken for muscle. Yet another mistake when attempting to identify the area is failure to remove the patient's undergarments. Merely raising the underclothing does not expose the area sufficiently and can constrict the area sufficiently to cause a low injection.

The patient should lie in a prone position with the toes pointed inwards or on their side with the upper knee flexed and upper leg forward. These postures help to relax the gluteal muscle.

The dorsalogluteal injection may be embarrassing for some outpatients and because of this the *deltoid and posterior triceps* area may be more acceptable. However, since these muscles are relatively small it is possible to involve the axillary or radical nerves (Fig. 11.21). The small mass of muscle may also be responsible for the incidence of post-injection pain and discomfort following injection

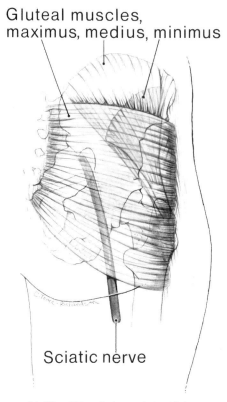

Gluteal muscles,
maximus, medius, minimus

Sciatic nerve

Figure 11.20. Site of dorsogluteal intramuscular injection demonstrating presence of sciatic nerve.

able and also dependent on the site of injection, the obesity of the patient and whether the patient is a child or an adult.

The patient is placed in a position appropriate for the site of injection as described previously. A small amount of air is drawn into the syringe, and this will be used at the conclusion of injecting into the muscle to ensure that all the drug is expressed from the lumen of the needle. This ensures that no irritating solution is deposited in nonmuscular tissue as the needle is withdrawn.

The site of injection is cleaned with a gauze swab moistened with an antiseptic solution. The skin is held taut by placing one hand flat on the muscle and spreading

into this site. The point of entry lies on the outer aspect of the arm below the acromion and above the level of the axilla. The patient may sit upright for this injection.

Another area which provides a large muscle mass in a relatively accessible area is the upper thigh, in particular the quadriceps. The area to avoid is the femoral triangle, containing the femoral artery, vein, and nerve (Fig. 11.22). These will only be encountered if the injection is too high.

Intramuscular Injection Techniques

The most common needle used for this injection is a 22-gauge, 1½-inch needle, although viscous solutions may require a 20-gauge needle. The length used is vari-

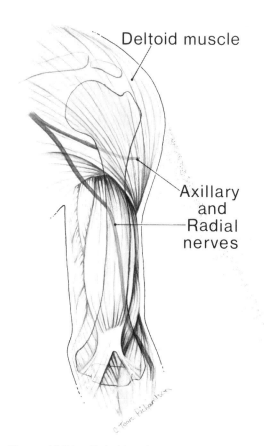

Deltoid muscle

Axillary
and
Radial
nerves

Figure 11.21. Deltoid and posterior triceps area for intramuscular injection demonstrating the presence of the axillary and radial nerves.

Femoral nerve, artery, vein

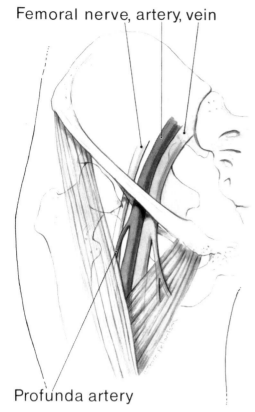

Profunda artery

Figure 11.22. The femoral triangle illustrating femoral artery, vein, and nerve.

the skin between the middle and index fingers. The needle is inserted at right angles to the skin (Fig. 11.19). Aspiration is then completed and if negative the solution is injected slowly. The needle is then swiftly removed and the area first held under pressure and then massaged with an antiseptic swab.

Bibliography

Adams RC: *Intravenous Anesthesia.* New York. Paul B. Hoeber, 1944.

Briscoe CE, Taylor PA: Morbidity following intravenous injections. *Anaesthesia* 29:290, 1974.

Dann TC: Routine skin preparation before injection. *Lancet* (2):96, 1969.

Pask A, Robson JC: Injury to the median nerve. *Anaesthesia* 9:94, 1954.

CHAPTER 12

Oral, Intramuscular, and Intravenous Sedation

Analgesia and sedation in the conscious patient through administering drugs orally, intramuscularly, or intravenously has allowed the modern dentist to overcome the biggest obstacle to providing dental care to the public: anxiety. Studies have shown that up to 50 per cent of the population in Western countries avoid routine dental treatment because of fear of denistry. Sedation techniques are both safer and more effective in gaining the patient's confidence in the dentist than general anesthesia when used to counter this fear. The key requirements for these techniques are the correct choice of route of administration and a knowledge of the pharmacology of the drugs used.

ROUTE OF ADMINISTRATION

The oral route of administration is regarded by many dentists as the safest route. This is partly because it is an uncomplicated procedure and partly because it is the traditional method of sedation. Overprescription of these drugs, however, has become an ever-increasing problem in recent years. Not only does this provide an avenue for willful or accidental drug abuse by the patient, but drug adverse reactions appear to be on the increase. One survey claims that 1 in 6 of all admissions to a hospital in England were due to one of these factors. The most severe type of adverse reaction is, of course, anaphylactic shock, admittedly less common *via* the oral route than with intramuscular or intravenous injection. Even with immediate medical attention, however, this is a life-threatening situa-

tion. If a patient is instructed to take the medication at bedtime the night before an appointment, then the possibility of the symptoms going unnoticed or help being unavailable is increased.

Overdosage or underdosage with oral drugs is associated with using empirical formulas for prescribing drugs. There are so many variables, ranging from the patient's individual metabolism to his emotional condition, that it is difficult to assay the correct sedative dose for any one person.

From the above, it becomes obvious that the safest way to administer a drug is to be present when the patient receives the drug and to titrate each drug against the patient. We are able to do this accurately using the intravenous or inhalation route, where the patient's response to the drug is continually monitored.

PHARMACOLOGY OF THE DRUGS USED FOR ANALGESIA, SEDATION, AND HYPNOSIS

There have been many classifications given for sedative and hypnotic drugs and there will doubtless be many more as new drugs are synthesized in the future. However, at present the following simple classification suffices.

I. Barbiturates
II. Nonbarbiturate sedative hypnotics
   A. Chloral hydrate
   B. Ethchlorvynol
   C. Paraldehyde
   D. Glutethimide
   E. Methaqualone

III. Antianxiety agents (minor tranquil-
izers)
   A. Meprobamate
   B. Benzodiazepines
IV. Narcotic analgesics
   A. Morphine
   B. Meperidine
   C. Fentanyl
   D. Alphaprodine hydrochloride
   E. Pentazocine
V. Antihistamines with sedative prop-
erties
   A. Phenothiazines
   B. Hydroxyzine
VI. Anticholingeric agents

Barbiturates

This group of drugs depresses the central nervous system in particular and can depress a wide variety of other biological functions. Depending upon dosage, the effects of these drugs may range from mild sedation to deep hypnosis, general anesthesia, and eventually to death (Table 12.1). They are especially effective in the reticular activating system and the cerebral cortex. Their probable action is by preventing transmission of impulses at the presynaptic nerve terminals. Respiration and cardiovascular depression is minimal when small sedative doses are utilized; however, with increasing doses, respiratory depression becomes a clinically evident feature. The site of this action is the reticular formation of the medulla, wherein is situated the neurogenic center for respiratory drive while awake. In sleep, the respiratory drive is controlled by the arterial concentration of carbon dioxide and the hydrogen ion in the respiratory center. In the hypnotic state, therefore, the breathing mechanism resembles that of normal sleeping. Increasing the dosage of barbiturates may depress the medullary respiratory center sufficiently that it no longer responds to increases in carbon dioxide concentrations. Since carbon dioxide itself is a general anesthetic agent the respiratory center will be depressed further. Respiratory control is then taken over by the primitive aortic and carotid bodies and is driven by hypoxia. Thus overdosage with barbiturate can lead to a hypoxic coma leading eventually to anoxia.

Extremely high concentrations of barbiturates are required before depression of the myocardium occurs.

Metabolism of the barbiturates is carried out by the liver and the breakdown products are excreted by the kidneys. The very long-acting barbiturates, however,

Table 12.1.
Classification of Commonly Used Barbiturates According to Duration of Action

	Generic Name	Trade Name
Ultrashort-acting	Thiopental	Pentothal
	Thiamylal	Surital
	Methohexital	Brevital
Short-acting	Cyclobarbital	Phandodorn
	Allylbarbital	Sandoptal
	Heptabarbital	Medomin
	Secobarbital	Seconal
Intermediate-acting	Amobarbital	Amytal
	Aprobarbital	Alurate
	Butabarbital	Butisol
	Allobarbital	Dial
	Pentobarbital	Nembutal
	Vinbarbital	Delvinal
Long-acting	Barbital	Veronal
	Mephobarbital	Mebarbal
	Metharbital	Gemonil
	Phenobarbital	Luminal

are excreted unchanged. Although apparently short acting, the rate of metabolism of thiopental sodium is relatively slow. The short duration is explained by the redistribution of the drug from the brain to the other tissues. Long term use of barbiturates can increase the enzymatic metabolism of the liver six-fold, which is a consideration where other drugs are being administered, since their metabolism will also be increased. Drugs such as the coumarins, phenytoin, and griseofulvin may thus require an increase in dosage for the same therapeutic effect.

The barbiturates are anticonvulsant and elevate the threshold of neurons to excitation. It should be noted, however, that the barbiturates are not analgesic but may indeed be hyperalgesic and for this reason they should not be given as a hypnotic where pain is present unless an analgesic is used concomitantly. This action is probably due to depression of higher central nervous system centers allowing control to revert to the more primitive systems of the central nervous system.

Although barbiturates are used to enhance sleep, the sleep produced is not a natural sleep in that there is a reduction in rapid eye movement (REM) and, therefore, a reduction in dream periods. The patient may, therefore, awaken feeling drugged and tired after a barbiturate-induced sleep.

In contrast, some patients may exhibit an idiosyncratic reaction to barbiturates and become more excited and apprehensive than sedated. This is thought to be due to a depression of normal inhibition.

Despite these drawbacks, the long-acting barbiturates will probably continue to be popular as oral sedatives and certainly pentobarbital with its high therapeutic index will continue as a drug of choice for intravenous sedation.

ULTRASHORT-ACTING BARBITURATES (THIOPENTAL, METHOHEXITAL)

Although the ultrashort-acting barbiturates are advocated by many as useful sedative agents in various techniques, they must be regarded as general anesthetic agents. Only those trained and experienced in general anesthesia who can recognize and treat any concomitant problems should be prepared to use these drugs for outpatient dentistry.

PENTOBARBITAL (NEMBUTAL)

The sodium ethyl methyl barbiturate derivative known as pentobarbital and marketed under the trade name Nembutal is the most commonly utilized of the barbiturate sedatives. Depending upon dosage, the effects of the drug may range from mild sedation to deep hypnosis and anesthesia. The systemic pharmacology of pentobarbital is quite similar to that of thiopental with the site of action felt to be the reticular activating system and cerebral cortex. Respiratory and cardiovascular depression is minimal when the small sedative doses are utilized; however, with increasing dosage, respiratory depression becomes a clinically evident feature. As with thiopental, respiratory depression is due to the depression of the neurogenic respiratory drive with reversion to medullary control, which is affected by the arterial concentration of carbon dioxide. Increasing dosage may depress the medulla to a point where respiratory control is taken over by the primitive aortic and carotid bodies and is driven by hypoxia.

It has been shown that minimal dosage of pentobarbital will create an antianalgesic effect due to the suppression of higher centers of inhibitory control and subsequent over-reaction to painful stimuli. Studies indicate that the duration of action of pentobarbital is approximately 90 minutes after an intravenously administered sedative dose.

Metabolism of pentobarbital sodium takes place in the liver, and the metabolic breakdown products are excreted by the kidneys. Pentobarbital sodium is bound to plasma proteins to a lesser extent than thiopental and, therefore, the greater proportion of the pentobarbital is excreted as the original drug in the urine.

The margin of safety between the sedative and toxic dose of pentobarbital is of such magnitude that this drug has gained much favor for intravenous sedation. It may be utilized as the sole drug for sedation or may be combined with a narcotic or a tranquilizer and its potentiating actions utilized allowing lower dosage of all drugs concerned.

The intravenous dose of pentobarbital may range from as little as 30 mg to as much as 200 mg, depending on the individual patient. Utilization of pentobarbital sodium by the intravenous route should be by slow incremental administration with observation for 1 to 2 minutes after each addition of the drug to provide the desired level of sedation. It must be remembered that pentobarbital is not an analgesic and, therefore, the patient may react inordinately to painful stimuli after an adequate level of sedation has been obtained.

In summary the barbiturates produce all signs of CNS depression from mild sedation to coma, depending on the dose and patient susceptibility. They are useful sedatives and hypnotics but not for long term insomnia. In addition to the "morning after" effect of dowsiness and depression when used over a short term, prolonged use leads to tolerance and dependence.

The Nonbarbiturate Sedative-Hypnotics

CHLORAL HYDRATE (NOCTEC)

Chloral hydrate is an excellent sedative-hypnotic, appearing as colorless or white hygroscopic crystals with a pungent odor. It is extremely irritating and, therefore, it use is limited to oral capsules or suppositories. Gastric irritation can be reduced by a glass of water or milk immediately after a capsule.

Chloral hydrate is rapidly absorbed from the intestinal tract and metabolized in the liver and kidney into its active form, trichlorethanol. This is eventually excreted via the kidneys and bile either free or in the conjugated glucuronide form. As the metabolic pathway is the same as that of ethanol and as both are central nervous system depressants, alcohol may significantly potentiate the hypnotic effect of chloral hydrate. Like the hydrocarbon anesthetic, it produces mild cerebral depression at therapeutic doses and can lead to depression of the respiratory and vasomotor centers at higher doses.

Its hypnotic effect is rapid, producing drowsiness within 15 minutes and sleep within an hour and it has found much favor in pedodontics when used in the suppository form. The usual pediatric dose is 50 mg per kg not to exceed 1 g.

ETHCHLORVYNOL (PLACIDYL)

As this is a condensation product of chloral hydrate, many of its properties are understandably similar. It is a clear yellow liquid from a pungent odor and a bitter taste and is presented in a capsulated form. Its main advantage over chloral hydrate is that it is less irritating to the gastric mucosa.

It is rapidly absorbed from the gastrointestinal tract, producing hypnosis in 30 minutes, and is metabolized in the liver. Since both chloral hydrate and ethchlorvynol may affect the prothrombin time, care should be taken when these are used on patients receiving coumarin or coumarin-like anticoagulants. Ethchlorvynol also may be potentiated by alcohol.

If used as an hypnotic premedicant for an adult dental outpatient, an adequate dose is 500 mg at bedtime.

PARALDEHYDE

Although a safe hypnotic with a high therapeutic index, paraldehyde is seldom used in dentistry. The main disadvantage is the offensive smell of paraldehyde, as it is excreted in the breath in its free form. It is an irritating, inflammable liquid and, although it can be given intravenously, it is more commonly administered orally since the taste is not unacceptable. Its onset and action are similar to those of chloral hydrate.

GLUTETHIMIDE (DORIDEN)

Although this drug is very similar in action to the barbiturates, they produce greater depression of the cardiovascular center. It was felt initially that this drug did not have the problems of tolerance and dependence associated with the barbiturates and therefore might replace them; however, these claims were found to be erroneous. In addition relatively large quantities of this drug were necessary to produce effects similar to the barbiturates. It is excreted *via* the bile and then resorbed in the small intestine, prolonging its action. The drug may interfere with the action of coumarin or coumarin-like drugs and the dosage of the drugs must be altered accordingly.

In dentistry, it may be given preoperatively as 500 mg the night before surgery and 500 mg 1 hour before the dental appointment.

METHAQUALONE

The effect of methaqualone is similar to that of the barbiturates, although it differs in that the cortex is depressed prior to the brainstem reticular formation. In low doses, sedation is produced while higher doses lead to hypnosis. The hypnotic effect is enhanced by barbiturates, chlorpromazine, glutethimide, alcohol, and other central nervous system depressants. This drug has found some popularity as a street drug mainly because of its reputation as an aphrodisiac. This latter property has yet to be substantiated and it is felt that it is the paresthesia which can be produced in the appendages of the body which have led to this claim.

Following oral administration, methaqualone is absorbed rapidly to produce drowsiness in 10 to 20 minutes and sleep in 30 minutes. It is metabolized by the liver and excreted as a glucuronide in the

urine and feces. As with most of the sedative hypnotics, caution should be used in patients with renal or hepatic dysfunction.

The standard oral hypnotic dose for an adult is 150 to 300 mg at bedtime and less in elderly or debilitated patients.

Antianxiety Agents (Minor Tranquilizer)

MEPROBAMATE

This drug is very similar to the barbiturates in its action and again was wrongly felt to have all the benefits of barbiturates without the problems of tolerance and dependence. This includes increased microsomal enzyme activity in the liver, which may affect the metabolism of other drugs. Meprobamate decreases the intraneural conductivity in the hypothalamus and spinal cord with little effect on the medulla or autonomic system.

It is a white, odorless crystalline powder with a bitter taste. Taken orally, it is rapidly absorbed from the gastrointestinal tract and reaches peak blood levels in 2 hours. All but 10 per cent of the drug is conjugated with glucuronic acid in the liver and excreted *via* the urine.

A wide variety of side effects have been reported, including drowsiness, ataxia, vertigo, visual impairment, nausea, and agranulocytosis. Once a popular sedative, it has been replaced almost entirely by the benzodiazepines.

In contrast to the overall depressant effect of the barbiturates the benzodiazepines act selectively in the limbic system. Following their administration neural activity decreases in the amygdala and the hippocampus, causing a sedative effect. Encouraged by the findings of opiate receptor sites in the CNS a search was launched for diazepine receptor sites. These were first identified in 1977 and have since been shown to possess stereospecific binding with good correlation between binding affinities and therapuetic doses. These receptor sites consist of a complex consisting of a γ-aminobutyric acid (GABA) receptor, a benzodiazepine receptor, and a chlorine ionophore. When the benzodiazepine receptor is activated the complex is changed such that the GABA receptor changes from a low to a high affinity. This is accomplished by blocking the actions of the GABA modulin, a protein which would otherwise lower the receptor affinity. Thus the benzodiazepines, when combined with their receptors, increase the inhibitory effects of GABA and produce sedation.

Having established that benzodiazepine receptor sites exist, research has been aimed at producing even safer benzodiazepines. In addition, using the same logic which led to the search for and discovery of the endogenous opiates, an endogenous benzodiazepine is now being sought, which would explain the presence of these receptor sites. Several substances such as purines, nicotinamide, thromboxine A2, a 15,000-dalton peptide and hormone have been linked to the endogenous benzodiazepines but none fulfill all the criteria.

BENZODIAZEPINES

The benzodiazepines act selectively on the limbic system, which controls emotional behavior, without causing the depressive cortical effects found with the barbiturates. This, in addition to their high therapeutic index, has allowed them to become the most highly prescribed group of drugs in North America.

Benzodiazepines are anticonvulsants and are the drugs of choice for status epilepticus. They also have muscle relaxant properties due to their effect on the brainstem reticular formation. This may account for their success in controlling gagging, although their sedative properties no doubt contribute to this effect. Their wide acceptance as sedatives, orally, intravenously, and intramuscularly, is partly due to their lack of effect on the respiratory and cardiovascular systems even in overdose quantities. The elderly, however, are very susceptible to the diazepines and care should be exercised when administering to the aged.

The first of the benzodiazepines to be marketed was chlordiazepoxide (Librium) which found great popularity as an oral sedative. This was superseded by diazepam (Valium) which had the added advantages of being more potent and when given intravenously it provided both sedation and amnesia. This combination makes diazepam an excellent intravenous sedative agent in dentistry since there is good sedation for 45 minutes to 1 hour and the amnesia is sufficient in most cases to obliterate the patient's memory of the local anesthetic injections if given during the first 5 minutes after induction. There will also be an apparent reduction in time for the patient, especially during the first hour of sedation. Other benzodiazepines have been synthesized, but none have matched the overwhelming success of diazepam.

The diazepines are absorbed efficiently from the gastrointestinal tract, with peak blood levels within 2 hours, metabolized in the liver, and excreted either in the original form or as their metabolite mainly by the kidneys. They have relatively long half-lives; chlordiazepoxide between 7 and 24 hours and diazepam between 8 and 48 hours. This, coupled with the fact that metabolites such as n-desmethyl diazepam are also sedatives, leads to prolonged recovery from a single intravenous injection and a formidable buildup in blood levels when these drugs are given orally over any length of time. From 4 to 6 hours after administration of a single dose of diazepam, there is a rise in blood level of the drug. Although this is accompanied by a clinically evident increase in sedative effect in practical terms, it is not of sufficient magnitude to cause concern in the dental outpatient. It has been suggested that the reason for the second peak in diazepam blood level is reabsorption from the small intestine following excretion of the bile from the gall bladder. This hepatic recycling effect has, to date, remained unproven.

Long term oral use of diazepam leads not only to tolerance of the drug but also to a state of depression in the female patient. For this reason, it is now suggested that oral diazepam be limited to 6 weeks' duration.

Although it is relatively non-toxic, lethargy and confusion may be noted, especially in the older patient. In extreme cases, this may be accompanied by muscle weakness or fatigue, ataxia, nystagmus, and dysarthria. Since benzodiazepines cross the placental barrier and appear in the milk of lactating females, it is suggested that intravenous diazepam should not be used for elective dentistry in pregnant or nursing females.

CHLORDIAZEPOXIDE (LIBRIUM)

Due to the superiority of diazepam as an intravenous sedative agent, the use of chlordiazepoxide is restricted to oral sedation prior to a dental appointment. It is supplied in 5-, 10-, and 25-mg tablets for this purpose and also in injectable packs for intramuscular and intravenous injection.

DIAZEPAM (VALIUM)

Diazepam is a colorless crystalline substance which, although insoluble in water, is soluble in alcohol and propylene glycol. In tablet form, it is supplied in 2, 5, and 20 mg. These may be prescribed for the anxious patient as a premedicant; an average dose of an adult is 5 mg the night before and 5 mg an hour before an appointment. The unpredictability of oral sedation, however, must be kept in mind.

For intravenous sedation, diazepam is supplied dissolved in propylene glycol at a concentration of 5 mg per ml. It appears as a clear yellow, viscous fluid but when diluted will precipitate out to form an emulsion. Because of this, the manufacturers state that it should not be diluted

with parenteral fluids before injection. The reasoning behind this is obscure since diazepam precipitates within the plasma almost on contact.

The variability in response to diazepam demands that the drug be titrated against each patient. Although the average sedative dose for an adult may be 10 to 15 mg, general anesthesia may be reached with less than 5 mg in an elderly patient. The rate of administration should be 2.5 mg per minute to enable the operator to assess the drug's effect. The two most commonly used clinical signs of adequate sedation are ptosis (drooping of the upper eyelid), altered speech (slurring of words or delayed response in answering questions). Blurred vision was initially reported to be a third sign but later investigations suggest that this was caused by the atropine used in the original study. Diazepam alone will not normally produce blurred vision at sedative dosages.

The irritant properties of the drug have been shown to be caused by both the solvent and the solute itself. A burning sensation following the course of the vein is, therefore, a frequent occurrence during administration. This symptom normally disappears after a few minutes. The irritation may lead to phlebitis, thrombosis, or thrombophlebitis when injected into small veins.

The possibility of general anesthesia due to careless titration still calls for the patient's abstinence from food or liquids for 6 hours before sedation. This is reinforced by studies which suggest that there is laryngeal incompetence during the first 5 minutes of intravenous diazepam sedation.

Prolonged recovery from intravenous diazepam requires that patients be accompanied home by a responsible adult following treatment; they must avoid activities demanding mental alertness and motor coordination such as moving machinery or driving for the rest of the day, and they should not plan to make important decisions that day. In exceptional cases, the patient may still feel the drug's effects the following day. Fortunately, they are normally aware of this impairment and should this occur they are advised that the foregoing precautions still apply. This delayed recovery is probably the greatest drawback to the use of intravenous diazepam and has led to the development of drugs which have a more rapid recovery rate.

FLURAZEPAM (DALMANE)

Although having sedative and muscle relaxant properties similar to other benzodiazepines, flurazepam is used mainly as a hypnotic. It normally induces sleep within half an hour, does not appear to reduce the REM as do the barbiturates, and may be useful to prescribe to a nervous patient the night before a dental appointment.

OXAZEPAM (SERAX)

This metabolite of diazepam is supplied as 10-, 15-, and 30-mg tablets and has anxiolytic and hypnotic properties similar to oral diazepam. Since the mean half-life of oxazepam at 7 hours is much shorter than that of diazepam (31 hours) it is a safer hypnotic, especially in the elderly.

With the impressive success of the benzodiazepines the search has continued for more effective members of this group of drugs. Table 12.2 demonstrates how the benzodiazepines have flourished. The basic properties of sedation, muscle relaxation, anticonvulsant and amnesia remain common to all to varying degrees. However, they are advertised according to their individual strengths. For example, flurazepam is marketed as a hypnotic while clonazepam is marketed as an anticonvulsant and diazepam is a sedative. Their greatest distinction, however, is their half-lives. The prolonged half-life of diazepam for example of up to 50 hours has led to very high blood level peaks after several days of use. Triazalam with the shortest half-life, 2 to 5 hours, may thus be regarded as a safer long term sedative. Initial clinical trials with triazolam suggest that it is an excellent oral hypnotic and oral sedative for outpatient dentistry. Its amnesic properties are also impressive. It is one of the few drugs marketed in a "geriatric" dosage (0.25 mg) in addition to the adult dose of 0.5 mg. The short half-life suggests a rapid recovery from the drug.

Narcotic Analgesics

MORPHINE

Morphine is the principal compound of the opium alkaloids and is the time-hon-

Table 12.2
Benzodiazepines

Drug	Dose	Half-Life
	mg	*hr*
Alprazolam (Xanax)	0.25–0.5	6–20
Bromazepam (Lectopam)	3–6	10–20
Chlorazepate (Tranxene)	15–60	30–60
Chlordiazepoxide (Librium)	15–100	5–30
Clonazepam (Rivotril)	1–10	24–48
Diazepam (Valium)	6–10	20–50
Flurazepam (Dalmane)	15–30	24–48
Ketazolam (Loftran)	15–36	1.5
Lorazepam* (Ativan)	2–3	10–15
Nitrazepam (Mogadon)	5–10	18–34
Oxazepam* (Serax)	30–120	5–20
Temazepam (Restoril)	15–30	8–22
Triazolam* (Halcion)	0.25–0.5	2–5

* No active metabolites.

ored narcotic against which all other narcotics are judged. Morphine is a potent analgesic agent which primarily affects the central nervous system pain centers and alters the perception of a painful stimulus reaching the central nervous system. Therapeutic doses of morphine sufficient to relieve mild to moderate pain induce relatively minimal respiratory depression. In larger doses, respiration is moderately to severely depressed because of lack of responsiveness of medullary centers to hypercarbia. Intraocular and cerebrospinal fluid pressure are elevated due to the increase in $PaCO_2$.

The incidence of nausea and vomiting after the administration of morphine is increased because of a stimulating action of morphine on the vomiting center of the medulla which is sensitized to vestibular movements. It is, therefore, best used in patients confined to bed. There is minimal cardiovascular depression with moderate to large doses of morphine; however, the drug has been found to be a potent histamine liberator and, as such, itching and urticaria may appear after the administration of morphine. It is, therefore, contraindicated in the asthmatic patient.

Gastric motility is decreased after administration of morphine, and the result of this is constipation. The smooth muscle of the biliary tract, including the sphincter of Oddi, is stimulated; however, the narcotic drugs, including morphine, are nevertheless used to alleviate the pain of biliary colic.

Pupillary constriction is noted after administration of morphine, and when this drug is utilized for premedication prior to anesthesia, the eye signs related to anesthesia depth are no longer valid. Pupillary constriction is a central and not a peripheral action, caused by stimulation of the pupillary constrictor fibers of the oculomotor nucleus.

Because of its long duration of action (approximately 4 hours) morphine cannot be considered an acceptable drug for outpatient sedation. The combined use of morphine and nitrous oxide-oxygen, however, is a valid technique for use as a general anesthetic in the hospital situation, and recent studies have shown that minimal cardiovascular depression is noted even after massive doses of morphine have been administered. Substitution of one of the shorter acting narcotic analgesics in the narcotic nitrous oxide-oxygen technique has allowed this to be adapted to the outpatient situation.

Morphine in the dental outpatient will generally be relegated to its use as postoperative analgesic and, as such, it is administered by the intramuscular route in doses of 8 to 15 mg. The advantages of potent analgesia and euphoria, together with an increased incidence of nausea and vomiting and other side effects, must be weighed against the need for analgesia.

With these considerations in mind, it will be found that morphine will be utilized usually only in the patient having undergone extensive surgery, such as maxillofacial surgery or removal of impacted teeth necessitating hospitalization.

Morphine is detoxicated in the liver by conjugation with glucuronic acid, and metabolites are excreted by the kidneys and the gastrointestinal tract. A small portion of the injected dose is eliminated unchanged in the urine.

MEPERIDINE (DEMEROL)

Meperidine, which is ethyl-1-methyl-4-phenol-piperidine-4 carboxylic acid, is structurally similar to atropine and is marketed in the United States under the trade name Demerol. It is a narcotic approximately $\frac{1}{10}$ as potent as morphine and has an action upon the central nervous system much like that of morphine. Moderate to severe pain can be relieved with meperidine, and side effects are generally less than after the use of morphine. Therapeutic doses of meperidine sufficient to relieve moderate pain produce only mild sleepiness with little or no euphoria or amnesia. The respiratory centers in the medulla are depressed in their reactivity to hypercarbia and, consequently, the cerebrospinal fluid pressure is increased. Hypotension and tachycardia are more commonly seen with meperidine than with morphine.

Meperidine has a direct relaxant effect on smooth muscle of the bronchioles and intestine and, in consequence, constipation rarely occurs. As with morphine, meperidine stimulates the sphincter of Oddi, and the pain of biliary colic may not be relieved by this drug.

Meperidine appears to release histamine; however, this release is not as striking as with morphine. Meperidine has a quinidine-like effect on the myocardium.

It has been claimed that meperidine, being structurally similar to atropine, causes dilated pupils after administration, while others claim vasodilatation. The classic eye signs of anesthesia are, therefore, unreliable when using this drug.

The side effects of meperidine are generally of a more minor nature than those seen after morphine; they may include sweating, nausea, vomiting, and confusion. Hypotension and arrhythmias are more common than with morphine. The duration of meperidine is approximately one-half that of morphine (2 hours rather than 4 hours) and, therefore, may be more useful for analgesia and/or anesthesia supplementation in the outpatient situation. Adult dosage ranges from 50 to 100 mg.

FENTANYL (SUBLIMAZE)

Fentanyl, a piperidine derivative, is a newer narcotic agent with a potency 100 times greater than morphine. The action of fentanyl upon the nervous system is morphine-like and apparently exerts its effect in the same major areas as morphine.

Fentanyl produces respiratory depression in the same manner as morphine and meperidine, namely, by lowering the sensitivity of the respiratory center to carbon dioxide levels. Fentanyl has relatively minor cardiovascular effects with changes much the same as seen after morphine. Fentanyl, like morphine, may induce bradycardia of a vagal nature, which is easily reversed with atropine.

Fentanyl, while a very potent analgesic, has a very weak emetic action and, therefore, differs markedly from morphine and meperidine. There is almost a total lack of histamine release after administration of fentanyl, which allows this drug to be given to the asthmatic patient.

Fentanyl produces stimulation of the gastrointestinal tract's smooth muscle, and while it does not produce as great a constipating effect as morphine, fentanyl's constipating action may be of a longer duration.

The very short duration of action of fentanyl (approximately 45 minutes) makes this drug the most useful of the mentioned narcotics for outpatient use, give in doses of 50 μg.

ALPHAPRODINE HYDROCHLORIDE (NISENTIL)

A constituent of several of the currently popular intravenous analgesia techniques is the narcotic alphaprodine hydrochloride. This drug appears to have a potency approximately twice that of meperidine and approximately one-fifth that of morphine. The systemic physiological effect of alphaprodine is quite similar to that of meperidine, and the basis for its use appears to be its shorter duration of action of approximately 45 minutes. The drug appears to be less nauseating. Respiratory depression is more evident in equipotent analgesic doses.

Intravenous dosage of alphaprodine will vary from 20 to 40 mg administered slowly intravenously, and it must be borne in mind that if other drugs such as the phenothiazines or barbiturates are concurrently administered this dosage may be reduced by up to one-half. Submucosal buccal injections result in uptake which parallels intravenous administration.

PENTAZOCINE (TALWIN)

Pentazocine is a benzazocine analgesic with sedative properties. Given either orally or parenterally, it is an antagonist to the opiates, but only has ⅟₅₀ the activity of nalorphine in this respect. It has been used successfully in clinical trials as an intravenous sedative but its analgesic properties are not sufficient to preclude the use of local anesthetics. The sedation produced following the intravenous administration of 30 mg of pentazocine is equivalent to that produced by 10 mg of diazepam but does not produce the marked amnesia of the diazepam. In an attempt to obtain the best from both drugs, a standard dose of pentazocine may be given followed by titration of diazepam.

Antihistamines with Sedative Properties

PHENOTHIAZINE DERIVATIVES

The most commonly utilized phenothiazine derivative in dentistry is promethazine, marketed under the trade name of Phenergan. Promethazine is thought to act by selective depression of the hypothalamus and reticular activating formations and the thalamic cortical projections resulting in depression of the centers for basal metabolism, body temperature, sleep and wakefulness, vasomotor tone, vomiting, and hormonal balance. The sedation obtained from promethazine does not include the element of euphoria, but rather it produces a state of indifference and lassitude. Promethazine exerts an antiemetic action by direct depression of the vomiting center itself. The cardiovascular effects of promethazine are basically parasympatholytic with resultant tachycardia and a rather profound peripheral dilatation due to adrenergic blockade. Cardiovascular effects are generally minimal, but there may be postural hypotension due to the vasodilated peripheral vascular bed. The effects of promethazine on the respiratory system are minimal.

Promethazine has a marked antihistaminic action which makes it an ideal drug to be used in combination with the narcotics, which are known histamine releasers. Summarized, the actions of histamine are: 1) contraction of smooth muscle in the intestine, ureter, and bronchioles; 2) depression of blood pressure; and 3) increased glandular secretion.

Depending upon dosage, any or all of these histamine effects may be counteracted by promethazine.

It has been demonstrated that promethazine used by itself provides no analgesic action and, indeed, may act as a mild antianalgesic, in other than dental pain. However, pulp testing after promethazine shows elevation of the pain threshold.

Promethazine has been shown to greatly potentiate the action of narcotics and barbiturates, and its use in many intravenous techniques is predicated upon this potentiation. It has been found that narcotic dosage can generally be reduced by approximately 50 per cent when combined with promethazine, and its potentiation factor must be kept in mind when administering postoperative analgesics to the patient who may have received promethazine either as a preoperative medication or during surgery.

Oral administration of promethazine results in slow uptake of the drug and delayed onset of action. However, after intramuscular or intravenous administration, effect is noted very rapidly. The duration of action of promethazine, regardless of route of administration, may be up to 24 hours, and this must be borne in mind when these drugs are administered to the outpatient.

The principal metabolic breakdown pathways for promethazine involve oxidation, with the metabolites being excreted in the urine.

Promethazine is most commonly utilized for intravenous sedation in combination with a narcotic or barbiturate and/or anticholinergic agent. When utilized in this manner, dosage range is 10 to 15 mg administered in incremental doses intravenously, watching carefully for the desired effect. Total narcotic dosage must be reduced proportionately to the dosage of promethazine administered.

HYDROXYZINE

Typical of this class of drugs and a common component of numerous analgesic techniques is the non-phenothiazine tranquilizer hydroxyzine hydrochloride, marketed as Vistaril or Atarax. Hydroxyzine is a low potency tranquilizer qualitatively similar to the phenothiazine tranquilizers. Because of increased atropine-like side effects, hydroxyzine has found only minor usage in anxiety states; however, with its lower potency it has become a useful drug in the dental outpatient.

The effect of hydroxyzine on the major systems of the body is quite similar to the more potent phenothiazine tranquilizers, but of a much more limited magnitude. Of importance to dentistry is hydroxyzine's sedative effect and marked antiemetic effect and its capability of potentiation of narcotics and barbiturates administered conjointly.

Administration of hydroxyzine has recently been limited to oral or intramuscular injections because of adverse local reaction after intravenous injection. Local reactions have varied from mild phlebitis to frank thrombosis, and the limitation of hydroxyzine to intramuscular injection has required that numerous intravenous analgesia techniques be modified. At present, we have modified any technique requiring the use of the intravenous hydroxyzine by the substitution of promethazine, which has resulted in a marked decrease in the number of local complications. The limitations of hydroxyzine hydrochloride to intramuscular use makes discussion of dosage

for intravenous analgesia academic. For historic interest only, it should be noted that hydroxyzine hydrochloride was administered intravenously in dosage ranging from 12 to 50 mg well diluted and slowly.

Current use of hydroxyzine with potentiation of concurrently administered narcotics or barbiturates allows reduction in the dosage of these drugs by 25 to 50 per cent.

Anticholinergic Agents

The belladonna derivatives atropine and scopolamine are utilized in many of the currently popular intravenous analgesia techniques.

Both atropine and scopolamine have an antisalivary action, with scopolamine having the greater effect. Both drugs have a vagolytic action; atropine's vagolytic action is of a much greater extent, and the increase in cardiac rate will generally be sustained for upwards of 45 minutes. Scopolamine, on the other hand, has a transient vagolytic action which may exert itself for only 10 to 15 minutes, after which the cardiac rate may fall to control levels or actually proceed to bradycardia.

Atropine possesses a mild medullary stimulant action which may help to alleviate respiratory depression caused by concurrently administered drugs. Scopolamine, on the other hand, is a medullary depressant, and its use is often predicated upon its ability to produce mild to moderate amnesia. Scopolamine administered concurrently with cardiodepressant drugs may tend to enhance the cardiorespiratory depressant effect of these drugs.

Adult dosage of either drug will generally be in the range of 0.4 to 0.6 mg administered intravenously. When utilizing these drugs in children, the basis for dosage should be approximately 0.1 mg per 10 kg of body weight.

Scopolamine, because of its ability to produce amnesia, should be utilized cautiously in the very young patient or the very elderly patient as disorientation and hallucinations occur.

INTRAVENOUS SEDATION TECHNIQUES

As will be obvious from the preceding list of drugs available for intravenous sedation and analgesia, many techniques have been evolved, each with its own advantages and disadvantages. Only the more common of these techniques will be described.

Methohexital

The use of methohexital in accord with S. L. Drummond-Jackson's technique of ultralight anesthesia for restorative dentistry involves the incremental injection of 1 per cent methohexital to maintain the patient in an ultralight level of anesthesia. The basis of this technique is the induction in the patient by an anesthetic dose of methohexital and then allowing the patient to return to the lightly sedated level. Additional 10- to 30-mg increments of methohexital are added as necessary to maintain this light sedation level. The use of local anesthesia with this technique is felt unnecessary and the ease of administration of methohexital has led many people to think of this technique as the panacea for restorative dentistry. It is obvious, however, that if a patient is not reacting to dental procedures without the use of local anesthesia, then they are entering the realm of general anesthesia; the dentist is, therefore, acting as an operator-anesthetist. In addition, this technique was designed for dental procedures of 10 to 20 minutes, which is much shorter than most dental procedures in North America require.

A safer procedure is to use local anesthesia but reduce the incremental doses of methohexital while ensuring that the patient retains all his reflexes throughout. Even then, however, the level of sedation is erratic, requiring continuous patient assessment and repeated drug administra-

tion. The borderline between sedation and general anesthesia is narrow in these cases and treatment should be kept to a minimum.

Pentobarbital

The use of pentobarbital as a single agent for sedation in the outpatient is a widely utilized technique. Pentobarbital is adminstered in 10- to 25-mg increments intravenously at a slow rate with observation of the resulting sedation and limitation of the amount of drug to only that required to place the patient in a lightly sedated condition.

Pentobarbital utilized intravenously as a single agent can provide excellent sedation and hypnosis, but it provides little or not analgesia and, indeed, may create a state of hyperalgesia wherein any attempt to accomplish a painful procedure may casue an exaggerated patient response. This is, however, one of the better drugs for the dentist to utilize when he is beginning his training in intravenous techniques as observations of the effects of a single drug can be accomplished without interference of multiple drug combinations.

The Jorgensen Technique

The intravenous psychosedation technique described by Dr. Neils Jorgensen, and termed by some the Loma Linda technique, involves the use of three drugs: pentobarbital, meperidine, and scopolamine.

The method involves the intravenous administration of pentobarbital at the rate of 10 mg every 30 seconds until the first cortical symptoms are noted. These symptoms may take the form of drowsiness, lightheadedness, diplopia, or a feeling of floating. When this baseline of sedation is reached, an additional increment of 10 per cent of the dosage required to initiate the baseline sedation is given. A second syringe containing 25 mg of meperidine and 0.32 mg of scopolamine diluted to a 5-ml volume with saline is then attached to the intravenous infusion tubing. The two drugs are administered, the dose being related to the total dosage of pentobarbital given.

The psychosedative effects of this drug combination can be excellent, with minimal disturbance to the physiological makeup of the patient (Fig. 12.1). Experimental pain studies have shown that this technique does not relieve experimentally induced tooth pain, but there is an elevation of the pain threshold to periosteal stimulation.

One of the drawbacks of this technique is the prolonged recovery of some patients, which may be as long as 5 to 6 hours before they can safely be allowed to leave the dental office. There is also the problem of using multiple drugs and thereby increasing the possibility of drug adverse reaction. In conclusion, the Jorgensen technique is suitable for dental procedures which may take several hours but recovery room facilities must be available and the problem of delayed recovery recognized.

The Shane Technique

The intravenous amnesia technique described by Sylvan M. Shane involves the utilization of four drugs: alphaprodine, hydroxyzine, atropine, and methohexital. In recent drug studies, it has been found that hydroxyzine hydrochloride may cause vascular inflammation after intravenous injection, and an alternative drug should be substituted in the regime. It is suggested that a suitable drug for substitution in this technique is promethazine, which can be administered intravenously with minimal local toxicity. The original technique for intravenous amnesia involved the administration of 30 mg of alphaprodine, 25 mg of hydroxyzine, and 0.4 mg of atropine injected slowly intravenously over a 2- to 3-minute period. The modified technique now involves

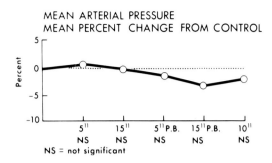

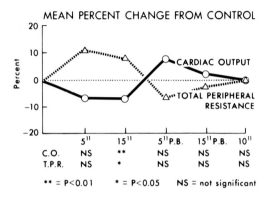

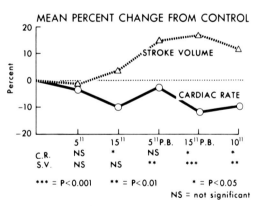

Figure 12.1. The effects of the Loma Linda technique on cardiovascular parameters. The data were recorded 5 and 15 minutes after induction, and then 5 to 15 minutes after an alveolar nerve block with 1.8 ml of lidocaine with 1:100,000 epinephrine added. The most dramatic change in cardiovascular parameters was produced by the 18 μg of epinephrine.

substitution of promethazine for hydroxyzine with the same dosage of 25 mg being utilized. Immediately after this drug combination has been injected and the full sedative effects of these drugs have been observed, a 10- to 20-mg increment of methohexital is injected intravenously and local anesthetic injections are performed while the patient is in the deeply sedated state.

The duration of the original drug combination will be approximately 1 to 2 hours and incremental doses of 10 to 20 mg of methohexital may be added during this time as necessary to maintain the controlled amnesic state.

Recent cardiovascular and experimental amnesia studies have shown that while this technique provides a significant degree of amnesia and sedation, there is moderate cardiovascular depression with this drug combination. While this depression may not be of sufficient magnitude to warrant discouragement of this technique, it must be realized that in the severely compromised cardiac patient, a depression of the cardiac output amounting to nearly 30 per cent is hazardous. Experimental analgesia studies have shown that this technique provides significant periosteal analgesia but has a very minor effect on tooth sensitivity.

Diazepam

Because of its high therapeutic index, its predictable sedative effect, and its remarkable amnesia, diazepam has become the most popular method of intravenous sedation in dentistry. Efforts to enhance its properties by combining it with other drugs have been attempted. In combination with short-acting barbiturates such as methohexital, the sedative and amnesic effects are increased; in combination with nitrous oxide the sedation can be prolonged and in combination with pentazocine sedation is both more profound and longer lasting. These are all embellishments, however, on a simple safe technique which has transformed intravenous techniques from the gray areas of general anesthesia to predictable controlled levels of sedation.

Synthesized by L. H. Sternbach and E.

Reeder in 1961, it has become the intravenous sedative of choice in many fields of medicine and dentistry. The drug is administered in its undiluted form beginning with one or two drops to ensure that the injection is not intra-arterial and that there is no adverse reaction to the drug. After 2 minutes incremental doses can be given at the rate of 2.5 mg (0.5 ml) over a 30-second period and a further 30 seconds allowed to elapse to assess the drug's effect. There are two signs of cortical effect, either of which may be taken as the end point for sedation: ptosis or altered speech (Fig. 12.2). One study which investigated the reliability of these signs found them to be relatively consistent with both novices and experienced operators rating the signs at approximately the same increment and with a good correlation between the two signs.

The average dose for the healthy adult is about 12.5 mg, but patient tolerance varies and the elderly especially are very susceptible. Induction, therefore, may take 5 minutes or more during which time topical anesthetics may be applied. On reaching the required level of sedation, local anesthetics are given as normal. In the initial years of use it was claimed by some that less local anesthetic was required when using diazepam. Since most patients will have no recollection of the

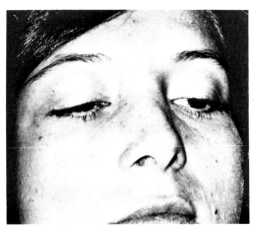

Figure 12.2.   Ptosis is obvious evidence of sedation.

locals if given in the first 5 minutes but will remember subsequent re-enforcing injections, there seems little point in economizing on local anesthetics at the expense of one of the more dramatic properties of the techiques.

The amnesic effect will continue throughout the procedure to a lesser extent but will still leave the patient aware that time has been condensed. This technique allows the operator to complete prolonged surgical or restorative procedures which previously would have required a general anesthetic.

ALTERNATIVE TECHNIQUES OF ADMINISTERING DIAZEPAM

Initially diazepam was administered using a single syringe containg 20 mg (4 ml). This technique, however, has been criticized by some since once the needle is removed there is no longer a patent vein that can be used in the event of an emergency. This may be overcome by the setting up of an intravenous drip before embarking on venipuncture on the opposite arm.

Despite warnings by the manufacturers that diazepam should not be mixed with a parenteral fluid before injection, many advocate the injection of the drug directly into the intravenous drip. There is no doubt that the diazepam does precipitate as it can be seen as a fine emulsion in the tubing. However, if diazepam is titrated into a breaker of serum, the precipitation can also be seen immediately. Clinically, there would appear to be no reason why diazepam cannot be administered by this method.

A more practical disadvantage to this technique is the apprehension that an intravenous drip can cause in an already nervous patient. If a patent vein is desired without the appearance of a continuous drip and without mixing it with a parenteral solution, the two syringe technique may be employed. After administering the diazepam from a 5-ml syringe through a 25-gauge butterfly needle, it is replaced with a 10-ml syringe containing a solution such as dextrose. Then 5 ml are used to flush diazepam from the vein and the remainder of the dextrose given over the following 30 minutes. Not only does this provide a patent vein over the first critical 30 minutes but the flushing action reduces the incidence of thrombosis and thrombophlebitis.

With the drugs described in this chapter it is obvious that the dentist has great flexibility in deciding which intravenous drug is suitable for a given patient or for a particular dental procedure. Supervised clinical experience, however, is necessary not only for the safety of the patient but for the benefit of the dentist to achieve confidence and competence in this important area. It is the responsibility of the dental profession and dental educators to provide such instruction at the undergraduate and continuing education levels.

Bibliography

Baird ES, Hailey DM: Delayed recovery from a sedative: correlation of plasma levels of diazepam with clinical effects after oral and intravenous administration. Br J Anaesth 44:803, 1972.

Brown PR, Donaldson D, Gray I, et al: Intravenous sedation in dentistry—a comparative study of pentazocine and diazepam. Dent Pract 21:2, 1970.

Caudill WA, Alvin JD, Nazif MM, et al: Absorption rates of alphaprodine from the buccal and intravenous routes. Pediatr Dent 4(1):168, 1982.

Donaldson D, Gibson G: Systemic complications with intravenous diazepam. Oral Surg 49:126, 1980.

Everett GB, Allen GD: Simultaneous evaluation of cardiorespiratory and analgesic effects of intravenous in combination with local anesthesia. J Am Dent Assoc 81:926, 1970

Healey, TE, Vickers MD: Laryngeal competence under diazepam sedation. Proc R Soc Med 64:85, 1971.

Hockings N, Ballinger BR: Hypnotics and anxiolytics Br Med J 286:1949, 1983.

Jorgensen NB, Leffingwell F: Premedication in dentistry. J S Calif Dent Assoc 21:25, 1953.

Kaufman RD, Agleh KA, Bellville JW: Relative potencies and duration of action with respect to respiratory depression of intravenous meperidine, fentanyl and alphaprodine in man. J Pharmacol Exp Ther 208:73, 1979.

Olsen RW: Drug interaction at the GABA receptors-ionophore complex. Annu Rev Pharmacol 22:245, 1982.

Smith AJ: Self-poisoning with drugs: a worsening situation. Br Med J 4:157, 1972.

CHAPTER 13

General Anesthesia in Dentistry

General anesthesia is the loss of ability to perceive pain associated with loss of consciousness. It is this latter feature that distinguishes general anesthesia from analgesia and conscious sedation. As consciousness itself is little understood, so too is the understanding of general anesthesia. Basically, however, there is a teleological concept of a sequential depression of the central nervous system from higher to lower centers; the most sensitive centers are the higher centers of learning.

General anesthesia has been a major feature of dentistry since the introduction of general anesthesia to the public by dentistry. Approximately ⅕ of all general anesthetics given in the United States are given for dentistry. That number, 5,000,000 general dental anesthetics, is not open to absolute confirmation, but with the development of dental insurance programs, better data have become available. For example, in southern California, approximately 250,000 general anesthetics are administered annually by oral surgeons. The annual report of activities is a requirement for membership in the Southern California Society of Oral and Maxillofacial Surgeons. Insurance carriers report approximately 500,000 anesthetics administered annually in dental offices. In addition to the patients anesthetized for dentistry in the office, numerous anesthetics are given in general dental offices and free-standing ambulatory care centers.

The mortality rate with dental anesthesia approximates that for outpatient anesthesia performed in free-standing ambulatory clinics; that is, one dental fatality in approximately 280,000 administrations. The annual mortality rate in dental offices reported by Berkowitz and Smith from actuarial data was 58 deaths. The mortality rate reported by the S.C.S.O.M.F.S. suggests a mortality rate of 3 in 1,250,000, but such figures are confused by the 30 deaths reported from intravenous sedation in 1977 by the American Society of Oral Surgeons. Nonetheless, despite the imperfect collection of data, the safety record suggests that general anesthesia for dentistry is a safe modality and has set an example to hospital anesthesia in patient care—an excellent record of a necessary service by the profession to the patient. As anesthesia is a requirement of many patients for dentistry, the dental student should understand anesthesia and its implications. In addition, many of the drugs administered for conscious sedation can easily be expanded to produce general anesthesia. The distinction between anesthesia and conscious sedation must be understood.

DEPTH OF ANESTHESIA

Although the concept of depth of anesthesia developed by Guedel is not now directly applicable to the anesthetic depths obtained by current general anesthetics, nonetheless it provides the basic concepts for anesthetic depth. In some respects it is a description of the side effects of anesthesia, effects which are significant. Anesthetic agents by definition are reversible, and thus the central nervous system effects of anesthesia are also reversible, but the side effects of anesthesia may produce prolonged or permanent effects.

Classic Guedel Signs

The signs and symptoms of anesthesia in the Guedel classification of depth and anesthesia are based upon the appearance or loss of specific physiological functions as depth increases. There is selective depression of the central nervous system, probably in phylogenetic order (Fig. 13.1).

It must be stressed that the most significant feature differentiating anesthesia from analgesia is that under analgesia there is no loss of consciousness and the patient can talk to the administrator. If this distinction is clearly understood, then analgesia remains a safe technique for the general dentist. The description given below is for diethyl ether anesthesia without opiate or atropine premedication. Other anesthetics and combinations of agents affect the classic signs.

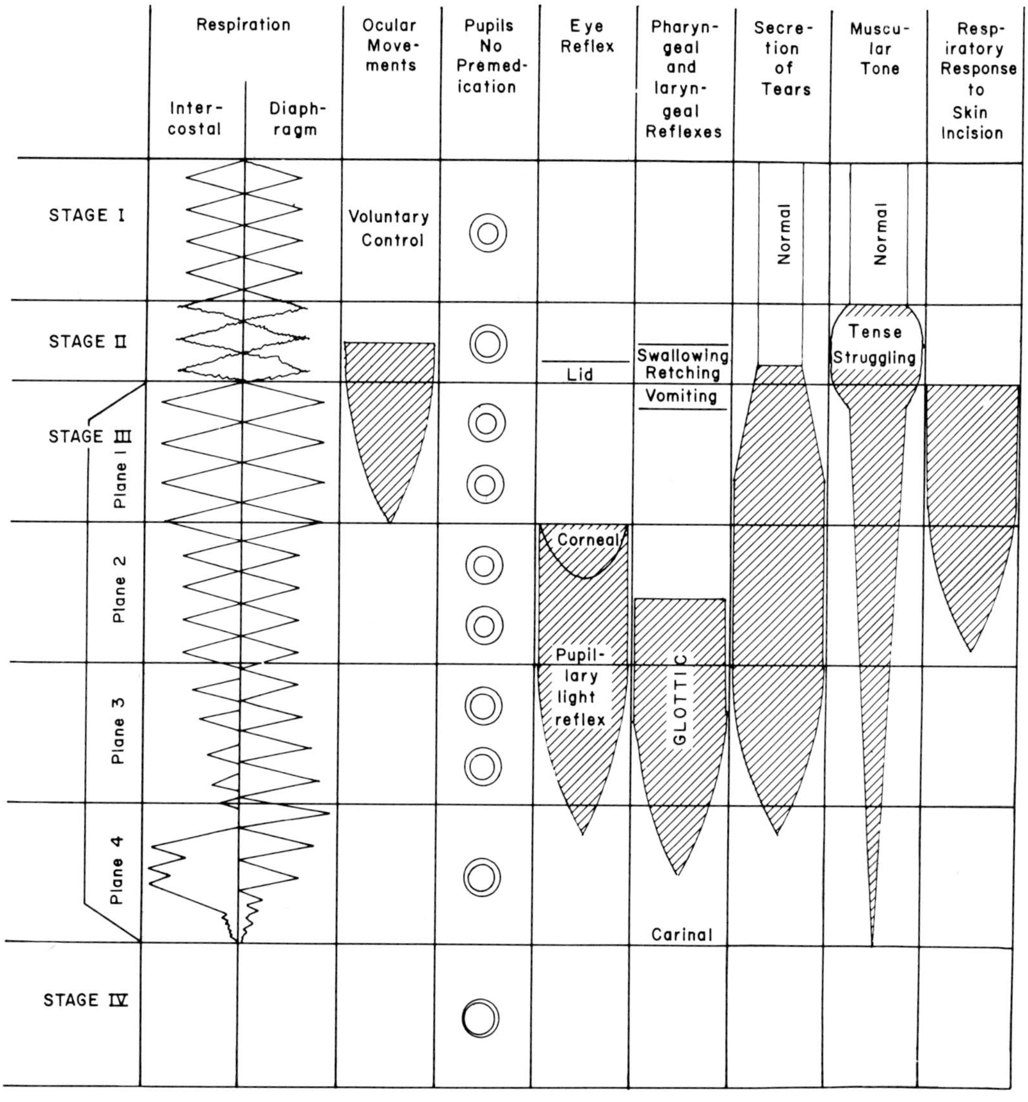

	Respiration (Intercostal / Diaphragm)	Ocular Movements	Pupils No Premedication	Eye Reflex	Pharyngeal and laryngeal Reflexes	Secretion of Tears	Muscular Tone	Respiratory Response to Skin Incision
STAGE I		Voluntary Control				Normal	Normal	
STAGE II				Lid	Swallowing / Retching / Vomiting		Tense Struggling	
STAGE III — Plane 1								
Plane 2			Corneal					
Plane 3			Pupillary light reflex	GLOTTIC				
Plane 4				Carinal				
STAGE IV								

Figure 13.1. The chart illustrates the classical signs of unpremedicated diethyl ether anesthesia as described by Guedel with the additional modification of the reflex signs by N. A. Gillespie.

STAGE 1

This is from the beginning of anesthesia to the loss of consciousness. It is defined as analgesia. There is depression of intellect, memory, and psychomotor functions, with loss of time and space orientation. Sensation of pain is absent, and usually the pain threshold is depressed. It may be that the patient's reaction to pain is altered and, if the patient is expecting an operative procedure, minor surgical procedures will be tolerated. The analgesia is more profound upon emergence rather than during induction. The loss of eyelash reflex is the best index of transition to Stage 2.

STAGE 2

The excitement or uninhibited response lasts from loss of consciousness to onset of automatic breathing. Stimulation during this period is undesirable, as uninhibited reaction occurs. The use of restraints is not indicated or the patient will react violently. The second stage is often noticed in emergence from anesthesia when delirium can occur. The pharyngeal and laryngeal reflexes are obtunded, though vomiting can occur. Breath holding, coughing, and swallowing are indicative of Stage 2. The loss of the lid reflex indicates transition to Stage 3.

STAGE 3

The stage of surgical anesthesia from the onset of a regular respiratory pattern to the cessation of respiration. It can be divided into four planes.

Plane 1

From onset of automatic respiration to cessation of eyeball movement. The eyeballs will oscillate slowly or become eccentrically fixed. Both eyes should be examined, as pupillary dilatation may persist. Reaction to light is still present and the pupil will dilate in response to surgical stimulus. There is secretion of tears throughout the period of plane 1. Tearing is a useful indication of plane 1, that required for outpatient oral surgery. The respiratory rate responds to surgical stimuli.

Plane 2

From cessation of eyeball movement to commencement of intercostal paralysis. Respiration is regular, the volume is diminished, and the respiratory responses to surgical trauma disappear. The pupils begin to dilate, and muscle tone lessens as anesthesia deepens. The corneal reflex disappears in the middle of plane 2, but should never be elicited. Pharyngeal reflexes are obtunded.

Plane 3

From commencement to completion of intercostal paralysis. Tidal volume is reduced, and inspiration is shorter than expiration. Jerky diaphragmatic movements appear and only abdominal movement is evident. There may be increased respiratory rate. The pupillary light reflex is abolished, as is the conjunctival. The laryngeal reflex is abolished.

Plane 4

Complete intercostal paralysis to diaphragmatic paralysis. Tidal exchange is inefficient, and respiration is termed paradoxical as the chest falls with inspiration because of complete intercostal paralysis. Tracheal tug is evident, as the trachea moves down with each inspiration. It is probably due to the unopposed action of the diaphragm displacing the hilum of the lung. The pupils are dilated and no longer react to light.

STAGE 4

The stage of onset of diaphragmatic paralysis to apnea and death. All reflex activity is lost, the pupils are widely dilated. Respiration and circulation fail in this period. If this plane is reached, then drastic action should be taken to reverse by ventilation with oxygen.

Other reflexes which are depressed by deep anesthesia are the carinal reflex and the traction reflexes from the peritoneum and mesentery.

Clinical Signs of Anesthesia

The signs of anesthesia with all anesthetic agents are related to the preceding description but are affected by their unique properties. The clinical signs of anesthesia are mainly due to progressive increase of muscular paralysis in eyeball muscles, intercostals, and diaphragm, together with progressive abolition of reflex responses.

Respiratory arrest with deep anesthesia must be distinguished from breath holding in response to stimulation which occurs with light anesthesia. Breath holding is evident at the end of inspiration when the glottis is closed; it may follow a cough or prolonged expiratory effort.

Of the agents used in dental anesthesia nitrous oxide has classical stages of anesthesia as described by Clement. However, it is now rarely given without supplemental agents, and balanced anesthesia alters the classic pattern.

The intravenous barbiturates and narcotic premedication usually depress respiration prior to induction of anesthesia, and the respiratory patterns are thus less clearly defined.

If halothane and methoxyflurane or the narcotics are used, the pupils are constricted with light planes of anesthesia. The influence of the anticholinergics upon the pupils should be recognized in evaluating depth of anesthesia.

With experience, it is possible to determine the depth of anesthesia with each agent, combination of agents, and situation. In dental anesthesia an attempt to initiate surgery before an adequate depth of anesthesia is achieved will often initiate problems. Deep anesthesia is, however, unnecessary and should be avoided.

The character of the operation, the operative situation, and the patient affect the level of anesthesia required. Each patient becomes an individual experiment, and the unique response of that patient determines the amount of anesthesia required. If the beginner is uncertain as to the level of anesthesia, it is usually advisable to defer the surgical stimulus while the anesthesia is lightened. When a classic response is obtained and a certainty as to depth has been made, then the operation can be restarted.

Auxiliary Aids to Depth of Anesthesia

These are *not* useful for clinical application in dental anesthesia.

ELECTROENCEPHALOGRAM

The changes in EEG show characteristic patterns for most general anesthetics. However, as other factors can more profoundly influence the EEG than the anesthetic itself, such as changes in the superior vena cava pressure, the usefulness of this method of monitoring the depth of anesthesia is doubtful.

Hypoxia is readily indicated during anesthesia by a decrease in amplitude and frequency of the waves. The influence of $PaCO_2$ in apparently increasing depth of anesthesia is also apparent in the electroencephalogram. The principal use of the electroencephalogram in monitoring is for an indication of hypoxia.

The changes in EEG in relation to depth of anesthesia indicate that the first level corresponds to Stage 1, the second shows high amplitude rhythmical waves and corresponds to Stage 2, the third level shows complex and irregular waves, and succeeding levels show increasing suppression until the seventh, which is characterized by complete absence of waves.

BLOOD LEVELS OF ANESTHETIC AGENTS

When equilibration has been reached, the depth of anesthesia is related to the tension of anesthetic within the arterial blood, as equilibration with the brain has been achieved. It requires 10 to 20 minutes of anesthesia to achieve this level. However, it is the individual cells' response to the concentration of the anesthetic agent which determines depth of anesthesia. There is no index of the response of cells to a given level of anesthetic; consequently, it is not possible to indicate truly a given depth of anesthesia with this method.

The failure of the ancillary methods of evaluating depth of anesthesia is evident by the failure of the servomechanism methods of anesthesia, linked to EEG and blood levels of anesthetic agents.

MINIMUM ANESTHETIC CONCENTRATION

The concept of *minimum anesthetic concentration* (MAC) was introduced by Saidman and Eger in 1964 and has been helpful in evaluation and comparison of the effectiveness and potency of inhalation anesthetic agents (Table 13.1).

Minimum anesthetic concentration is defined as that alveolar concentration which will prevent a gross skeletal muscle response to a standard surgical stimulus and incision, in 50 per cent of patients. It is known as the MAC 1 for an agent at 1 atmosphere pressure. As MAC is related to the oil/water solubility, it has been found to be a useful investigational tool, which allows comparison of the potency of different anesthetic agents. It must be emphasized that it is not to be used as an index for the administration of anesthe-

sia, especially in dental anesthesia. It usually requires a minimum of 18 minutes for equilibration before determination, which is much less than the time required for the performance of the routine dental anesthetic.

An inverse relationship between MAC and oil/gas partition coefficient has been demonstrated, MAC $\times$ oil/gas partition coefficient = constant. MAC is decreased 10 to 20 per cent by metabolic acidosis, but $PaCO_2$ does not alter MAC. Hypoxia does not effect MAC until PO_2 falls to 30 mm Hg, a fall of 20 per cent. As might be expected, hemorrhage and hypothermia decrease the level of MAC. It is not affected by the duration of anesthesia, hypo- or hypercarbia, or mild hypoxia.

Of all the factors evaluated among inhalation agents, lipid solubility has the strongest positive correlation with anesthetic potency. Thus, methoxyflurane (oil/gas partition coefficient 825) and halothane (oil/gas partition coefficient 224) with their high lipid solubility are extremely potent anesthetics, while cyclopropane (oil/gas partition coefficient 11.8) and nitrous oxide (1.4) are rather less potent agents.

Narcotic premedication (morphine) reduces MAC only slightly for halothane while 70 per cent nitrous oxide reduces MAC for fluoroxene from 3.4 per cent to 0.8 per cent. In view of these findings 70 per cent nitrous oxide is routinely administered with potent volatile agents such as halothane or methoxyfluorane for dental anesthesia. By so doing, less volatile agent is required with the following advantages: 1) decreased cost of anesthesia, 2) increased speed of recovery, 3) decreased cardiovascular and respiratory depression. These advantages outweigh the theoretical disadvantage of decreased oxygen concentration as hypoxia does not occur with 25 to 33 per cent oxygen during anesthesia with spontaneous respiration. Narcotic premedication is not considered clinically significant in reducing MAC and has largely been abandoned for this

Table 13.1
Minimum Anesthetic Concentration

Anesthetic	% atm in O₂	% atm in N₂O
Methoxyflurane	0.16	0.07
Halotane	0.75	0.29
Isoflurane	1.15	0.50
Enflurane	1.68	0.57
Nitrous oxide	110	

purpose. Recovery time is prolonged following anesthesia preceded by narcotic premedication, an undesirable feature in ambulatory patients.

VOLATILE ANESTHETIC AGENTS

Inhalation agents (volatile or gaseous) had until recently been considered by anesthetists to be generally safer than intravenous agents for general anesthesia as respiration was a simple method of elimination of the anesthetic agent and reversal of anesthesia. Intravenous agents are generally more depressing in their activity on the cardiorespiratory system. It is now, however, appreciated that all the volatile agents are in part metabolized, although enflurane and isoflurane are minimally metabolized. However, an additional factor is the presence of trace contamination of the atmosphere, and intravenous agents do not suffer from this problem. Consideration of the of intravenous agents not only for induction of an-

esthesia but as the principal agent then must be made (Fig. 13.2).

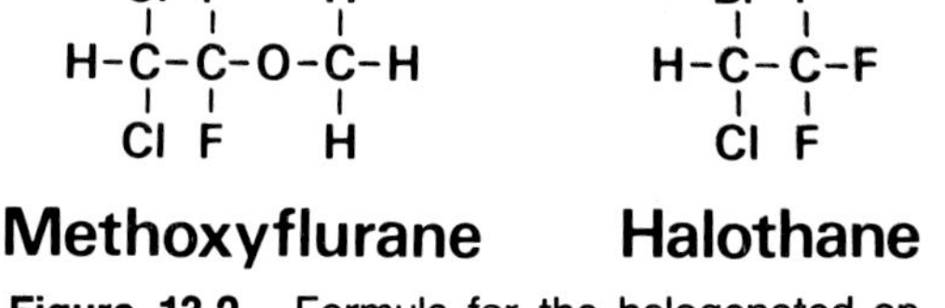

The explosion hazard in the presence of inflammable agents is great in dental anesthesia as there are many sources of ignition present: 1) inadequate conduction protection in dental offices; 2) sparks created by friction of dental forceps and elevators on teeth; 3) use of dental drills; 4) use of open-flamed Bunsen burners or spirit lamps; and 5) use of electrocautery. Because this hazard is better avoided, explosive agents such as diethyl ether are not indicated for dental anesthesia. Until the introduction of the halogenated hydrocarbons, the intravenous agents enjoyed great popularity because they are not explosive.

Volatile general anesthetic agents for dental anesthesia should have the following properties: 1) nonflammable; 2) potent enough to produce adequate anesthesia without hypoxia; 3) ability to be vaporized in adequate amounts with available apparatus; 4) have rapid induction and recovery times; and 5) produce few unpleasant side effects in ambulatory patients (e.g., nausea and vomiting) (Table 13.2).

Isoflurane

Enflurane

Methoxyflurane

Halothane

Figure 13.2. Formula for the halogenated anesthetic agents in current use.

Halothane (Fluothane)

The boiling point of halothane is 50.2°C; thus, adequate and accurate vaporization is readily possible in either the copper kettle or Fluotec vaporizer.

Halothane mixtures of up to 50 per cent in oxygen are not inflammable or explosive. However, use of halothane in the presence of an open flame (such as Bun-

Table 13.2
Properties of Halogenated Agents

Property	Halothane	Isoflurane	Methoxyflurane	Enflurane
Boiling point (°C)	50	49	105	57
Vapor pressure 20°C (mm Hg)	243	238	23	180
Blood/gas	2.4	1.4	13	1.9
Oil/gas	236	98	825	99
Stabilizer	Yes	No	Yes	No
MAC (human)	0.74	1.15	0.16	1.7

sen burner or spirit lamp) is contraindicated as free bromine, a toxic element, is liberated.

Halothane is stored in amber bottles, as exposure to light causes it to decompose to volatile acids. Thymol added as a preservative is responsible for the characteristic odor of halothane vapor.

Halothane has a softening effect on rubber, which is of no significance in newer anesthetic machines. However, on older equipment all dome valves had to be replaced because of decomposition in the presence of halothane. In vaporizers without check valves damage to the seals on flow meters can result, the leak-back occurring when the machine is not in use.

Soda lime and halothane do not react with each other. Therefore, halothane can be safely used in carbon dioxide absorption systems without formation of toxic decomposition products.

UPTAKE, DISTRIBUTION, ELIMINATION

Halothane has a blood/gas partition coefficient of 2.36. Because it is relatively insoluble in blood, it is not taken up rapidly in large quantities from the lung alveoli; therefore, alveolar tension quickly reaches inspired tension of halothane, and induction of anesthesia is rapid.

During recovery the majority of halothane is excreted by exhalation from the lungs. Since its blood solubility is rather low, this process progresses fairly rapidly. Metabolic end products of halothane (trifluoroacetic acid, bromide) have been found in the urine, and it has been calculated that 10 to 25 per cent of inspired halothane is metabolized in the body. There is an increase in serum bromides which may cause postoperative depression following prolonged anesthesia.

PHARMACOLOGY

Cardiovascular System

The principal effects of halothane on the cardiovascular system are peripheral vasodilation, hypotension, bradycardia, and arrhythmias. These changes are directly proportional to the contentration of the inspired halothane mixture and to the depth of anesthesia.

Bradycardia is attributed to increased vagal tone which can be readily reversed by reducing the halothane concentration. Intravenous atropine is also effective, but it is not recommended as it often produces ectopic cardiac rhythm. Premedication with atropine does not significantly reduce the incidence or degree of bradycardia.

Decreased stroke volume, arterial pressure, and cardiac output are the result of direct myocardial depression. Sympathetic ganglion blockade with peripheral, splanchnic, and cerebral vasodilation occur. The resulting hypotension may be associated with increased pulmonary resistance. Lack of increase in blood catecholamines during deeper anesthesia with halothane partially prevents compensation for the hypotensive state. Hypotension is usually most severe during induction of anesthesia when higher concentrations of halothane are used. Blood pressure responds to decreased halothane concentration or administration of a vasopressor. During dental anesthesia with halothane, rises in blood pressure due to surgical stimulation under light anesthesia have regularly been recorded, and hypotension has not been a problem.

"Halothane shakes" is a common feature seen during recovery from halothane anesthesia. Intense shivering, occasionally accompanied by cyanosis, occurs, especially in robust persons. Vasodilatation and body cooling during anesthesia cause the shivering. The markedly increased muscular activity during shivering utlizes greater amounts of oxygen and accounts for any cyanosis. If cyanosis develops, oxygen should be administered.

Although catecholamine levels are not increased, the myocardium has greater irritability during halothane anesthesia. There are many causative factors in the production of ventricular cardiac arrhythmias with halothane including anesthetic induction, endotracheal intubation, hypercarbia, surgical stimulation during light anesthesia, intravenous atropine, and use of epinephrine. Progression to ventricular fibrillation may occur if ventricular arrhythmias go undetected or untreated. Dental patients in whom anesthesia was induced with thiopental show a significant reduction in the incidence of cardiac irregularities.

Respiratory System

Secretions are not stimulated by inhalation of halothane vapor, and atropine premedication is not indicated for its drying effect. Most clinicians do not consider halothane a bronchodilator, but rather a benign vapor, nonirritating to bronchioles and unlikely to initiate bronchospasm.

During surgical anesthesia pharyngeal and laryngeal reflexes are obtunded. Placement of a nasopharyngeal tube and adequate oral packing for procedures in the mouth are facilitated.

Respiration is depressed in a regular fashion in direct proportion to the depth of anesthesia. As anesthesia deepens, tidal volume is decreased and respiratory rate increases (tachypnea). Because of the dead space tachypnea is not able to compensate for the decrease in tidal volume. Respiratory arrest precedes cardiac arrest and is reversible by positive pressure ventilation with 100 per cent oxygen.

Surgical stimulation during light anesthesia for oral surgery usually causes increases in tidal volume despite the increased respiratory rate. Blood gas analysis shows adequate ventilation during halothane-nitrous oxide-oxygen dental anesthesia.

Central Nervous System

Halothane is a poor analgesic, and anesthesia is enhanced by the addition of nitrous oxide to the inspired mixture. A slight drop in cerebral oxygen comsumption occurs during halothane anesthesia; however, no evidence of hypoxia has been shown when cerebral blood flow was diminished during hypocarbia.

Other Systems

Relaxation of masticatory muscles occurs rapidly, allowing direct laryngoscopy or placement of a mouth prop between the teeth. Induction can be carried to adequate depth to allow endotracheal intubation without aid of a muscle relaxant.

Mucus, saliva, and gastric secretions are not stimulated. The incidence of postoperative nausea and vomiting is low.

Central fixation of pupils and cessation of lacrimation, together with return of regular respiration, indicate surgical anesthesia for oral procedures. When a nasopharyngeal tube is used, its placement uncomplicated by coughing, breath holding, or reflex movement is further evidence of adequate surgical anesthesia. With increasing depth of anesthesia there is a regularly progressive decrease in blood pressure and heart rate and an increasing tachypnea.

CLINICAL CONSIDERATIONS

Halothane is ideally suited for supplementation in dental anesthesia because induction is rapid and recovery quickly follows termination of the agent. Nausea and vomiting are seldom seen in unpremedicated patients. Halothane as an adjuvant to nitrous oxide-oxygen for dental anesthesia is less depressant on the cardiovascular and respiratory systems than the barbiturate (methohexital, thiopental)-nitrous oxide-oxygen sequence.

Premedication is not generally given ambulatory patients prior to halothane anesthesia. Secretions are not stimulated and so atropine is not required for this purpose. Bradycardia is not prevented by the usual doses of atropine. Intravenous atropine given just prior to induction of anesthesia can induce ventricular cardiac arrhythmias. Narcotics are not given as they have little effect in reducing the minimum anesthetic concentration, and they contribute to postoperative nausea and vomiting. Narcotic, barbiturate, and tranquilizer premedicants potentiate hypotension and respiratory depression during anesthesia and prolong recovery time.

Induction of anesthesia can be accomplished either with a barbiturate (methohexital or thiopental) or by inhalation of nitrous oxide and oxygen followed by introduction of halothane. Thiopental apparently protects the myocardium against arrhythmias which occur during induction when nitrous oxide and oxygen are used alone. However, significant cardiovascular depression following thiopental or methohexital induction persists into the recovery period. Decrease in mean arterial blood pressure is greatest following methohexital and appears to be due to its specific effect on lowering peripheral resistance. For this reason, if a barbiturate is to be used for induction prior to halothane supplementation for dental anesthesia, thiopental is preferable to methohexital.

Injection of epinephrine has been advocated during dental anesthesia to reduce hemorrhage attending oral surgical procedures. Katz et al. have suggested that use of 1:100,000 to 1:200,000 concentrations of adrenaline is safe during halothane provided 1) the patient has no preexisting cardiac disease or thyrotoxicosis, 2) he is adequately ventilated, and 3) a dose of 10 ml per 10 minutes or 30 ml per hour of the dilute solutions for an average adult is not exceeded. The use of adrenaline during halothane anesthesia requires continuous monitoring of the patient by cardiac stethoscope or electrocardiograph for detection of serious arrhythmias and the availability of digitalis, β-adrenergic blockers, lidocaine, Dilantin, and a defibrillator for treatment of those arrhythmias which develop. An acceptable alternative for hemostasis of the injection of 1:20,000 phenylephrine (Neosyne-phrine), which lacks arrhythmia potential.

Methoxyflurane (Penthrane)

Methoxyflurane is a clear, colorless liquid which has a characteristic fruity odor that is objectionable to some patients. It is stored in amber bottles with a preservative to prevent decomposition by sunlight. With a boiling point of 104.65°C at atmospheric pressure and a low vapor pressure (23 mm Hg at 20°C), methoxyflurane is difficult to vaporize. A maximum of only 4 per cent can be vaporized in the copper kettle and 3.0 per cent in the vaporizers which are temperature- and flow-controlled.

Methoxyflurane is nonflammable under clinical conditions in concentrations up to 4 per cent. Since induction concentrations are rarely carried above 3 per cent, explosion hazards are not present.

Soda lime does not react with methoxyflurane and it can be used safely in rebreathing carbon dioxide absorption systems.

UPTAKE, DISTRIBUTION,
ELIMINATION

The Ostwald partition coefficient for methoxyflurane in rubber is 742 at 25°C. Therefore, it is highly soluble in the rubber parts (tubing, reservoir bag) of the anesthetic apparatus. Approximately 25 to 33 per cent of the methoxyflurane vaporized is absorbed by rubber and fails to reach the lung alveoli during induction of anesthesia. On termination of the methoxyflurane, that which had diffused into rubber re-enters the anesthetic system. The blood/gas solubility coefficient for methoxyflurane is 13.0. Since it is very soluble in blood and large amounts are absorbed by rubber, it takes a relatively long time for alveolar concentration to equal inspired concentration; therefore, induction time is prolonged.

Once anesthesia is terminated, 55 per cent of the methoxyflurane is excreted by respiration. Approximately 45 per cent of inhaled methoxyflurane is metabolized, and the ethyl ring is broken, releasing fluorine and carbon dioxide. The fluoride radical has been detected for up to 3 days in the body. Small amounts of methoxyflurane continue to be released from fat for 24 or more hours and can be detected on the patient's breath during this time. Only about 0.1 to 0.3 per cent concentration is usually required for maintenance of anesthesia when combined with nitrous oxide-oxygen.

PHARMACOLOGY

Cardiovascular System

Methoxyflurane has a primary depressant effect on the myocardium. Hypotension is a result of decreased stroke volume, cardiac output, cardiac rate, and decreased vascular resistance. All parameters of renal hemodynamics are affected less by methoxyflurane than by halothane. Plasma catecholamines are not increased significantly by methoxyflurane. The degree of cardiovascular depression occurs in proportion to the concentration of the drug delivered to the patient, and it can be reversed by reducing the concentration.

Respiratory System

Progressive depression of respiration ocurs in relation to increasing concentrations of the drug. Tidal volume is affected more than the respiratory rate. Dental patients are adequately ventilated with spontaneous respiration for outpatient oral surgery procedures.

Methoxyflurane is nonirritating and does not stimulate secretions; use of atropine for drying effect is not indicated. Pharyngeal and laryngeal reflexes are adequately obtunded during surgical anesthesia.

As it is eliminated by the lungs over a prolonged period following recovery, the odor of methoxyflurane lingers on the patient's breath. This odor is often perceived as a noxious one by the patient and undoubtedly contributes to the increased nausea and vomiting, compared with patients anesthetized with halothane.

Central Nervous System

Methoxyflurane has good analgesic properties, making it well suited for dental analgesia.

Other Systems

Masticatory muscles relax early in induction, allowing placement of a mouth prop. Extreme shivering is often seen following methoxyflurane anesthesia, particularly in young healthy adults, and is presumably due to decrease in body temperature as a result of peripheral vasodilation. Pupil changes are insignificant as they become constricted and centrally fixed early in the induction before surgical anesthesia. Masticatory muscle relaxation usually occurs before pupil fixation and, unlike halothane, is not a reliable sign of surgical anesthesia.

CLINICAL CONSIDERATIONS

As only minimal amounts of methoxyflurane can be vaporized, it is important that a vaporizer be able to deliver maximal concentrations required during induction in order to shorten this period. The copper kettle and Pentec vaporizers are best suited for this purpose. Use of a vaporizer which can deliver only a low concentration markedly prolongs induction of anesthesia.

The use of atropine premedication is not routinely advocated. Secretions are not stimulated by methoxyflurane. Recent studies indicate no significant effect of atropine premedication on mean arterial pressure, as the increase in cardiac rate is offset by a proportional fall in stroke volume due to the decreased ventricular filling time (Fig. 13.3).

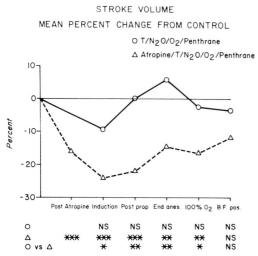

STROKE VOLUME

MEAN PERCENT CHANGE FROM CONTROL

O T/N$_2$O/O$_2$/Penthrane

△ Atropine/T/N$_2$O/O$_2$/Penthrane

	Post Atropine	Induction	Post prop	End anes.	100% O$_2$	B.F. pos.
O		NS	NS	NS	NS	NS
△	***	***	***	**	**	NS
O vs △		*	**	**	*	NS

Figure 13.3. The effect of atropine medication on stroke volume should be noted; the reductions with atropine are significant. (Reprinted with permission from Allen, G. D., Everett, G. B., and Kennedy, W. F., Jr.: Cardiorespiratory effects of general anesthesia in outpatients: the influence of atropine. *J Oral Surg* 30:576, 1972.)

Seventy per cent nitrous oxide is routinely used with methoxyflurane to reduce the MAC and attendant cardiovascular and respiratory depression. Oxygen-methoxyflurane anesthesia is not advocated and is unsatisfactory for dental procedures.

Paralleling the effects seen with halothane, use of a barbiturate for induction prior to methoxyflurane produces greater depression of cardiovascular parameters for a longer time than following nitrous oxide-oxygen induction. The cardiovascular depression produced by methoxyflurane for similar surgical anesthesia levels is less than that seen with halothane supplementation of nitrous oxide-oxygen. Severe hypotension is occasionally seen following barbiturate induction. Because of methohexital's greater specific depressant effect on peripheral resistance, thiopental is preferred if barbiturate induction is used. Mean induction times for outpatient dental anesthesia have been shown to be 8 minutes as opposed to a mean of 5 minutes with halothane. Anesthesia should be maintained with the smallest concentration necessary to render the patient free of movement or reflex activity (usually 0.1 to 0.3 per cent with 70 per cent nitrous oxide). The nephrotoxicity of methoxyflurane is discussed separately.

Enflurane (Ethrane)

Enflurane possesses many of the properties of an ether, such as muscle relaxation, and has been used extensively in general surgery. It is a nonflammable agent with a boiling point of 56.6°C and a vapor pressure of 180 mm Hg at 20°C. It is stable and does not react with soda lime and is thus compatible with closed-circuit anesthesia. No stabilizer is added; it does not decompose with light; it has a musty odor. Some of the properties of the agent indicate that it is unsuitable for use in outpatient dental anesthesia.

Suitably constructed vaporizers have been made for use with enflurane, and no deleterious effect upon the equipment has been noted with the agent.

UPTAKE, DISTRIBUTION, ELIMINATION

The drug is rapidly taken up, which speeds induction. Excretion is rapid and aids recovery. It should be noted that despite the low blood/gas solubility coefficient, less than that of halothane, induction is not fast. This in part may be attributed to the anxieties produced by the occurrence of overt seizures at concentrations in excess of 4 per cent. Thus, although vaporizers will deliver concentrations of 7 per cent, in clinical practice this is rarely used, and thus induction is slowed.

PHARMACOLOGY

Cardiovascular Effects

In clinical studies, sudden drops in blood pressure occur with the administration of enflurane. The sudden drops in blood pressure are preceded by the loss of the P wave of the ECG, which merges into the QRS complex. The dysrhythmia does not seem to affect ventricular rhythm, but the fall in blood pressure is clinically significant and somewhat alarming when the agent is being administered.

With spontaneous respiration, the cardiovascular effects are much less, and the elevation in carbon dioxide releases endogenous catecholamines which maintain the blood pressure. Concomitantly, however, the elevation in carbon dioxide causes an additional fall in total peripheral resistance to 30 per cent below control level.

It would seem then that the cardiovascular effects of enflurane do not lend themselves to outpatient dental anesthesia. In particular, the sudden alarming drop in blood pressure which occurs could cause problems, particularly in a patient with a relatively fixed cardiac output, where there would be no increased cardiac output due to the elevation of carbon dioxide.

The cardiac rhythm is extremely stable during enflurane anesthesia. Indeed, if exogenous epinephrine is to be used, it is the safest of the halogenated anesthetic agents. If exogenous epinephrine is to be injected, it is better injected with lidocaine rather than saline, as the incidence of ventricular arrhythmias under these circumstances is much reduced.

Respiratory System

At all levels of enflurane anesthesia, respiratory depression is a prominent feture. Indeed, it would be inappropriate in most situations to allow spontaneous respiration with enflurane early in anesthesia, due to the rapid rise in carbon dioxide levels. In dentistry, the elevation of carbon dioxide would be evident, as spontaneous respiration is routine.

Because the agent is an ether, it is a useful drug to administer to asthmatics.

Central Nervous System

At all concentrations in the MAC region of 1.86 per cent, there is seizure activity noted on the electroencephalogram. If, in addition, careful observation is made of the hands and feet, fine motor activity can also be noticed at all concentrations. The effect of carbon dioxide on the seizure activity would appear to be protective. Thus, if carbon dioxide level is elevated with spontaneous respiration, the seizure activity will disappear. If the carbon dioxide is maintained at a steady level, the seizure activity remains. If then nitrous oxide is added to the inspired mixture, the seizure activity becomes worse. Decreasing the carbon dioxide level as with hyperventilation increases seizure activity.

It possesses good muscle-relaxant properties. As the drug is a fluorinated compound, it is partially metabolized. Metabolism, however, is minimal and only 2.4 per cent of the administered enflurane is metabolized, releasing free fluoride ions. There are increased fluorides noted in the urine on the first day following operation.

CLINICAL CONSIDERATIONS

Enflurane will depress the heart and stimulate the central nervous system. Lowering carbon dioxide promotes seizures and in 50 per cent of the volunteers studied frank seizures were noted. Postoperatively there was slowing of the electroencephalogram in 50 per cent of volunteers for several days. No permanent effect was noted. It should be noted that α waves also occurred with halothane, and thus this cannot be considered a problem.

Enflurane, with its propensity to develop seizure activity, although not damaging would nonetheless be alarming in an outpatient situation. The tendency to sudden drops in blood pressure, and the inability of the drug to produce as rapid an induction as halothane, would limit its use in outpatient anesthesia. It does, however, have a role to play in patients in whom exogenous epinephrine is to be injected, when it is the safest of the agents to be administered. Enflurane can be recommended for major oromaxillary surgery.

Isoflurane (Forane)

This halogenated ether is a structural isomer of enflurane. The boiling point is 48.5°F, and the vapor pressure parallels that of halothane; the agent is thus readily vaporized. There is no preservative required and thus no chemical reactions within the circuit to the rubber or soda lime. It is extremely stable and is not affected by light.

UPTAKE, DISTRIBUTION, ELIMINATION

It is the least soluble of all the halogenated hydrocarbons, with a blood/gas solubility coefficient of 1.4. Consequently it should be the agent which produces the most rapid induction of anesthesia. However, the mild pungency of the vapor prevents a rapid rate of increase of the vapor during induction, and consequently induction is somewhat slower than with halothane and parallels that of enflurane. For induction of anesthesia 1.5 to 3.5 per cent isoflurane is required, and for maintenance 0.7 to 2.1 per cent. It should be given with nitrous oxide for induction. Isoflurane is rapidly excreted and recovery therefore is rapid.

PHARMACOLOGY

Cardiovascular Effects

There is minimal depression of myocardial function or cardiac output with anesthetic doses of isoflurane. There is some increase in cardiac rate with consequent decrease of stroke volume. Peripheral resistance is lowered by decreased resistance to muscle blood flow, but with anesthetic concentrations there is little change in blood pressure or cardiac rate. Patients appear to be able to tolerate high concentrations of isoflurane over the range of 1 to 2 MAC without depression of myocardial function, as opposed to en-

flurane and halothane in which some depression does occur. Particularly, however, cardiac rhythm is stable; rarely are ectopic rhythms seen with isoflurane.

Respiratory System

There is a dose-related depression of respiration. The $PaCO_2$ rises, while the response to inspired carbon dioxide is depressed. Respiration is depressed considerably more than with halothane. Indeed it is difficult to maintain spontaneous respiration with isoflurane even during induction of anesthesia, when attempts are made to rapidly increase concentration of the agent. Controlled respiration with the agent would seem to be indicated.

Central Nervous System

The MAC of isoflurane is 1.15, whereas with 70 per cent nitrous oxide in oxygen the MAC falls to 0.5. It will, if given 30 per cent above the MAC, depress movement in the majority of humans. The electroencephalogram correlates with the concentration, and there does not appear to be any indication of seizure activity as with enflurane.

Because of the resistance of isoflurane to biodegradation, there is no hepatotoxicity, and liver injury has not been demonstrated. Similarly no change is noted in renal function, although there is a decreased renal blood flow with increased concentrations. The agent is the least metabolized of all halogenated hydrocarbons. Metabolism is only $\frac{1}{10}$ of that of enflurane, that is, 0.17 per cent.

Clinical Experience

The pungency of the vapor makes induction of anesthesia slow, and concentration must be increased slowly. The use of intravenous induction and the addition of nitrous oxide to isoflurane make for better induction. An index of depth of anesthesia for surgical levels is the cessation of eyeball movement with centering of the eye. The stability of the response of the cardiovascular system is noted by the minimal changes in blood pressure which occur and the absence of changes in cardiac rhythm. Falls in blood pressure occur slowly, even with increasing concentrations. There appear to be no sudden drops in blood pressure as occur with enflurane. A notable feature, however, is the early onset of respiratory depression.

Toxicity

It is now established that in acute clinical concentrations, anesthetic agents can be toxic. In addition there is a potential hazard of chronic exposure to low concentrations of these toxic substances. Until recently, the volatile anesthetics were considered to be inert substances which were totally eliminated from the body. There is now evidence that the inhalation hydrocarbon inhalation anesthetics are metabolized in the body.

METABOLISM OF VOLATILE AGENTS

The biodegradation of the volatile anesthetic agents has raised problems of possible toxic effects, particularly on the liver and kidney, of anesthetic metabolites and the possibility of sensitization of individuals to anesthetics. The combination of free radicals with large protein fractions to form antigenic molecules is a reasonable concern.

The development of enzyme induction of anesthetic agents is a recognized entity, and thus, such drugs will stimulate not only their own metabolism but that of simultaneously administered drugs.

There are three significant features in drug metabolism. Most drugs are nonpolar and therefore lipophilic or relatively water-insoluble. During metabolism, a drug becomes more polar and thus more water-soluble, and therefore more readily excreted from the body. Drug metabolism usually results in a compound which has

pharmacological activity which is unrelated to the parent compound, thus the concept that drug metabolism is a detoxification process. Finally, some drugs require biotransformation to produce a pharmacologically active compound.

The pharmacological processes in the liver and kidney by which the drugs are metabolized are oxidation and conjugation.

BIOTRANSFORMATION AND TOXICITY

In regard to toxicity the duration of administration of drug is more more significant than the actual concentration given. Thus, if a drug is given at 1× MAC concentration for 10 hours, this is much more toxic than if the drug is given at 10 × MAC for 1 hour. The drugs administered for anesthesia are metabolized, and the majority produce no toxic products. Others are biotransformed to nontoxic metabolites, but some of the intermediate stages may be toxic, while finally other drugs may produce a highly toxic metabolite which does not necessarily have to pass through a toxic intermediate. The metabolism is usually related to enzymes. Biotransformation is dependent upon the microsomal mixed function oxidase enzyme system, and the liver contains the majority of these enzymes. Cytochrome P-450 is the most important component of drug transformation. Volatile anesthetics are metabolized in this enzyme system. It is significant then that the form of biotransformation of the volatile anesthetics may indicate a relationship to untoward toxic effects. Thus, halothane metabolism could possibly produce an intermediate metabolite which is hepatotoxic. The nephrotoxicity of methoxyflurane is probably due to the metabolic product, organic fluoride, although intermediate agents may be important.

Halothane

The carbon-fluorine bound in halothane is readily broken, while the carbon-chloride and bromine are more slowly broken apart in the liver. The free bromine release may account for the hangover that is noticed following prolonged halothane anesthesia. The products accumulate rapidly in the liver, and leave slowly, to be excreted in the urine. Between 10 and 25 per cent of the administered halothane is metabolized. The metabolites are trifluoroacetic acid and trifluoroacetylethanolamide which are final metabolites and considered nontoxic in the amounts formed. Unlike methoxyflurane, halothane does not produce free fluoride ions.

There is a current theory that hepatitis associated with halothane administration is related to allergy. Little scientific documentation exists for the theory, despite evidence that multiple or second halothane administrations produce hepatitis and challenge tests have produced hepatitis. However, it is known that halothane is biotransformed, and the metabolites may cause problems.

There is a high mortality in humans with hepatitis associated with halothane administration. The younger age group, however, would seem to present no concern, and infants and children with undeveloped microsomal enzyme systems are at a very low risk for anesthesia-related hepatotoxicity. Halothane is preferred in pediatric clinics, and the younger age groups present no problems in this regard.

Repeated exposure to halothane is a possible problem and in some areas it is not recommended that it be administered within one month of a prior exposure. Certainly history of unexplained jaundice following past exposure is a contraindication to anesthesia with a halogenated agent. Obesity is a factor, as the obese patient metabolizes inhalation anesthetics more than a normal patient and presents as a simple dose-response relationship. The middle aged patient also metabolizes more halothane than the younger group, while genetic factors seem to influence metabolism in middle aged female. A cautious practitioner would avoid halothane in the presence of obesity, female sex, middle age, and repeat anesthesia.

Methoxyflurane

Methoxyflurane is biodegraded, and sodium pentobarbital will produce an increased deposition of fluoride in the bones after methoxyflurane. Free fluoride is released in great quantities, and will produce a polyuric renal insufficiency. No question exists that methoxyflurane is nephrotoxic. In the healthy patient undergoing a relatively minor operation, any agent will be acceptable. However, if there is a suggestion of cardiac or renal disease, then in such instances renal injury could result and it is wise to avoid methoxyflurane. The renal lesion associated with methoxyflurane administration is dose-related and dependent upon the amount of inorganic fluoride released by biodegradation. Low-dose methoxyflurane anesthesia usually produces only moderate increases in inorganic fluoride concentration, and these are unassociated with renal insufficiency. There are, however, variations, and minimal concentrations together with susceptibility could produce nephrotoxicity. In addition, the interaction of methoxyflurane with tetracycline and gentamycin is established. This is a great concern and should be considered if antibiotics are to be used concomitantly. If methoxyflurane is to be administered, it should be limited to special situations where low dosage is assured, such as in obstetrical analgesia or surgical procedures of short duration, particularly less than 2 hours.

Enflurane

Metabolism of this ether is minimal use. Only 2.5 per cent of free fluorides are released. It should be appreciated, however, that this is greater than with halothane, and in patients with renal disease, enflurane is not indicated.

Isoflurane

This is the least metabolized of all the halogenated hydrocarbons. Virtually no biodegradation occurs with the agent, only 0.17 per cent of the agent being retained after cessation of anesthesia. If toxicity of inhalation agents are a concern, then this must be the drug of choice.

CHRONIC TOXICITY

The presence of operating room pollution has been established, and OSHA has recommended that the trace concentrations of the volatile anesthetic agents in the operating room be reduced to acceptable levels. Small amounts of halothane and methoxyflurane have been detected in end expired air of anesthetists and nurses up to 30 hours after exposure. Concentrations of methoxyflurane have been detected in end expired air of patients for as long as 18 days after anesthesia.

FACTORS OTHER THAN ATMOSPHERIC POLLUTION

There could be a residual in equipment of the volatile agent. The rubber-gas and soda lime partition coefficients are significant in that they will take up the volatile anesthetic agents. The concentration and amount are dependent upon the surface area exposed and the time at which it is exposed. This will contribute to chronic toxicity, and further could expose subsequent patients to unexpected amounts of volatile anesthetic agents.

The solvents in the operating room and other contaminant gases have been regulated, and trace contamination with these solvents can initiate toxic responses.

A significant problem is that radiation may combine with these toxic agents and compound the problem.

FACTORS IN PRODUCTION OF TOXICITY

The agents may be directly toxic, such as chloroform or methoxyflurane, they may increase metabolism, or they may produce hypersensitivity. For a drug to produce hypersensitivity, an antigen must be formed. The drug must be large enough or a reactive molecule to be capable of combining with proteins. Skin rashes, eosinophilia, arthralgia, fever, or other signs of hypersensitivity are seen. There is a history of previous exposure to an antigen and once established, hypersensitivity is usually long standing.

The long-standing exposure of operating room personnel to trace amounts or low concentrations in the atmosphere is indeed evidence against hypersensitivity by chronic exposure; otherwise there would be a much higher incidence of toxicity than is reported. There is, of course, still the problem of enzyme induction and drug interaction, which are unknown quantities. The toxicity with trace contamination is noted in that cell division may be affected, as with nitrous oxide, and there is the potential for teratogenetic effects or increased numbers of spontaneous abortions. The immune response could be altered, and could account for the increased number of suicides in anesthesiologists. Central nervous system alteration has also been noted with evidence of headache and irritability in exposed personnel.

Although the case is not proven, nonetheless it is prudent to lower the concentrations of trace contaminants to achievable levels.

Vaporizers

The provision of an adequate means of vaporization is essential to the clinical application of the volatile anesthetic agents.

The demands of modern anesthetic practice have brought many changes from these early attempts at vaporization of volatile anesthetic agents. An anesthetic vaporizer should be reasonably accurate and efficient. Regular incremental changes in concentration should be possible, and required concentrations should be available to achieve adequate depths of anesthesia. Temperature changes caused by latent heat of vaporization decrease vaporization and require compensation. The rate of flow, surface area over which or through carrier gas is passed and temperature of the liquid affect the vapor concentration. Vaporizers such as the *copper kettle* (for ether, halothane, methoxyflurane), the *Fluotec* (for halothane), and the *Pentec* (for methoxyflurane) have been developed to meet these demands in continuous flow anesthetic systems (Fig. 13.4).

A knowledge of the vapor pressure of a volatile agent enables the anesthetist to calculate quickly the inspired concentration being delivered to the patient by a "bubble-through" type of vaporizer such as the copper kettle (Fig. 13.5). The principle of the copper kettle is that the vaporizer is constructed of a highly conductive metal. When attached directly to an anesthetic table-top of similar material, it has a large heat reservoir available which will prevent the temperature in the vaporizer from falling because of the latent heat of vaporization. A known flow of oxygen is then bubbled through the liquid anesthetic agent at room temperature. Taking halothane as an example, its vapor pressure is 241 mm Hg at 20°C. If a flow of 100 ml of oxygen is passed through the

COppER KETTLE

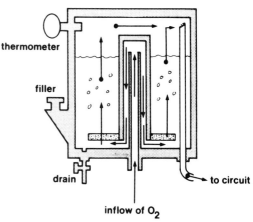

Figure 13.5. The gas flows in a copper kettle are shown; a measured quantity of volatile anesthetic agent is added to the diluent gases.

copper kettle vaporizer, then as the vapor pressure is 241/760 mm Hg or approximately ⅓ atm, 100 ml of oxygen will pick up 50 ml of halothane (i.e., a total of 150 ml of 33⅓ per cent halothane or 50 ml of pure halothane vapor). If this quantity (50 ml of pure halothane vapor) is added to 5 liters per minute flow of nitrous oxide-oxygen mixture, the patient will receive an inspired concentration of 1 per cent (50/5000) halothane. Similarly, if 200 ml of oxygen are bubbled through the copper kettle and then added to a 5-liter nitrous oxide-oxygen per minute flow, the patient will receive 2 per cent halothane vapor.

Anesthetic vaporizers each have a degree of inaccuracy in the concentration they deliver at various settings on their dials. In some vaporizers this inaccuracy occurs in a regular, predictable manner, while in others the inaccuracy is unpredictable, particularly in the higher ranges. The performance of a vaporizer should be known, it should be regularly recalibrated to assure continued accurate performance, and it should be used only in the type of anesthetic system for which it was designed.

There have been several accidents with

TEMPERATURE CONTROLLEd VApORizER

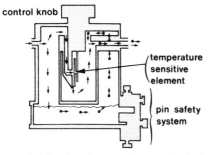

Figure 13.4. In a temperature-controlled vaporizer, a variable percentage of the gas stream is diverted through the temperature-sensitive control over the liquid agent.

vaporizers, but developments in the more modern vaporizers should prevent them. The copper kettle originally had no indication of a maximum safe filling level. Recent models have a side filler and this prevents the kettle from being overfilled. An incorrect agent could be added to a kettle vaporizer, and for this reason many no longer purchase the kettle type vaporizer. A pin safety system has been advocated for this form of vaporizer and is available on the more recent temperature controlled vaporizers which can be filled only by the agent for which they are designed. Bubble-through vaporizers can be a problem if a silicone lubricant or sealant is used on the vaporizer. Bubbling can occur and foam can be carried over into the breathing system and kill the patient. Older vaporizers are mounted in series, rather than parallel, and thus both can be opened at the same time and contaminate the other. Agent selector switches have been developed to prevent simultaneous administration of vapors.

INTRAVENOUS ANESTHESIA

In the main, inhalation agents are eliminated by the lungs, and overdose can be rapidly cleared by supporting respiration. However, the intravenous agents depend largely upon biotransformation in the liver for reversal of their effects, a much slower process. Should a complication occur, a period of resuscitation, often prolonged, is required while the drug undergoes metabolic detoxification. Therefore, the use of intravenous agents requires the same degree of skill in managing the airway and recognizing and treating complications as does the administration of other types of anesthetic agents.

Intravenous anesthesia for office dental procedures has long been a popular practice because of the pleasantness, rapidity, and seeming simplicity of induction. Although the hazards of intravenous agents have also been recognized for many years, the brevity of procedures has given this

technique a margin of safety. Since significant decrease in blood oxygen tension occurs following intravenous anesthetic induction with barbiturates, supplemental oxygen or nitrous oxide-oxygen is mandatory.

Once the needle is inserted into a vein, it should be left in place with an intravenous drip throughout the operation. The veins of the cubital fossa are best avoided as movement of the elbow may cause infiltration of the drugs subcutaneously or into the brachial artery. It is unnecessary to try to start an intravenous infusion in a struggling child before an inhalation induction. If the procedure is to last more than a brief period, an intravenous line can be established after anesthetic induction is completed and vasodilatation has occurred.

Use of intravenous agents does not eliminate the requirement to establish and maintain a patent airway throughout the procedure.

The ultrashort-acting barbiturates have proven useful in general anesthesia, especially for their ability to achieve rapid induction. Such compounds include the thiobarbiturates (thiopental, thiamylal) and the oxybarbiturates (methohexital). Since their principal actions are similar, their general properties should be considered. Methohexital and thiopental are the most widely used barbiturates in dental anesthesia.

Barbiturates

The barbiturates are derivatives of barbituric acid. Substitution of the oxygen atom on carbon 2 of the barbiturate nucleus with sulfur produces thiopental, a rapid acting, highly lipid-soluble compound. Similarly, methylation of nitrogen atom 1 in methohexital is responsible for its affinity for lipids (Fig. 13.6).

Aqueous solutions of the barbiturates are strongly alkaline (pH 11). The alkaline barbiturate solutions are highly irritating to arterial vessels, and intra-arterial injec-

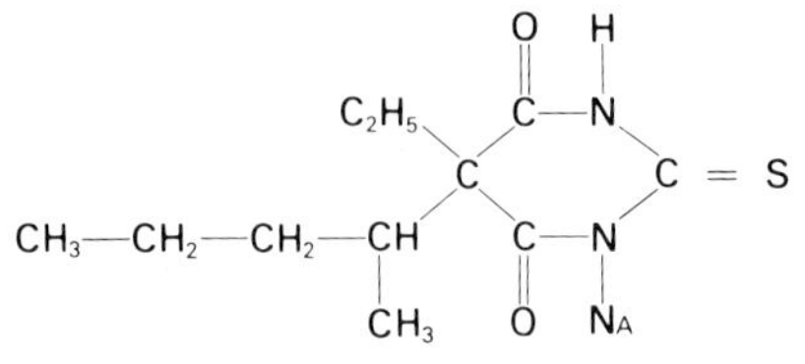

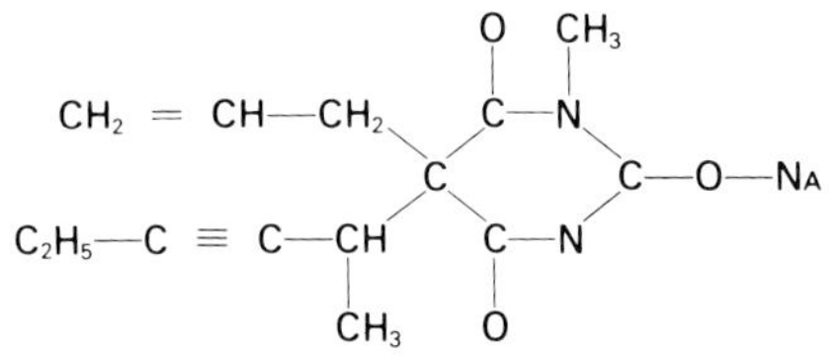

Figure 13.6. The ultrashort-acting barbiturates are lipid soluble and do not readily dissolve in water. They are available as sodium salts to facilitate intravenous administration when the pH is 11.

tion provokes an intense arteriospasm which requires emergency treatment. Alkaline barbiturate solutions are not "self-sterilizing" and can support bacterial growth. Therefore, long term storage of prepared solutions is not recommended.

The ultrashort-acting barbiturates have the potency to produce a full range of effects, depending on the dose given. These effects include sedation, hypnosis, anesthesia, coma, and death.

ANESTHETIC ACTION

The initial activity of a dose of barbiturate is on the ascending reticular activating system (RAS).

Plasma concentration of the barbiturate does not appear to be the controlling factor in producing a given depth of anesthesia. There is no consistent relationship between plasma barbiturate levels and electroencephalographic patterns (Table 13.3). Cerebral oxygen consumption is decreased during barbiturate anesthesia. There is little or no analgesic effect on afferent sensory impulses. In fact, in doses insufficient to cause anesthesia there is an antianalgesic effect. Increased response to pain may occur.

Patients given a larger initial dose of barbiturate will recover consciousness with a higher blood level of the drug and will require larger subsequent increments to maintain anesthesia than will patients who receive smaller induction doses. For example, a patient given an induction dose of 500 mg of thiopental and a total of 2.0 g including subsequent increments for maintenance of anesthesia will regain consciousness with a blood level of about 20 mg per 100 ml. On the other hand, another patient given an induction dose of 250 mg and a total of 1.0 g of thiopental may awaken with a blood level of 10 mg per 100 ml. This phenomenon is termed acute tolerance, the mechanism of which remains unclear.

RESPIRATORY EFFECTS

A hypnotic dose of barbiturate depresses the neurogenic control, so that respiration is maintained by the chemical drive. Anesthetic levels of barbiturate cause additional depression of both chemical and hypoxic controls. Further increase in dose abolishes both neurogenic and chemical controls, so that respiration is maintained solely by the hypoxic stimulus. Rate and depth of respiration also decrease progressively. Brief apnea may occur after rapid injection of a large induction dose.

Rhythmic respiratory movements decrease progressively as increasing levels of barbiturate affect the brainstem. Disruption of the rhythmic cycle of respiration may cause laryngospasm because of irregular firing of respiratory neurons stimulating the muscles controlling vocal cord openng, closure, and inspiratory, expiratory movements. Laryngospasm is most likely due to inability of barbiturates to block afferent sensory impulses from the pharyngeal and laryngeal areas in the

Table 13.3
Methohexital Blood Levels Throughout Oral Surgery Anesthesia and at Recovery

Patient	Time (R. Recovery)											
	2	3	4	5	6	7	8	9	10	11	12	R
					min							
A	0.00	0.00	0.00		0.44		0.51		1.47			0.77
B	0.00	0.00			1.70		1.65		1.73		0.11	1.35
C	0.00	0.00	0.45		2.00		3.06		4.6			3.20
D	0.34	0.34	1.12		1.62		1.31					1.36
E	0.00	1.40	0.66		1.08		3.32					2.48
F	2.48	1.29	1.00		0.72		0.73					0.90
G	4.98	1.54			0.64		1.16				1.01	1.31
H	0.00	0.00	0.59		1.23		1.41		3.38		2.41	2.41
I	0.31	0.94	0.58		0.80		0.66					0.83
J	0.00	0.00	2.69		2.05		2.54		2.17			2.18
Mean	0.81	0.55	0.79		1.23		1.64		2.67		1.18	1.68
S.D.	1.65	0.66	0.81		0.58		1.01		1.30		1.16	0.83
N	10	10	9		10		10		5		3	10

From Donaldson, D. and Allen, G.D.: Unpublished data.

presence of surgical stimulation or contamination with foreign material. Bronchospasm is most likely to occur in the asthmatic patient who is given thiopental, and it may be due to the presence of the sulfur atom.

CARDIOVASCULAR EFFECTS

Anesthetic concentrations of barbiturate depress the activity of the hypothalamic autonomic center which causes mild decrease in the force of myocardial contraction. Depression of the medullary vasomotor center produces mild dilatation of muscle and skin blood vessels with a slight decrease in total peripheral vascular resistance. Direct action of barbiturates on the heart may also depress myocardial contractility. Barbiturate anesthesia does not sensitize the myocardium to the arrhythmic effects of catecholamines. There is an increase in cardiac rate, probably on a reflex basis due to peripheral vasodilatation. While there is decrease in stroke volume, cardiac output and mean arterial pressure are maintained by the increased rate of contraction.

OTHER EFFECTS

Most barbiturates suppress seizure activity by raising the threshold to excitation of cortical neurons, independent of their sedative or anesthetic effects. However, methohexital has been shown to produce seizure activity, and it is not recommended for use in known epileptic patients.

Vomiting after barbiturate anesthesia is uncommon. However, laryngospasm, struggling under too light anesthesia, recent ingestion of food or fluids prior to anesthesia, or gastric dilatation may contribute to vomiting.

In anesthetic concentrations barbiturates produce very little muscle relaxation.

UPTAKE, DISTRIBUTION, AND ELIMINATION

Barbiturates rapidly reach peak concentration in the brain (approximately 30 seconds), and unconsciousness ensues.

Approximately two-thirds of an injected dose of barbiturate is bound to plasma proteins (principally albumin) and not available for diffusion into the tissues. Equilibration takes place between the unbound portion and the tissues, and it is dependent partly upon the pH of the blood. Respiratory acidosis due to carbon dioxide retention causes increase in depth of anesthesia with a given dose of barbiturate.

Termination of anesthetic action, often within 5 to 10 minutes, is not primarily by biotransformation but by redistribution within the body. The slow release of the drug from fat depots causes prolonged recovery and the hangover effect after multiple-dose barbiturate anesthesia.

Metabolic degradation of the thiobarbiturates (thiopental) occurs by oxidation and desulfuration, principally in the liver. The electroencephalogram will show changes for 24 hours. The oxybarbiturates (methohexital) are deactivated only in the liver. There is no drug which safely reverses or antagonizes the actions of the barbiturates.

SELECTION OF PATIENTS FOR INTRAVENOUS BARBITURATE ANESTHESIA

Careful selection should be made to avoid unsatisfactory anesthesia or complications.

Technical Considerations

Patients with poor or absent superficial veins are unsuitable candidates for intravenous techniques. Patients with cervical or oral swellings or severe retrognathia may develop rapid intractable respiratory obstruction without warning after an induction dose of barbiturate. Robust, muscular, or alcoholic patients may require doses approximating toxic levels to produce anesthesia, and muscle relaxation even for insertion of a mouth prop may be inadequate. Endotracheal intubation during barbiturate anesthesia requires the use of a muscle relaxant in all patients.

Drug Interactions

Other depressant medications (especially alcohol) combine with barbiturates to produce enhanced central nervous system depression. Normal doses of barbiturates given to patients taking monoamine oxidase inhibitors for the treatment of mental depression or hypertension have caused severe barbiturate intoxication. Such medications are best recognized by a careful preanesthetic history.

Medical Conditions

The use of any barbiturate is absolutely contraindicated in patients with a history of acute intermittent or latent porphyria.

Patients with respiratory diseases such as active bronchial asthma, acute respiratory infection, and chronic bronchitis are not suitable candidates for barbiturate anesthesia.

Patients with the various muscle diseases (muscular dystrophy, myotonia congenita, dystrophic myotonia) are poor risks for barbiturate anesthesia.

Renal or hepatic insufficiency may not be absolute contraindications to barbiturate anesthesia. However, interference with metabolism and elimination of the barbiturates usually indicates cautious administration of smaller doses. Such patients are seldom candidates for barbiturate anesthesia for nonemergent dental procedures.

Idiosyncratic or allergic reactions have been reported following administration of both methohexital and thiopental. Previous history of such a reaction contraindicates further use in the patient.

Advantages

Induction of barbiturate anesthesia is pleasant and rapid; the patient often requests it. If supplemented with other agents, it is suitable for short procedures. Oral secretions are not stimulated, and the incidence of postanesthetic nausea and vomiting is low compared to other agents. Barbiturates do not sensitize the myocardium to the effects of catecholamines, making it possible to inject local anesthesia with epinephrine without increased risk. There is no explosion hazard and no atmospheric pollution with trace contaminants of expired gases.

Disadvantages

Significant respiratory depression or apnea can occur with large doses of barbiturate. Little or no analgesia or an "antianalgesic" effect occurs. There is poor muscle relaxation making anesthesia of muscular patients difficult and endotracheal intubation impossible without use of a relaxant. There is an increased incidence of laryngospasm especially in the presence of "light" anesthesia or stimulation or contamination of the pharynx. Cardiovascular depression can be significant in hypovolemic or debilitated patients. Prolonged depression and delayed recovery follow multiple doses of barbiturate for maintenance of anesthesia. There is no antagonist; once the barbiturate is given, it cannot be removed.

THIOPENTAL SODIUM (PENTOTHAL)

Thiopental is a yellow amorphous powder with an odor resembling hydrogen sulfide. Thiopental sodium is soluble in water, and it is usually prepared in a 2.5 per cent solution (25 mg per ml) which has a pH of approximately 10.8. The solution is relatively unstable and should be used within 24 to 48 hours after preparation.

Induction of Anesthesia

Thiopental induction produces significantly greater depression of mean arterial pressure and stroke volume than inhalation induction with nitrous oxide-oxygen, and this depression produced by the barbiturate persists into the recovery period. Such considerations are important in selection with impaired cardiovascular systems.

Recovery time after a single dose of thiopental is longer than after a comparative dose of methohexital. Thus, methohexital is more widely used in outpatient dental anesthesia where rapid recovery is an important consideration.

An intravenous test dose of 50 mg (2 ml of a 2.5 per cent solution) of thiopental may be administered to observe the patient's response. An induction dose of thiopental (2 to 3.5 mg per kg body weight) is given over a 15- to 30-second interval. Shortly after the injection of the barbiturate the patient will yawn and close his eyes. At this time it is often possible to insert a mouth prop, but surgical manipulations may precipitate struggling, coughing, or laryngospasm. Additional inhalation or intravenous anesthetic agents are added to provide smooth maintenance of anesthesia for the surgical procedure.

Thiopental Supplementation

Following induction with a thiobarbiturate as described above, nitrous oxide and oxygen are administered in a ratio of 7:3 by a nasal mask. Use of a nasopharyngeal tube is not recommended as pharyngeal reflexes are poorly obtunded. A mouth prop and oropharyngeal pack are placed. A local anesthetic may be injected to anesthetize the operative site. Surgery is begun, and the level of anesthesia is maintained by administering additional 50 to 100 mg increments of thiopental as required. At the conclusion of surgery 100 per cent oxygen is administered for 2 to 3 minutes after which the patient is allowed to breathe room air. The airway is maintained until the patient has recovered his protective reflexes. Return of a positive Bender face-hand test, an indicator of recovery from anesthesia, can be expected 30 to 45 minutes after termination of surgery.

Intermittent supplementation of anesthesia with thiopental produces significantly greater cardiovascular and respiratory depression when compared with purely inhalation techniques such as halothane, nitrous oxide, and oxygen. The cardiovascular changes persist into the recovery period. Because repeated doses of barbiturate can cause eventual saturation of lean tissue and fat depots with prolonged recovery and physiological depression, lengthy anesthesia (greater than 30 minutes) with this technique for outpatients is not recommended.

Thiopental as Sole Agent

A single induction dose of thiopental may produce adequate anesthesia for simple, brief procedures such as uncomplicated removal of one or more teeth in the same quadrant or incision and drainage of an abscess. Operating time can be saved if the mouth prop is placed before injection of thiopental. An oropharyngeal pack is always placed, strong suction must be at hand, and oxygen must be given. If operating time exceeds the duration of effect of the induction dose, nitrous oxide and other agents must be added to minimize the total amount of subsequent increments of thiopental and the associated cardiorespiratory depression.

METHOHEXITAL SODIUM (BREVITAL)

Methohexital sodium is a white powder which is readily soluble in aqueous solution. It is generally prepared in a 1 per cent solution (10 mg per ml) for intravenous injection.

The site of action and effects on the central nervous system of methohexital are similar to those of thiopental. While methohexital is approximately three times as potent as thiopental, methohexital is more rapidly metabolized and its effects on the central nervous system are of shorter duration. The electroencephalogram will show changes following methohexital for up to 6 hours. Recovery following single or repeated doses of methohexital is more rapid following thiopental.

Methohexital produces significantly greater depression of the cardiovascular system than thiopental when used to supplement nitrous oxide-oxygen anesthesia. However, a 50 per cent increase in heart rate after methohexital administration tends to compensate for a large decrease in total peripheral resistance and stroke volume.

The effects of methohexital on respiration are similar to those of the other barbiturates. Significant increases in arterial carbon dioxide tension indicate the extent of respiratory depression.

Hiccoughing is more likely to occur following an induction dose of methohexital than other barbiturates. Numerous explanations for the phenomenon were originally suggested: too rapid administration, too slow administration, old or new solutions, use of dextrose, saline, or distilled water as a solvent, or the use of atropine premedication. It is due to direct stimulation of the midbrain by the barbiturate and, occasionally, occurs with thiopental. It is more common if promethazine is used as a premedication.

Because of its shorter recovery time, methohexital has become the most popular ultrashort-acting barbiturate in outpatient dental anesthesia.

Methohexital Induction

A test dose of 20 mg (2 ml of a 1 per cent solution) is given, and the patient's response is observed. Severe pain in the injection site or distal to it may indicate extravasation of the barbiturate solution or intra-arterial injection which requires immediate management. After the patient's response is observed, an induction dose of methohexital is given in 15 to 30 seconds. A dose based on body weight (1.0 to 1.4 mg per kg) is generally used, at a rate of 1 mg per second. Loss of the eyelid reflex, as end point of induction, is an accurate prediction in 50 per cent of patients. The mouth prop is inserted, and additional inhalation or intravenous agents are given as indicated to maintain anesthesia.

Methohexital Supplementation

As soon as the induction dose has taken effect, nitrous oxide and oxygen in a 7:3 ratio are administered by nasal mask. A mouth prop and oropharyngeal pack are placed, and local anesthesia may be injected into the operative site. After surgery is begun the level of anesthesia is maintained with periodic supplemental 10- to 20-mg doses of methohexital as required. At the end of the procedure, 100 per cent oxygen is given for 2 minutes, and the airway is maintained until the patient regains protective reflexes. Recovery may be expected in 20 to 30 minutes, faster than following thiopental-supplemented anesthesia, but significantly delayed compared to inhalation agents.

Methohexital can be prepared in a 0.2 per cent solution (2 mg per ml) and used as a continuous drip for induction or maintenance of anesthesia. The level of anesthesia may be more consistent with this technique, but constant vigilance of the anesthetist is mandatory. Inadvertent massive overdose of methohexital can easily occur if the anesthetist should become preoccupied with another problem. As the sequence of events in outpatient anesthesia is often rapid, the continuous intravenous infusion of methohexital does not meet the technical requirements of safety and cannot be recommended.

Because the anesthesia produced by methohexital does not obtund pharyngeal and laryngeal reflexes, laryngospasm is a constant hazard with this technique. An oropharyngeal pack should always be in place to prevent pharyngeal contamination, strong suction must be available, and the anesthetist must be experienced in management of the airway.

Methohexital as Sole Agent

The use of intermittent doses of methohexital as the sole agent for "ultralight" anesthesia for restorative dentistry has been popularized by Drummond-Jackson in Great Britain. Unfortunately, arterial hypoxemia, respiratory obstruction, and contamination of the trachea are common sequelae of this technique which may oc-

cur undetected, to the detriment of the patient. Methohexital should always be supplemented with oxygen and used as sole agent only for brief procedures to minimize total dose and cardiorespiratory depression and prevent prolonged recovery (Fig. 13.7).

ETOMIDATE

This intravenous induction agent has recently been released for use in the United States. There has been a decade of clinical experience in Europe. The drug is unrelated to previous induction agents and has the advantage of not being a barbiturate. The drug is dissolved in propylene glycol as a 0.2% solution, 2 mg per ml; this vehicle has reduced the venous

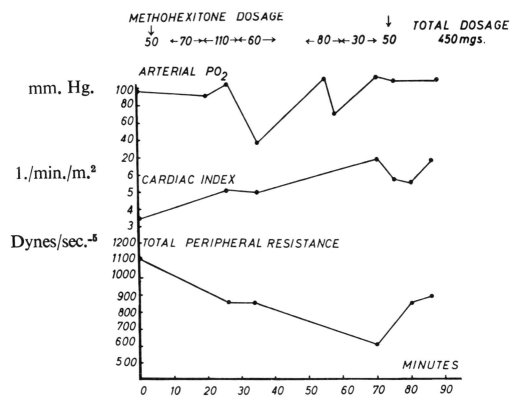

Figure 13.7. The relationship of cardiac output, expressed as cardiac index, total peripheral resistance, and arterial oxygen tension to methohexital dosage and anesthetic time. The failure of the cardiac output to respond to hypoxia is evident. (Reprinted with permission from Robinson, J. S., Wise, C., Heath, M. J., and Tomlin, P. J.: Responses to intermittent methohexitone. *Br Dent J* June 3, 1969.)

irritation which occurred with the aqueous solution.

Teratogenetic effects have not been noted in animals, and there is no histamine release demonstrated with the agent. It is rapidly distributed and metabolized in the liver and the inactive metabolite excreted by the kidneys. The usual anesthetic induction dose is 0.3 mg per kg. At this dosage hypnosis is evident without analgesia. Induction occurs as rapidly as with an intravenous barbiturate, and recovery from a single dose occurs in 3 to 5 minutes.

Heart rate is slightly increased, the mean arterial pressure falls 15 per cent, there is a 17 per cent fall in total peripheral resistance, while coronary profusion is increased. Myocardial oxygen consumption is reduced 14 per cent. Studies on the respiratory effects indicate minimal and short-lived depression in the rate of respiration and minute volume, although these changes are less than with the intravenous barbiturates. EEG changes parallel those with thiopental, but more burst suppression episodes are noted.

The advantages of the drug are that it will cause minimal cardiovascular depression and respiratory effect, and there is a wide margin of safety between the induction dose and the lethal dose, as studied in rats. Of major significance is the fast recovery and elimination. Recovery is related to dosage, but the character of recovery good. There is little hangover and the patient is much more alert than following an intravenous dose of barbiturate.

Adverse reactions noted are pain on injection, reported by 30 to 80% of patients. It can be reduced by the administration of a small dose of narcotic or local anesthetic before its administration. Injection into a large vein reduces the incidence of pain. Involuntary muscle movements and myoclonus have been noted in 10 to 60 per cent of patients, and patients do move in response to stimulation. Its

major disadvantage for the outpatient, however, is nausea and vomiting that occurs in approximately 30 per cent of patients. Postoperative venous thrombosis is common.

Its use for outpatient anesthesia has been noted, and an attempt to produce sedation with doses of etomidate, 0.1 mg per kg, combined with diazepam, did produce satisfactory intravenous sedation which required supplementation with local anesthesia. The patients clenched their jaws following injection of etomidate, and a mouth prop was necessary for placement of the local anesthesia. Another suggested use of etomidate in dentistry has been for sedation with continuous intravenous etomidate for postoperative patients following oromaxillary fixation.

The margin between sedation and anesthesia is small. In one study verbal contact was frequently lost with the patient when sedation was attempted. It confirms that the agent is an anesthetic agent and should only be utilized by those who are able to control the airway in all circumstances.

MUSCLE RELAXANTS

The terminus of the nerve within the muscle is known as the neuromuscular junction and is made up of the nerve terminal, synaptic cleft or gap, and the muscle receptor site. The effector substance at the neuromuscular junction is acetylcholine, synthesized by choline acetylase and stored in vesicles at the nerve terminus. Resting membrane potential, is due to the relative concentrations of ions on either side of the cell membrane. Potassium (K^+) and chloride ions (Cl^-) predominate on the inside with sodium (Na^+) and chloride (Cl^-) ions on the outside. A nerve impulse, arriving at the nerve terminal, causes a decrease in the potential across the cell membrane. Concurrent with the initial depolarization, the permeability of the cell membrane to potassium (K^+) and sodium (Na^+)

ions is altered, changing the relative potential difference across the cell membrane. Restoration of the postsynaptic membrane to the resting level is complete when potassium has been returned to its intracellular position and sodium has been pumped back out of the cell (Fig. 13.8).

The enzyme acetylcholinesterase, stored within the shoulders of the muscle end plate, is responsible for the removal of acetylcholine. The released acetylcholine is broken down into choline and acetic acid by the action of acetylcholinesterase.

Neuromuscular Block

There are two principal types of neuromuscular blockade, both of which seem to exert their effect in the region of the postsynaptic membrane. When a drug is administered which allows depolarization but interferes with repolarization, the neuromuscular block produced is referred to as a depolarization block. A typical example of a depolarizing blockade drug is succinylcholine.

A drug preventing the passage of acetylcholine from the presynaptic membrane to the postsynaptic membrane in sufficient quantity to elicit an action potential is referred to as a nondepolarizing blockade agent. A typical example of a drug causing this nondepolarizing blockade in d-tubocurarine.

NONDEPOLARIZING NEUROMUSCULAR BLOCKING AGENTS

d-Tubocurarine

d-Tubocurarine is a quaternary alkaloid which produces a competitive blockade by combining with the cholinergic receptor at the postsynaptic membrane and denying acetylcholine access in the normal manner (Fig. 13.9). Because of its chemical nature it does not cross the blood-brain barrier or cross the placental barrier. It is redistributed to inactive receptor sites throughout the body, where it is eventually detoxicated. Urinary excretion may account for 50 to 70 per cent

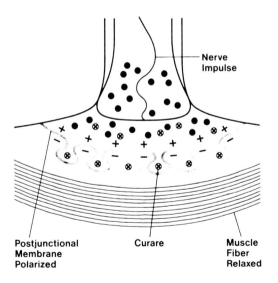

Resting Muscle End Plate

Figure 13.8. Acetylcholine passes across the end plate to the sole plate, changing the polarization of the membrane and stimulating the muscle fiber.

Action of Curare

Figure 13.9. The action of the nondepolarizing muscle relaxant, curare, is indicated. The curare prevents passage of the acetylcholine across to the membrane, preventing polarization.

of the injected dose. There is no central action on the central nervous system, but it does partially block the sympathetic ganglia, causing some lowering of systemic blood pressure. The partial blockade of autonomic nerves accounts for the antiarrhythmic properties of curare.

It acts classically at the motor end plate of skeletal muscle, producing muscle relaxation in the following sequence: ptosis, diplopia, relaxation of muscles of the face and jaw followed by limbs, anterior abdominal wall, intercostal muscles, and finally diaphragmatic musculature.

It is given as 3 mg per ml in a dosage of 15 to 30 mg, 30 mg being required for endotracheal intubation. After intravenous injection, the effective duration of action is 30 minutes, though repeated administrations result in a cumulative effect. It can produce its effect if given intramuscularly.

Gallamine Triethiode (Flaxedil)

Its action is similar to that of curare. It has marked vagal blocking properties which result in tachycardia. It is contraindicated, however, in patients with existing tachycardia. It is totally excreted by the kidney and therefore should not be used in patients with severe renal disease. It is administered as 20 mg per ml, and 80 mg of gallamine are equivalent to 15 mg of d-tubocurare. An effective duration of action is 20 minutes.

Pancuronium (Pavulon)

It can be used at induction for intubation, 1.5 mg being given under these circumstances. Supplementary doses of 0.5 to 1 mg are then given. Duration of action is greater than with curare, and the last dose given should never be more than 0.5 mg. Onset of action for maximum effect is usually 2 to 3 minutes. It has the advantage that in atropinized anesthetized patients, little or no cardiovascular changes are noted.

REVERSAL OF NONDEPOLARIZING BLOCKADE

In order to overcome or reverse this type of blockade, an increased concentration of acetylcholine must be presented at the postsynaptic membrane. The most common method for accomplishing an increase in acetylcholine is by the inhibition of acetylcholinesterase activity, thus allowing the buildup of acetylcholine at the postsynaptic membrane.

Neostigmine (Prostigmine)

This agent has a prolonged action which is in excess of that of curare, being excreted unchanged by the kidney. It is given in 0.5-mg increments to a total of 2.5 mg. If given in overdose, an excess of acetylcholine can build up at a muscle end plate and produce a dual block owing to the accumulation of acetylcholine. The prior injection of 1.2 mg of atropine is required to block the muscarinic activity of the agent. It should be given with extreme care to asthmatic patients in whom it can produce bronchospasm.

The action of neostigmine on the myocardium can cause bradycardia and even cardiac arrest, while troublesome increased activity of the bowel and bladder can be blocked by large doses of atropine. The excess excretions, especially salivary, cannot be completely inhibited.

If a nondepolarizing drug is given, then it should be routine to administer an anticholinesterase drug, preferably neostigmine, in order that the muscle-relaxing properties of curare are covered by the antagonist during the period of recovery.

DEPOLARIZING NEUROMUSCULAR BLOCKING DRUGS

Succinylcholine

It is clinically related to acetylcholine and is a quaternary ammonium compound. Succinylcholine produces a depolarizing block in the same manner as acetylcholine but repolarization is delayed until the succinylcholine is metabolized (Fig. 13.10). It is taken up by all skeletal muscle end plates. Succinylcholine is broken down by the enzymes plasma cholinesterase or psuedocholinesterase, which abound in the plasma. Breakdown is quite rapid and with a normal response to succinylcholine, relaxation is usually evident for 3 to 6 minutes. In approximately 1 in 3,000 people, an atypical cholinesterase enzyme is present and breakdown of succinylcholine is greatly retarded, resulting in prolonged paralysis with normal doses of the drug.

There has been no central effect or any effect on the myocardium demonstrated, but it does affect cardiac conduction and can cause bradycardia and even cardiac arrest. The administration of atropine, 0.6 mg prior to the second injection of succinylcholine, is said to be protective against cardiac arrest, but the authors have seen cardiac arrest occur in this situation. The occurrence of bradycardia is more obvious in children.

A preferred technique is to administer gallamine, 20 mg, or curare, 3 mg, prior

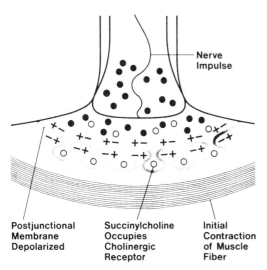

Action of Succinylcholine

Figure 13.10. Succinylcholine will depolarize the postjunctional membrane and occupies the cholinergic receptor until it is removed and metabolized.

to the succinylcholine, as it has a protective action directly on the myocardium.

Succinylcholine has a direct action on the blood vessels, resulting in increase of systolic and diastolic blood pressure. Because of the release of potassium cardiac arrythmias can occur. Salivary secretions are increased and ocular pressure is increased following administration. The fasciculations noted after injection are due to the contraction of single or groups of motor units leading to visible skeletal muscle contractions. These contractions are most evident in the neck and face. Postrelaxant muscle pains are common after the use of succinylcholine. The majority of the fasciculations and muscle pains can be eliminated by administration of a small dose of nondepolarizing muscle relaxant 2 to 4 minutes prior to administration of the relaxant dose of succinylcholine; however, this technique can contribute to postoperative apnea. It is preferable to use a smaller dose or a dilute solution of succinylcholine, 0.2 per cent instead of the usual 20 mg per ml solution, or to administer the drug at a slower rate which will contribute to a lower incidence of postoperative muscle pain. Postoperative muscle pain is seen most frequently in active patients with minimal operative trauma, typical of outpatient dental anesthesia.

In the average adult, 40 to 60 mg of succinylcholine will produce paralysis adequate for endotracheal intubation, giving a 3- to 5-minute period of apnea. Ventilation with 100 per cent oxygen or allowing the patient to breathe 100 per cent oxygen for 2 minutes prior to intubation will prevent the falls of oxygen tension which occur during the period of apnea, especially if intubation is delayed. A 10 to 20 mg dose of succinylcholine can produce some degree of muscular paralysis and is often recommended by the administrators of intravenous anesthesia to obtund or depress laryngeal reflexes when laryngeal spasm becomes evident. The injection can be given sublingually or intramuscularly, if a suitable vein is not available, and may be chosen in small children.

Large doses of succinylcholine in excess of 1 g can result in prolonged action or production of prolonged apnea. Owing to dual block, the depolarizing character of the block changes and becomes nondepolarizing in nature and a curare-like block develops.

The action of succinylcholine on enzyme systems has resulted in its implication in the production of malignant hyperpyrexia.

Succinylcholine is used in dentistry for intubation and should be available during administration of all general anesthetics, in order to terminate laryngeal spasm. It is an essential part of the anesthetist's armamentarium for emergency use.

MONITORING

The most valuable method is the activity of the reservoir bag. It can be misleading and therefore other techniques are necessary. In the unconscious patient, inspiratory force, that is the negative pressure developed against an occluded airway, can be used; however, other drugs will affect this. The nerve stimulator probably offers the best compromise, though it still must be used properly in conjunction with clinical judgment.

ENDOTRACHEAL ANESTHESIA

The many indications for endotracheal anesthesia are dependent upon the anesthetist and the practice followed. Thus, many oral surgeons intubate every patient for oral surgery under general anesthesia, apart from the most simple procedures. Others consider the hazards to outweigh the advantages. The indications for endotracheal anesthesia are:

1. Inability to maintain an airway.

2. When intermittent positive pressure ventilation is to be used for a prolonged period; otherwise distention of the stomach by inflation with gas may occur.

3. Operations about the head and neck where the airway will be compromised.

4. Operations about the head and neck where the anesthetist will be remote from the operating area.

5. In the case where a full stomach renders the hazard of vomiting, regurgitation, and inhalation of the vomitus a serious hazard, and only a cuffed endotracheal tube will guarantee the freedom of the airway from aspiration of infected material.

6. If the airway is compromised before induction of anesthesia, problems with the airways are likely to arise during the operation.

7. Treatment of respiratory failure or if toilet of the tracheobronchial tree is indicated.

8. Protection against pulmonary aspiration.

9. Airway management in advanced cardiopulmonary resuscitation.

Mechanical Hazards

1. Obstructed tubes: always examine before use.

2. Kinked tubes: angle of mouth, back of pharynx, surgeon, connector.

3. Tubes can be cut.

4. Separation of connectors: slip off and become disconnected under drapes.

5. Improper diameter: large—trauma and edema; small—obstruction to respiration.

6. Improper length of tube: endobronchial intubation and atelectasis of opposite lung if tube too long; tube may slip out of trachea with inspiration if length is too short.

7. Foreign bodies: check mouth for chewing gum, tobacco, loose teeth, partial dentures; check tip of endotracheal tube after passage through nose for blood clots, adenoidal tissue, or mucosa.

Complications

1. Laryngitis: vocal cord congestion, submucosal hemorrhage.

2. Edema: of vocal cords, epiglottis, supra- or subglottic areas.

3. Laryngeal ulceration followed by granuloma formation.

4. Ecchymosis: cords, plate, tonsils, tongue.

5. Tracheitis.

6. Tracheal stenosis.

Since significant morbidity is associated with endotracheal intubation, it should not be undertaken without a valid indication. Several hazards of intubation of the trachea unique to dental anesthesia are as follows:

1. Use of a muscle relaxant for intubation may result in prolonged apnea. The difficulties of providing artificial ventilation in a dental office must be appreciated. Intravenous administration of succinylcholine for relaxation during intubation may result in severe muscle fasciculations. Postoperatively, muscle pain may be greater than pain from the operative site.

2. Laryngeal edema may occur postoperatively, especially in children. Since the outpatient may be dismissed and at home before its onset, early narrowing of the larynx may not be detected. Delayed recognition may lead to fatality.

3. Movements of the head occur during anesthesia for dental procedures. Movement of the endotracheal tube within the larynx and trachea can also occur with production of trauma and subsequent scarring or stenosis.

4. The nose can be traumatized during passage of a nasal endotracheal tube. Mucosal injury may be associated with profuse epistaxis. Patients with repaired cleft palates or velopharyngeal flaps should not have endotracheal tubes placed through the nose.

5. Deeper anesthesia is usually required for the passage and maintenance of an endotracheal tube than for the dental procedure.

6. The additional time needed for placement of an endotracheal tube in outpatient practice may exceed the time required to complete the dental procedure.

For routine outpatient anesthesia for brief procedures (less than 30 minutes) there is usually not an indication for endotracheal intubation. However, for prolonged restorative procedures intubation of the trachea is always advisable. If it is known in advance that endotracheal intubation will be required for a given dental procedure, especially in children, a strong argument can be made for treating that patient and providing recovery care in a hospital environment.

OUTPATIENT DENTAL ANESTHESIA

Outpatient dental anesthesia requires the same standard of care as administration of anesthesia in the hospital. Inadequate provision of personnel or equipment for outpatients on economic grounds is indefensible.

Personnel

The "team approach" should be considered in outpatient dental anesthesia. The administrator of dental anesthesia, be it dentist or anesthesiologist, is responsible for the anesthetized patient. The employment of a nurse-anesthetist does not absolve the doctor of this responsibility. The ideal situation for outpatient dental anesthesia is thought to be a trained dental anesthesiologist or physician anesthesiologist trained in dental anesthesia to administer the anesthetic and another dentist to perform the operative procedure. Because of a lack of sufficient trained dental anesthesiologists at the present time, the team approach is an acceptable alternative. Training of the personnel on the team is the responsibility of the doctor in charge. Each person should know his job, respond instantly to the requests of the doctor, and be able to assume the job of another member of the team if necessary. The minimum personnel required in the team approach to dental anesthesia are:

1. *Operator.* As the licensed professional person (dentist) he is responsible for the anesthesia and the total care of the patient. Although it is a dual responsibility, limited availability of qualified anesthesiologists makes it a necessity.

2. *Jaw supporter and monitor.* This person maintains the airway by holding the nasal mask or nasopharyngeal tube in place and supporting the mandible. The patient is monitored by observing respiration, blood pressure, pulse, or heart rate. Changes in concentration of oxygen, nitrous oxide, and volatile agent and administration of intravenous agents may be made on the order of the operator. (In some states this practice is considered illegal).

3. *Chairside assistant.* The assistant provides adequate suction to clear secretions, blood, and debris from the oral cavity, holds retractors, and passes instruments as required.

4. *Circulating nurse.* This person must be available to assist any of the other members of the team, obtain additional instruments or drugs, and be otherwise available in the operatory at all times.

None of the members of the anesthetic team should have duties which take them out of the operatory or otherwise distract them from their primary efforts on the team.

Modifications

Differences in the approach to outpatient anesthesia *vs.* hospital practice are involved mainly with reducing recovery time and in competition for the airway. Recovery time is reduced by using little or no premedication, utilizing techniques of airway control (such as nasal mask or nasopharyngeal tube rather than endotracheal intubation) which require lighter planes of anesthesia, using agents with fairly rapid recovery time, and keeping the length of procedures to a minimum. Competition for the airway is resolved in most cases not by endotracheal intuba-

tion, but by controlling the airway with good jaw position, well-placed oral packs, and use of nasal mask or nasopharyngeal tubes so that good ventilation is maintained and access to the operative field is not compromised.

Many dentists supplement the general anesthetic with local anesthesia. Because the operative site is pain-free, it is suggested but unproven that minimal amounts of other agents are required to render the patient amnesic and unaware of his surroundings during the procedure. There are disadvantages to combining local anesthesia with sedative hypnotic combinations of inhalation or intravenous agents. Local anesthesia of the tongue and palate, if required for the operative procedure, may allow aspiration of foreign material from the mouth in the sedated patient, and untoward reactions to the local anesthetic agent and epinephrine may not be quickly recognized in the sedated or obtunded patient. The only proven value is the efficiency of early postoperative pain relief.

Operating Position

There are five basic positions for outpatient dental anesthesia: 1) seated, legs down; 2) seated, legs up; 3) semi-supine; 4) supine; 5) Trendelenburg (Fig. 13.11).

The interest created in the position of the patient by investigation into sudden, unexplained death in dental patients in Great Britain has prompted much speculation and research into the effect of various positions on cardiorespiratory physiology. The Trendelenburg and supine positions aid venous return to the heart from the lower extremities and perfusion of the cerebral vasculature. In the Trendelenburg position respiration is compromised because the abdominal viscera are forced by gravity against the diaphragm, interfering with its normal descent during inspiration. There is an increased risk of silent regurgitation of stomach contents in both positions. Many intubate the trachea in every case to control the airway

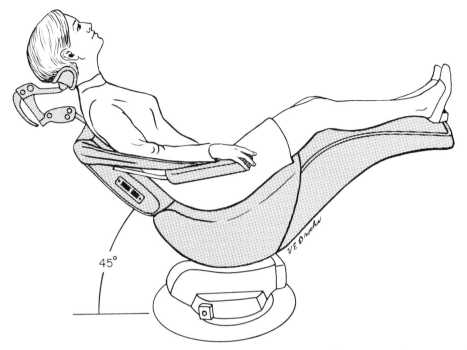

Figure 13.11. Position of patient in the contour dental chair is of importance in proper airway maintenance. The 45° position is the best compromise between cardiovascular and other considerations.

and protect against aspiration of foreign material. However, the hazards of intubation may outweigh the advantages in dental outpatients. Because of minimum interference with normal cardiovascular and respiratory physiology and maximum protection against silent regurgitation of stomach contents, the semi-supine position is favored for induction and maintenance of dental anesthesia in adults. In children inhalation anesthesia is induced with the child seated and his legs crossed "Indian style" to minimize kicking and struggling (Fig. 13.12).

In the outpatient, the hands should be placed in the pocket or in the lap so that they do not fall during induction of anesthesia, and are in a position of rest. Tight belts should be avoided, and the brassiere should be loosened. It is of advantage often to leave the brassiere in place to hold the chest stethoscope. There should be no foot rest on the dental chair as the patient can readily push against this into the position of opisthotonus. The patient may consider a lap strap a restraint but the simple explanation that it will prevent his falling on the floor should satisfy his objections. It is important to note that the absence of a lap strap is detrimental to medicolegal defense. Care must be taken to lubricate the corners of the lips if the mouth is to be stretched, and to watch the eyes for damage by the operator's hands or instruments.

Operative Requirements

The operator's desire for a more comfortable working position may dictate a particular patient position. For example, it is often easier to perform restorative dentistry on the mandible when it is parallel to the floor, or on the maxilla with the head tilted well back. However, many oral surgeons, because they operate on patients in the supine position in hospital operating rooms, are used to this position

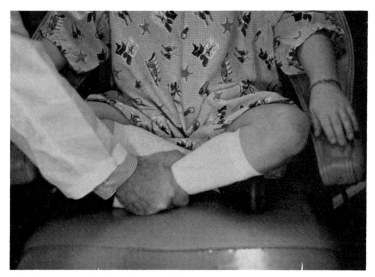

Figure 13.12. Child seated in dental chair. The gently placed hand on the ankle maintains the upright position and aids control if excitement occurs during induction.

for surgical procedures and prefer it in all settings. If the operator's choice of patient position places unreasonable physical demands on the person responsible for controlling the airway, compromises cardiorespiratory function, or places the patient at risk for pulmonary aspiration of foreign material, endotracheal intubation must be considered essential for that patient. In general, the semi-supine position provides the best working conditions for most procedures, minimal alteration of cardiovascular and respiratory function, and maximum protection against regurgitation of gastric contents in the patient without an endotracheal tube.

Regurgitation and Aspiration

Vomiting is an active process, generally occurring during the second stage of anesthesia. Laryngeal reflexes are active, and pulmonary aspiration does not always occur. Regurgitation of stomach contents is a passive event, generally occurring during surgical planes (Stage 3) of anesthesia when laryngeal reflexes are depressed or absent, and pulmonary aspiration is a definite threat. In the supine position gravity flow allows material from either the oral cavity or stomach to be inhaled into the tracheobronchial tree. The use of intravenous agents and "ultralight" anesthesia is no protection against pulmonary aspiration. Numerous studies have demonstrated soiling of the larynx in patients anesthetized or even sedated with various intravenous agents, including diazepam, methohexital, narcotics, and ketamine. The Trendelenburg position, where gravity causes foreign material to flow away from the larynx and pool in the nasopharynx from which it can be removed, prevents pulmonary aspiration, but compromises spontaneous respiratory movements and is a difficult operating position for most dentists. The semi-supine position enlists the aid of gravity in preventing regurgitation, the forerunner of pulmonary aspiration.

Cardiovascular and Respiratory Effects

Positioning for maximum cardiovascular function under anesthesia requires elevation of the legs to improve venous return to the heart and lowering of the head to increase perfusion of the cerebral vasculature. However, such a position allows the abdominal viscera to fall against the diaphragm and interfere with normal respiratory excursions. It has been demonstrated that an optimal balance of ventilation and perfusion occurs when the dental patient is in the semi-supine position.

During an investigation into sudden death in dental patients in Great Britain, fainting under anesthesia was proposed as a cause of fatal cerebral anoxia. It was proposed that once a patient fainted, there was a persistent tendency for repetitive faints for several hours. Further research has demonstrated no fainting during general anesthesia in dental patients. However, Forsyth showed severe cardiovascular depression in dental outpatients who fainted before induction of anesthesia. Although anesthesia was deferred, severe depression of cardiac output and stroke volume persisted for over 1 hour. Since cardiac rate and mean arterial pressure, the parameters usually monitored in clinical situations, rapidly returned to normal, the prolonged aftereffects of fainting probably go unnoticed. Therefore, it is advised to defer anesthesia following a syncopal attack for at least 2 hours, if not until another day.

Protection of the Airway

Protection of the airway is the most essential part of outpatient dental anesthesia technique, and it should be the primary mission of all members of the anesthetic team. Whenever an airway problem develops, the operator should stop his procedure until the problem is resolved. The assistants should not let their position or activities interfere with the airway at any time.

AIRWAY MAINTENANCE

With a nasal mask it is easier to work with the patient in the upright position as the mandible is held more easily forward. The posture of "sniffing the morning air" with the cervical spine flexed forward and the head extended provides the best airway patency. The mandible is brought forward by applying manual pressure behind the angle. However, excessive pressure against the mandible may be a cause of postoperative discomfort, and misdirected pressure against the carotid body can cause vagal stimulation and bradycardia, and is best avoided. Support of the mandible is particularly important when the lower teeth are being operated upon. Pressure on the mandible by the operator causes an up-and-down movement of the unsupported jaw, increased stimulation of the patient, and intermittent airway obstruction. In general, the mandibular teeth are operated on first as procedures in the maxilla impose less interference with airway maintenance. Consequently, anesthesia can be lightened toward the latter part of the procedure, reducing recovery time. A support on the dental chair for the elbows or forearms of the chin holder assists in preventing fatigue. If the chin holder requires relief because of difficulty in maintaining the airway or during a long operation, endotracheal intubation should be a consideration.

NASOPHARYNGEAL TUBE OR MASK

The nasopharyngeal tube will often overcome an airway problem that is due to partial nasal blockage, mouth-breathing, tongue, or pack position. A major advantage in dental anesthesia is that the oral pack can be positioned against the nasopharyngeal tube to provide a better seal with the mouth open, than can a nasal mask. Of course, the nasopharyngeal tube can cause nasal trauma or cardiac arrhythmia during passage or become blocked with mucus, tissue, or blood.

Velcro can be used to fasten the nasal tube or mask to the head of the patient. The strap should be applied with care to avoid pressure to the eyes or other structures.

OROPHARYNGEAL PARTITION

The gauze 4 × 4-inch pad is a suitable and readily available material. It is refolded into a 2 × 8-inch pack, moistened with saline, and a string is attached which is left outside the mouth for easy removal. Recent litigation has made it advisable to use gauze with a radiopaque marker. Once the initial pack has been placed, it should be changed as frequently as needed or additional packing placed to prevent blood soaking through and reaching the pharynx. When the nasal mask or nasopharyngeal tube is used, proper placement of the pack is between the soft palate and the base of the tongue to avoid stimulating the pharyngeal tissues which can cause coughing and laryngospasm in the lightly anesthetized patient. A sponge is a suitable alternative for many operators, and has been shown to reduce leakage of anesthetic gases (Fig. 13.13).

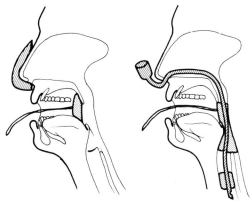

Figure 13.13. On the *left* the correct placement of an oropharyngeal partition for outpatient anesthesia is noted. The pack extends between soft palate and base of tongue but does not encroach upon posterior surface of epiglottis or pharyngeal tissues where glossopharyngeal stimulation and gagging could result. *Right*, placement of oropharyngeal pack about the endotracheal tube. It is placed firmly in both piriform fossae and the vallecula. The tail or a string lies outside the mouth.

MOUTH PROP

There are many types of mouth props available for dental anesthesia. The dental anesthetist should choose a mouth prop which has a sufficiently broad surface area so that pressure is not exerted on a single tooth, a variety of sizes available to allow adequate opening of the jaws, and a chain or cord attached for easy removal. They should be able to be sterilized in an autoclave. Two popular and widely used mouth props which meet these criteria are the Goldman and the McKesson. A special feature of the Goldman prop is that an oral pack may be placed between the upper and lower limbs of the prop (Fig. 13.14).

The prop can be placed between the jaws before the patient goes to sleep or

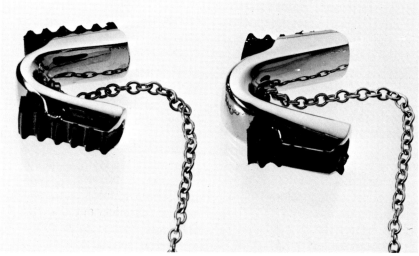

Figure 13.14. The Goldman mouth prop, which allows for placement of the pack between the surfaces abutting the teeth.

after induction of anesthesia. For a brief intravenous anesthetic for the removal of one or two teeth, the mouth prop may be placed before induction of anesthesia to save operating time. However, patient dislike of having the mouth propped open while awake and difficulty of establishing nasal breathing with an open mouth are contraindications to placing the mouth prop before inhalation induction. If the prop is to be inserted after the induction of anesthesia, a sufficient depth should be reached so that force is not necessary to insert a mouth prop. There is no indication to forcefully open the mouth with a Ferguson or Moult ratchet, except in an emergency, as damage to teeth or lips can result. In procedures where both sides of the mouth will be operated upon, especially under light anesthesia, a second mouth prop should be available for placement before the first prop is removed, so the jaws cannot start to close and require forceful reopening.

OPERATIVE REQUIREMENTS
Oral Surgery

Oral surgery procedures for dental outpatients are usually brief, involving the removal of one or more teeth or minimal soft tissue surgery. Since elevation of teeth or the mucoperiosteum is a very painful procedure, adequate depth of anesthesia is an important consideration. Pain at the operative site may be blocked by injection of local anesthesia. Addition of small increments of inhalation (particularly nitrous oxide) and intravenous agents (barbiturates, narcotics) produces an amnesic, obtunded patient during the procedure with minimal physiological depression. Endotracheal intubation is seldom required for airway control during short oral surgery procedures. The nasal mask usually provides a good vehicle for inhalation of gases, except when the anterior maxilla is the operative site; then the nasopharyngeal tube is indicated to allow clear access. Mouth prop, oropharyngeal packing, and strong suction are all necessary to keep the airway free of secretions, blood, and tooth and bone fragments.

REDUCTION OF BLOOD LOSS IN ORAL AND MAXILLOFACIAL SURGERY

The major factor in reduction of blood loss is surgical technique, however, there are some features of anesthesia which will reduce bleeding. A slight head-up tilt will reduce venous pressure and hemorrhage, while vasodilatation due to hypercarbia and hypoxia can increase bleeding. In addition the depression of respiration may also elevate intrathoracic pressure and raise central venous pressure. The general anesthetic agent does not affect hemorrhage during surgery, however; use of a local anesthetic with vasoconstrictor can be most effective.

A useful practice is the development of deliberate hypotension during anesthesia. The risks are minimal in comparison to the risks of an unnecessary blood transfusion. Important features to note in developing deliberate hypotension is that the oxygen-carrying capacity of the blood before surgery be adequate, which necessitates an adequate hemoglobin level before surgery. Blood loss can be reduced in many oral and maxillofacial surgery operations from 3,000 ml to as low as 250 ml. The techniques are varied and have been shown to be safe. Monitoring must be meticulous, and the blood pressure maintained within strict limits. The technique should be rapidly reversible. Elevation of the inspired oxygen tension throughout the operative procedure is necessary to compensate for the lowered blood pressure.

The level aimed for is usually one-third reduction of the systolic blood pressure, that is from 120 to 80 mm Hg. This leaves a margin of safety and adequately reduces blood loss. The margin of safety is necessary, as the critical closing pressure of the smaller arterioles is unknown except for the kidney. In the kidney a critical closing pressure of 60 mm Hg is present, whereas in the brain it may be as low as 30 mm Hg.

The two techniques of deliberate hypotensive anesthesia currently in vogue are accepted as safe.

Increasing depth of anesthesia: The depth of anesthesia is increased by an inhalation agent, and the patient is paralyzed with curare, which also may lower the blood pressure. The blood pressure is further lowered by using intermittent positive pressure ventilation. Thus by elevating the mean intrathoracic pressure venous return is decreased. It has the advantage that when the intermittent positive positive pressure ventilation stops the blood pressure will rise. Its major disadvantage is that it is not always successful in reducing blood pressure, particularly in the young vigorous patient.

The use of agents to directly lower the blood pressure: Ganglion blockade with Arfonad is a useful technique for hypotensive anesthesia. It is given intravenously, 500 mg in 500 ml. In combination with general anesthesia it will satisfactorily lower the blood pressure, although tachyphylaxis may develop.

Sodium nitroprusside (Nipride) has a direct action producing peripheral vasodilation, and is made up in a 5% dextrose solution. It must be fresh—less than 4 hours old. It is given in a dose which must not exceed 10 μg per kg per minute. It has the major advantage that the activity starts and stops promptly. It is necessary to use an infusion pump or microdrip to regulate the administration of the continuous infusion. It is extremely successful and it will produce a definitive drop in blood pressure. The major disadvantage is that cyanide toxicity will develop over a prolonged period. It is imperative when using sodium nitroprusside that there be continuous intra-arterial monitoring of the blood pressure.

Cranioplasty

These patients may have had prior prolonged operations and cosmetically look normal, but the airway may be distorted. Operations usually last 5 to 10 hours and there are a spectrum of abnormalities, which range from a constricted nasopharynx with airway obstruction to gross facial distortion with no airway problem. The worst situation is the Treacher-Collins syndrome, in which intubation may be difficult or even impossible. In hemifacial microsomia and oculo-auriculovertebral dysplasia, intubation may be extremely difficult. In addition to these syndromes there are many kinds of facial clefts and encephaloceles. These patients share common psychological problems and are treated frequently as mentally retarded, although in some there is evidence of high intelligence. There is a high incidence of deafness, which adds to the problem of multiple operations and hospitalizations.

It is important not to oversedate these patients preoperatively, as airway obstruction may develop. Intravenous induction is contraindicated, and intubation with a National Catheter reinforced endotracheal tube, not an anode tube, is indicated. The problem with the regular anode tube is that extubation may occur spontaneously. The tube is usually wired to the nasal septum or the gum. It is imperative that the airway and tube be secured at all times. If disconnect or problems occur the surgeon should be notified instantly.

Restorative Dentistry

Most restorative dentistry procedures are prolonged as multiple restorations are usually placed in all quadrants. Short restorative procedures may be done with a nasopharyngeal tube in place, provided an oropharyngeal pack is placed and strong suction is available to prevent soiling of the pharynx and larynx with dental debris. Anesthetist fatigue can be a factor in airway control for long procedures; therefore, endotracheal intubation is indicated. Because there is usually a need to check dental occlusion, the nasoendotracheal tube is preferred. An intravenous infusion is always started, and the induction phase is never hurried.

The eyes should be covered with gauze shields. During anesthesia secretion of tears ceases; closing the eyelids prevents drying of the eyes and keeps dental debris from entering and causing corneal abrasion. The open nostril should also be occluded to prevent entrance of debris. The lips are lubricated.

During prolonged operations gastric secretion continues and accumulates. It is wise to place a nasogastric tube prior to packing to prevent postoperative regurgitation of stomach contents. The gastric tube is even more essential if the teeth are wired shut following surgery.

A pack is always placed to prevent foreign material from pooling around the endotracheal tube. In addition to its operative indications, the rubber dam is an additional method of protecting the airway from dental debris.

Deeper anesthesia is required for procedures on the lower teeth as pressure on the mandible is transmitted to the endotracheal tube which stimulates the trachea and may cause coughing. Therefore, the lower teeth are restored first. Pressure on the maxillary teeth is not transmitted to the endotracheal tube, so the anesthesia can be lightened when maxillary procedures are done last. The patient will regain protective reflexes and consciousness sooner.

If a prolonged procedure is planned, two operators are advisable. The two dentists can alternate periodically so that fatigue does not lengthen the operation unnecessarily.

In preparing patients for anesthesia, it is useful to have a secure head drape and eye lubricant and eye pads. The throat pack should be lubricated with a water-

soluble jelly. During surgery, it is important to avoid leaning on the chest, pressing on the connectors and, above all, disconnecting the endotracheal tube. Lubrication will reduce labial edema. Inform the anesthetist when using local anesthetics and epinephrine.

Pediatric Patients

The majority of outpatient dental anesthesia for restorative dentistry is performed on children. Anesthesia for the pediatric patient differs from that for the adult. The major difference concerns the anatomy of the airway.

ANATOMICAL DIFFERENCES

The relatively large head of the child causes the neck to be flexed forward when in the supine position. Therefore, elevating the child's head on a pillow is not necessary when manipulating the airway or placing an endotracheal tube. Growth of the child progresses with age, and the larynx increases in anterior-posterior diameter from 7 mm at 3 days of age to 23 mm at 20 years. In adults the glottis is the narrowest portion of the airway while in the child the cricoid ring is the narrowest area. The posterior plate or lamina of the cricoid cartilage is inclined posteriorly in the child, and the larynx assumes a funnel shape in this area. Therefore, passage of the tube through the glottis of the child does not guarantee that it will pass unimpeded into the trachea. The larynx is located opposite the second cervical vertebra and is "tucked" under the mandible. This position of the larynx combined with a large tongue makes direct vision of the glottis for intubation difficult. The epiglottis is U-shaped and is inclined at 45° to the anterior pharyngeal wall, as the hyoid bone is intimately associated with the thyroid cartilage. The child's vocal cords are half cartilaginous, and the vocal processes of the arytenoid cartilages are inclined inferiorly and medially. This gives a concave shape to the larynx when viewed from the lateral aspect.

The large, floppy epiglottis and other anatomy of the small child's airway require that the epiglottis be elevated during laryngoscopy with either the curved or straight blade. The variations in the pediatric larynx require that a large selection of sizes of endotracheal tubes always be available. The first view of the larynx should be for determination of the proper endotracheal tube size. The size selected should fit loosely within the trachea to avoid trauma or ischemia to the mucosa with subsequent airway problems after extubation.

PSYCHOLOGICAL APPROACH

The person administering the anesthetic should talk to the child. Various distractions can be used to make inhalation induction enjoyable for the young patient. Since children often sense an adult's true feelings, a genuine enjoyment of children and confidence in one's ability to provide a smooth induction do much to establish rapport. Careful preparation of the child during the preoperative visit, as well as reassurance of anxious parents whose feelings of fear the child often perceives, will eliminate the need for premedication. The problem of the incorrect dosage of premedication which often results in a delerious, hyperactive child or in the oversedated child with significant cardiovascular or respiratory depression is thus avoided.

TECHNICAL CONSIDERATIONS

If the small child is anesthetized in the dental chair, it may be advantageous to place him in a car safety seat which is attached to the regular dental chair. Use of this device elevates the child so the head of the child reaches the chair head rest. Another method is to have the child sit on a cushion or "booster" chair.

Children should not have a mouth prop placed before induction. This not only produces apprehension, but it is conducive to mouth-breathing. Flooding of the child's face with nitrous oxide from a mask held over the child's forehead is a pleasant method of starting the induction if venipuncture or intravenous induction is resisted.

Nasopharyngeal tubes must be passed with care to avoid trauma to the large masses of adenoidal tissue which may be present. The length of nasopharyngeal tubes should be checked before and after placement to ensure their patency, and to avoid irritation of the epiglottis and inadvertent placement into the larynx.

At the conclusion of the operation the child should be carefully observed until his protective reflexes are returning and he responds to stimuli. Then he can be carried from the dental chair in the "head down" position facing the attendant, so that the airway and patient color can be observed. This position also aids in flow of secretions, blood, or debris out of the mouth rather than backward into the airway. The child is placed in the "position of safety" in the recovery room, semi-prone with the head down, the jaw supported if necessary and the knee flexed.

AGENTS AND PREMEDICATION

No available anesthetic agent is satisfactory for all children. However, since psychological disturbances seldom occur when ketamine is used in children, this agent has frequent use in pediatric anesthesia. Ketamine can be given intramuscularly by the nursing staff, and the child's antipathy is directed toward them rather than the doctor. If the child will tolerate a venipuncture, intravenous administration of ketamine produces a shorter duration of action, and reduces the recovery time for outpatient procedures. For the unmanageable child, rectal thiopental, (40 mg per kg), is an acceptable method of inducing anesthesia and requires no prior premedication. The readily available premeasured paste is a convenience. The child is told the temperature is being taken.

NEUROLEPTANESTHESIA

"Neuroleptic" is a term that characterizes a pharmacological phenomenon in which there are 1) somnolence without total unconsciousness, 2) psychological detachment from the environment, 3) retained ability to follow commands, and 4) diminished motor activity. When nitrous oxide and oxygen are added, true anesthesia is produced and the term neuroleptanesthesia is used.

Droperidol and fentanyl are available in a fixed combination (2.5 mg and 0.05 mg, respectively, in each milliliter) for intravenous or intramuscular administration as Innovar.

Pharmacology

The effect of Innovar is basically a summation of the effects of the two constituent drugs, droperidol and fentanyl. The action of fentanyl is quite similar to morphine. There is an increase in the pain threshold and alteration of the psychic response to pain. Droperidol causes blockade of selected areas of the basal ganglia and the limbic system.

Central nervous system effects include analgesia with little or no hypnosis, general quiescence, and reduced response to environmental stimuli. Pharyngeal and laryngeal reflexes are obtunded. Droperidol produces adrenergic blockade while fentanyl produces parasympathetic stimulation. Fentanyl has only a mild emetic action, while droperidol is a powerful antiemetic. Extrapyramidal reactions including Parkinson-like signs, dystonia, dyskinesia, and akathisia may be produced by droperidol.

Fentanyl is a powerful respiratory depressant; large doses result in apnea. Muscular rigidity of the thoracic and abdominal walls may occur by a direct excitatory effect on spinal reflexes. Droperidol has virtually no effect on the respiratory system.

The cardiovascular system is altered by the α-adrenergic-blocking action of droperidol which decreases blood pressure. The threshold to epinephrine-induced cardiac arrhythmias is raised significantly by droperidol. Fentanyl causes some slowing of heart rate because of its parasympathomimetic action, but it has little direct effect on the myocardium. The duration of action of fentanyl is approximately 45 minutes while that of droperidol is 6 to 8 hours.

Use in Anesthesia

With the exception of obtundation of pharyngeal and laryngeal reflexes, the qualities of neuroleptanalgesia would seem ideally suited for outpatient dental anesthesia. However, when the duration of action of the two components of Innovar are considered, the lengthy effect of droperidol (6 to 8 hours) makes early dismissal of the outpatient from the office or clinic unwise.

Innovar is more readily suited to the hospitalized patient where postoperative recovery can be supervised without the need for early ambulation. Since amnesia is often incomplete, the patient may have unpleasant memories of the events during the operation. Addition of nitrous oxide-oxygen overcomes this problem. Use of a muscle relaxant may be necessary for endotracheal intubation and to abolish skeletal muscle rigidity. Since the effect of droperidol is prolonged, supplemental doses of fentanyl (0.05 to 0.1 mg) alone can be given at indicated intervals for procedures lasting over 45 minutes. The effects of fentanyl are gone 45 to 60 minutes after the last dose, but droperidol may exert α-adrenergic-blocking action for several hours after administration making bed rest in the supine position necessary to avoid hypotension.

The recovering patient will tolerate an endotracheal tube for extended periods, and analgesic requirements are reduced. Nausea and vomiting are uncommon. There may be confusion, inability to concentrate, and mental depression. If extrapyramidal signs occur, they may be abolished with diphenhydramine (25 mg), atropine (0.5 mg), or benztropine (1 to 2 mg) given intravenously. The patient is not alert but is easily aroused, and will take deep breaths or cough on command.

DISSOCIATIVE ANESTHESIA

The dissociative state is one in which the patient becomes mentally separated from his external environment. Substances related to hallucinogenic drugs such as LSD or phencyclidine (PCP) produce such effects. A phencyclidine derivative, ketamine, introduced in clinical anesthesia in the middle 1960s, produces operating conditions in which the patient appears to be awake with his eyes open and exhibits occasional movements. However, profound analgesia and amnesia are present, and the patient feels detached from everything including his own extremities.

Pharmacology

Ketamine exerts its dissociative effects by interruption of cerebral association pathways and depression of the thalamo-cortical tracts while the reticular activating and limbic systems and the medullary centers are spared. Profound analgesia occurs, but visceral pain is poorly obtunded.

The cardiovascular system is stimulated during ketamine anesthesia. Increases in mean arterial pressure, cardiac rate, and cardiac output are the result of direct effect of ketamine, Cardiovascular responses may be modified by administration of diazepam prior to induction.

The airway is easily maintained, Pharyngeal and laryngeal reflexes are minimally depressed, but soilage of the trachea has occurred during controled studies. There is initial stimulation followed by minimal respiratory depression with normal doses of ketamine. Decreases in airway resistance may occur in patients with bronchospastic pulmonary disease who are given ketamine. Overdose causes apnea.

Skeletal muscle tone may be normal or increased. Movements which occur during ketamine anesthesia are usually purposeless. Use of a muscle relaxant may be necessary. Intraocular pressure may increase as a result of increased tone of extraocular muscles.

There is little disturbance of the gastrointestinal tract and a low incidence of nausea and vomiting. Hepatic and renal function are not altered. Secretions are not affected.

Use in Anesthesia

Ketamine is available in 10, 50, and 100 mg per ml concentrations for parenteral administration. Induction of anesthesia is accomplished by intravenous (1 mg per kg) or intramuscular (10 mg per kg) injection. Following intravenous administration onset of action occurs within 1 to 2 minutes. Onset after intramuscular injection is 3 to 5 minutes with duration of 2 to 25 minutes. Addition of nitrous oxide and oxygen and injection of local anesthesia into the operative site reduces the incidence of patient movement for subsequent increments (0.5 mg per kg) of ketamine, depending upon the length of the procedure. Although pharyngeal and laryngeal reflexes remain intact or are even hyperactive with laryngospasm in some patients, the trachea can become contaminated with foreign material. Placement of an oropharyngeal pack or an endotracheal tube and the availability of strong suction are mandatory. When the induction dose of ketamine was limited to 1 mg per lb intramuscularly, followed by nitrous oxide, oxygen, and local anesthesia, the average recovery time in pediatric outpatients from completion of the procedure to discharge from the clinic was 30 minutes.

Recovery from ketamine anesthesia is often complicated by hallucinations, psychomotor activity, delerium, or "bad dreams." These reactions may last from minutes to hours. In many cases these "bad trips" are remembered vividly by the patient and may recur afterwards as flashbacks. The episodes are less likely to happen in children, especially if the patient is allowed to awaken undisturbed and unstimulated in a quiet, darkened recovery area. Outpatient use of ketamine is usually reserved for children less than 12 years of age to minimize these psychic complications.

Precautions

Because of stimulation of the cardiovascular system, ketamine is contraindicated in patients with hypertension, atherosclerotic heart disease, or history of cerebrovascular accident. Patients with a history of psychiatric illness should not be placed at risk for a hallucinogenic episode with ketamine.

Ketamine Analgesia

This is a popular technique used in obstetrics and pediatric dentistry. A state of analgesia is said to be produced by the administration of either 2 mg per kg intramuscularly or 0.2 mg per kg intravenously. It would appear to be a successful technique, but analgesia may be an inappropriate term. Experience would seem to indicate that supplemental regional analgesia is necessary both for obstetrics and dentistry if this technique is used, and it would appear to be ketamine sedation. No controlled studies have been published regarding this technique, and the hazards of ketamine anesthesia may occur even with this small dosage.

Bibliography

Allen GD, Everett GB, Kennedy WF, Jr: Cardiorespiratory effects of general anesthesia on outpatients: methohexital, nitrous oxide-oxygen, halothane. J Oral Surg 28:814, 1970.

Allen GD, Hayden J: The influence of the semisupine position on silent regurgitation. Anesth Progr 12:12, 1975.

Allen GD, Kennedy WF Jr, Everett GB, et al: A comparison of the cardiorespiratory effects of methohexital and thiopental supplementation for outpatient dental anesthesia. Anesth Analg 48:730, 1969.

Allen GD, Kennedy WF Jr, Tolas AG, et al: Comparative cardiovascular effects of general anesthesia for outpatient oral surgery. J Oral Surg 26:784, 1968.

Allen GD, Ricks CS, Jorgensen NB: The efficacy of the laryngeal reflex in conscious sedation. J Am Dent Assoc 94:901, 1977.

Allen GD, Sims J: Full mouth restoration under general anesthesia in pedodontic practice. J Dent Child 34:488, 1967.

Allen GD, Ward, RJ, Tolas AG, et al: Cardiovascular responses during general anesthesia of dental outpatients. J Oral Ther Pharmacol 1:602, 1965.

Bourne JG: The common fainting attach: a danger in dental chair anesthesia. Br Dent J 119:62, 1965.

Burchiel KJ, Stockard JJ, Calverley RK, et al: Relationship of pre- and postanesthetic EEG abnormalities to enflurane-induced seizure activity. Anesth Analg 57:509, 1977.

Calverley RK, Smith NT, Jones CW, et al: Ventilatory and cardiovascular effects of enflurance anesthesia during spontaneous ventilation in man. Anesth Analg 57:610, 1978.

Carson IW, Moore J, Balmer JP, et al: Laryngeal competence with ketamine and other drugs. Anesthesiology 38:128, 1973.

Churchill-Davidson HC: A philosophy of relaxation. Anesth Analg 52:495, 1973.

Cohenour K, Gamble JW, Metzgar MT, et al: A composite general anesthesia technique using ketamine for pediatric outpatients. J Oral Surg 36:594, 1978.

Cousins MJ, Mazze RI: Methoxyflurane nephrotoxicity: a study of dose-response in man. JAMA 225:1611, 1973.

Douglas HJ, Eger EI, II, Biava CG, et al: Hepatic necrosis associated with viral infection after enflurane anesthesia. N Engl J Med 296:553, 1977.

Driscoll EJ, Christenson GR, White CL: Physiologic studies in general anesthesia for ambulatory dental patients. J Oral Surg 12:1496, 1959.

Drummond-Jackson, SL: Intravenous anaesthesia. Soc. Adv. Anaesth. Dent. London, England, 1967.

Dunsworth AR, Thornton WE, Byrd DL, et al: Evaluation of cardiovascular and pulmonary changes during diazepam-meperidine anesthesia. J Oral Surg 33:18, 1975.

Dykes MHM, Gilbert JP, Schur PH, et al: Halothane and the liver: review of the epidemiologic, immunologic, and metabolic aspects of the relationship. Can J Surg 15:217, 1972.

Eger EI, Saidman LJ, Brandstater B: Minimum alveolar anesthetic concentration: a standard of anesthetic potency. Ancsthesiology 26:756, 1965.

Ferstandig, LL: Trace concentrations of anesthetic gases: a critical review of their disease potential. Anesth Analg 57:328, 1978.

Forsyth WD, Allen GD, Everett GB: An evaluation of cardiorespiratory effects of posture in the dental outpatient. Oral Surg 34:562, 1972.

Goldman V: Intravenous anaesthesia for the ambulant patient. S Afr Med J 43:74, 1965.

Hagen JO, McCarthy FM: General anesthesia for the ambulatory patient: the anesthetic team. J S Calif Dent Assoc 37:224, 1969.

Healy TE, Vickers MD: Laryngeal competence with diazepam sedation. *Proc R Soc Med* 64:85, 1971.

Hubbell AO: Methohexital sodium anesthesia for oral surgery. *J Oral Surg* 18:295, 1960.

Jenkins LC: Chronic exposure to anaesthetics: A toxicity problem. *Can Anaesth Soc J* 20:104, 1973.

Katz RL: Monitoring of muscle relaxation and neuromuscular transmission. In Crul J, Payne JP (eds): *Monitoring in Anaesthesia.* Amsterdam, Excerpta Medica, 1970, p 125.

Katz RL, Katz GJ: Complications associated with the use of muscle relaxants. In Foldes RR (ed): *Clinical Anesthesia. Muscle Relaxants.* Philadelphia, F. A. Davis, 1966, p 121.

Katz RL, Matteo RS, Papper EM: The injection of epinephrine during general anesthesia with halogenated hydrocarbons and cyclopropane in man. II. Halothane. *Anesthesiology* 23:597, 1962.

McCarthy FM: Facts and fallacies regarding general anesthesia in dental offices. *J Oral Surg* 19:492, 1961.

McPeek B, Mathieu H, Guralnick WC: Fact or fancy—a reasoned view of halothane. *J Oral Surg* 32:8, 1974.

Meyer RA, Allen GD: Halothane in outpatient dental anesthesia. *Oral Surg* 24:760, 1967.

Meyer RA, Allen GD, Hooley JR: Methoxyflurane in outpatient oral surgery. *Oral Surg* 21:594, 1966.

Scaramella J, Allen GD, Goebel WM, et al: Lidocaine as a supplement to general anesthesia for extraction of third molars. *Anesth Prog* 26:118, 1979.

Smith JD, Allen GD, Perrin EB: A comparison of visual and auditory assessments of recovery from general anesthesia. *Oral Surg* 23:596, 1967.

Stevens WC, Cromwell TH, Halsey MJ, et al: The cardiovascular effects of a new inhalation anesthetic, Forane, in human volunteers at constant arterial carbon dioxide tension. *Anesthesiology* 35:8, 1971.

Tolas AG, Allen GD, Ward RJ, et al: Comparison of effects of methods of induction of anesthesia on cardiac rhythm. *J Oral Surg* 25:54, 1967.

Wise CC, Robinson, JS, Heath MJ, et al: Physiological responses to intermittent methohexitone for conservative dentistry. *Br Med J* 2:540, 1969.

CHAPTER 14

Postoperative Care

Postoperative care of the patient begins when the operation finishes, whether or not the patient is awake. The administrator of the anesthesia or analgesia is responsible for the patient until discharge from the recovery area.

Serious complications or death have occurred in the postoperative period following both anesthesia and conscious sedation. Therefore, the recovering patient must be actively managed by trained personnel and not left to the care of friends or relatives in the dental office.

OBJECTIVES

The objectives of proper postoperative care include: 1) maintenance of a patent airway until protective reflexes return; 2) support of adequate ventilation (oxygen uptake, carbon dioxide elimination); 3) protection of the recovering patient from injury; 4) maintenance of stable vital signs; 5) "objective" judgment as to when the patient has recovered; 6) appropriate management of complications; 7) postoperative pain relief.

These objectives are most appropriately met when the dental patient is cared for by well-trained personnel in adequately equipped, spacious surroundings and where a systematic approach is followed on a daily basis.

INITIAL RECOVERY PHASE

As soon as the operator has completed the operation, the oropharyngeal packs are removed and the mouth and pharynx are suctioned clear of hemorrhage, secretions, and debris. The bite block is removed after gauze packs are placed over any surgical sites. All anesthetic gases are turned off and 100 per cent oxygen is administered for 2 to 3 minutes to counteract the effects of diffusion hypoxia (if nitrous oxide was used) and to provide the patient with an oxygen reserve. If an endotracheal tube is in place, it is usually best removed after the patient is sufficiently awake that protective reflexes have returned.

When the patient has active reflexes, the decision can be made by the doctor responsible to move the patient to the recovery area. In some offices or clinics the operatory is used as the recovery area, and the outpatient is allowed to remain in the contour dental chair during the recovery period. Separate recovery space is used in other clinics, so that the operatory may be more efficiently utilized for surgery.

If the patient is to be moved to a separate recovery area, transport may be by wheelchair, mobile surgical chair/table, or a stretcher. It is also acceptable practice to allow the awake patient to walk with assistance to the recovery area. Muscle contraction induced in the lower extremities by walking aids venous return and helps maintain an adequate cardiac output while the patient is erect. Two persons should assist the patient in walking to the recovery room, one in front who can support the patient under each axilla and on whose shoulders the patient can rest his hands, and one behind the patient who can grasp the patient by belt or waist.

A child who is not yet fully awake should be carried by the anesthetist to the recovery area with his head down and facing the anesthetist (Fig. 14.1).

When awake and able to follow com-

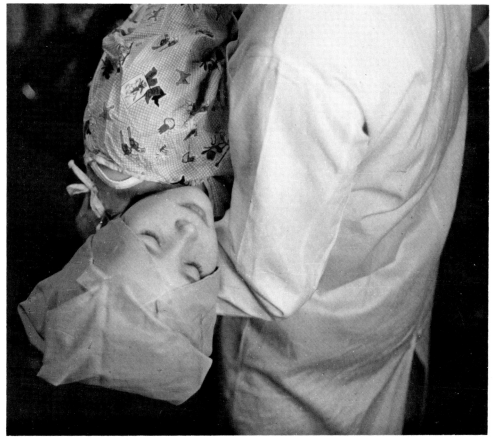

Figure 14.1. A child should be carried head down and facing the anesthetist to the recovery room. It aids close observation of the airway and gravity helps prevent foreign bodies or the tongue from falling into the airway.

mands the patient should be encouraged to cough and deep breathe. This assists clearing of any retained secretions in the tracheobronchial tree and helps re-expand peripheral atelectatic areas of the lungs.

The personnel caring for recovering dental patients, whether they be R.N.s, L.P.N.s, or trained dental assistants, should have unique training. They should be able to establish and maintain an airway by manual or mechanical means, be skilled in the use of suction apparatus, and able to administer oxygen by bag and mask or resuscitator. They must possess good judgment in knowing when to call for assistance in the management of a problem. Certification in basic life support by the American Heart Association is highly desirable if not mandatory. One person may often easily manage several recovering patients in the same area, but should not be distracted by the demands of duties elsewhere. Constant vigilance over the recovering patient is paramount.

The requirements of an adequate recovery area include sufficient space to allow personnel to attend the patient, a cot for the patient preferably with side rails, monitoring equipment, a good light source, strong suction, oxygen and equipment to administer it, equipment such as a Ferguson gag to force open the patient's jaw in an emergency (Fig. 14.2), and a method of communication if an emergency arises.

Most of the postoperative problems in recovering dental patients are secondary

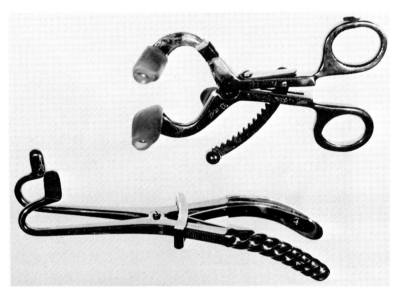

Figure 14.2. The Ferguson gag with Ackland jaw (*bottom*) can be used to pry open the tightly clamped jaw in an emergency. The jaws should be placed behind the teeth to avoid damage. It is recommended for care outside the charge of the anesthetist. The Moult mouth prep (*top*) is used to maintain an open mouth during oral surgery.

to an inadequate airway and are usually avoidable by proper technique. The patient should be placed in the "position of safety," semi-prone with a pillow under the chest (Fig. 14.3). In this position gravity aids the maintenance of the airway (the mandible falls forward not backward) and allows secretions, blood, or vomitus to flow out of the mouth, not pool in the pharynx. The patient should lie facing the recovery room attendant for adequate observation. Most airway problems can be managed by proper patient positioning, strong suction, and the administration of oxygen. The administration of succinylcholine or other drugs to manage laryngospasm is seldom indicated and not recommended unless the personnel have the talent necessary to maintain ventilation.

A written record should be kept during recovery. Blood pressure, pulse, respirations, other pertinent observations, any complications, and their treatment should be duly recorded by the attending personnel either as a continuation of the anesthetic record or on a separate form. All

such records should become part of the patient's chart for future reference and for medicolegal reasons.

An objective method of assessing recovery is highly desirable in outpatient anesthesia practice. Bender and Jaffe devised the "hand-face" test, and Smith *et al.* compared visual and auditory methods of assessing recovery from general anesthesia. Allen and Tolas, using the Phystester, an apparatus originally developed to evaluate intoxication in automobile drivers, found that 50 per cent of the patients who were awake and appeared clinically "recovered" from general anesthesia could not perform simple visual or verbal maneuvers. Trieger *et al.* developed a graphic methd of assessing visual and motor skills which seems accurate and simple to use in a clinical setting. Regardless of the patient's ability to perform on a sensorimotor examination after anesthesia, however, it is deemed advisable that the patient not leave the office unaccompanied by a responsible adult or be allowed to drive an automobile or operate

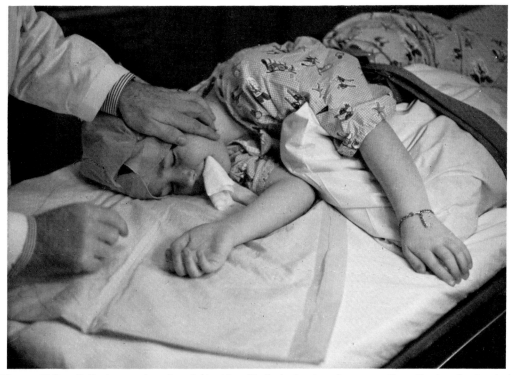

Figure 14.3. Patients are placed on their side with their chest resting on a pillow, the head extended and the arms placed so as not to place a strain on the brachial plexus.

machinery for the rest of the day. The patient should be advised not to make important decisions for 24 hours postoperatively.

When ready to leave the office or clinic, the patient is generally given postoperative instructions regarding care of the surgical site. Any of a number of symptoms which may indicate a complication of anesthesia, such as fever, dyspnea, chest pain, persistent cough, or wheezing should be indicated as needing report. Such patients should be seen again and evaluated for a pulmonary complication.

EARLY POSTOPERATIVE PROBLEMS

Numerous problems can arise in the dental outpatient recovering from anesthesia or intravenous sedation. Because outpatients are selected on the basis of good physical status, most complications are due to mechanical difficulties or in- attention to proper technique rather than pre-existing systemic disease. Therefore, knowledge of these potential problems before they occur may prevent their occurrence or facilitate their management.

Respiratory Problems

The most common complications involve the respiratory system.

AIRWAY OBSTRUCTION

The airway can be obstructed by the tongue falling back against the posterior wall of the pharynx. This can be prevented by adequate manual support of the mandible. Foreign bodies within the airway can cause mechanical airway obstruction. The inhalation of dental calculus during or after operation is a seldom appreciated cause of postoperative respiratory complications. Direct laryngoscopy should be done at the conclusion of operation to detect and remove foreign material. The improper placement of an oropharyngeal airway in the patient recovering from anesthesia can produce airway obstruction. Stimulation of pharyngeal or paralaryngeal tissues in the lightly anesthetized patient by the airway can induce coughing or laryngospasm, or displace the tongue posteriorly against the pharyngeal wall.

LARYNGOSPASM

Laryngospasm can be initiated by foreign bodies, by the oral airway, or on extubation. The patient's lungs should be well oxygenated at the conclusion of anesthesia as laryngospasm is made worse by hypoxia. The endotracheal tube should be removed while the patient is still deeply anesthetized or after he has active reflexes. Vocal cord closure is more likely to occur during Stage 2 of general anesthesia. It is helpful to slowly deflate the cuff of the endotracheal tube and, as it is withdrawn, exert positive pressure on the reservoir bag in order to blow out of the airway any foreign material resting on or near the vocal cords.

RESPIRATORY DEPRESSION

Ventilatory inadequacy can occur as a result of overdosage of narcotics, barbiturates, muscle relaxants, or inhalation anesthetic agents. Ventilation should be assisted or controlled until adequate spontaneous respiration returns. These is no need for an endotracheal tube if the airway can be maintained by simpler means. A narcotic antagonist or reversal of a nondepolarizing muscle relaxant may be appropriate in certain patients.

PULMONARY ASPIRATION

Foreign material from either the stomach or oral cavity can be aspirated into the tracheobronchial tree if adequate precautions are not taken during recovery. Stomach contents should be minimal or absent if an appropriate fast was observed by the patient prior to anesthesia. However, gastric emptying is variable and dependent upon multiple factors not always within control of the anesthetist. Regurgitation is a passive process and usually occurs during a surgical plane of anesthesia when the patient is supine, allowing vomitus to flow by gravity into the pharyngeal area. Vomiting is an active process occurring during Stage 2 of general anesthesia or when the patient has regained consciousness. It does not require the aid of gravity in the supine patient to bring vomitus into the pharyngeal area from which it can enter the larynx. If the patient has been intubated for anesthesia, the endotracheal tube should be left in place until protective reflexes have returned. If pulmonary aspiration occurs, it will be signaled by violent coughing, wheezing, and cyanosis. Active measures must be instituted immediately to prevent morbidity or mortality.

SUBGLOTTIC EDEMA

Pressure of a tightfitting endotracheal tube or prolonged inflation of a high-pressure cuff is thought to cause this problem. Both irritation and ischemia of subglottic tissues may occur, particularly after a lengthy procedure. Movement of the oral endotracheal tube occurs with respiration and is also irritating to laryngotracheal tissues. Use of a nasal endotracheal tube and a well-placed pharyngeal pack prevents tube movement with respirations. Subglottic edema is more likely to occur in small children because of relatively minor amount of intratracheal edema can significantly reduce the diameter of the child's airway. Subglottic edema can occur several hours after the termination of anesthesia. The onset of subglottic edema is heralded by inspiratory stridor or croupy respirations, tachypnea, sternal retractions, use of accessory neck muscles for inspiratory efforts, and flared nares. Cyanosis is a late and ominous sign preceding total airway obstruction. The patient should be diagnosed early and treated in a respiratory intensive care unit. Treatment includes humidified air, steroids, nebulized bronchodilators, and consideration of tracheotomy.

ATELECTASIS

During anesthesia it is common for many small peripheral lung alveoli to be underventilated or blocked by secretions, causing them to collapse. Atelectatic areas should be re-expanded postoperatively by encouraging the recovering patient to frequently cough and deep breathe. An entire lobe or lung may collapse during anesthesia if one mainstem bronchus (usually the right) is intubated, preventing ventilation of the opposite lung. The severe pulmonary shunting and hypoxemia that immediately result are easily recognized after intubation when breath sounds are absent in the collapsed lung and there is asymmetrical chest expansion with inspiration. Treatment consists of repositioning of the endotracheal tube into the trachea so that both lungs are well ventilated. Aspirated solid foreign material may lodge in a bronchus or bronchiole and cause atelectasis of distal lung alveoli. Bronchoscopy is often required for the removal of such material. Atelectasis is a cause of early postoperative fever and, if not successfully treated, will progress to pneumonitis or lung abscess.

Cardiovascular Problems

Pre-existing cardiovascular disease will predispose to complications in the postoperative period. Previously undiagnosed coronary artery disease is more likely in patients over 40 years of age, especially males, and in patients with diabetes mellitus. Unexpected cardiovascular problems may develop in such patients.

HYPOTENSION

Hypotension and cardiovascular instability occur at the conclusion of an operation when the patient's cardiovascular system is subjected to stresses it is poorly equipped to handle. Cardiovascular tone and reflexes are obtunded by anesthesia. If the posture of the patient is altered, pooling of blood can occur in vascular beds, venous return decreases, and cardiac output is depressed, causing a significant decrease in blood pressure and tissue perfusion. Therefore, the patient must not be moved during deep anesthesia unless the supine position is maintained to ensure adequate venous return to the heart. If the patient is sufficiently awake so that skeletal muscle movement can occur and he can walk from the operatory, then contraction of lower extremity muscles during walking assists venous return to the heart. However, the practice of forcing the patient from the dental chair or table before return of adequate cooperation in walking is dangerous. A portable stretcher should be used to move the patient in that case.

Other causes of hypotension which should be recognized at the end of operation include inadequate replacement of fluid deficits or blood loss, severe pain, vasovagal responses, rapid removal of carbon dioxide which accumulated during anesthesia, and gastric dilatation from gases or oxygen inadvertently forced into the stomach. In the anesthetized or recovering patient who is too obtunded to complain of chest pain, persistent hypotension may be the only evidence of myocardial infarction until an electrocardiographic tracing is obtained.

CARDIAC ARRHYTHMIAS

Irregularities of cardiac rhythm may be atrial or ventricular in origin and rapid or slow. Rapid or irregular contractions of the myocardium interfere with normal filling and pumping action and compromise cardiac output and coronary artery perfusion. Ventricular arrhythmias can progress to ventricular fibrillation. Diagnosed pre-existing arrhythmias are usually under control with medication, such as digitalization for atrial fibrillation, and they generally indicate significant underlying cardiac disease. Arrhythmias occurring de novo under anesthesia may be due to the anesthetic agent, surgical stimulation under light anesthesia, blood gas abnormalities (hypoxemia, hypercarbia), previously undiagnosed heart disease, or metabolic disease. At the end of operation when anesthesia is terminated the patient should have few arrhythmias other than those that were pre-existing unless the airway is compromised or hypotension is not corrected. The majority of cardiac arrhythmias in the postoperative period occur without obvious cause, are transient, and require no treatment. There is often more risk in treating a brief arrhythmia than in merely observing it. If an arrhythmia persists and/or the patient's condition deteriorates, an electrocardiogram should be made and consultation requested immediately.

PULMONARY EDEMA

The onset of pulmonary edema is recognized by distended neck veins, cyanosis, severe dyspnea, tachypnea, cough producing pink frothy sputum, tachycardia, and moist rales and expiratory wheezes. Patients with cardiovascular disease, especially during prolonged operations and vigorous overreplacement of intravenous fluids, are particularly at risk. Such patients should be recognized and hospitalized before operation, adequately digitalized, and not fluid overloaded during operation. Treatment of pulmonary edema should be conducted in a coronary care unit and consists of sitting the patient up to reduce dyspnea, diuretics, morphine, aminophylline, and, in some cases, endotracheal intubation and mechanical ventilation.

MYOCARDIAL INFARCTION

Severe or prolonged lowering of mean arterial pressure during operation seriously compromises coronary artery perfusion and may cause myocardial ische-mia or infarction. Patients with pre-existing coronary artery disease are particularly susceptible. If the recovering patient is not awake sufficiently to complain of the characteristic chest pain of myocardial infarction, its presence should be suspected when sudden, severe hypotension or persistent ventricular arrhythmias occur. The oscilloscope does not always display the characteristic injury pattern in the S-T segments, so a full 12-lead electrocardiogram should be taken and consultation sought immediately.

HEMORRHAGE

Rebound vasodilatation which follows vasoconstriction produced by locally injected epinephrine or lapses in surgical technique may cause bleeding during the recovery period. Significant oozing should be treated by the surgeon. Blood loss in excess of 15 per cent of total blood volume may require replacement, if the patient remains unstable in spite of vigorous fluid replacement.

Neurological Problems

FAILURE TO REGAIN CONSCIOUSNESS

The outpatient who fails to rapidly regain consciousness after the termination of the operation is a source of considerable anxiety to attending personnel. The problem is less acute if a well-staffed recovery area is available, and it is commonplace in hospital practice where rapid recovery is not a requirement. Attempts to arouse the patient by physical means may prove injurious. Pharmacological effects of analeptics (e.g., Ritalin, Bemegride) are usually only transitory, increase cerebral oxygen consumption, may cause convulsions, and are not worth the risk. Specific antidotes for various drugs (narcotic antagonism and curare reversal) should be considered only after a careful appraisal of the reasons for the patient's failure to recover. Recent work would seem to indicate that physostigmine is a nonspecific analeptic to sedation with some inhalation and intravenous agents. Its time course has not yet been determined. The following features should be considered in evaluating such patients.

1. *Anesthetic agents.* Some of the volatile inhalation anesthetic agents (e.g., methoxyflurane) have a prolonged action and must be terminated well before the end of operation. Even halothane or enflurane must be terminated several minutes before the end of surgery so that recovery is not prolonged. Excessive use of barbiturates and narcotics will prolong recovery time. Usually the patient can be maintained on nitrous oxide-oxygen during the placing of sutures or carving of amalgam restorations at the end of operation. The surgeon and anesthetist should communicate so that the conclusion of the procedure is anticipated by all concerned.

2. *Physiological disturbances.* Inadequate ventilation causes carbon dioxide retention. The cerebral vasodilatation and edema induced by hypercarbia delay recovery; in fact, hypercarbia itself has narcotizing effects on the central nervous system. A period of hypoxia or hypotension can have similar effects. Although controlled ventilation with lowering of arterial carbon dioxide tension will not delay return of consciousness, it can delay the return of spontaneous respiration. Significant alterations of core body temperature during anesthesia (hypo- or hyperthermia) should be noted. Children are particularly susceptible to excessive loss of body heat under anesthesia if they are not adequately protected with warm blankets or drapes. Rectal temperatures should be monitored during prolonged cases such as extensive restorative dentistry or major maxillofacial surgery, particularly if blood replacement is needed.

3. *Surgery.* Complications of surgery such as shock or fat or air embolism can delay recovery. Development of metabolic acidosis can occur during anesthesia if poorly controlled diabetics are subjected to operation.

4. *Pre-existing conditions.* Poorly controlled or unrecognized renal or hepatic disease can alter metabolism or slow excretion of drugs used in anesthesia and prolong their effects. Misuse of insulin or failure to recognize adrenal insufficiency due to chronic exogenous administration of corticosteroids are potential problems during and after anesthesia. The careful completion of a preoperative history will alert the clinician to such conditions.

POSTANESTHETIC EXCITEMENT

The thrashing, combative patient emerging from anesthesia is a challenge to attending personnel. The patient must be protected from injury and the cause determined in order to provide rational treatment. The practice of giving all patients a narcotic or diazepam without further investigation is to be deplored. A significant condition may be overlooked which can contribute to postoperative morbidity.

A common cause of excitement during emergence from anesthesia is hypoxia. A partially obstructed airway of diffusion hypoxia can cause this effect without cyanosis, especially in the elderly patient. Excitement should always be considered to be due to hypoxia until proven otherwise and adequate oxygen administered.

Scopolamine can cause excitement, particularly in children and the elderly. It can be treated by physostigmine, 2 mg, in the adult. Barbiturates in the presence of pain have an antianalgesic effect and cause considerable agitation. Ketamine, especially when the patient is not kept in quiet surroundings during recovery, can cause hallucinations and a stormy emergence.

Young children often awake crying and thrashing as a by-product of their underlying anxiety about the procedure. They need only be gently restrained to prevent injury.

In prolonged cases where excessive intravenous fluids were administered, overdistention of the urinary bladder can cause agitation in the recovering patient. If percussion and palpation of the lower abdomen discloses an enlarged bladder, it can be decompressed by passing a Foley catheter if the patient cannot void.

The chronic alcoholic patient often exhibits excitement or combativeness during recovery. Small doses of diazepam, 5 to 10 mg, or chlordiazepoxide, 25 to 100 mg, given slowly intravenously often have a calming effect on these patients.

Severe pain from the surgical site, particularly in the presence of barbiturate anesthesia, may cause agitation or excitement. Injection of local anesthesia before the end of the procedure will provide a pain-free interval during recovery without the respiratory or cardiovascular depression associated with use of narcotics for pain relief at this time. The patient who awakens with intermaxillary fixation in place is likely to be combative or agitated unless carefully warned preoperatively.

The proper management of postanesthetic excitement requires advance planning so that assistance is immediately available on a prearranged signal. The patient can then be restrained and protected from injury while the cause of excitement is adequately investigated and properly treated.

Gastrointestinal Problems

NAUSEA AND VOMITING

Approximately 5 per cent of all patients given a general anesthetic will vomit in the postoperative period. The incidence seems to be greater among females than males. A careful history preoperatively may reveal patients who have vomited after every general anesthetic they have received and are predisposed to the problem. Persistent nausea and vomiting are particularly troublesome in outpatients because of interference with adequate hydration and the administration of medications on return home. Factors other than predisposition can cause postanesthetic nausea and vomiting.

1. *Fasting.* An "adequate" period of abstention from food and liquids must be observed prior to anesthesia. Unfortunately, gastric emptying time can be prolonged by factors such as fear or anxiety, narcotic medications, shock, or trauma, making it difficult to predict accurately when the stomach is empty. It is prudent to ask outpatients to observe a 4- to 6-hour fast prior to anesthesia. Patients must be closely questioned regarding any intake of food, fluids, or water prior to starting anesthesia as many patients fail to grasp the importance of fasting and do not follow preoperative instructions.

Fasting is not a prerequisite for conscious sedation, indeed it may often cause nausea postoperatively.

2. *Anesthetic agents.* Halothane, barbiturates, and nitrous oxide-oxygen are associated with a low incidence of nausea and vomiting.

3. *Anesthetic technique.* Anesthesia in which hypoxia, hypercarbia, or excessive coughing or struggling occur increases postoperative nausea and vomiting.

4. *Narcotics.* The opiate derivatives have been associated with vomiting in 25 per cent of patients, which limits their usefulness as anesthetic supplements and premedication, particularly in outpatients.

5. *Operation.* If blood, mucus, or other secretions are allowed to enter the stomach, their rejection in the postoperative period can be expected. Proper oral packing and suctioning during and after operation should prevent such material from reaching the stomach.

6. *Gastric distention.* Anesthetic gases may be forced into the stomach during induction of anesthesia or during a period of airway obstruction. Nitrous oxide will diffuse into the gut during conscious sedation; if there is a closed loop of bowel present, this too is a factor causing disten-

tion. Distention of the stomach by such gases may cause vomiting on recovery, as well as arrhythmias and hypotension. It is suspected by observing tachycardia and tachypnea and by a hypertympanitic note to percussion in the epigastric region. The distended stomach should be decompressed by passage of a nasogastric tube.

Postoperative nausea and vomiting, if persistent, require treatment with antiemetic medication. Rectal administration of trimethobenzamide (Tigan), 200 mg, or prochlorperazine (Compazine), 25 mg, in the adult or appropriately smaller doses in the child is usually effective.

Other Postanesthetic Problems

CONJUNCTIVITIS

Secretion of tears ceases during Stage 3 of general anesthesia. The eyelids should be taped in closed position or covered with eye pads. In operative dentistry under general anesthesia dust particles of tooth enamel or amalgam can enter the unprotected eye, causing irritation or abrasion of conjunctiva or cornea. Conjunctivitis also results from the drying effect of anesthetic gases flowing across the open eye.

PRESSURE LESIONS

Improper positioning of extremities causes traction or pressure on peripheral nerves which may cause paresis or paresthesia. Prolonged pressure of anesthesia equipment about the face or other areas of the body causes tissue ischemia or necrosis.

HEADACHE

Headache is usually considered a minor sequel to general anesthesia. Its incidence has been estimated as high as 50 per cent. Postanesthetic headache assumes more importance in outpatients who expect to be fully ambulant and reasonably comfortable soon after recovery from an anesthetic. Although preoperative anxiety is thought to be a contributing factor in headache, outpatients are often not premedicated in order to reduce recovery time. Preoperative assurance by the anesthetist or surgeon can help allay anxiety and reduce incidence of headache. Patients anesthetized with controlled ventilation have fewer headaches than those who breath spontaneously. The increased cerebral vasodilatation which accompanies hypoxia, hypercarbia, and halothane anesthesia undoubtedly is a factor in headaches. Elevation of the head, application of cool, moist towels to the forehead, reassurance by attending personnel and mild, nonnarcotic analgesics are all helpful in relieving headache. Narcotics are contraindicated as they can aggravate a headache by increasing intracranial pressure. Persistent or increasingly severe headache may indicate an expanding intracranial lesion. Neurosurgical consultation should be sought, especially if there is a change in level of consciousness or the appearance of focal or lateralizing neurological signs.

MUSCULOSKELETAL PAIN

Following a bolus injection of succinylcholine for muscle relaxation there is a brief period of generalized muscle fasciculations which is equivalent to violent physical exercise. Postoperatively, the patient may complain of rather severe pain in the chest, back, and abdominal muscles for 1 to 2 days. Muscle pain in the chest wall may mimic the pain of myocardial infarction. Reassurance of the patient and mild analgesia with salicylates or codeine are helpful. Muscle fasciculations with succinylcholine can be prevented by injecting a small dose of a nondepolarizing relaxant prior to succinylcholine administration or by giving succinylcholine by intravenous drip rather than by bolus injection. Under deep anesthesia, abnormal patient positioning can overstretch ligaments or tendons and be another source of postoperative discomfort which is better prevented than treated.

URINARY RETENTION

During anesthesia for prolonged procedures, excessive amounts of intravenous fluids may be administered. If the urinary bladder fills beyond normal capacity, the normal reflex which stimulates the detrusor muscle and initiates voiding is abolished. The older male patient with bladder neck obstruction secondary to an enlarged prostate gland is especially susceptible. If standard measures such as standing to void or application of warm moist compresses to the perineal area are not successful, the bladder can be decompressed with a single catheterization. Normal voiding usually returns after this unless the patient had significant pre-existing bladder neck obstruction.

SORE THROAT

Sore throat is an almost universal sequel to general anesthesia. The irritating and dry effects of inhaled gases on pharyngeal mucosa and the trauma of laryngoscopy, endotracheal intubation, and placement of gauze pharyngeal packs are all contributing factors. Most postanesthetic sore throats resolve within 24 to 48 hours. Gargling with warm salt water or a commercial mouthwash with mild topical anesthetic properties, avoidance of solid foods, and use of mild analgesics such as aspirin are usually all that is necessary to ease the patient's discomfort.

Late Complications

Responsibility for the care of the outpatient does not end when the patient leaves the office or clinic after recovery from anesthesia and surgery. Although perhaps less likely to occur in fully ambulatory outpatients after minor or brief procedures than in hospitalized patients after major surgery, the same types of complications can occur in either group. Therefore, before being discharged after recovery, outpatients should be instructed to report any untoward reactions or symptoms of illness to the responsible personnel as soon as possible. Common symptoms after outpatient procedures include fever, dehydration, persistent cough or dyspnea, and flu-like symptoms. Such symptoms may indicate a significant underlying disease process requiring diagnosis and treatment.

FEVER

Elevated body temperature could be due to the infectious process associated with dentoalveolar abscesses of nonvital teeth. Incision and drainage of abscesses and removal of involved teeth should cause rapid resolution of such infection and febrile response. However, persistent fever should alert the clinician to a significant complication. Pulmonary complications, wound infection, urinary tract infection, and thrombophlebitis are well known causes of fever in postoperative patients.

PULMONARY

Atelectasis, which is the most common reason for fever in the first 24 postoperative hours, may progress to pneumonitis if unrecognized and untreated. Calculus, tooth fragments, or other foreign material, if aspirated into the tracheobronchial tree, may obstruct a bronchus or bronchopulmonary segment and produce a lung abscess.

DEHYDRATION

Fasting before anesthesia and surgery, inadequate fluid replacement during operation, and persistent nausea or vomiting postoperatively in the outpatient combine to produce a significant deficit of body fluids. Decreased circulating blood volume causes orthostatic hypotension. Blood pressure drop in the ambulatory patient produces further nausea which interferes with intake of fluid and necessary medications, thus perpetuating the vicious cycle of dehydration. Such patients require antiemetic medication, usually given rectally, and improved oral intake, or they need to be hospitalized where intravenous therapy can be provided.

EMBOLIC PHENOMENA

Patients with significant venous insufficiency, venous disease, or history of thrombophlebitis in the lower extremities are at increased risk of thromboembolism postoperatively. During anesthesia and surgery venous stasis in the lower extremities can occur if preventive measures are not taken. Such patients should have their legs elevated during operation. Ace wraps or elastic stockings can assist in prevention of venous pooling in the legs. Early ambulation after surgery further increases venous return from the lower extremities and decreases the likelihood of thrombus formation. Propagation of thrombi in the deep venous system of the legs places the patient at significant risk for embolism to the lungs. Thrombophlebitis or phlebothrombosis may be heralded by calf tenderness and swollen, red and tender veins, or it may be completely asymptomatic. Pulmonary embolism is characterized by sudden dyspnea, tachypnea, tachycardia, and a loud pulmonic second heart sound. The classic symptoms of chest pain, cough, and hemoptysis usually indicate pulmonary infarction, but occur in less than 10 per cent of pulmonary emboli. Preventive measures as described above should reduce or eliminate most such complications in dental patients, whether hospitalized or not.

THE FLU

Following anesthesia and operation on outpatients, occasional patients will complain of fever and chills, myalgia, cough, and sore throat. Such complaints should not be dismissed. The patient should be seen to rule out a significant complication, particularly a pulmonary problem. Symptomatic treatment over the telephone without patient examination is to be condemned.

HEPATITIS

A patient who develops an unexplained fever, particularly after halothane anesthesia, should be investigated for hepatocellular damage.

Pain Relief

Surgical procedures and other operative manipulations in and about the mouth and maxillofacial region are expected to result in significant pain for many patients. Unfortunately, pain is not a predictable phenomenon. The patient's response to pain may be governed by inherent ethnic or sociological considerations, previous experience, preoperative patient education, the extent and severity of the procedure, and the patient's individual pain threshold and physical status. Indeed, it may vary in the same patient. Therefore, postoperative pain and the need for its relief should be assessed on an individual basis for each patient.

One-third of postoperative patients do not require potent analgesic medications and will respond favorably to placebos. However, no patient should be refused pain-relieving medication when there is a legitimate need. Narcotic analgesics should be prescribed in dosage and number so that extra pills are not surplus after the need for pain relief ceases.

Postoperative complications, such as alveolar osteitis, often signal their onset with increasingly severe pain. Such patients should be seen and the complication treated rather than continuing symptomatic treatment with stronger analgesics.

Establishment of good rapport between the surgeon or anesthetist and the patient ahead of time reduces patient anxiety, which is important in modifying the pain response. Patients who are told honestly what to expect in terms of swelling, jaw stiffness, pain, and its relief will be better prepared and respond with less anxiety in the postoperative period. Sincere concern for and gentle reassurance of the patient postoperatively also do much to augment analgesic medications. Knowledge of the practitioner's availability by telephone after office hours helps to allay anxiety even though a phone call to the doctor is not made.

Time-honored methods for pain relief in dentistry include the use of local anesthesia, application of ice packs to surgical areas, use of analgesic medications, placement of sedative dressings, and psychic support of the patient. The general condition of the patient has an effect on the magnitude of pain and its relief. Adequate nutrition, fluid intake, metabolic function, and rest are all parts of a necessary foundation on which to base a rational regimen of postoperative pain relief.

The immediate postoperative period is generally the time of greatest pain after dental procedures. Use of regional local anesthesia allows the patient to recover from sedation or general anesthesia in a pain-free state. If the patient's need for relief can be anticipated, it is helpful to take an oral analgesic before the numbness subsides. The transition from anesthesia to postoperative pain will be more gradual and better tolerated.

NONADDICTIVE ORAL ANALGESICS

Aspirin (acetylsalicylic acid) is the standard analgesic drug against which others are compared. It produces satisfactory relief of mild pain in recommended doses of 600 mg every 3 to 4 hours in adults, with proportionally smaller doses for children. Doses larger than 600 mg may prolong, but will not increase, the analgesic effect. Aspirin has significant anti-inflammatory and antipyretic effects which may enhance the analgesic effect in a patient with an infectious or inflamma-

tory process. If taken in excess, aspirin causes significant blood loss from the gastric mucosa. It also inhibits platelet function and enhances the anticoagulant activity of coumadin. Combining aspirin with an antacid has the theoretical advantages of reducing gastric upset and hastening absorption from the stomach and onset of analgesia, but controlled clinical trials have failed to substantiate such claims. Analgesic combinations containing aspirin, phenacetin, and caffeine possess no advantages over aspirin alone. However, aspirin and codeine do have additive analgesic effects.

Acetaminophen is a *para*-aminophenol derivative with analgesic and antipyretic properties similar to aspirin. It does not possess anti-inflammatory effects, however. A similar compound is phenacetin which is de-ethylated in the body to form acetaminophen, the metabolite responsible for its analgesic effect. Abuse of preparations containing phenacetin has caused renal papillary necrosis. Renal damage has not been associated with acetaminophen, but acute overdosage can result in fatal hepatic necrosis if not promptly treated. Usual analgesic doses of acetaminophen are similar to those of aspirin. Advantages claimed for acetaminophen over aspirin include lack of gastrointestinal irritation, no inhibition of platelet activity, and no enhancement of anticoagulant medications. Acetaminophen is also available in codeine preparations.

PROSTAGLANDIN INHIBITORS

This group of nonsteroidal anti-inflammatory agents possess potent analgesic properties. It is important that they be started prior to the development of the pain or discomfort, and therefore a loading dose should always be given at the beginning of therapy. Many studies have shown them to be more potent than the aspirin-like compounds. They may be classed then as four moderate analgesics. Examples are zomepirac (Zomac), 100 mg;

tolmetin (Tolectin), 200 mg; naproxen (Naprosen), 250 mg; and ibuprofen (Motrin), 400 mg. It must be appreciated that these drugs show cross-tolerance, and therefore reactions to one may produce reactions to another.They are a useful drug in reducing the amount of inflammatory response to dental trauma and subsequent pain.

ADDICTIVE ANALGESIC PREPARATIONS (TABLE 14.1)

Codeine is the standard narcotic analgesic available for oral administration. Oral doses are usually well tolerated by most patients, and gastric absorption is adequate and predictable. Doses of 30 to 60 mg are effective in relieving mild to moderate pain for 3 to 4 hours. Larger doses may prolong the period of analgesia, but they do not increase the analgesic effect. Codeine is frequently combined with aspirin or acetaminophen which significantly increases the analgesic effect. Codeine is the least expensive of the narcotic analgesics. Because it produces very little euphoria it is less likely than other narcotics to be addicting. However, prolonged use often causes constipation. Nausea and vomiting occurring with codeine and other narcotics are caused both by a local irritating effect on gastric mucosa and central stimulation of the vomiting center. Thus, parenteral administration of a narcotic is just as likely as oral administration to cause nausea and vomiting in a susceptible patient. Patients experiencing this untoward effect with one narcotic are as liable to experience it with all other narcotics.

Other narcotic analgesics are available for oral administration. Meperidine (Demerol) and morphine are poorly or unpredictably absorbed from gastric mucosa and are not often used for pain relief in outpatients. Hydromorphone (Dilaudid), oxymorphone (Numorphan), and oxycodone (Percodan) produce good analgesia when taken orally. Unfortunately, their ability to produce euphoria makes them popular among drug abusers, and their use in outpatients should be limited to brief periods for severe pain only.

Propoxyphene (Darvon, Dolene) was developed as a mild analgesic which was thought to be nonaddictive. Unfortunately, its effectiveness is little better than aspirin or acetaminophen, and it has produced addiction with chronic use.

Pentazocine (Talwin) is a weak narcotic antagonist, but has good analgesic properties. It is available alone or in combination with aspirin for oral use, but nausea and vomiting are extremely common. Chronic use is also capable of causing addiction.

Intramuscular or intravenous administration of narcotics for postoperative pain relief following outpatient dental procedures is seldom indicated. Patients undergoing traumatic or extensive procedures which cause severe pain probably should be hospitalized where parenteral administration is routinely available. Parenterally administered narcotics are more liable to produce hypotension, particularly with postural changes. Persistent nausea and vomiting may result, a distinct liability in an outpatient who expects to be fully ambulatory shortly after recovery from a dental procedure. It is thought that the incidence of hypotension and respi-

Table 14.1.
Analgesic Equivalents

Drug	Dose	
	Oral	Intra-muscular
	mg	*mg*
Alphaprodine (Nisentil)		30
Codeine	60	65
Diamorphine (heroin)		3.0
Fentanyl		0.1
Hydromorphone (Dilaudid)	1	1.5
Meperidine (Demerol)		100.0
Methadone (Dolophine)		8.0
Morphine		10.0
Oxycodone (Percodan)	5	
Oxymorphone (Numorphan)		1.5
Pentazocine (Talwin)	50	60.0

ratory depression is similar among the various narcotics when equipotent doses are given. However, if a parenteral narcotic analgesic is indicated for the dental outpatient, fentanyl (Sublimaze) may be the drug of choice. Fentanyl in a 0.05-mg dose has analgesic activity equivalent to meperidine, 50 mg, produces no significant hypotension or respiratory depression, and has a duration of activity of only 45 minutes, all distinct advantages in the recovering outpatient.

Use of narcotic antagonists is not recommended routinely, especially in outpatients. Their effect may end before the narcotic has been completely metabolized. If an outpatient is sent home after administration of a narcotic antagonist, respiratory depression may recur after the patient arrives at home and is unattended by skilled personnel. They have the disadvantage of terminating the analgesic effect, as well as the respiratory depression, produced by the narcotic. Narcotic antagonists, nalorphine (Nalline) and levallorphan (Lorfan), are also agonists and can cause respiratory depression. Naloxone (Narcan) is an N-allyl derivative of oxymorphone which has the advantage of not possessing agonist properties. Its duration of action is dose dependent, lasting 1 to 5 hours in doses of 0.2 to 0.6 mg intravenously. When given in the absence of a narcotic, it does not cause respiratory depression, pupillary constriction, or psychomimetic effects. The use of fentanyl with its shorter duration of action probably precludes the need for narcotic antagonists in outpatients unless dose miscalculation results in acute severe respiratory depression during anesthesia.

PROLONGED REGIONAL BLOCK ANESTHESIA

The use of regional block or infiltration anesthesia in combination with general anesthesia or sedation will produce a patient who recovers in a pain-free state. Patients who undergo traumatic surgical procedures such as excision of deeply impacted teeth, repair of facial fractures, wide excision of malignant tumors, or osteotomies of the maxilla or mandible often awaken from anesthesia with severe pain requiring heavy and frequent doses of narcotics for relief. Such doses may cause respiratory and cardiovascular depression, nausea, and vomiting. Lidocaine (Xylocaine) or mepivacaine (Carbocaine) combined with adrenaline provides up to 2 hours of analgesia when injected into the operative site or for regional nerve block. However, the combination of tetracaine (Pontocaine) 0.15 per cent, dextran 6 per cent, and adrenaline 1:200,000 or bupivacaine (Marcaine), 0.25 to 0.75 per cent, when administered for regional nerve blocks, produces up to 13 hours of postoperative analgesia. Such patients are alert, comfortable, able to cough, deep breathe, and ambulate, and do not experience the nausea or respiratory and cardiovascular depression associated with narcotic analgesia.

Bibliography

Allen GD, Everett GB: Postanesthetic complications after inpatient general anesthesia for odontectomy: report of case. *J Oral Surg* 30:433, 1972.

Allen GD, Meyer RA: An evaluation of the analgesic activity of meperidine and fentanyl. *Anesth Progr* 20:72, 1973.

Allen GD, Tolas AG: Assessment of recovery by means of the Phystester: preliminary report. *J Oral Surg* 31:592, 1973.

Beecher HK: The powerful placebo. *JAMA* 159:1602, 1955.

Brock RC: Studies in lung abscess. *Guy's Hosp Rep* 96:141, 1947.

Cooper SA, Beaver WT: A model to evaluate mild analgesics in oral surgery outpatients. *Clin Pharmacol Ther* 20:241, 1976.

Cooper SA, et al: Comparative analgesia potency of aspirin and ibuprofen. *J Oral Surg* 35:898, 1977.

Egbert LD, et al: Reduction of postoperative pain by encouragement and instruction of patients: a study of doctor-patient rapport. *N Engl J Med* 270:825, 1964.

Fink BB: Diffusion anoxia. *Anesthesiology* 16:511, 1955.

Greenfield W, Granada MG: The use of a narcotic antagonist in the anesthetic management of the ambulatory oral surgery patients. *J Oral Surg* 32:760, 1974.

Jaffe J, Bender MB: Perceptual patterns during recovery from general anesthesia. *J Neurol Neurosurg Psychiatr* 14:316, 1951.

Koch-Weser J: Acetaminophen (medical intelligence). *N Engl J Med* 295:1297, 1976.

Lasagna L: The clinical evaluation of morphine and its substitutes as analgesics. *Pharmacol Rev* 16:47, 1964.

Laskin JL, et al: Use of bupivacaine hydrochloride in oral surgery—a clinical study. *J Oral Surg* 35:25, 1977.

Meyer RA: Blood volume considerations in oral surgery. *J Oral Surg* 29:617, 1971.

Meyer RA, Chinn MA: Prolonged postoperative analgesia with regional nerve blocks following oral surgery. *J Oral Surg* 26:1821, 1968.

Riding JE: Postoperative vomiting. *Proc R Soc Med* 53:671, 1960.

Smith JD, et al: A comparison of visual and auditory assessments of recovery from general anesthesia. *Oral Surg* 23:596, 1967.

Trieger N, et al: An objective measure of recovery. *Anesth Progr* 16:4, 1969.

Trieger N, Rubinstein S: The current status of halothane. *J Oral Surg* 31:595, 1973.

Tyrrell MF, Feldman SA: Headache following halothane anesthesia. *Br J Anaesth* 40:99, 1968.

Vandam LD: Clinical pharmacology of the narcotic analgesics. *Clin Pharmacol Ther* 3:827, 1962.

Walker DG: Prevention and treatment of postoperative pulmonary complications. *J Oral Surg* 30:813, 1972.

Weil TM: Fever and postoperative patient. *J Oral Surg* 31:201, 1973.

CHAPTER 15

Selection of Pain Control Modality

The selection of any pain control modality assumes that the practitioner has available a complete armamentarium of pain and anxiety control methods. These might range from psychological measures through local anesthesia to general anesthesia. The selection of the technique is dependent upon the patient's medical and dental condition. If general anesthesia is considered necessary to perform good dentistry, then as for any other surgical procedure, it is an important health consideration. If the practitioner is limited in his scope of pain control to a single technique, then numerous failures will occur, and the desired level of pain control will not be individually achieved (Fig. 15.1).

A frequent problem that arises is inability to achieve satisfactory local anesthesia together with conscious sedation. Under these circumstances it is tempting to expand conscious sedation by combinations of local anesthesia, inhalation sedation, and intravenous sedation that may be general anesthesia. There is a wide margin of safety between conscious sedation and general anesthesia. However, this margin is breached by the introduction of combination techniques to which euphemistic descriptions are attached, indicating a level of anesthesia which is less than general anesthesia. Until such time as separation of these levels has been scientifically defined, general anesthesia is best left to be administered by those with complete training in general anesthesia. If general anesthesia is indicated, the facility should be the equal of any available for anesthesia regardless of location and the surgical requirement should be met

with a minimum of medication. In many instances the team approach provides an excellent method of caring for the dental patient.

The importance of psychological measures in pediatric pain control cannot be overemphasized, in particular, attention to the parent. The presence or absence of a parent can often determine the outcome of the induction of any form of pain control. Communication is an important part of patient care, and nowhere more evident than in the pediatric patient.

OPERATIVE FEATURES IN SELECTION OF PAIN CONTROL MODALITY

Unfortunately, hospital dentistry, with the availability of good general anesthesia, has not expanded to the level of need. Thus, the dentist is often limited in his choice of pain control techniques. It is better to abandon any particular treatment than to endeavor to expand the pain control techniques beyond the limits of training.

Operative Requirements

The purpose of pain control is to provide surgical access. The surgical necessity may dictate which technique will be chosen to allow the surgery to be performed with a minimum of trauma and in the shortest time.

ORAL AND MAXILLOFACIAL SURGERY

A prolonged procedure or if there will be extensive bone trauma will require a

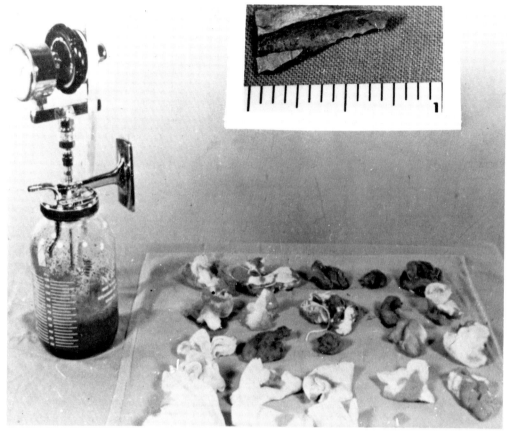

Figure 15.1. It is not always possible to predict the problems which may occur during surgery, and selection of techniques may ultimately prove to be in error. This blood loss occurred in a vestibuloplasty which was performed on an outpatient. The anesthesia was administered by nasal mask and lasted 2 hours, 20 minutes. The fragments of denture were found at laryngoscopy when the operation was concluded.

profound sedative technique. Extensive surgical incisions and the possibility of postoperative hemorrhage and multiple sutures may require careful postoperative supervision. If epinephrine is the vasoconstrictor then reactionary hemorrhage is possible up to 48 hours postoperatively.

Deliberate hypotension may be essential in maxillofacial operations to allow a successful surgical outcome. Surgical exposure is an essential requirement in many cases.

It is considered that direct monitoring of arterial blood pressure is essential below 80 mm Hg, and maintenance of a pressure below this can result in impairment of kidney function.

In the majority of instances general anesthesia is indicated. An anesthesiologist familiar with the techniques of oral and maxillofacial surgery will provide more satisfactory anesthesia than the occasional anesthetist. It is possible to perform many major oral surgery techniques with conscious sedation in combination with local anesthesia, but is limited by the trauma and duration. An operating table is uncomfortable for periods in excess of 1 hour.

With intermaxillary fixation postoperative vomiting should be avoided. The techniques followed must prevent carbon dioxide accumulation, a major facor in postoperative vomiting. Antiemitic agents have not proven totally effective but premedication with antiemetic agents should be considered. Induction of anesthesia with thiopental and maintenance with nitrous oxide-oxygen relaxant or nitrous oxide-oxygen with enflurane or isoflurane is probably best and will allow liberal use of locally injected epinephrine for vasconstriction. A nasogastric tube placed during the operative procedure will prevent accumulation of secretions in the stomach. Postoperative pain relief with narcotics should be combined with an antiemetic agent.

Neuroleptanesthesia is an alternative technique for this form of surgery as vomiting is negligible. However, the psychological problems and irrational behavior with droperidol must be considered. Postoperative ventilation must be carefully observed.

EXODONTURE

A majority of exodonture cases can be performed with safety by any of the techniques suggested. The brevity of the procedure will decrease the risk. It is important to ensure that foreign bodies do not enter the airway as there are many reports of foreign material entering the airway with local anesthesia unsupplemented by any form of sedation. A pharyngeal pack with radioopaque marker is recommended to conform with legal requirements.

RESTORATIVE DENTISTRY

Ideally this type of case can be performed with conscious sedation in combination with local anesthesia. The need for repeat visits may suggest that a general anesthetic technique be used to perform the restorative work in one session. Fragments of tooth or foreign material may enter the airway, and the placement of a prosthesis under anesthesia can be a hazard in the recovery period if it becomes dislodged and enters the airway. Two lim-

iting factors to be considered in duration of operation are that microscopic trauma can be detected following endotracheal intubation of 2 hours; macroscopic trauma is evident after 6 hours. The need for catheterization of a full bladder will be evident in an operative procedure of 4 to 6 hours. In small children where movement of an oral endotracheal tube could be a hazard, it is probably better to limit the operation to 2 hours. If a nasal endotracheal tube is used, perhaps 6 hours is a maximum (Fig. 15.2). It is doubtful if several short anesthetic procedures are less of a hazard, particularly with the availabilty of expert recovery facilities. However, the psychological and the financial status of the patient will be major considerations.

PEDIATRIC DENTISTRY

The problems in pediatric dentistry are the small airway in a small operative field, in addition to achieving psychological support. When the child is between 2 and 5 years of age, conscious sedation frequently fails, and to rely on communication with a child who is frightened and drugged is a tenuous concept. If conscious sedation cannot be achieved, then it is best to use general anesthesia and this necessitates a separate anesthetist. A technique to consider is ketamine in either subanesthetic or anesthetic doses. The airway is not guaranteed, but provided the airway is safeguarded, then intramuscular ketamine might avoid the hazards of endotracheal intubation.

The blood volume of the pediatric patient is small and in combination with a relative anemia and high metabolic rate reduces the margin of safety for anesthesia. The requirements of anesthesia and total patient care under such circumstances outweigh the surgical requirement. The object is to achieve maximum dental care within an acceptable time limit, even though the quality of dentistry may be compromised.

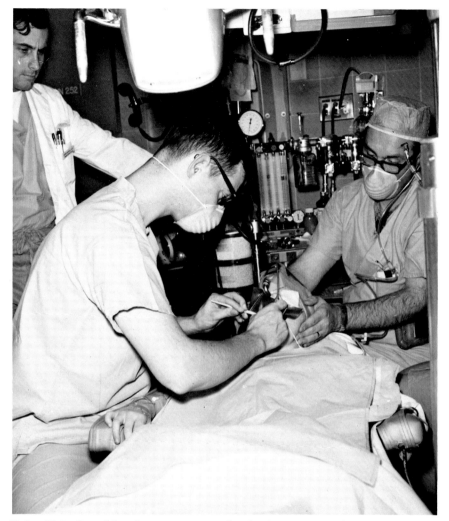

Figure 15.2. Distortion of the airway may occur despite the presence of an endotracheal tube. The operator's arm does not press on the chest of the patient.

Duration

The length of time for operative procedures with conscious sedation has not been delineated. Patient stress should be considered in sessions in excess of 4 hours. The use of conscious sedation expands the possibility of dentistry at one session. The limiting factor may be the ability of the dentist to perform adequately for prolonged periods.

In general anesthetic techniques there are guidelines which could be followed providing for the safety of the patient. The

skill, facilities, and experience of the individual operator provide unique variations in the time schedule. Thus for outpatient office anesthesia, the maximum duration should be 20 minutes.

For outpatient hospital practice, the duration should be less than 40 minutes. The surgical facilities are comparable but the margin of safety is increased because of the available facilities for resuscitation and outpatient recovery.

For procedures in excess of 60 minutes the hospital setting is probably best. Prolonged anesthesia usually requires endotracheal anesthesia. The possibility of irritation of the larynx during prolonged operations with subsequent postoperative laryngeal edema is a hazard. The simplest method of ensuring that undetected postoperative problems do not arise is for the patient to be admitted to the hospital following surgery and kept under continuous supervision overnight (Fig. 15.3).

It is possible to provide outpatient general anesthesia with endotracheal intubation, and not admit the patient to the hospital. Under these circumstances the anesthetist must ensure that a responsible adult is able to supervise the postoperative welfare of the patient. In addition it is important to explain the problems that could arise to the guardian, and to provide the patient with a written statement of the procedure. The occurrence of any untoward event during the anesthesia would indicate admission to the hospital for observation.

Many of the problems of prolonged anesthesia can be related to the time for which the patient is removed from a normal environment. Hypoglycemia, renal function, retention of water and sodium, metabolic acidosis, and potassium loss can be altered by the duration of the anesthe-

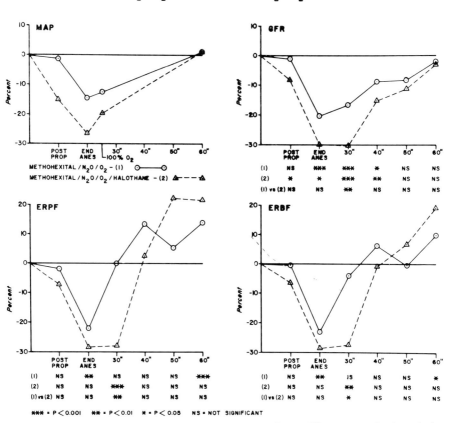

Figure 15.3. The renal effects and mean arterial pressure of two different anesthetic techniques are shown. The study demonstrated the difference between brief anesthesia and that lasting over an hour. In short anesthetics, the renal effects parallel only those of the blood pressure, whereas in prolonged anesthesia, there are increases in efferent arteriolar vasoconstriction further decreasing effective renal plasma flow and increasing glomerular filtration.

sia. The changes in respiratory pattern together with loss of humidity can result in miliary atalectasis, a common accompaniment of prolonged anesthesia. Changes in the immune response of white cells are noted with anesthesia, the degree being related to duration of exposure.

Facilities

It is imperative that all the necessary facilities for patient care should be available in the office. These facilities should conform to minimal standards to allow emergency treatment of patients. They are unrelated to the form of pain control chosen, but rather predicated upon the fact that the patient is under the care of a doctor. Thus oxygen, a means for its delivery, and emergency medical drugs must be available in the office, regardless of the pain control modality.

General anesthesia requires facilities which are the equal of those available in hospital practice. Thus, oxygen, anesthetic machine, intravenous equipment and drugs, monitors, and resuscitative equipment including laryngoscope and ECG defibrillator are required (Fig. 15.4).

The number of trained personnel needed depends on the type of pain control modality. The operator performing local anesthesia alone will probably manage with a single assistant. If conscious sedation is performed, a single assistant and a circulator would be needed. If in-

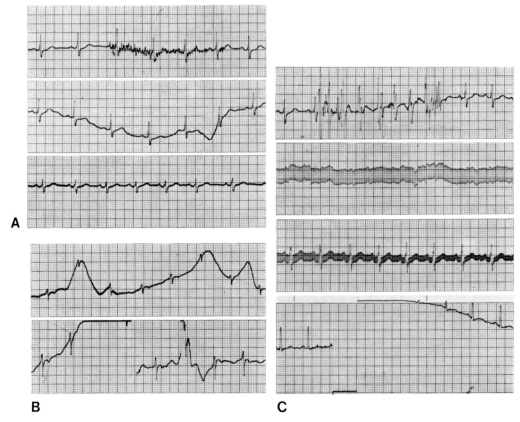

Figure 15.4. When using ECG monitors for outpatient anesthesia an understanding of their deficiencies is essential. *A*: involuntary movement (I), voluntary movement (II), poor skin prep (III); *B*: loose electrode (I), dried out electrode (II); *C*: poor connection (I), broken lead wire (II), bad ground (III), static electricity (VI). (Courtesy Graphic Controls Corporation, Buffalo, N.Y.)

travenous conscious sedation is used, consideration of the use of a separate assistant to monitor respiration should be given. The absence of the reservoir bag as a monitor of respiration adds an additional hazard to intravenous conscious sedation. Three assistants plus the operator, who may or may not be in charge of the anesthesia, should be in the room when general anesthesia is administered.

THE UNIQUE PATIENT

While each patient is unique, with an individual response to medication, certain groups present common problems (Fig. 15.5).

Extreme Anxiety

For this group, pain control usually requires chemical sedation, be it inhalation or intravenous. There are many for whom

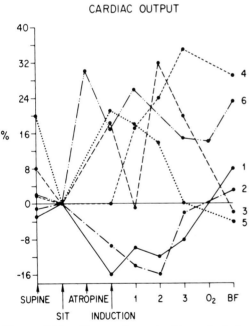

CARDIAC OUTPUT

Figure 15.5. The cardiac output in a single individual subject to six different techniques of pain control illustrate the wide variety of effects following such treatments: *1*, nitrous oxide; *2*, methoxyflurane-oxygen; *3*, the Jorgensen technique; *4*, diazepam, 10 mg; *5*, methohexital, 1 mg per kg; *6*, halothane, nitrous oxide-oxygen following atropine, 0.4 mg, and thiopental, 3 mg per kg.

intravenous induction is essential; inhalation techniques require patient cooperation.

General anesthesia with intravenous induction may be indicated. Excess salivation is common, and the preoperative placement of a bite block further increases salivation. Anticholinergics are indicated to diminish the possibility of laryngeal spasm subsequent to a barbiturate induction. The bite block should be placed either after induction or during administration of the intravenous medication.

Elderly Patient

Incidental disease is more common and therefore more potential problems exist. Nitrous oxide-oxygen conscious sedation will provide oxygen supplementation, and elevation of the oxygen tension is a useful additional safety feature. Many of these patients suffer with hypertension, a disease in which there is a labile blood pressure and any form of sedation is useful in stabilizing the blood pressure.

The administration of general anesthesia in the office could be hazardous. The potential benefits of admission to the hospital should be considered for the elderly, as there may be little financial penalty. The decreased emotional tone may be of great benefit in reducing the anesthetic requirement.

There is an increased cardiovascular hazard, a low blood volume, a depressed cough reflex, and a stiff chest. As there is already decreased cerebral oxygenation, any untoward incident during anesthesia can further compromise cerebral function. Age alone is a factor, but an assessment of physiological aging should be made. If the above factors indicate potential problems during anesthesia, then inpatient anesthesia is warranted.

Pediatric

In children supplementation of local anesthesia with some form of conscious sedation is imperative. Psychological support may be all that is required, but rarely can this be accomplished in a child who has suffered previous trauma. The desire to ensure a successful outcome results in the concept of extending analgesia, particularly nitrous oxide, by decreasing the oxygen concentration. It is a hazard.

Children are emotionally labile with an increased metabolism, and there is an absolute and relative need for increased anesthesia. Although the margins of safety are greater, there are still hazards in that immature enzyme systems can result in prolonged apnea with muscle relaxants.

Because of increased metabolism, temperature changes are more common in the child. For general anesthesia constant temperature monitoring is essential and consideration should be given to regulation of the ambient temperature. Inhalation of dried gases can result in water loss throughout the procedure. In combination with atropine, hyperpyrexia may proceed to convulsions. The high mortality rate necessitates prompt treatment with oxygen and diazepam. Malignant hyperpyrexia should be treated promptly by appropriate measures.

In pediatric anesthesia postoperative airway problems are common. The larynx is narrowest in the area of the cricoid ring, and unique pediatric equipment is an essential.

Movement of the oral endotracheal tube is a problem. Passage of the nasotracheal tube through infected adenoidal tissue can frequently cause serious bacteremia.

There are advantages in children of selecting outpatient anesthesia, ranging from improvement in psychological attitudes to a decreased chance of cross-infection.

Patient Sex

A chaperone is essential for all female patients under conscious sedation. Operation on a pregnant woman should be deferred to the second trimester, in order to secure the pregnancy. In the first trimester, the stress of anesthesia can produce an abortion, and in the last trimester anesthesia or sedation could induce premature labor. Any drug administered in the first trimester could be implicated in the production of teratogenetic effects.

Emergency Procedures

Conscious sedation is useful, as psychological means of producing relaxation are less successful with an unfamiliar patient. The use of general anesthesia requires at least 4 hours of fasting. This does not preclude the possibility of vomiting, but allows normal stomach emptying and attention to the hazard. The possibilities of silent regurgitation must always be considered, and the use of an inhalation technique is preferable. The semi-supine position tends to minimize silent regurgitation.

Administration of general anesthesia immediately following a failed local anesthetic should be discouraged. The production of excess endogenous catecholamines together with the epinephrine of the local anesthetic can sensitize the myocardium to arrhythmias. Operation should be deferred.

METHODS OF PAIN CONTROL

The individual response of the patient determines the effect of any pain control technique. Maintenance of peripheral resistance is significant in the response of the patient to subsequent stress; the 22 per cent fall in peripheral resistance following epinephrine is noteworthy. Major changes in peripheral resistance follow halothane and methohexital. Changes in blood pressure are minimal. Falls in oxygen tension occur with methohexital. Elevations of cardiac output follow atropine.

Psychological Methods

The use of psychology and hypnosis forms a part of every operator's armamentarium. It may not be a deliberate technique, but the approach to the patient is predicated upon a desire to reduce the degree of anxiety in the patient and achieve some measure of pain control. If hypnosis is possible, and it can be rapidly induced, then this may well be the safest form of pain control available. Inhalation sedation may be used to speed induction.

The reason for not using psychological techniques is due to their uncertainty of action and the need to expedite the operation. However, psychological support considerably reduces the need for chemical sedation, and should be used on every occasion.

Local Anesthesia

Local anesthesia is an essential part of all forms of conscious sedation. Local anesthesia supplementation is considered by many as an essential component of general anesthesia as it decreases the noci-ceptive reflexes. There are obvious benefits of local anesthesia as postoperative pain is reduced and awakening is more comfortable. There is a risk with local anesthesia, as Malmin indicates. In 1977 five children died in California from overdose of local anesthetic. The use of an aspirating syringe and a maximum dose based on weight, not number of cartridges, reduces the risk.

It has been recommended that 200 μg of epinephrine can be administered to patients with cardiovascular disease. Recent studies indicate major cardiovascular changes with amounts of epinephrine as small as 20 μg. The cardiovascular changes increase in parallel with the dose of epinephrine administered, while the central β stimulation persists for 90 minutes, and the peripheral α effect for 120 minutes. This imbalance occurs during the period when the patient is leaving the office (Fig. 15.6).

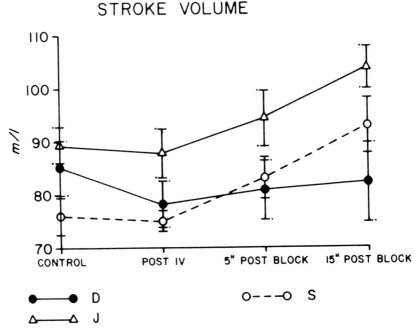

Figure 15.6. The stroke volume is noted after three different sedation techniques. In the D technique diazepam, 0.15 mg per kg, followed by 1.8 ml of 2 per cent lidocaine was used. In the J, (Jorgensen) technique and in the S (Shane) technique, 2 per cent lidocaine with 18 μg of epinephrine followed the intravenous medication. The increase in stroke volume was approximately 25 per cent following this small dose of epinephrine. (Reprinted with permission from Allen, G. D., Everett, G. B., Forsyth, W. D., and Kennedy, W. F.: The cardiorespiratory effects of epinephrine and local anesthetics for dentistry. *Anesth Prog* 20:152, 1973.)

The American Dental Association and the American Heart Association in 1966 indicated that the endogenous effects of epinephrine were greater than the effects of exogenous epinephrine. There is no support by recent research for this concept. The study by Tolas confirms the elevation of circulating epinephrine due to exogenous sources and not as a consequence of stress.

Oral Medications

Uncertain in absorption, and unpredictable in effect, the advantage of the oral technique is simplicity of administration. The technique will fail in 50 per cent of patients, and regurgitation is an ever-present hazard. Hydroxyzine and pentobarbital elixir are frequently prescribed and their efficacy would appear to be parallel. They may be of value in reducing nausea in some patients in whom a subsequently administered narcotic is to be given. The oral medication of choice is alcohol. Alcohol is absorbed from the stomach, its onset in 20 minutes is more certain, and it has stood the test of time as a reliable hypnotic in the correct dose, 3 oz of 80 proof alcohol being recommended for the adult. Hypoglycemia can occur in response to alcohol in children.

A most significant aspect of oral premedication is the responsibility of administering the oral agent prior to the arrival of the patient at the office. Any untoward response will be the responsibility of the prescribing dentist. The drugs may also be administered in suppository form, and promethazine, 25 mg, is commonly used.

Intramuscular and Subcutaneous Techniques

Intramuscular injection of a drug should always be preferred to subcutaneous injection. The better blood supply to the muscle ensures a more satisfactory uptake. Injections into the deltoid produce a more rapid response than injections into the lower limbs. However, the muscle bulk of the deltoid is much less than the lower limb and injection can damage the circumflex nerve. The gluteal region can be hazardous, as drugs can track down between the muscle layers and damage the sciatic nerve. The anterolateral aspect of the thigh is the preferred site. In an emergency an injection into the tongue will produce almost as rapid a response as injection into a vein.

Intramuscular techniques are unsatisfactory, as the drug is given in bolus form, not to a baseline but to produce a predetermined response based on weight. Excessive dosage and delay in recovery are problems with intramuscular techniques. The technique of injecting narcotics into the buccal mucosa should be noted as injection of alphaprodine in this area produced blood levels comparable to intravenous administration. Simultaneous injection of promethazine into the buccal mucosa will produce tissue necrosis and is contraindicated.

Inhalation Analgesia

Nitrous oxide-oxygen inhalation analgesia forms the basis of conscious sedation techniques. The use of inhalation techniques provide a source of oxygen in case of emergency and to supplement inhalation of air when intravenous techniques are used. A nitrous oxide-oxygen inhalation sedation machine should be available in all dental offices where pain control is practiced. The homeostatic mechanisms of the body are largely improved by the inhalation of nitrous oxide-oxygen, and the use of nitrous oxide-oxygen for compromised cardiovascular patients has been promoted. Many studies have been performed evaluating the efficacy of nitrous oxide-oxygen for analgesia in coronary patients and indicate the safety of the technique. Nitrous oxide does not directly depress left ventricular performance in normal subjects, but there are slight changes in blood pressure and heart rate with analgesic levels of nitrous oxide. There is a dose-related response to the level of nitrous oxide. Changes in blood pressure are probably due to reductions in systolic blood pressure and suggests that nitrous oxide has significant effects on the peripheral vasculature. It suggests that nitrous oxide reduces aortic impedance to a greater extent than peripheral vascular resistance. It would appear that nitrous oxide reduces the cardiac afterload, the systolic pressure, without concomitantly reducing coronary perfusion pressure, diastolic blood pressure. Nitrous oxide-oxygen provides a relaxed comfortable patient capable and willing to accept extended treatment with the assurance of a pleasant dental experience. It provides an easily controllable level of sedation with rapid reversal of effects. While the sedation is not as profound as that with intravenous techniques, the essential safety feature of easy reversibility makes this a technique applicable to nearly all dental procedures except those requiring profound sedation.

The volatile analgesic agent methoxyflurane can add a further dimension to inhalation analgesia, provided accurate vaporizers are utilized. It is a profound analgesia expanding the technique to allow operation without local anesthesia. The other advantage is that methoxyflurane can be given with 100 per cent oxygen.

Intravenous Sedation

The use of the intravenous route for sedation provides a controllable means for relief of anxiety in the dental patient. Provided the injection is given slowly, it is possible to achieve a baseline to a definite end point; oversedation should not occur. Sedation is usually more profound than with inhalation techniques, although reversal cannot be readily accomplished. A major disadvantage of the intravenous technique is the delay in recovery in many patients, and therefore intravenous techniques are usually chosen for more prolonged procedures.

The techniques can range from single drug usage to polypharmacy. Simple sedation can be provided by the use of an intravenously administered barbiturate, though antianalgesia has been demonstrated with these drugs.

Diazepam (Valium) administered intravenously is useful and has a brevity of action which makes it particularly suitable for oral surgery. Sedation and amnesia for up to 30 to 45 minutes have been demonstrated. The amnesia is most profound between 5 and 15 minutes, and the local anesthetic should be given at this time. Note that intramuscular diazepam does not produce effective sedation or amnesia. The drug should be administered either intravenously or orally (Fig. 15.7).

The safest intravenous technique available is a combination of drugs as developed by Jorgensen, utilizing pentobarbital, meperidine, and scopolamine. It is a technique employing multiple drugs yet acceptable to produce suppression of anxiety and apprehension. Cardiovascular upset is minimal, though little analgesia is noted. Local anesthesia is an essential part of this technique. There are many variations on the Jorgensen technique. The principal object is the titration of an initially administered drug to produce definite clinical signs as a baseline for relief of anxiety. At this end point a further dose of narcotic is given not to produce analgesia but to increase euphoria.

Another technique suggested is the Shane technique, using alphaprodine, hydroxyzine, and atropine with subsequently administered methohexital. It provides analgesia with profound sedation. Studies indicate that cardiovascular depression is a significant feature of this technique and it should not be used in any but the most healthy patients (Fig. 15.8).

There are numerous other techniques utilizing such agents as phenergan, meperidine, alphaprodine, fentanyl, and diazepam singly and in various combinations. The evidence would indicate that in the presence of a narcotic, aspiration of

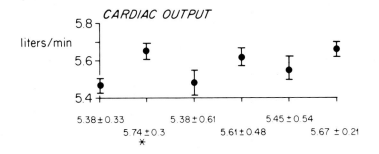

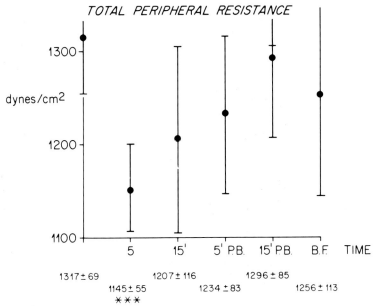

Figure 15.7. The cardiac output and total peripheral resistance changes seen after diazepam, 0.15 mg per kg, and a mandibular block with 1.8 ml of 2 per cent lidocaine are shown. The fall in total peripheral resistance at 5 minutes is noteworthy. (Reprinted with permission from Allen, G. D., Everett, G. B., and Butler, L. A.: Human cardiorespiratory and analgesic effects of intravenous diazepam and local anesthesia. *J Am Dent Assoc* 92:744, 1976.)

saliva or regurgitated stomach contents is an ever-present hazard, and respiratory depression can occur. Oxygen should be available.

Monitoring of respiration is essential. Several recent fatalities have been due to unnoticed respiratory failure following intravenous techniques.

Alternatives to General Anesthesia

Inability to achieve satisfactory operating conditions with conscious sedation has led to a search for alternate means of patient care without a separate anesthe-siologist. The desire to avoid a separate anesthetist is not only economic but due to a shortage of personnel adequately trained to administer the techniques. Nothing can replace the skilled person in patient care, and thus many of the alternatives may be more hazardous than general anesthesia. Many anesthetists consider that endotracheal general anesthesia is the most satisfactory way of managing compromised patients. Alternatives with their potential for inadequate operating conditions and subsequent attempts to expand the alternative are much more

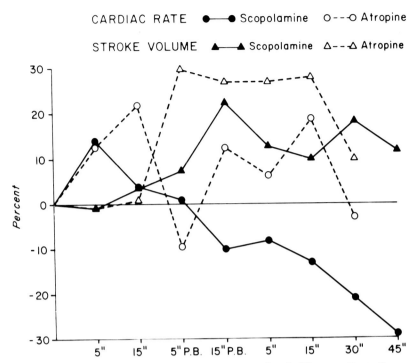

Figure 15.8. In the Shane technique, note should be made of different effects if scopolamine or atropine is used. A profound secondary bradycardia results with scopolamine and lowers cardiac output.

hazardous than a prepared general anesthetic in which a skilled person is solely responsible for the sedation (Fig. 15.9).

The alternatives to general anesthesia presuppose that the dentist performing such alternatives will have the necessary skills to perform competent cardiopulmonary resuscitation and have all the necessary equipment for general anesthesia, as the alternatives can easily become general anesthesia. The techniques described are all intravenous, though in many instances supplementation with inhalation agents such as nitrous oxide-oxygen is used. Supplementation with nitrous oxide-oxygen is a safety feature in that there is visual monitoring of respiration, and increases in the oxygen administered to the patient can overcome the falls in oxygen tension which occur due to respiratory depression. Elevation of carbon dioxide, while in themselves nonphysiological, are not contraindications to a technique. It is fashionable to consider that these techniques are not general an-

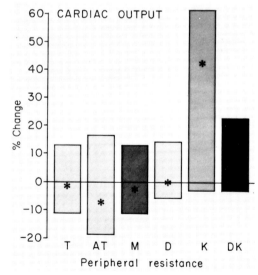

Figure 15.9. The cardiovascular effects of a single dose of intravenous anesthetic are shown. *, changes in blood pressure. The changes noted are the following: T, thiopental, 3 mg per kg; AT, thiopental, 3 mg per kg following atropine, 0.4 mg; M, methohexital, 1 mg per kg; D, diazepam, 0.4 mg per kg; K, ketamine, 2.2 mg per kg; and DK, ketamine, 2.2 mg per kg following diazepam, 0.15 mg per kg.

esthesia. This has not been demonstrated, and it is incumbent upon the users of these techniques to demonstrate scientifically that this is a safe technique and not general anesthesia with all the concomitant hazards.

METHOHEXITAL

The use of methohexital for intravenous anesthesia has developed because of its brevity of action as compared to thiopental. The techniques described initially used thiopental, and either of the agents used properly will produce the satisfactory level of what is considered ultralight anesthesia, wherein the patient is considered to be within 10 mg of methohexital away from being fully awake. The technique is described as ultralight anesthesia or the minimal increment technique by the Society for the Advancement of Anaesthesia in Dentistry (SAAD). Clinically there is a state of amnesia produced by minimal doses of methohexital, supplemented with or without nitrous oxide-oxygen, which is not general anesthesia. The patient moves in response to stimu-

lation and would appear to be in stage 2 of the Guedel classification but vomiting is not present because an intravenous agent is used. Nonetheless studies indicate the hazard of laryngeal soiling with methohexital as the sole agent for dental anesthesia. The Trendelenburg position appears less advantageous than the semi-supine position for dentistry, in view of the hazards of silent regurgitation and the cardiorespiratory advantages of the semi-supine position (Table 15.1). Review of Intravenous Anesthaesia SAAD indicates that the minimal increment technique is not applicable to the type of dentistry performed in many centers in the United States. In a study of the technique it was found that the dose required for placement of a rubber dam was often in excess of that required for a definitive procedure performed by the SAAD group.

It must be emphasized that the methohexital technique has a good safety record. It remains, however, to be scientifically shown as a unique form of anesthesia, which can be distinguished from general anesthesia (Fig. 15.10).

Table 15.1
The Advantages and Disadvantages Attributed to the Trendelenburg and Semisupine Positions are Compared

	COMPARATIVE ADVANTAGES AND DISADVANTAGES	
	ADVANTAGES	DISADVANTAGES
SEMISUPINE POSITION	15% improved respiratory efficiency. Easier to maintain airway and, therefore, decreased incidence of endotracheal intubation with inherent risks. Decreased incidence of silent regurgitation.	Increased incidence of inhalation of foreign material once it enters the pharynx. Decreased venous return. Increased danger of sequelae from vasovagal phenomenon because of decreased venous return.
TRENDELENBURG POSITION	Increased venous return. Decreased incidence of danger from vasovagal faint. Decreased possibility of aspiration of foreign debris because of "sump" configuration.	14.5% reduction in vital capacity because of impaired diaphragmatic excursion and restricted volumetric lung expansion secondary to increased pulmonary blood volume. Increased possibility of aspiration secondary to increased incidence of regurgitation. Difficult to maintain the airway in absence of endotracheal intubation.

NEUROLEPTANALGESIA

The combination of fentanyl with droperidol used in neuroleptanesthesia and analgesia is not recommended for outpatient use. It will supplement many inadequate regional blocks. The combination will produce profound analgesia and allow many operations to be performed. The duration of action of droperidol is 6 hours and has certain unique disadvantages in that the patient feels remote with an increasing anxiety, even though no complaint is made. Respiratory arrest is an ever-present hazard, as supplementation with fentanyl will produce narcotic depression. For outpatient dental anesthesia half the dose of the mixture, 1 cc per 50 pounds of body weight, is given together with supplementary fentanyl.

It may have a role in outpatient oral surgery, where to achieve the depth of anesthesia by conventional methods would be hazardous. It may be indicated for the strong healthy man in whom anesthesia difficulties are anticipated. It must be stressed, however, that only someone who is fully capable of taking care of the airway and providing artificial ventilation of the patient should consider its use.

KETAMINE

Ketamine has been extensively investigated in inpatient hospital practice. The studies in dental anesthesia are not definitive. The delay in recovery of patients having received ketamine combined with the hypertensive response indicates it is not a satisfactory drug for outpatient anesthesia. The bizarre psychological problems encountered in some patients suggest it is better avoided in adults. Cardiovascular problems can in part be overcome by the prior administration of diazepam (Fig. 15.11).

It is possible to use analgesic doses of ketamine for pain control in children. In this instance a dose of 2 mg/kg intramus-

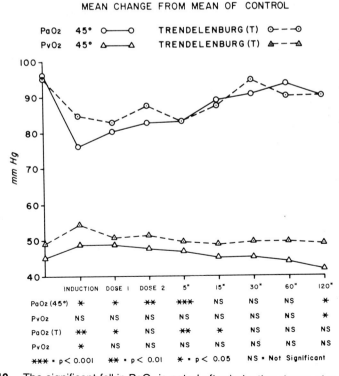

Figure 15.10. The significant fall in PaO_2 is noted after induction doses of methohexital.

cularly is given, which produces lack of response in the patient. Supplementary local anesthesia must then be administered. Recovery is still a problem.

The laryngeal reflexes are obtunded by anesthetic doses of ketamine, and no studies have been made as yet of the effects on the airway of these analgesic doses of ketamine.

OPIATES

Meperidine is the most commonly used narcotic for outpatient sedation in dentistry. The dose range from 50 to 100 mg in the adult is sufficiently wide to allow titration until development of a significant response. Hypotension and tachycardia are common side effects of meperidine, and it is not the drug of choice in the cardiac patient. Fentanyl, because of its duration of action of only 45 minutes, appears to be a more satisfactory drug. Euphoria is not evident unless combined with another hypnotic or tranquilizing drug.

CONCLUSION

Thus it is evident that with these techniques general anesthesia can supervene.

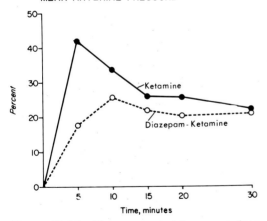

MEAN ARTERIAL PRESSURE

Figure 15.11. The mean arterial pressure rises following ketamine can be modified by diazepam, 0.15 mg per kg, 5 minutes before 2.2 mg per kg ketamine. (Reprinted with permission from Allen, G. D., Boas, R. A., and Everett, G. B.; Modification of cardiovascular effects of ketamine by diazepam. *Anesth Prog* 21:8–11, 1974.)

If the absence of protective reflexes is a measure of general anesthesia, then all of these drugs can produce, albeit only short-lived, a degree of general anesthesia.

Indications for General Anesthesia

The attempt to use general anesthesia when other forms of sedation fail is hazardous, but a planned general anesthetic is of minimal risk to the patient. Extreme anxiety may require general anesthesia, or the patient may have neurological deficits which prevent the patient from controlling movement. Major procedures are an indication for general anesthesia where prolonged operations are uncomfortable and stressful for the patient. Adverse reactions to local anesthesia or infection at the operative site may indicate the need for general anesthesia.

Cardiorespiratory disease can be an indication for general anesthesia as loss of airway even for a brief period can result in inadequate oxygenation.

A hemorrhagic diathesis can be a hazard with local anesthesia as the blind placement of a needle into tissue could result in the development of a hematoma at the site. Bleeding may be difficult to control whereas under general anesthesia careful hemostasis is possible. The use of an oral endotracheal tube in such patients can be relatively atraumatic.

Congenital abnormalities may necessitate general anesthesia, as anatomical distortion prevents satisfactory local anesthesia from being developed.

Balanced Anesthesia

The triad of balanced anesthesia is sedation, analgesia, and relaxation. The components are achieved in various ways, and each particular aspect can be stressed dependent upon the surgical requirement of a particular operation. Thus, during intra-abdominal operations, surgical relaxation is the prime requirement. During dental anesthesia, the prior requirement is analgesia. Maximal relaxation may be required for the placement of a nasoendotracheal tube or the mouth prop and thereafter relaxation is not required.

The individual activity of a drug should be considered, rather than the mass action of the majority of anesthetic or analgesic agents. Initially, nitrous oxide was used as a fully potent anesthetic agent. Using the McKesson secondary saturation technique, it was possible to achieve sedation, analgesia, and relaxation with nitrous oxide. The current use of nitrous oxide exemplifies the correct use of a drug where the nitrous oxide is used for analgesia and sedation, and relaxation is achieved by a muscle relaxant. The muscle relaxant-nitrous oxide techniques and the nitrous oxide-oxygen regional anesthetic techniques probably afford the best examples of balanced anesthesia. The safety records of these techniques appear to bear out their advantages.

PREMEDICATION

Classically, premedication was thought to reduce the amount of anesthetic agent required for production of anesthesia. Studies of minimum anesthetic concentration (MAC) have shown that the reduction of anesthetic requirement by opiate/anticholinergic premedication is minimal. The premedicant will produce preoperative sedation, but it will not significantly reduce the amount of total anesthetic required.

BARBITURATES

The barbiturates are used for induction of anesthesia. They do not produce anesthesia without the penalty of severe cardiorespiratory depression. They are antianalgesics and should be used only for sedation.

ANTICHOLINERGICS

Scopolamine will produce tranquilization and is the anticholinergic of choice if sedation is required. Glycopyrrolate has a significant advantage in that secretions are decreased without cardiovascular effects.

ATARACTICS

Can be used for sedation, but the intravenous use of hydroxyzine is limited due to thrombophlebitis.

DIAZEPAM (VALIUM)

Diazepam is an extremely useful drug for sedation because amnesia is total, and yet consciousness is not lost. It produces minimal cardiorespiratory depression. The effect on the cardiovascular system, however, is more prolonged than that produced by thiopental if used for induction of anesthesia (Fig. 15.12).

NITROUS OXIDE

Nitrous oxide is the classic agent used for production of analgesia. Studies of MAC have shown it to be an important part of all anesthetic combinations, allowing reduction in the requirement for more potent anesthetic agents. In modern anesthesia, nitrous oxide is used as a carrier gas and analgesic agent in all balanced anesthetic combinations. It produces analgesia with minimal cardiovascular de-

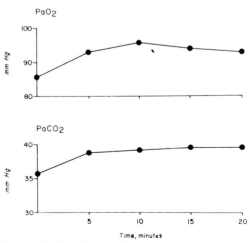

Figure 15.12. No significant respiratory depression is seen with diazepam.

pression. Although nitrous oxide added to anesthetic combinations produces cardiovascular depression, it is less than the cardiovascular depression caused by the more potent agent required to produce the same level of surgical anesthesia.

INTRAVENOUS NARCOTICS

Intravenous narcotics will produce satisfactory analgesia during dental anesthesia. The agent of choice would appear to be fentanyl, which has a duration of action of 45 minutes. Doses of 0.05 mg of fentanyl in dilute solution will not produce hypotension in the normal adult and, unless combined with other more potent anesthetic agents such as halothane or methoxyflurane, will not produce respiratory arrest. An intravenous narcotic should be given in a dilute solution in order that the dose may be titrated. Because the duration of action of morphine is 4 hours and meperidine 3 hours, their intravenous use is rarely indicated in dental anesthesia. On an equipotent basis, the cardiorespiratory depression produced by morphine is less than that produced by meperidine. Meperidine tends to produce hypotension, which is not a feature of intravenous morphine.

Non-narcotic analgesics used as alternatives, such as butorphenol (Stadol) and nalbuphine (Nubane) do not appear to offer any additional advantage.

GENERAL ANESTHETICS

Methoxyflurane, isoflurane, and enflurane have analgesic activities. Halothane is a poor analgesic agent. In selecting general anesthetics, attention should be paid to the possible toxic effects of these agents. As an example it is useful to avoid halothane in the alcoholic as liver disease and prior hepatitis are common.

LOCAL ANESTHETICS

The analgesia produced by local anesthesia is significant and is considered by many to reduce the need for inhalation agents. Studies do not confirm this; the significance of the analgesia is the postoperative pain relief rather than the current effect. Overdose with local anesthetic can occur, and the vasoconstrictor in the solution does have a systemic effect. The concept of harmful effects of nociceptive reflexes particularly in dentistry has not been demonstrated. Inhibition of local reflexes is a major factor in the production of relaxation.

Methoxyflurane, isoflurane, and enflurane are ethers and thus relaxation is good.

MUSCLE RELAXANTS

Muscle relaxants have no central anesthetic action. If patients are anesthetized with nitrous oxide-oxygen and a muscle relaxant, sedation may be minimal, and care must be taken that they do not recall the event. In outpatient dental anesthesia, succinylcholine is the agent of choice for its brevity of action. There have been reported cases of patients receiving succinylcholine who have developed prolonged apnea in an outpatient setting. Such an occurrence poses problems to the anesthetist not fully equipped to maintain ventilation. Gallamine can be used in the dental office, as its duration of action may only be 20 to 30 minutes. If the operative procedure is prolonged, the relaxation will diminish by the time the patient leaves the chair. An advantage of gallamine over succinylcholine is that neostigmine or tensilon can be used to reverse the muscle relaxation.

INTRA-ANESTHETIC HAZARDS

In selecting anesthetic agents the hazards of drug interaction must be considered.

Epinephrine

The halogenated hydrocarbons used in anesthesia—methoxyflurane, halothane, isoflurane, and enflurane—sensitize the myocardium to epinephrine. Enflurane sensitizes the myocardium least and is the agent of choice when using vasoconstrictors. Halothane has been studied by Katz, who indicated a dosage level of 100 μg of epinephrine in the first 10 minutes to a total of 300 μg in the first hour.

Succinylcholine

Pseudocholinesterase is part of the metabolic pathway for both succinylcholine and some of the local anesthetics. Thus local anesthetics can prolong the action of succinylcholine, a combination used frequently in dental anesthesia. The second dose of succinylcholine can produce bradycardia, leading to cardiac arrest. The use of intravenous atropine before the second dose of succinylcholine is recommended, but is not universally successful in the prevention of drug-induced arrest.

Digitalis

Intravenous digitalis during anesthesia, or prior to induction of ancsthcsia, can predispose to cardiac arrhythmias. The anesthetic most likely to cause these problems is halothane.

Atropine

Intravenous atropine in combination with halothane can produce dangerous cardiac irregularities. It should be used only when indicated and never indiscriminantly.

Analgesics

Anticholinesterases and the narcotic antagonists can prolong the action of analgesics. Severe respiratory depression can develop if anticholinesterases and antagonists are used in combination with narcotics.

Rectal Anesthesia

The most commonly used rectal anesthetic is thiopental. Made up as a paste by Abbott, the dose is 40 mg per kg of body weight. This is a smooth, safe way of inducing anesthesia in the child. The distraught child presented for restorative dentistry will often submit to placement of a rectal thermometer. It requires that the anesthetist stay with the patient from the time of the rectal insertion. The patient still needs an intravenous infusion and full anesthetic care. Induction can proceed with nitrous oxide-oxygen and a relaxant.

INFLUENCE OF DISEASE ON SELECTION

Those diseases which will influence the type of conscious sedation administered are noted. In relating disease and the selection of pain control modalities, the use of local anesthesia alone is not necessarily the technique of choice. Outpatient treatment should be considered prior to other modalities of care. Five per cent of patients admitted to the hospital contract infections, and in children particularly the hazards of cross-infection while in the hospital are significant. It has been estimated that 20 per cent of the patients while in the hospital develop iatrogenic disease. If dentistry can be performed on an outpatient basis, not only does it provide economic and psychological benefits, but there is a real protective aspect in limiting the incidence of cross-infection.

Cardiovascular Diseases

Cardiovascular disease is a universal problem. All patients admitted for outpatient anesthesia over the age of 45 years receive an electrocardiogram and chest X-ray as a routine hospital practice. The investigations are not confined to this group, but indicate the extent of potential cardiovascular problems. All patients presenting for dental care should have a blood pressure recording, as the incidence of hypertension in the population is significant. The pain control modality or surgery could precipitate a cardiovascular crisis in this group of patients (Fig. 15.13).

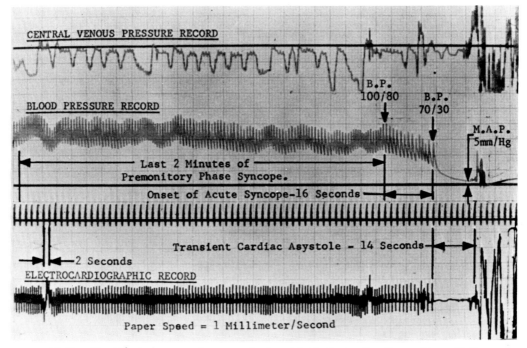

Figure 15.13. The blood pressure changes prior to a faint indicate alterations with ventilation and a transient asystole is recorded. Recovery of cardiovascular parameters following a faint does not occur for at least 2 hours, or even that same day. (Reprinted with permission from Allen, G. D.: Minor anesthesia, *J Oral Surg* 31:330, 1973.)

Of significance are the medications taken by the patient. These can range from anticoagulants to antihypertensive medications so preoperative evaluation of the patient is of major significance. The digitalis group of drugs may produce sinus pause and arrest, and consideration should be given to inpatient care.

LATENT CARDIOVASCULAR DISEASE

The insidious nature of cardiovascular disease is such that detection is often impossible. The patient will complain of early fatigue with disinclination for any increase in activity further compounded by a lack of fitness. Continuous aching in the legs may indicate ineffective or inadequate circulation, and the complaint of a tight collar is often an early indication of latent cardiovascular problems. Under such circumstances the dentist should proceed with care. No particular technique is contraindicated; rather it is an indication for careful monitoring.

CORONARY INFARCTION

Various estimates of reinfarction have been made, but the earlier the operation is performed following the infarct the greater the risk. After 6 months, the incidence declines to 10 per cent, and after 2 years the patient is considered in the same group as the general population. The technique of choice in these patients would be local anesthesia without epinephrine, supplemented by nitrous oxide-oxygen. In the first 6 months after an infarct up to 75 per cent of patients reinfarct following operation and hospital admission is indicated. A consultation with anesthesia is advisable, and general anesthesia with endotracheal intubation is often indicated to achieve good oxygenation throughout the procedure.

HYPERTENSION

The important feature is to stabilize the blood pressure throughout the procedure. Adequate levels of anesthesia prevent sudden rises in response to trauma. The incidence of arrhythmias in hypertension is increased, and thought should be given to treating the hypertension with diazoxide (Hyperstat) or hydralazine (Apresoline). The use of nitrous oxide-oxygen sedation has an additional advantage in that it increases the oxygen tension.

ARRHYTHMIAS

In this group, prior medical consultation should have been obtained, and stabilization of medication achieved. The level of anesthesia should prevent hypertensive responses as these may further precipitate re-entry arrhythmias and exaggerate pre-existing arrhythmias. Premature ventricular contractions (PVCs) are not a serious problem, and often benign. Mild sedation will normally produce beneficial effects in such patients, and reduce the incidence of problems. However, if six PVCs occur in 1 minute, then the patient should be considered to have a pathological problem.

ANTICOAGULANT THERAPY

If the patient is heparinized, then admission to the hospital should be considered. The selection of the pain control modality is less important than the ability to provide hemostasis. The oral anticoagulants combine with free protein, and there is less protein to bind subsequently administered medications. The patient may be more sensitive to intravenously administered agents such as barbiturates.

Respiratory Diseases

It is not essential to perform outpatient anesthesia on this group of patients; hospitalization may be indicated.

COMMON COLD

No patient with a common cold should receive treatment, particularly anesthesia, except in an emergency. Ten days to 2 weeks should elapse after the symptoms have subsided to allow the respiratory mucosa to return to normal.

NASAL BLOCKAGE

If nasal blockage is permanent, then the problems of using a nasal mask are greatly increased. The nasal vasoconstrictors will not affect bone or cartilage; inspection of the airway will reveal the problem. Do not use a nasopharyngeal tube to clear the passages as the nasopharyngeal tube itself may become blocked. Following intravenous induction of a sedative technique, a full face mask can be used to reach any depth of anesthesia for a brief operation, or oral endotracheal anesthesia can be used.

RESPIRATORY OBSTRUCTION

Patients with respiratory obstruction should be anesthetized in a hospital setting. The choice of anesthesia is usually some form of regional block, but if mild obstruction is present then nitrous oxide-oxygen halothane anesthesia is useful. Severe respiratory obstruction indicates endotracheal anesthesia or tracheostomy. A 13-gauge cricothyroid needle should be available as should all facilities for emergency tracheostomy.

EMPHYSEMA

In the emphysematous patient there is a loss of elasticity in the lung. If exercise tolerance is good, then there is no problem and any form of conscious sedation is applicable. Air trapping and expansion of loculated pockets by nitrous oxide may impair ventilation. The semi-supine position is of benefit for such patients, in order that they may use their abdominal musculature to aid in expiration.

BRONCHOSPASM

Some constriction of the airway suggests that the operation should be deferred until the patient is free of acute disease. Bronchial asthma is an intermittent disease. Antispasmodics should be continued; Benadryl is a useful premedication, and aminophylline may be given intravenously or orally as a preoperative measure. Induction of conscious sedation should be smooth. In many patients the placement of a nasal mask may induce bronchial asthma, and care should be taken to ensure that the patient understands the techniques in order to prevent alarm. Epinephrine in the local anesthetic is of benefit. Intravenous conscious sedation may be the method of choice, and diazepam is better than a barbiturate. If general anesthesia is to be performed, nitrous oxide-oxygen halothane is the technique of choice, with intubation using succinylcholine if needed.

CHRONIC BRONCHITIS

Chronic bronchitis is a combination of respiratory obstruction and intrapulmonary disease. Exercise tolerance is a measure of the seriousness of the problem and determines the choice of outpatient care. The patient's routine medication should be continued and anesthesia induced without premedication; atropine or scopolamine will dry secretions. Preoperative respiratory therapy should be considered. The lungs should be as free from disease as possible. Supplementary oxygen should be given if intravenous techniques are followed, and if general anesthesia is indicated, then nitrous oxide-oxygen halothane is indicated. The postoperative problem is the major consideration and determines the need for hospital care. The careful monitoring of blood gases is indicated in severe disease.

RESPIRATORY CRIPPLE

The respiratory cripple is recognized by dyspnea at rest with the lowered arterial oxygen tension and a high arterial carbon dioxide tension. These patients should be admitted to the hospital for dental care, and consideration given to the use of general anesthesia or anesthesiological sup-

port. The hazard is that supplementary oxygen in the presence of a respiratory depressant will result in elimination of the anoxic drive to respiration. Subsequently respiratory arrest leads to further carbon dioxide retention, and carbon dioxide narcosis supervenes. Careful monitoring of blood gases and respiration is required and no attempt should be made to perform outpatient anesthesia or conscious sedation.

Metabolic Disorders

In this group are considered the several genetic problems and the problems of pharmacogenetics. Many patients with congenital abnormalities involving the airway, such as Klippel-Feil or Pierre Robin syndrome, present for dental treatment. Ideally, such patients would receive anesthesia only with local anesthetics, supplemented possibly by nitrous oxide-oxygen sedation. In selecting further pain control modalities, it would be preferable to avoid intravenous conscious sedation, as meticulous titration of the dosage must be followed in order to avoid respiratory arrest. If further measures are required, then in selecting general anesthesia a determination should be made as to the difficulty of intubation. Prior to anesthesia, determine for how long attempts will be made to persevere with nasal intubation before proceeding to oral intubation. If oral intubation is unsuccessful after a reasonable time, then consideration in this group should be given to tracheostomy. It would be preferable with the patient anesthetized to perform necessary extractions, and no attempt would be made to perform definitive dentistry without the endotracheal tube in place.

ELECTROLYTE CHANGES

The diseases in which electrolyte changes can be suspected are noted in Table 15.2. If electrolyte changes are suspected, a serum electrolyte evaluation

Table 15.2
The Diseases in Which Electrolyte Changes May Be Suspected Alert the Operator to Possible Changes in Drug Response

Obesity
Heart disease
Renal disease
COPD (chronic obstructive pulmonary disease)
Peripheral vascular disease
Endocrine
Arthritis
Hepatic dysfunction
Diabetes

should be made and corrected before any form of conscious sedation, otherwise drug distribution may be affected. The potassium level is significant in its ability to change cardiovascular responses. Any form of therapy is indicated, but it would be useful to provide electrocardiographic monitoring of the patient throughout the procedure.

PHARMACOGENETICS AND DISEASE

Numerous genetic disorders promote pharmacological problems. These range from abnormal pseudocholinesterase levels which affect the metabolism of the muscle relaxants, abnormal binding of plasma proteins, hereditary changes associated with structural defects such as aortic stenosis, hyperkalemia, myotonia congenita, and other hereditary disorders such as malignant hyperpyrexia and hepatic porphyria. The problem is best resolved with the anesthesiologist and pediatrician who are aware of the problems.

MONGOLOID AND OBESE CHILD

Airway maintenance in such patients may be difficult, and oversedation in the office must be avoided. Inhalation sedation may not be satisfactory, and intravenous techniques are necessary to achieve satisfactory levels.

CYSTIC FIBROSIS

Inhalation sedation may result in rises in pressure in closed cysts of the lung.

The enlargement of these cavities could cause further respiratory embarrassment. Anticholinergic drugs in such patients will dry secretions and result in further mucous plugs. Hospitalization is indicated.

LIVER AND RENAL DISEASE

There is no single satisfactory assessment of liver function, and an index of liver function is best obtained from several features: the presence of antigen B, a prothrombin of less than 80 per cent, a transaminase twice normal, albumin less than 3.5 per cent, and a good history.

Nitrous oxide-oxygen sedation would be the most satisfactory form of conscious sedation. If the level of relief required is not obtained, then hospital admission should be considered.

Hematological Problems

The majority of problems associated with these diseases are surgical. Confirmation that laboratory values are within acceptable limits must be made. If coagulation defects are present a hematoma at the venipuncture site may be a problem. If intubation is performed, pharyngeal or laryngeal hematoma may develop, while nasal endotracheal intubation and nasopharyngeal tubes are contraindicated. Supplemental local anesthetic techniques may result in hemorrhage at the site of needle placement. This group of patients would be better treated in a hospital with carefully administered general anesthesia.

Sickle cell disease is a very common problem in the community under anesthesia. Sickling should be suspected if jaundice, anemia, osteitis, and crises occur elsewhere in the body. The death rate under anesthesia in sickle cell trait is 0.19 per cent and with the disease itself, 4 per cent. Consideration should be made as to whether all the population at risk should have a sickle test performed before anesthesia. Thus both trait and disease are significant problems. Any decrease in oxygen tension will result in abnormal binding; the molecule is distorted and the cell ruptures. In addition, the sickle cell does not carry oxygen well, and acidosis increases this propensity. Oxygen saturation, not the oxygen tension, is important.

If the surgery is elective, then it should be delayed until the hemoglobin is over 8 g. Preoperative transfusion should be avoided if possible, otherwise bone marrow suppression develops. In addition, over 6 per cent of the patients will develop hepatitis or have hepatitis from transfusion. To avoid acidosis, the patient should be kept warm throughout the operation. Avoid meperidine in these patients.

Nervous System Diseases

Inhalation techniques are useful. In anesthesia, relaxants should be avoided as their action may be uncertain with spinal disorders: if the motor neuron is intact the reflexes remain normal. In neuronal diseases which affect the nerve roots or peripheral nerves, there are depressed reflexes with mild motor and sensory involvement. Progressive muscular weakness develops. Examples are seen in nutritional and diabetic neuropathies. Before administering conscious sedation the levels of the nervous disease should be delineated, in order that any postoperative problem may not be attributed to the conscious sedation.

The introduction of new drugs to anesthesia poses problems for epileptic patients, in that many of the new drugs may initiate epileptic type seizures. Such drugs as ketamine, a derivative of phencylidine, cause spontaneous muscular movements. Enflurane will frequently cause epileptic type bursts on the EEG and at all concentrations slight muscular movements in the hands and feet. Methohexital is potentially a convulsant despite being a barbiturate, as it is a methylated compound. Numerous cases of epileptic seizure have been reported following methohexital, and the drug is used to activate the EEG to diagnose epilepsy.

Endocrine Disorders

The problems of adrenal suppression and thyroid, hypo- or hyperactivity, are understood. However, selection for the diabetic poses problems due to the varying nature and severity of the disease.

The diabetic treated by diet alone, or oral antidiabetic agents, can be cared for in the office with any technique indicated. It is the insulin-dependent diabetic who poses problems in selection. If the diabetes is controlled with a single injection of long acting insulin, then the potential problem is allowing the diabetes to get out of control during the surgical procedure. It would be better if the patient were treated with local anesthesia alone or inhalation conscious sedation. The margin of safety is reduced for intravenous techniques, and would be best avoided. If general anesthesia is considered, then intravenous barbiturates supplemented with nitrous oxide-oxygen would be a satisfactory technique. The unstable diabetic poses problems even in hospital care. The only satisfactory way of handling the diabetic is to admit the patient for serial blood sugars, and titrate intravenous insulin as required. The blood sugar should be monitored in the insulin-dependent diabetic, as should the electrolytes. The diabetic is usually out of control postoperatively, and it is important to care for the patient accordingly.

Muscular Diseases or Myopathies

Muscular diseases pose major anesthetic hazards as mucle relaxation is affected. The classical signs of depth of anesthesia are dependent on muscle relaxation. These patients normally require respiratory assistance, and the anesthetist then is concerned with return of spontaneous respiration. The use of inhalation agents is preferred.

MUSCULAR DYSTROPHY

Muscular dystrophy is due to excess acetylcholinesterase distribution throughout the muscle or inadequate available enzymes and subsequent reduced membrane sensitivity. Connective tissue overgrowth and excess muscle protein production occur; abnormal meta-myoglobins are present. The typing of muscular dystrophy is based upon age and distribution. The Duchenne type occurs in males under 3 years of age and affects the pelvis and shoulder girdles. The facioscapularhumeral is slower in onset and begins in early childhood, affecting the limb girdle.

POLYMYOSITIS

Polymyositis is associated with dermatomyositis, and the patient often exhibits malignancy. Special care is needed in this instance, as the polymyositis group are improved by steroids.

Muscle End Plate Diseases

The two muscle end plate diseases considered below exhibit problems in general anesthesia. Dystrophia myotonica, which may be a myopathy, is included in this group. Conscious sedation poses no problems.

MYASTHENIA GRAVIS

The muscle weakness in myasthenia gravis can be overcome by the administration of anticholinesterase, e.g., neostigmine (Prostigmine) 30 to 60 mg q.i.d., pyridostigmine (Mestinon) 12 to 200 mg b.i.d., or, briefly, endrophonium (Tensilon) 10 mg, a test evaluation only. The hazards of the disease are compounded by the potent drugs which are necessary for treatment. The muscle relaxants, in particular curare, may result in permanent apnea. The recommended technique of anesthesia is to give neostigmine as required intravenously. Avoid the opiates as neostigmine potentiates the action and duration of opiates. Use inhalation anesthetic techniques and avoid or decrease the amount of thiopental for induction of anesthesia, as this

may produce severe respiratory depression. Intubate the patient without a relaxant and maintain spontaneous respiration throughout the operation. Careful observation in the postoperative period is essential.

DYSTROPHIA MYOTONICA

Patients with dystrophia myotonica are unable to relax sufficiently following a hand grip, for example. The muscles atrophy, and in consequence respiratory insufficiency develops. In addition to general muscular problems, atrophy occurs in the heart muscle and testicles, and the patients are bald, have cataracts, and mental deterioration. They are classically hypersensitive to thiopental, one of only two absolute contraindications to thiopental. With myotonica the patient becomes rigid with succinylcholine.

Porphyria

This disease is transmitted to the offspring *via* a Mendelian dominant gene. It is found only in people of Scandinavian or South African Dutch descent. Multiple segmental demyelination occurs in the central nervous system, and if sufficiently severe the axon may become involved. In addition, central lobular necrosis of the liver occurs. Uroporphyrins may be present but are not pathognomonic as they occur in other diseases. Porphobilin is always present in the acute disease; it is colorless but darkens if left in the light. Porphobilin is also present in the latent disease.

CONGENITA

This form is found in males; excess porphyrins are present, and so photosensitivity is present. There is no central nervous system involvement, abdominal symptoms are noted, and no porphobilinogen is present in the urine. The barbiturates do not affect these patients.

CUTANEA TARDA

This occurs later in life and is similar to congenita, but no gross mutilations develop. Porphyrins are present in the urine but no porphobilinogen.

ACUTE INTERMITTENT

There is no photosensitivity but porphobilinogen is present in the urine. The diagnosis of the disease is difficult, as it is classically known as "the little simulator." The distribution is dependent on the presence of demyelinated nerves. A patient may feel a little off-color, mental changes are indefinite, and insomnia is frequent. Colicky abdominal pain, together with vomiting and constipation, occur. Muscle weakness and paralysis develop and the red-colored urine which develops on standing is classical. Mortality rate is 25 to 30 per cent, usually owing to respiratory paralysis which will reverse in 2 to 3 months if the patient is maintained on ventilation. It is recommended that barbiturates be avoided. This is another absolute contraindication to thiopental. Avoid curare as its antidote, neostigmine, may possibly demyelinate the nerve. Regional anesthetics are best avoided because of medicolegal hazards. For pain, chlorpromazine with meperidine is recommended.

Unusual Diseases

It would be important for the person facing a patient with the diseases of unusual nature to review the problems of these diseases. The article by A. E. P. Jones on unusual syndromes, and the textbook *Anesthesia and Uncommon Diseases* by Katz and Kadis, are useful compendiums for such problems.

Bibliography

Allen GD, Sim J: Full mouth restoration under general anesthesia pedodontic practice. *J Dent Child* 34:488–492, 1967.

Allen GD, Everett GB, Forsyth WD, et al: The cardiorespiratory effects of epinephrine and local anesthetics for dentistry. *Anesth Prog* 20:152, 1973.

Allen GD, Everett GB, Kennedy WF, et al: Individual response to total spectrum of pain control in dentistry. *Anesth Prog* 22:144, 1975.

Allen GD, Everett GB, Butler LA: Human cardiorespiratory and analgesic effects of intravenous diazepam and local anesthesia. *J Am Dent Assoc* 92:744–747, 1976.

Caudill WA, Alvin JD, Nazif MM: Absorption rates of alphaprodine from the buccal and intravenous routes. *Pediatr Dent* 4:168, 1982.

Dixon RA, Thornton JA: Tests of recovery from anaesthesia and sedation: intravenous diazepam in dentistry. *Br J Anaesth* 45:207, 1973.

Driscoll EJ, Smilack RH, Lightbody PM, et al: Sedation with intravenous diazepam. *J Oral Surg* 33:32, 1972.

Forsyth WD, Allen GD, Everett GB: An evaluation of cardiorespiratory effects of posture in the dental outpatient. *Oral Surg* 34:562, 1972.

Giuffrida JG, Bizzarri DV, Saure AC, et al: Anesthetic management of drug abusers. *Anesth Analg* 49:272, 1970.

Guntheroth WG, Abel FL, Mullins GL: Blood pressure and cerebral blood flow in shock: The case against the Trendelenburg position. *Circulation* 26:725, 1962.

Healy TEJ, Robinson JS, Vickers M: Physiological responses to intravenous diazepam as a sedative for conservative dentistry. *Br Med J* 3:10, 1970.

Jones AEP, Pelton DA: An index of syndromes and their anaesthetic implications. *Can Anaesth Soc J* 23:207, 1976.

Kannel WB, Schwartz MJ, McNamara PM: Blood pressure and risks of coronary heart disease: The Framingham Study *Dis Chest* 56:43, 1969.

Katz J, Kadis LB: *Anesthesia and Uncommon Diseases*, ed. 2. Philadelphia. W. B. Saunders, 1982.

Katz RL, Weintraub HD, Papper EM: Anesthesia, surgery and rauwolfia. *Anesthesiol Biol* 25:142, 1964.

Levinson BW: States of awareness during general anesthesia. *Br J Anaesth* 37:544, 1965.

Lundy JS: Balanced anesthesia. *Minn Med* 9:399, 1926.

Lyttle JJ: Anesthesia morbidity and mortality survey of the Southern California Society of Oral Surgeons. *J Oral Surg* 32:739, 1974.

Malmin O: *The Shot that Kills.* Hicksville, N. Y. Exposition Press, 1974.

McCarthy FM: Safer practice. *SAAD Digest* 2:4, 1973.

Medicolegal: Two dental deaths. *Br Med J* 341, 1975.

Perlroth MG, Hultgren HN: The cardiac patient and general surgery. *JAMA* 232:1279, 1975.

Quinn TW, Kendrick TP, Pfeffer RC: The surgical anesthesia team, in the dental clinics of North America. *Anesth Analg* April 1973.

Rubin A, Allen GD, Everett GB: Induction of general anesthesia with diazepam or thiopental: A comparison of the cardiorespiratory effects. *Anesth Prog* 25:39, 1978.

Schemel WH: Unexpected hepatic dysfunction found by multiple laboratory screening. *Anesth Analg* 55:810, 1976.

Taggert P, Hedworth-Witty R, Carruthers M, et al: Observations on electrocardiogram and plasma catecholamines during dental procedures: the forgotten vagus. *Br Med J* 2:787, 1976.

Tarhan S, Moffitt EA, Taylor WF, et al: Myocardial infarction after general anesthesia. *J A M A* 220:1451, 1972.

Tolas AC, Pflug AE, Halter JB: Arterial plasma epinephrine concentrations and hemodynamic responses after dental injection of local anesthetic with epinephrine. *J Am Dent Assoc* 104:41, 1982.

Trieger N, Jacobs AW, Loskota WJ, et al: A comparison of psychomotor and breathalyzer determined alcohol effects on the "cocktail party drinker." *Anesth Prog* 19:116, 1972.

CHAPTER 16

Accidents

Accidents are unforeseen events which occur because of improper technique, malfunction of equipment, or other unpredictable phenomena. Such events can happen during the administration of dental anesthesia or analgesia. Many untoward incidents under conscious sedation parallel those under anesthesia. If unrecognized or untreated, they can be embarrassing at best, or lead to significant morbidity or mortality. Legal considerations may also be involved.

Fortunately, most such accidents are preventable. However, the person administering anesthetics must slavishly adhere to the principles of accurate history taking and physical examination, proper patient evaluation and preparation, maintenance of accurate equipment in good working order, accuracy in drug administration, continuous observation and monitoring of the patient during anesthesia, and adequate postoperative care. Consultation should be sought without delay whenever treatment of any accident is beyond the scope of the responsible person.

RESPIRATORY SYSTEM

Contamination of the lungs during tooth extraction under general anesthesia was once a leading cause of pulmonary abscess. Tooth fragments, fillings, dental calculus, and blood were aspirated into the lungs. Properly placed oropharyngeal packs and strong suction during surgical procedures in the mouth under anesthesia have greatly reduced if not eliminated this problem. Gauze packs should be tagged with a string hanging from the mouth and a radiopaque marker to prevent their being lost in the pharynx. A loosely placed pack will allow leakage of blood and debris, and if placed too far posteriorly can completely obstruct the airway unless the patient is intubated. Before using a tonsil suction in the mouth or pharynx, the suction tip should be firmly attached to prevent its loss in the pharynx (Fig. 16.1).

The use of endotracheal tubes introduces certain inherent risks, both major and minor (Table 16.1). Endotracheal in-

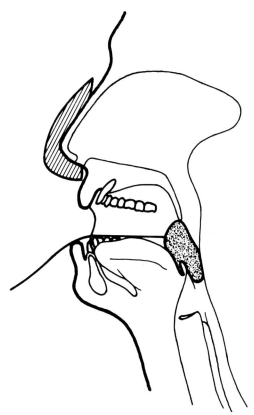

Figure 16.1. A misplaced or a pharyngeal partition can slip into the pharynx causing respiratory obstruction. The string allows easy removal of the pack and readjustment.

Table 16.1
Mortality and Morbidity in Endotracheal Intubation

Deaths during attempted intubation
  Only 2 ASA Class I (*Anesthesiology* 1973)
  2 of 36 anesthetic deaths (*Med J Aust* 1970)
Morbidity categories
  Aspiration
  ECG abnormalities
  Mechanical problems
  Trauma

In studies of anesthetic deaths, endotracheal intubation is a significant cause of death, while many categories of morbidity are associated with and following intubation.

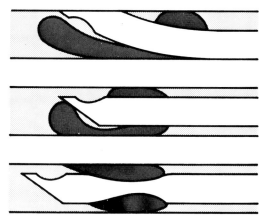

Figure 16.2. The cuff on an endotracheal tube can be overinflated or distend in the wrong direction and may occlude the lumen of the tube. An endotracheal tube does not guarantee a satisfactory airway.

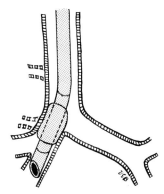

Figure 16.3. Unintentional endobronchial intubation due to intubation of the right mainstem bronchus. Additional problems can occur if a cuff occludes the right upper lobe bronchus even in normal placement of the tube. Occlusion of the apical lobe bronchus may be due to an abnormal origin of the bronchus.

tubation does not guarantee the airway. The tube may kink, partially or completely blocking the airway. The most common site for this is at the junction with the metal connector. Endotracheal tubes have collapsed on inflation of the cuff, completely occluding the lumen (Fig. 16.2). Old endotracheal tubes which have lost strength and elasticity should be discarded. Endobronchial intubation, which usually occurs down the right mainstem bronchus, may be prevented by visually checking for equal bilateral lung expansion and auscultating both sides of the chest following intubation (Fig. 16.3). Failure to recognize endobronchial intubation will cause massive collapse (atelectasis) of the unventilated lung.

Nasal masks must be carefully placed to avoid occlusion of the nares. Nasopharyngeal and endotracheal tubes can become obstructed by adenoidal tissue, mucus plugs, or clotted blood.

Technical difficulties with anesthetic apparatus cause respiratory problems. Carbon dioxide accumulates in nonrebreathing anesthetic systems in which expiratory valves are not free of resistance or are improperly placed in circuit, adding to dead space. Failure to appreciate the rebreathing which occurs when a bag or bellows and an incircuit vaporizer are incorporated into a demand-flow anesthetic machine has resulted in death. Flow-meters should be checked regularly for accuracy and to prevent sticking. A switch-over mechanism or alarm system prevents exhaustion of nitrous oxide or oxygen during an anesthetic. Auxiliary oxygen tanks should be available in case of emergency. Cylinder connections and wall outlets, if properly installed, prevent the wrong gas from being delivered. The use of standard color codes and wall plug-in sizes eliminates the mistaken delivery of nitrous oxide through an oxygen flow meter. Soda lime in rebreathing circuits should be promptly replaced when exhausted as indicated by its color change.

Contamination of nitrous oxide tanks with toxic impurities (nitric oxide, nitrogen dioxide, nitric acid) leading to serious pulmonary reaction, methemoglobinemia, and death has been reported. A chemical reaction in the lungs similar to that following aspiration of gastric acid occurs with inhalation of acidic nitrous oxide impurities. Treatment includes oxygenation, administration of bronchodilators and steroids, and lavage of the tracheobronchial tree with dilute bicarbonate solution. Methemoglobinemia is treated with methylene blue (2 mg per kg intravenously). Fourtunately, high safety standards in the modern industrial preparation of anesthetic gases makes such events rare.

Respiratory arrest has occurred after too rapid administration of diazepam. Intravenous doses of diazepam should be given at a rate not to exceed 2.5 mg per minute. Ethylene glycol, a component of intravenous diazepam solution, as well as the diazepam itself, has effects on respiration. The plunger on a chairside intravenous barbiturate administration set has been accidentally depressed by the pressure of the surgical assistant's thigh, discharging a large bolus of the barbiturate into the patient's vein, causing apnea. Such accidents are prevented by careful attention to proper technique.

CARDIOVASCULAR SYSTEM

Accidental anesthetic overdose constitutes a serious insult to the cardiovascular system as most anesthetic agents are direct myocardial depressants. The concentration and identity of intravenous agents must be verified prior to injection. Vaporizers should be cleaned and recalibrated periodically as recommended by the manufacturer. Flow meters should constantly be observed during anesthesia to check the adequacy of oxygen concentration and gas flow. Adequate stabilization should be provided for vaporizers of volatile agents to prevent spillage of liquid agents into the anesthetic circuit. Cardiac arrest following introduction of liquid halothane into a patient's lungs from a tipped-over Fluotec vaporizer has been reported. Aside from such catastrophies, most overdoses respond to support of blood pressure and maintenance of adequate ventilation with oxygen until the effects of the drug have been reversed.

Vascular complications, while seldom life-threatening, are nonetheless troublesome side effects of intravenous sedation and anesthesia when they occur. Intra-arterial injections are an ever-present danger as the cubital fossa is the most frequently chosen intravenous site. The close proximity of arteries and veins in this area, as well as the danger of the patient flexing his arm under light anesthesia or sedation increases the likelihood that the needle may enter an artery. An intraarterial injection under sedation or anesthesia is all the more unfortunate as it may not be immediately recognized and treated because the patient is not able to complain of the intense pain. The pH of most barbiturate solutions, for example, is greater than 10, provoking an intense vasospasm in the injected artery. Intense pain, blanching of the extremity, and loss of the arterial pulse distal to the site of puncture occur.

Thrombophlebitis may be a late complication of intravenous therapy, occurring several hours to days later. Intravenous meperidine, diazepam, and glucose-containing solutions are common offenders. An intravenous polyethylene catheter left in place longer than 12 hours is irritating to the vein. Preventive measures include dilution of irritating drugs prior to injection, buffering glucose intravenous drip solutions with bicarbonate, use of metallic needles, addition of small amounts of heparin and hydrocortisone to intravenous drip solutions running several hours or more, and use of a large vein.

The introduction of air into a vein can

be a life-threatening situation. An air embolus entering the ventricles of the heart causes cardiac arrest. All air bubbles must be removed from intravenous tubing before starting an infusion. Air trapped in syringes must be removed before injecting intravenous drugs. The size of an air embolus necessary to reach the heart before dissolving in venous blood has been variously estimated to be in excess of 20 ml. Air embolism to the heart is recognized by hearing the classic mill-wheel murmur in the precordial stethoscope. Treatment requires immediate positioning of the patient right side up to isolate the air bubble in the right atrium before aspirating.

Inadvertent extravascular injection of intravenous fluids or drugs usually causes no permanent disability. Skin sloughs rarely occur unless drug concentrations are higher than normally used intravenously or extremely large extravasations cause undue pressure. Elevation, moist heat, and injection of procaine to relieve pain and hyaluronidase to spread the extravasation are usually adequate treatment. Careful intravenous technique avoids most of these problems.

PERIPHERAL NERVES

Proper positioning of the patient prior to anesthesia usually prevents injury to peripheral nerves. Abnormal shoulder or arm position may compromise the brachial plexus or individual nerves (median, radial, ulnar) of the upper extremity (Figs. 16.4 and 16.5). Prolonged pressure of a full-face or nasal mask can cause paresthesia of the infraorbital or supraorbital nerves. Postanesthetic paresis of the buccal branch of the facial nerve has occurred from full-face mask pressure (Figs. 16.6 and 16.7).

Careful technique is a must to avoid sciatic nerve injury in intragluteal injections. The upper, outer quadrant of the buttocks should be used but does not preclude the drug tracking down between fascial planes and reaching the sciatic nerve. No more than 5 ml should be injected at a given site. Selection of the vastus lateralis muscle on the lateral aspect of the thigh is preferable for intramuscular administration.

Prior to induction of anesthesia, the patient's legs should be uncrossed to avoid pressure and ischemia of the pretibial

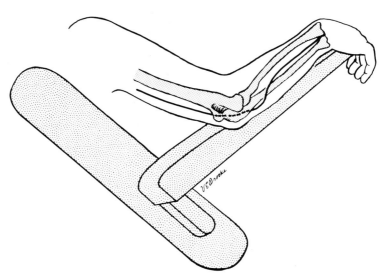

Figure 16.4. Ulnar nerve damage may result if the arm lies on the edge of the arm rest in an unsupported position.

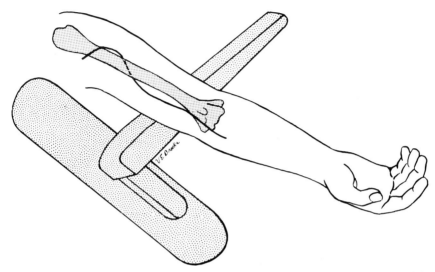

Figure 16.5. A supinated arm can lie on the arm rest, and resultant damage to the radial nerve can cause wrist drop.

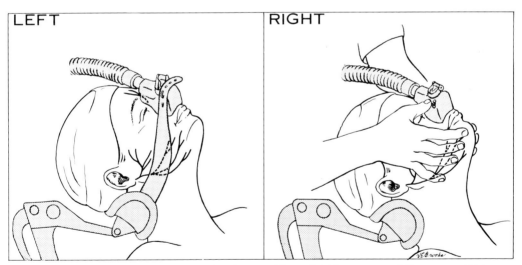

Figure 16.6. *Left:* the facial nerve can be damaged by a tight harness, and the supraorbital nerve by a firm bridge on the nasal mask. *Right:* damage to the facial nerve can also occur by finger pressure in supporting the jaw.

area. Prolonged pressure on the common peroneal nerve with the legs crossed during anesthesia can cause motor weakness of the dorsiflexor muscles of the foot and foot drop (Fig. 16.8).

General awareness by all in the operatory of the potential dangers of positional abnormalities in causing peripheral nerve injuries is the best safeguard against their

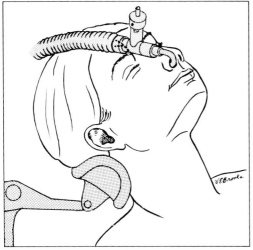

Figure 16.7. An unsupported endotracheal or nasopharyngeal connector can damage the supraorbital nerve.

occurrence. During induction and throughout anesthesia until the patient has regained consciousness and is cooperative, adequate restraints also help in preventing injury.

Provided there is no pre-existing neurological disease, the prognosis for peripheral nerve palsies is good. Neurosurgical or orthopedic consultation is generally advisable when a peripheral motor or sensory deficit occurs.

CENTRAL NERVOUS SYSTEM

Complications involving the central nervous system are just are likely to follow general anesthesia as spinal anesthesia. Local anesthesia is not without such risks either. Diplopia, blindness, spinal paralysis, cranial nerve deficits (especially the abducens nerve), and meningitis are among reported complications. Many central nervous system accidents are secondary to anoxia, emphasizing the importance of adequate ventilation during anesthesia.

Convulsions under general anesthesia are likely to occur in febrile conditions when body temperature rises above

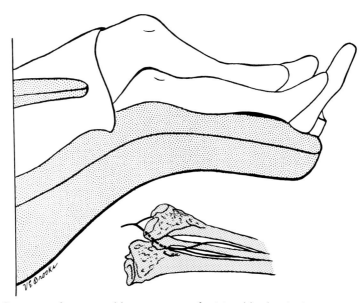

Figure 16.8. Pressure of a crossed leg can cause foot trouble due to temporary paralysis of the common peroneal nerve.

103°F. Children are particularly susceptible. Body temperature (preferably rectal for better accuracy) should always be checked prior to anesthetic induction when sepsis exists. General anesthesia for elective procedures should be cancelled in the presence of high fever. Febrile patients have greater oxygen requirements because of the increased metabolic rate. Higher oxygen concentrations should be provided under general anesthesia. If convulsions occur, they are managed by ventilation with 100 per cent oxygen, intravenous injection of diazepam (5 to 10 mg over 1 to 2 minutes), and reduction of body temperature with cooling blankets, rectal enemas with tepid water, and rectal administration of a combination of aspirin and acetaminophen. The effect of extreme rotation of the head and neck on cerebral blood flow has been investigated (Fig. 16.9). Rotation of the head more than 60° in the presence of vascular or cervical spine abnormalities significantly compromises perfusion of the brain (Fig. 16.10). Sudden accidental release of the dental chair headrest can cause acute stretching of the cervical spinal cord. Quadriplegia has resulted from such an event (Fig. 16.11).

MUSCULOSKELETAL SYSTEM

Pre-existing conditions such as cervical arthritis or recent neck or back injuries can be aggravated under sedation, particularly while seated in the dental chair. Exacerbation of whiplash injury under general anesthesia for oral surgery in the dental chair has occurred. Normal protective muscle splinting is relaxed under general anesthesia. Elective procedures should be deferred until clearance is obtained from the orthopedic surgeon.

Overzealous forward elevation of the mandible displaces the condyle out of the glenoid fossa. Dislocation of the temporomandibular joint preferably should be avoided, or recognized and reduced before the patient regains consciousness. Dislocation of the temporomandibular joint can cause rupture of the ligaments surrounding the joint and hemorrhage within the synovial space. Persistent pain and/or arthritic changes in the condyle or a myofascial pain dysfunction syndrome may plague the patient.

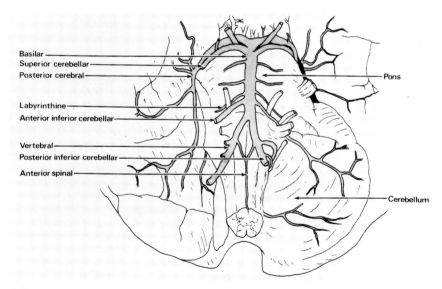

Figure 16.9. The blood supply to the base of the brain derives from the vertebral arteries. In the healthy patient either vessel may supply up to 100 per cent of the required blood supply; problems can occur if one vessel is diseased.

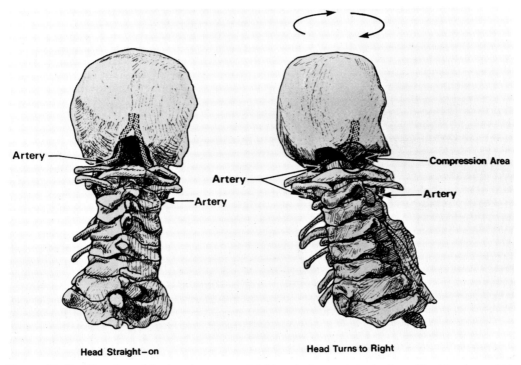

Figure 16.10. Rotation of the head can completely occlude a vertebral artery. The blood supply to the base of the brain is provided by the contralateral artery.

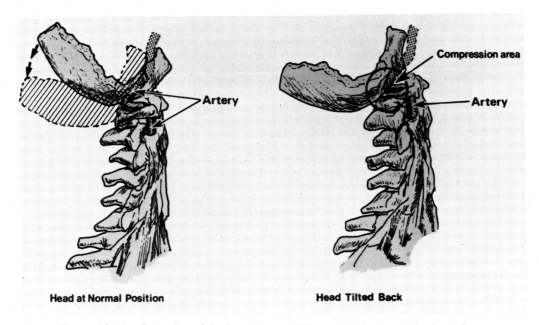

Figure 16.11. Extension of the head can partially occlude both vertebral arteries.

Succinylcholine, a depolarizing muscle relaxant, is commonly used in dental anesthesia to aid in endotracheal intubation, to break laryngeal spasm, or to manage the "resistant" patient in the dental chair. Cramping or aching of chest and abdominal muscles often occurs following intravenous injection of succinylcholine if muscles fasciculate, equivalent to brief violent exercise. Muscle fasciculations can be avoided by an intravenous drip of succinylcholine rather than a single intravenous dose, or by prior injection of a small amount of nondepolarizing muscle relaxant. The symptoms usually resolve within 24 to 48 hours without treatment other than mild analgesics.

Dual neuromuscular blockade, both depolarizing and nondepolarizing, occurs after repeated doses of succinylcholine, particularly if more than 500 mg are given. The prolonged apnea must be treated by controlled ventilation until return of adequate spontaneous respiration. Attempts at reversal of dual blockade with neostigmine or other anticholinesterases are controversial and may prolong rather than reverse muscle relaxation.

Plasma cholinesterase, responsible for hydrolysis of succinylcholine and aminobenzoic acid ester local anesthetics (procaine), is significantly reduced or totally lacking in 0.03 (1 in 2820) of the population. Prolonged apnea follows even small doses of succinylcholine. A prior history of prolonged apnea during general anesthesia or toxic reaction to small amounts of procaine should alert the clinician to this entity.

GASTROINTESTINAL TRACT

Vomiting during anesthesia can lead to pulmonary aspiration, a life-threatening emergency. Prevention of vomiting necessitates 4 or more hours of fasting prior to elective surgery. Outpatients, especially children, should be questioned concerning their last intake of food and drink to verify that preanesthetic instructions have been followed. Various factors, including gastric contents which are solid or have high osmotic pressure, fear, pain, and narcotics delay emptying of the stomach.

Regurgitation is a passive event and can occur even with nitrous oxide-oxygen when the cardiac sphincter may be rendered incompetent. Vomiting is caused by active muscle contractions and is most likely to occur during induction or emergence from anesthesia. Rapid, deep swallowing usually precedes the onset of vomiting. The patient must be placed immediately in a head-down position with the head turned to the right, particulate matter manually cleared from the mouth and pharynx, and strong suction applied to remove liquid gastric contents. The lungs must be examined for evidence of pulmonary aspiration. Danger to the respiratory tract is that of either complete mechanical blockage by solid food or invasion of the bronchial tree with liquid gastric contents containing hydrochloric acid.

Postoperative vomiting, while less serious, is an uncomfortable and debilitating nuisance for the outpatient. Females, children, and anxious patients are the most susceptible. The swallowing of blood from the mouth, periods of hypoxia, and narcotic premedication are contributing factors. Dehydration caused by preoperative fasting may lead to postoperative nausea and vomiting and emphasizing the importance of adequate intravenous fluid replacement during and following oral operations. Treatment consists of adequate hydration (oral or intravenous), antiemetic drugs (e.g., benzquinamide or prochlorperazine, rectally or intravenously, carbonated soft drinks: 7-Up or ginger ale) or antacids to neutralize gastric acidity.

Positive pressure ventilation in the presence of partial airway obstruction or during laryngospasm may cause inflation of the stomach with a large amount of anesthetic gases. Gastric distention can cause increased vagal reflex activity with slowing of the heart rate, cardiac arrhythmias, hypotension, regurgitation, or vomiting. The condition is recognized by epigastric fullness and hypertympanic note to percussion of the abdomen. A nasogastric tube is passed to decompress the stomach and relieve the condition.

Hiccups (singultus) following injection of thiopental or methohexital interferes with adequate ventilation because of intermittent clonic spasm of the diaphragm, with bronchoconstriction and glottic closure. Stimulation of the posterior pharyngeal wall at the level of the second cervical vertebra with a rubber suction catheter, the placement of a nasopharyngeal tube, or ephedrine, 5 mg intravenously twice, stops hiccuping.

Accidental bowel or bladder evacuation may happen during anesthesia, particularly following struggling, hypoxia, or convulsions. A routine visit to the lavatory before anesthesia is a helpful preventive measure.

EYES

Lacrimation ceases during surgical anesthesia or if an anticholinergic drug is given. If the surface of the cornea is dry, it is more susceptible to abrasions from foreign objects. Contact lenses must be removed prior to induction. The eyelids should be taped shut or protected with eye pads during dental operations under sedation or general anesthesia to guard against airborne tooth or filling fragments, blood, or other debris. Prolonged pressure of a full-face mask on the eyes has caused thrombosis of the central retinal artery and blindness. Atropine, scopolamine, or manipulations that increase intraocular pressure should be avoided in patients with glaucoma.

EARS

Protect the ears from excessive pressure of head drapes or the straps of full-face or nasal masks. Necrosis of the cartilage of the ear has resulted from prolonged pressure.

NOSE AND THROAT

Have the patient blow his nose prior to inhalation induction to remove mucus and foreign objects. Children may have placed beans or small stones in their nasal passages. These could fall into the pharynx and be aspirated into the lungs under anesthesia.

Nasal hemorrhage results from forcing a nasopharyngeal or nasoendotracheal tube past an obstruction which damages the nasal mucosa. Most hemorrhage problems are avoided by recognizing existing nasal passage obstructions during the preoperative examination, use of a smaller size tube, and gentle manipulation. Occasionally, anterior or posterior nasal packing is required for excessive or persistent hemorrhage. This is more likely to be necessary in elderly patients whose atherosclerotic vessels lack the ability to contract normally or in young children with adenoidal hyperplasia (Fig. 16.12).

Nasal intubation should not be done in patients with repaired cleft palates or velopharyngeal flaps. The distortion of normal anatomy in such patients increases the likelihood of significant trauma to their nasal passages by intubation through the nose.

Necrosis of the skin of the tip of the nose has occurred secondary to undue or prolonged pressure by a nasoendotracheal tube. Care should be taken to properly tape and support such tubes in position to avoid this problem (Fig. 16.13).

Accidental placement of an endotracheal tube beneath the pharyngeal mucosa, subcutaneous emphysema with mediastinal involvement, and retrobulbar hemorrhage have been reported following traumatic attempts at endotracheal intubation. Such problems are best avoided by gentle techniques under direct laryngoscopy.

MOUTH

Prior to sedation or anesthesia all removable prostheses or appliances should be taken from the patient. Loose teeth should be carefully noted and avoided during induction and intubation. Loose teeth or removable appliances can be dislodged, swallowed, or aspirated if appropriate precautions are not taken. An object aspirated into the lungs must be retrieved as soon as possible by a skilled bronchoscopist to prevent atelectasis or lung abscess. Foreign bodies which are swallowed and enter the stomach should

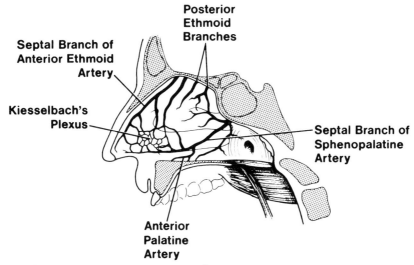

Figure 16.12. The blood supply of the nasal septum forms Kiesselbach's plexus, an area of confluence of multiple branches of external and internal carotid circulation. This area is easily traumatized during passage of a nasal tube and can cause a nosebleed.

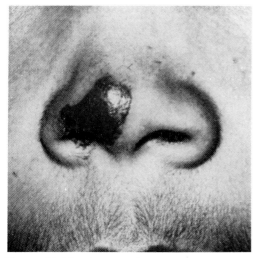

Figure 16.13. Necrosis of the ala nasi due to pressure of the endotracheal tube connector as it passes posteriorly. Pressure points should be avoided or padded. (Reprinted with permission from Barkin, M. E., and Trieger, N.: An unusual complication of nasal-tracheal anesthesia. *Anesth Prog* 23:57, 1976.)

be located by X-ray and their progress observed until they are completely passed through the intestinal tract in the feces. Most objects readily pass through the intestine, but occasionally a sharp object, such as a root canal reamer, causes pain

or perforation. Laparotomy is then indicated for direct surgical removal.

Sound natural teeth or fixed bridgework can be damaged by traumatic laryngoscopy or overzealous use of the ratchet mouth prop. This is most likely to occur when anesthetic induction or intubation is attempted by an unskilled anesthetist upon a patient with severe mandibular retrognathia or when jaw opening is limited by swelling and trismus secondary to an acute infection. Recognition of such patients preoperatively should alert the inexperienced anesthetist who is not equipped to deal with such problems.

RECOVERY CARE

Rapid recovery will minimize the incidence of accidents, the most dangerous problems being respiratory. Recovering patients must be actively supervised. Outpatients must be fully recovered, ambulant, and have a responsible adult present to drive them home following intravenous sedation or general anesthesia. An objective method of measuring recovery is helpful in documenting that a patient is sufficiently recovered to leave the office. Accidents outside of the office or clinic can be minimized by admonishing the patient not to drive a motor vehicle or work with machinery for the rest of the day.

POSTANESTHETIC HEADACHE

Headache is usually considered a minor sequel to general anesthesia. However, for the ambulant office patient, where preoperative anxiety without premedication increases the incidence, it has been shown to occur in 50 per cent of outpatients. Hypercarbia is undoubtedly a factor as patients anesthetized with controlled ventilation have fewer headaches than those who breathed spontaneously. Increased cerebral vasodilatation during halothane anesthesia was directly related to the incidence of headache.

Elevation of the head, mild non-narcotic analgesics, application of cool, moist towels to the forehead, and reassurance are helpful. Narcotics may aggravate a postanesthetic headache as they increase intracranial pressure.

MISCELLANEOUS PRECAUTIONS

A patient under the influence of sedation or general anesthesia is unable to give information concerning his identity or the procedure to be performed. While hospitalized patients wear identification bracelets, outpatients generally do not. Verification of the patient's identity, availability of the correct chart and X-rays, and consent for the planned procedure should be confirmed before beginning anesthesia. Operating on the wrong patient, performing an incorrect procedure, or giving the patient a drug to which he is allergic are then avoided.

All patients should be gowned and draped. The accidental soilage of street clothes by blood, vomitus, or other debris is embarassing and better avoided.

Syringes and bottles containing drugs should be correctly labeled with name, concentration, and date of preparation.

Anesthetic induction should not be started until it has been verified that oxygen is available, the anesthetic vaporizer has been charged, strong suction is ready, and all drugs and equipment are ready to use. At least one assistant should be present during anesthetic induction to assist the anesthetist or help restrain the patient and as a chaperone for female patients.

The patient who is struggling while under the influence of sedation or general anesthetics must be protected from injury. Use of safety belts or manual assistance may be necessary to keep the patient from falling out of the dental chair or dislodging intravenous needles. Fractures, tendon or ligament injuries, or torn vessels are best avoided. Transfer of the recovering patient from the operatory to the recovery area must be done with adequate assistance to avoid a fall. Patients who are not fully awake should not be forced to walk, but rather placed in a wheelchair or stretcher for transfer.

SUMMARY

Numerous accidents can happen to patients of the unwary. Knowing these potential problems and following careful technique and the necessary precautions will minimize the incidence of accidents. As sedation impairs the perception of the patient, iatrogenic accidents can occur even in those patients who are conscious.

Bibliography

Albright RL, Babett JA: Poisonous effects of the impurities of nitrous oxide. *J Oral Surg* 26:643, 1968.

Barkin ME, Trieger N: An unusual complication of nasal-tracheal anesthesia. *Anesth Progr* 22:57, 1976.

Blanc VF, Tremblay NAG: The complications of tracheal intubation. *Anesth Analg* 53:203, 1974.

Blitt CD: Complete obstruction of an armored endotracheal tube: case report. *Anesth Analg* 53:4, 1974.

Cascorbi HF: What are the health hazards for anesthesiologists? *Anesth Analg* 57:293, 1978.

Churchill-Davidson MD, et al: Dual neuromuscular block in man. *Anesthesiology* 21:44, 1960.

Coplans MP, Smith NL: Inhalation during dental anesthesia. *Lancet* 1:596, 1964.

Curry JT, Zallen RD: Reduction of thrombophlebitis associated with indwelling catheters. *J Oral Surg* 31:636, 1973.

Driscoll EJ: The dentist and the explosion hazard. *J Oral Surg* 11:26, 1953.

Driscoll, EJ, Gelfman SS, Sweet JB, et al: Thrombophlebitis after intravenous use of anesthesia and sedation: its incidence and natural history *J Oral Surg* 37:809, 1979.

Everett G, Hornbein TF, Allen GD: Hidden hazards of the McKesson Narmatic anesthetic machine. *Anesthesiology* 32:73, 1970.

Hall SC, Ovassapian A: Apnea after intravenous diazepam therapy. *JAMA* 238:1052, 1977.

Hitchen JE, Wiener AP: Unexpected obstruction of a nasotracheal tube: report of case. *J Oral Surg* 31:722, 1973.

Killey HC, Kay LW: *The Prevention of Complications in Dental Surgery*, ed 2. New York, Churchill Livingstone, 1977.

Lamoreaux LF, Urbach KF: Incidence and prevention of muscle pain following the administration of succinylcholine. *Anesthesiology* 21:394, 1960.

Meyer RA, Allen GD: Blood volume studies in oral surgery: II. Postoperative complications and the state of hydration. *J Oral Surg* 26:800, 1968.

Miller R, Arthur A, Stratigos GT: Intra-arterial injection of a barbiturate. *Anesth Prog* 23: 25, 1976.

Munson WE: Cardiac arrest: hazard of tipping a vaporizer. *Anesthesiology* 26:235, 1965.

Rosenberg M, Bolgla J: Protection of teeth and gums during endotracheal intubation. *Anesth Analg* 47:34, 1968.

Salems MR, Baraka A: Treatment of hiccups by pharyngeal stimulation in anesthetized and conscious subjects. *JAMA* 202:126, 1967.

Schiano AM, Strambi RC: Frequency of accidental intravenous injection of local anesthetics in dental practice. *Oral Surg* 17:178, 1964.

Scott GW: Inhalation and chest infection following dental extraction. *Guy's Hosp Rep* 101:77, 1952.

Scott M, Brechner VL: Retrobular hemorrhage from nasotracheal intubation. *Anesthesiology* 20:717, 1959.

Smith RH, et al: Subcutaneous emphysema as a complication of endotracheal intubation. *Anesthesiology* 20:714, 1959.

Snow JC, et al: Corneal injuries during general anesthesia. *Anesth Analg* 54:465, 1975.

Toole JF: Effects of change of head, limb and body position on cephalic circulation. *N Engl J Med* 279:307, 1968.

Topazian RG: Accidental intra-arterial injection: a hazard of intravenous medication. *J Am Dent Assoc* 81:410, 1970.

Tsueda K, et al: Hazards to anesthetic equipment during maxillary osteotomy: report of case. *J Oral Surg* 35:47, 1977.

CHAPTER 17

Pain

We now live in an "enlightened age" of medical science where major breakthroughs in basic research relate to practical clinical applications of discoveries. The quantity and quality of life has been truly appreciated. Prevention of diseases by immunizations, improved health conditions, antimicrobial therapy, and newer antineoplastic drugs has increased the length and quality of life. Until recently, a neglected facet of modern medicine was an integrated approach to the clinical management of chronic pain. With the recognition that chronic benign pain is a disease in itself, we can now direct our attentions to the subjective topic of the pain experience.

In an age in which man has harnessed the atom and has walked on the moon, there is still no single form of therapy that is completely safe and effective in the treatment of chronic benign pain. Many contemporary approaches to treatment of chronic pain have their roots in antiquity. Many cultures and civilizations still utilize techniques such as herbs, acupuncture, heat, cold, and massage as the basis for pain treatment in both chronic and acute pain. With the development of our modern pharmaceutical interventions, we have abandoned many of these primitive techniques. Acute pain is readily dispensed with by clinical availability of these drugs. Though these modern analgesics, anti-inflammatory agents, and psychotropic drugs are remarkably specific and effective for acute pain, they have failed the test of time in treatment of chronic benign pain. Applying the acute pain model to the chronic pain state has resulted in numerous polysurgical and drug treatment failures. This explains the advent of pain clinics (which are an outgrowth of nerve block clinics and other solely somatic oriented approaches). This is not to say that chronic pain is a psychological disease *per se*, but to emphasize that invasive somatic techniques are insufficient to optimally control chronic pain.

The development of the interdisciplinary approach to treatment of chronic pain has been a much needed outgrowth involving virtually all health care specialists working together sharing their respective knowledge and therapies. Not only is chronic pain controlled on this multiple interdisciplinary level, but we have also gained better insights on how to *prevent* the chronic pain experience.

Prior to the interdisciplinary approach, when an individual had a chronic pain problem, therapy was predicated upon the therapist's speciality. A person seeing a primary care specialist (internist, general or family practitioner, pediatrician, etc.) would probably receive systemic analgesics and tranquilizers; an anesthesiologist would perform a nerve block; a neurosurgeon would do neuroablative procedures; a psychiatrist might prescribe drugs plus psychotherapy or psychoanalysis; a psychologist might attempt hypnosis, biofeedback, or psychotherapy. All of these therapies are valid, it is only the timing and integration of all these disciplines for maximum effectiveness that was lacking.

Clinical research has made it apparent that one cannot separate mind and body and expect optimum results in pain control. Interest has been renewed in hypnosis, acupuncture and its modern corollary, electroacupuncture, in treatment of pain. Transcutaneous electrical nerve stimulation (TENS) and medical self-help care (biofeedback, autogenics, meditation) have also become popular. Part of the mysticism of the past is becoming the science of the present and the future with respect to these unorthodox modalities. The use of electrical stimulation for pain is not really new. It was first employed by Pedanius Discordides, a Greek surgeon with Nero's armies, who used a torpedo fish as a source of electricity. The ancient acupuncture needle has created a new concept of pain control generically called stimulation-produced analgesia (SPA). With these rebirths and the rerecognition of muscle pain syndromes, a noteworthy dent has been made in the management of chronic pain. Understanding that stress and psychological factors play an important role in a patient's tendency to attain and maintain the chronic pain state has also contributed much to our understanding of the total pain experience; thus, a more rational treatment plan can now be instituted when both somatic and psychological evidence are addressed.

The goal of this chapter is to provide exposure to modern dimensions in pain control and emphasize both physical and psychological examination as they relate to treatment of chronic pain. This chapter is not intended to be a complete work on chronic facial pain.

THE NATURE OF PAIN

What is pain or, more correctly, what is the pain experience? It is not merely a noxious sensation on "pain receptors" that causes pain to be registered at higher central nervous system function. The total pain experience encompasses that noxious sensation, the psychological makeup of that person, and the subsequent behavioral *reaction* to it.

In defining pain, a complex phenomenon involving soma and psyche comes into play. Any dentist or physician who wishes to wholly define a personal, private sensation of this nature should be knowledgeable in all disciplines of medicine, dentistry, and psychology. Currently, the medical profession does not have a specialist in chronic pain as we do in the acute pain model (i.e., surgeon for acute appendicitis, dentist for an acute abscessed tooth). But it is apparent that a specialty in chronic pain is slowly emerging from the ranks of the interdisciplinary study of pain, perhaps to be known as algology.

One must also be exact in what situation one defines the pain. For example, pathological pain is frequently compared to experimental pain, but numerous investigators have reported inconsistencies when comparing results of these situations. The experimental condition is self-limiting, portends no continuing or chronic pain, may be terminated if too adversive, and is associated with little or no anxiety. Chronic nonexperimental pain, on the other hand, is not self-limiting, tends to become worse with time, cannot be terminated, and has various degrees of accompanying anxiety and/or depression.

Classically, most definitions of pain rely almost exclusively upon a neurophysiological substrate and have omitted the vast contributions of psychological and psychiatric pain literature. The enlightened pain therapist is well aware of the hazards of a purely mechanistic approach as witnessed by numerous neuroablative procedures which have failed the test of time. Since pain is not only a noxious stimulus but also a psychological experience, chronic pain must be defined not only from the somatic, neurophysiological viewpoint, but also from the psychological perspective. When attempting to define chronic pain, the psychological factors are even more important, as they do not accurately fit the acute pain model definition. This will be elaborated upon in the subsection on psychological aspects of pain. It is to be hoped that a new and more comprehensive definition of pain will be forthcoming from the scientific research of numerous interdisciplinary pain groups.

Most medical dictionaries define pain in similar language for the acute pain experience. *Dorland's Illustrated Medical Dictionary* states that "pain . . . is a more or less localized sensation of discomfort, distress, or agony, resulting from the stimulation of specialized nerve endings. . . . It serves as a protective mechanism insofar as it induces the sufferer to remove or withdraw from the source." This is an accurate description for the acute pain model, but does not entirely describe chronic pain. Currently, chronic pain is associated with poor localization, specific neuroanatomical pathways, such as phantom limb pain and other central pain phenomena. Clinically, chronic pain of diverse anatomical location is frequently referred to as protopathic or global in nature. "The stimulation of specialized nerve endings" is correct when referring to acute pain from free nerve endings of dental pulpal origin, but what of referred pain to the gums, teeth, and adnexa from muscular and neural sources, remote from the orofacial area of pain complaint?

Acute pain does serve as a "protective mechanism to warn us that something is wrong," but in the chronic pain patient, pain serves very little, if any, useful function for the patient's immediate protection and safety. Discomfort, distress, or agony are very relative, affective experiences, although they may also reveal some clues to the etiology of the various components of the verbal complaint of pain. This is the view of the McGill pain questionnaire of Melzack and Torgerson in which they have categorized 102 terms most commonly used to describe the verbal report of pain into three general classes:

1. *Sensory, qualitative descriptors* in terms of temporal, spatial, pressure, thermal, and other properties. These verbal reports are of pain being "pounding" "spreading," "crushing," "burning," "aching."

2. *Affective quality descriptors* in terms of tension, fear, and various autonomic properties: for example, "exhausting," "awful," "nauseating."

3. *Intensity of the total* pain is expressed in terms such as: "agonizing," "excruciating," "miserable."

While *acute pain* does serve as a protective mechanism to seek help for that particular problem, chronic pain may exist long after the source of the original insult is gone, for example, phantom pain and causalgic pain states. Neural blockade with anesthetics may or may not define the etiology and if the anesthetic does not stop the pain, what then is the "source"? There are no known clinical tests to elicit the necessary data, such as there are in a blood sugar test for diabetes or a creatinine test for renal failure, to determine the subjective magnitude of the total pain experience.

PAIN AS A SENSATION

Pain professionals find it helpful to distinguish between a *painful sensation* (awareness of nociceptive stimulus) and the pain *experience* (the total subjective identification with pain). The total pain experience dictates how a particular person will *react* to a noxious stimulus. A broader definition of the pain experience may be a complex psychophysiological experience with several functional components: sensory-discriminative perception, suffering-motivational, and visceral somatic reflexes.

Pain as a "pure" sensation is mediated by pain receptors which are called nociceptors. Three types of nociceptors are currently identified: 1) high threshold mechanoreceptors, 2) heat nociceptors, and 3) "polymodal" nociceptors which are responsive to both thermal and mechanical noxious stimuli. With the activation of these pain receptors, afferent information is sent *via* the peripheral nerves and the neuraxis to be processed by the higher centers for both a physiological response and its modifications by the subjective interpretation of the pain experience.

The classical "pain pathway" is thought to involve large diameter, high conductive velocity, thinly myelinated A-δ fibers which mediate the "first pain." This "first pain" is rapid in onset, sharp, and generally well localized. Shortly thereafter, the "second pain" fibers of small diameter, unmyelinated, and slow conduction are activated; these are referred to as C fibers. These fibers have been shown to account for the aching, burning pain of long duration and poor localization, and seem to account for the affective and autonomic reaction to painful stimuli. The nociceptor afferent fibers of the trigeminal system supply cutaneous and subcutaneous tissue, viscera, and muscle and other deeper structures, subsequently relaying this information to the brainstem trigeminal nuclear complex. The complex pathway beyond this brainstem area will not be discussed in this chapter except to mention that the complex nature of the ascending and descending excitatory and inhibitory pathways and their interconnections remain a source of controversy and continuing research. However, recent work on descending pathways involved in antinociception will be discussed in the subsection "Stimulation-Produced Analgesia" (SPA).

The current physiological theories of pain generally fall into several major categories: specificity, pattern, gate control, and biochemical theories of pain.

The *specificity theory of pain* relies heavily on the fact that there are specific known peripheral fibers that function as nociceptive transmitters; *i.e.*, the A-δ and C fibers. This simplistic, straight-through action system to the central nervous system and somatosensory cortex lacks explanation of a specific role for the specialized nociceptors described previously, the physiological descending control systems, and the psychological reactions to the noxious stimulation.

The *pattern theory of pain* is based upon the concept that pain perception results from stimulus intensity and central summation (probably located in the dorsal horns of the spinal cord). This rejects the notion that there are specialized peripheral nerve endings and pain fibers. Painful stimuli do not exist, only stimuli that are painful. The clinical expression of pain is a result of the summation of the spacial and temporal pattern of input.

The Melzack and Wall *gate control theory* retains certain concepts of both the specificity theory and the pattern theory. Their theory proposes a dorsal, spinal gating mechanism in the substantia gelatinosa which modulates sensory input. The delicate balance of small fiber input (A-δ and C fiber) and large diameter input (A-β) when in balance results in no pain perception. Increased activity of large diameter fibers closes the gate and prevents the synaptic transmission to the centrally projecting (transmission) T cells. In contradistinction, the small diameter fibers open the gate and facilitate T cell activity when stimulus intensity is sufficient. Also, a central control trigger influences the gate by activating the efferent dorsal lateral funiculus (DLF) pathways and the afferent ascending dorsal column of the spinal cord. These activate selective brain processes that influence the modulating properties of the gate control system. The T cells activate the neural system that constitutes the action system responsible for both response and perception.

Melzack *et al.* viewed the specificity theory as making unwarranted psychological assumptions, but have accepted *specialization* (*i.e.*, A-δ and C fibers), and the rejected pattern theory as it seems to conflict with neurophysiological evidence of the specific nociceptors.

A recent *biochemical theory of pain* proposed by Lindahl implicates an alteration of the pH in a nerve or in the vicinity of a nerve or nerve ending. Elevated hydrogen ion concentrations exist in septic abscesses and are rendered painless when neutralized by alkaline solution injections. Tuberculous abscesses are neutral pH, but an injection of acidic solution will provoke pain. The nucleus pulposus and a herniated disc is acidic in nature, as are gastric ulcers, painful hematomas and fractures, malignant and aching tumors, ischemic pain (as in coronary insufficiency), and claudication. This may also be an attractive model for the study and treatment of pain.

It becomes apparent that many pure physiological explanations of pain have both validity and shortcomings in explaining pain phenomena. The psychological aspects of the pain experience will be explored in the next section.

PSYCHOLOGICAL ASPECTS OF PAIN

Far beyond the current physiological theories of pain lies the enormous amount of information obtained on psychological and behavioral aspects of pain. The goal of this section is to review those psychological areas which are important in the clinical management of chronic pain. Health care scientists speak of "thresholds of pain" as associated primarily with physiological functions and "tolerances" primarily in terms associated with the psychological variables, such as attitudes and motivation.

Numerous earlier experimental studies in pain devised to separate these two variable components have been questioned recently in view of the "sensory decision theory" (signal detection theory) which separates the cognitive factors from sensory variables. It appears to be more accurate than a pure threshold methodology as it accounts for willingness, and for subjective bias of an experimental subject in reporting the pain experience. It is hoped that this approach will give clearer data as to the various roles of the physiological and psychological aspects of experimental pain and will thus exert its influence on the management of clinical pain.

Numerous early life experiences (and operants) play a major role in an individual's subjective perception of pain. For example, animals raised in a selective pain-free environment in early life show marked insensitivity when exposed to noxious stimuli in later life. The family's total experience regarding pain and resultant attitudes are readily transmitted to their offspring. They are, perhaps, the most important factors in determining the degree of anxiety or lack of it related to expectant and actual dental treatment. Subsequently, this may be reinforced in either a positive or negative direction depending upon an individual's early dental experiences. Children of mothers with high anxiety scores exhibited more negative dental behavior during extractions than those children of mothers with low anxiety scores.

Pain tolerance is subject to the social influences of models. If this modeling process is a negative one, the results will generally be negative, just as any other of life's psychosocial learning processes. The interaction of the practitioner with the patient is of no less importance, since the practitioner is a model and a source of pain experience. The mere substitution of the word "discomfort" for the word "pain" portends minimal discomfort or no pain at all. This, of course, depends heavily on one's perception of dental pain and the skill of the interested and skilled practitioner. Numerous experimental studies using the word "pain" vs. more "neutral" terms have conclusively demonstrated neutral terms to have a more favorable outcome on children's behavior before, during, and after dental procedures.

In experimental design, subjects' abilities to control the pain experience has been shown to reduce anxiety and the amount of pain experienced. When a subject can voluntarily terminate a noxious stimulation, the results are generally more favorable. This application of control can be accomplished in the clinical situation with a well-informed patient who has at least partial control over a potentially painful procedure. It is well-known that reduction of anxiety increases pain tolerance and attenuates the physiological responses of sympathetic hyperactivity: increased cardiac rate, increased blood pressure and respiration, palmar diaphoresis, and muscular tension. It is also known that an intimate relationship exists between pain and anxiety, and many pain therapists recognize that treatment of one often provides relief of the other. A pure somatic mechanistic approach to pain is fraught with failure and compounds the clinical problems.

In the acute pain model, the noxious stimulus is identified and appropriate action is taken to terminate or control both pain and anxiety. However, for most chronic pain patients, the stimulus cannot be identified, which results in more anxiety since the fear of the unknown leads to an even more distressing pain experience. With time, many chronic pain patients will exhaust their sympathetic hyperactivity and pass into a more vegetative state with various signs and symptoms. This is characterized by feelings of helplessness, hopelessness, hysteria, hypochondriasis, and despair, with subjective complaints of sleep disturbance (initial, interval, and terminal insomnia), changes in appetite (loss or increase of weight), irritability, decreased interest, loss of self-esteem and libido, erosions of personal relationships with family and friends, as well as increased somatization of complaints. The acute pain patient then passes into the stage of a complicated pain problem and finally a chronic benign pain syndrome with all the negative consequences. The actual clinical situation may be viewed as a continuum from acute to chronic pain and elements of depression and anxiety coexist to varying degrees.

It has become increasingly clear that anxiety, reactive depression, and the somatic complaint must all be treated simultaneously if one is to be successful in treating the chronic pain patient. The philosophy of the well-organized interdisciplinary pain clinic should be to treat the chronic pain patient holistically without entering the arena of mind/body controversy. As in acute pain and anxiety, chronic pain is often treated effectively by treating the depression which may be left long after the initial noxious stimulus has regressed. This reactive depression exists to varying degrees in virtually all chronic pain patients and must be recognized to effect optimal therapy. In a simplistic fashion, it may be helpful to obtain a history concerning the chronic pain patient's depression in terms of losses (Table 17.1). Losses imply having had something which was positive that has been replaced by negative traits. A skilled practitioner will be able to derive much useful information, if these questions are asked in the context of comparing the present clinical situation to a time when the patient was healthy.

Most chronic pain patients do not present with the complaints of depression or anxiety, but do complain of pain and other organic symptoms. The clinician must be trained to elicit these subtle clinical expressions of depression in order to achieve optimal results.

Table 17.1
Clinical Expressions of Depression in Terms of Loss

1. Self-esteem
2. Hope
3. Emotional stability
4. Interest
5. Normal sleep
6. Libido
7. Energy
8. Appetite
9. Motivation
10. Family/friends
11. Vocation/avocation

Those patients who verbalize symptoms of depression seem to respond well to antidepressant medication. When combining psychological and pharmacological therapies, pain tolerance appears to increase while anxiety appears to decrease.

The most commonly used drugs are of the tricyclic group and to a lesser degree monoamine oxidase inhibitors. The dimethylated tricyclics (doxepin, amitriptyline, imipramine) tend to cause more central nervous system reuptake of serotonin and more sedation than the monomethylated group (protriptyline, desipramine, nortriptyline). The monomethylated tricyclics tend to facilitate greater uptake of norepinephrine and result in greater central nervous system stimulation. As a general rule, the dimethylated tricyclics are used more in agitated depression, the monomethylated tricyclics in retardant depressions. For further and more detailed clinical use of these psychotherapeutic drugs, their side effects, and complications, information is readily available in full disclosure inserts, the *Physicians' Desk Reference*, and other textbooks.

Experimental evidence from a wide variety of work seems to implicate the serotonergic neurons in the brain and descending pathways within the spinal cord involved in antinociception and the potentiation of the analgesic effects of opiate-like drugs. Evidence suggests that increased central nervous system activity of serotonin is associated with analgesia and potentiates narcotic analgesics, whereas decreased central nervous system serotonin activity is correlated with hyperalgesia and decreased responses to narcotic analgesics. Clinical studies involving use of tricyclics to increase serotonin reuptake in clinically depressed patients have shown it to be effective. The clinical use of serotonin precursor loading is used currently both for agitated depression, for sedation, and to augment the effects of opioid stimulation-produced analgesia. Reported in the literature is the use of L-tryptophan loading (3 to 6 g per day in divided doses) which has been supplemented with pyridoxine and nicotinamide to facilitate conversion to serotonin. It must be taken on an empty stomach, as it competes with other amino acids for central nervous system uptake. Therefore, tryptophan has been called "nature's tranquilizer" by it supporters and is found naturally in meat, bananas, avocados, pineapples, and dairy products.

The outcome of pain therapy depends on the training a pain therapist has received, his or her total perspective of what pain is, and understanding what the patient behaviors mean in their particular clinical situations. If organic causes have been ruled out by appropriate workups, frequently the naive practitioner will utilize the catch-all phrase: "psychogenic pain." At very best, this may be used as a positive reinforcer; at worst, as another insult to the chronic pain patient. When this tentative diagnosis has been reached by the process of excluding factors, the patient may, at least, be spared the numerous somatic techniques that are mutilative, destructive, irreversible, and frequently of questionable benefit. Even minimally invasive techniques, such as trigger point injection, acupuncture, and TENS (transcutaneous electrical neural stimulation), should be used with caution as they tend to separate, or deny, any psychological variables of the patient's chronic pain. These useful techniques, though not always curative in themselves, lend a nondestructive approach to the patient if utilized properly. These techniques may be viewed as a vehicle for appropriate adjunctive, psychological investigative therapy. It need not be labeled formally as psychotherapy, since it represents a therapeutic blend of both psychological and somatic techniques (holistic dentistry/medicine) in our industrialized world of mechanized health care.

PSYCHOGENIC PAIN

When numerous medical and surgical workups show a disparity between the patient's subjective complaints and the objective findings, the diagnosis of "psychogenic pain" frequently arises. When observing new patients with various forms of pain behavior, many practitioners fall into this trap. Since there is no identifiable noxious stimulus to cause the pain, it must therefore be in the patient's head. From the patient's perspective, it is pain, and to insist upon this diagnosis *alone* by exclusion adds more psychological problems to the patient's already burdensome list. Chronic pain is a dynamic interaction of somatogenic factors and anxiety, depression, and emotional variables. By imposing the label "psychogenic" on the patient, the therapist communicates "unreal, imaginary, unwarranted pain" and that the patient can readily dispose of the pain by himself or by psychotherapy. The use of the "psychogenic" diagnosis alone may be counterproductive to the patient's overall therapy and rehabilitation.

Psychophysiological pain, or pain of psychosomatic origin, is defined as: "a chronic exaggerated state of the normal physiological expressions of emotion with repressions of the individual's subjective feelings." It has been shown that long standing visceral states can eventually lead to structural changes and pathology, tension headaches and bruxism being prime examples. In the case of chronic bruxism, muscular dysfunction with hyperactive and occlusal contact leads to microtrauma and pain which intensifies muscular hyperactivity, protective immobilization, disuse atrophy, fibrous reactions, contracture, and disability. The vasospasm created by the pain and muscle spasm may lead to further secondary vasospasm by ischemia and, again, generate the fibrous reaction and contracture resulting in functional disability. Discussion with the patient about stress and anxiety reduction to relieve the symptoms is noninvasive and nondestructive, but is productive and may be the treatment of choice. It is simply not therapeutically effective to tell patients that there is nothing objective in their diagnostic

workup and then to tell the anxious patient he will have to learn to live with his pain. Situational adjustment and antianxiety drugs by themselves are insufficient. A total program of "how to relax" should be offered which may include biofeedback, hypnosis, guided imagery and/or meditation, depending on a critical analysis of how that particular individual has previously learned new skills in the past. Conditioned relaxation is not inherent and must be learned. Intellectual knowledge of these relaxation techniques is insufficient since they must be coupled with actual experience for eliciting the desired neural response. Knowledge of conditioned relaxation coupled with practice results in somatic understanding. This understanding by the body's cognitive centers spells "ease," not "disease."

Hypochondriacal pain may be viewed as a corollary to psychophysiological reactions. Obsessive concerns over tension headaches and myofunctional stomatognathic pain, will produce and/or exaggerate the symptoms. Psychophysiological pain and hypochondriasis may frequenlty coexist and reinforce each other in a destructive cyclical pattern. These patterns may exist because of simple suffering related to the unknown cause of the physical complaint to frank cognitive breakdown and psychoses. This represents a challenging psychotherapeutic problem but, when dealt with appropriately, may prevent or attenuate ongoing organic disease.

Hysterical conversion reactions to pain are frequently associated with the head and neck regions. They are frequently associated with conversion of anxiety into somatic symptoms which may be of symbolic nature. Once a conversion has been made there may be little clinical expression of anxiety and depression, and it is usually discovered by the psychologist during testing and inteview.

Use of the term "psychogenic pain" without a clear understanding by patient and therapist as to its meaning can further reinforce guilt, anger, anxiety, depression, and a host of other negative psychophysiological variables. Use of the term "psychogenic pain" can be an iatrogenic cause of further disease and not palliative in any sense. This does not mean that psychogenic factors are nonexistent and must be denied, but rather that they must be carefully utilized in the total concept of treating the mind and body of pain patients. It is much more humane and therapeutically positive to discuss and explore the psychological and behavioral variables that affect the nature of a patient's pain complaint. Overtly adding the "psychogenic" label to a patient brings into an already gray area conflicts which may defeat the course of optimal therapy. When exploring these variables, it must be kept in mind that the acute pain model is limited in temporal terms of seconds and minutes, while the chronic pain experience is manifested in terms of many months and years in which patients inevitably learn and condition themselves. The stimulus and response discrepancies of chronic pain patients should be appreciated since they are a source of valuable information for planning and prescribing further therapy. Since they are a behavioral reflection of that person's total pain experience, they should never be taken lightly or dismissed. Emotional distress is as real to a patient as any acute painful incident. A patient who is encouraged and allowed to participate in a therapeutic partnership will progress more rapidly in goal attainment.

Chronic pain patients in many clinical situations are *passive* recipients of numerous somatic therapies prescribed without benefit of active patient participation. Passivity encourages "sick behavior" by reinforcing feelings of helplessness, hopelessness, anxiety, anger, and further depression. "Well behavior" is an essential requirement necessary to ensure optimal results in long term therapy. Reinforcing "well behavior," while ignoring "pain behavior," is fundamental to effecting optimal pain rehabilitation.

Once the chronic pain syndrome is recognized and accepted as a total mind/body experience by both patient and therapist, then realistic goals which provide the necessary reinforcers can be set to ensure proper motivation and optimal pain relief. These are the same principles of learning which those health care practitioners who utilize operant conditioning and behavior modification techniques have shown to be effective. Many may argue that treating these behavioral symptoms alone may leave patients in chronic pain, but they no longer verbalize it. This is true, but this is in a positive direction, as it reduces and/or eliminates part of the symptomatology that heavily contributes to the chronic pain experience. In fact, it may well be the therapy of choice before attempting any somatic or pharmacological approach. If appropriately done in a clinical situation, it will further reinforce patients by giving them a new sense of self-worth as they progress from sick to well behavior. Rewards for goals achieved also help to mobilize the patient who is both mentally and physically deconditioned. Appropriately prescribed physical activity also helps recondition the body and mobilize the intrinsic healing powers inherent in all individuals. The same is true with the psychological factors. If you do not reward the patient for pain behavior, but do for well behavior, positive learning and conditioning occur, effecting maximal patient benefits.

THE PAIN EXPERIENCE

We prefer to think of chronic pain as a spectrum of subjective experiences involving physical, perceptual, cognitive, and emotional factors. As seen in the sections on the pure physiological mechanisms of pain and the psychological aspects of pain, it becomes increasingly clear that mind and body are inseparable. Thus, appropriate meaningful pain management inextricably involves both somatic and psychological approaches. This is the essential function of an interdisciplinary pain group and evolution of the total pain therapist (algologist).

When chronic pain is viewed from this holistic perspective, it becomes countereffective and countertherapeutic to consider whether the patient has "real or imaginary pain," "physiological or psychological pain" or even more counterproductive to label the pain syndrome "legitimate or illegitimate."

PREVENTING CHRONIC OROFACIAL PAIN

Although prevention of *acute* orofacial pain is a mandatory responsibility of the dental practitioner, prevention of the chronic pain experience is no less so.

In the same way that an allergic history to local anesthetics, sedatives, and inhalation agents is routinely conducted, dental patients should be evaluated psychologically to ensure that a dental procedure does not provide a convenient focus for the chronic pain experience. Untimely procedures conducted on anxious or agitated patients are often important etiological factors in the development of temporomandibular joint pain dysfunction syndromes.

Much can be learned from careful observation of patients. Sensitive issues may be *verbally* denied but subtly affirmed by body language, such as postural changes, flushing or blanching, eye blinks, or flickers. "Accidental" remarks and bouts of inappropriate crying or laughter may also be indicative of psychopathological dysfunction.

A review of psychological systems should include evaluation of cognitive perceptive factors, such as the perceived locus of control. "Externalizers" believe that they are innocent victims of a problem imposed by some unknown malevolent external force, and that only an outside agent (dentist or physician) can cure it. "Internalizers," on the other hand, feel that they themselves are responsible for their pain and, therefore, that they alone

have the ability to overcome it. Because expectations concerning the success or failure of therapy often become self-fulfilling prophecies, past experiences with pain or pain therapies may also be relevant. While a positive attitude on part of the therapist may be beneficial, we discourage promotion of unrealistic positive expectations, for when unfulfilled, they can sabotage further therapy.

Patients who complain that they have obtained less than optimal therapeutic results should not be quickly dismissed by saying: "You are crazy," or "It's all in your head" Such patients are almost certain to develop chronic pain-related problems. Had these patients been properly prepared prior to therapy, they might have easily avoided chronic pain problems.

Sir William Osler, the father of American medicine, once stated: "It is more important to know what sort of a patient has a disease than what sort of disease a patient has." The body does have a mind, and the two are inseparable. In the case of the chronic pain experience, dental therapy directed exclusively to the body is usually only palliative at best, and iatrogenic at worst.

CHRONIC PAIN PATIENT CHARACTERISTICS

Many years of experience with chronic benign pain patients has shown recurrent characteristic patterns that are now recognized by most pain therapists. Certainly, not all of these characteristics exist in each and every patient. They are viewed here as a spectrum that will channel the dental practitioner's attention to the milieu in which these patients attempt to survive.

Table 17.2 represents a formidable list of characteristics, all of which must be recognized and considered in pain management to ensure optimal relief of symptoms and rehabilitation. All of these characteristics are delicately intertwined and affect each other in numerous ways. Since the key to optimal chronic pain manage-

Table 17.2.
Chronic Pain Patient Characteristics

1. Addictions and dependencies:
   Narcotics
   Tranquilizers
   Other drugs
   Surgery
   Health care professionals
   Family/friends
2. High stress levels
3. Depression
4. Abnormal MMPI
5. Hostile/manipulative
6. Impotency/frigidity
7. Pain talk obsession
8. Poor surgical risk and prognosis
9. Physical and emotional deconditioning
10. Marital/family conflicts
11. Poor vocational prognosis
12. Permanent disability
13. Active litigation

Table 17.3
Acute Pain Model

1. Brief and usually self-limiting
2. Useful pain
3. Appropriate cure:
   Medical
   Surgical
4. Appropriate medications:
   Narcotics
   Other analgesics
   Antianxiety (tranquilizers)
   Cortisone and anti-inflammatory
   Tender loving care (TLC)
5. No permanent disability

Table 17.4.
Chronic Pain Model

1. Prolonged duration:
   Conditioning
   Litigation
   Isolated polytherapies
   Partial relief and exacerbations
2. No appropriate cure
3. Pain without significance
4. Acute pain medications inappropriate:
   Narcotics cause addiction and psychological dependence
   Analgesics lead to organ damage
   Antianxiety tranquilizers frequently cause frigidity, impotence, depression
   Cortisone and anti-inflammatories are frequently ineffective
   TLC may lead to reinforced pain behavior
5. Permanent disability

ment depends upon a "total person" approach, these characteristics must be discovered in the history and physical examination. If they are not pinpointed, important links will be missed and suboptimal pain management will result. Because of previous and ongoing factors involved in treating the chronic pain experience, this perspective must be taken. Most of these patients have obviously *failed the acute pain model* with numerous polysurgical and polypharmaceutical interventions, and now must be reviewed from the total interdisciplinary approach.

ACUTE VS. CHRONIC PAIN MODEL

The usual approach to the study of pain and its management is to briefly review the characteristics of acute (Table 17.3) and chronic pain (Table 17.4). These are not absolute, but represent the extremes of ends in the spectrum of an ongoing experience.

For management of acute or short term pain, modern dentistry and medicine have developed numerous effective drugs and procedures to attenuate those noxious stimuli. Since, by definition, acute pain is of brief duration and self-limiting, these agents and techniques provide the necessary temporary relief while the body heals itself.

When appropriately administered, nerve blocks and other modern anesthetic techniques (discussed elsewhere in this text) spare patients undergoing operative dental procedures the slightest degree of discomfort. Postoperative pain and discomfort can be minimized or eliminated by acupuncture, hypnosis, narcotics, nonnarcotic analgesics, and/or minor tranquilizers.

We are all aware that acute pain is an appropriate signal telling us something is wrong and that definitive action is taken to eliminate it by various techniques. Yet these highly developed and sophisticated approaches that have proven so successful in acute pain management are ineffective and fail the test of time in the treatment of long term or chronic pain.

Chronic pain, unlike acute pain, does not get better by itself. In fact, it usually gets worse with time, and the patient has acquired many of the chronic pain patient characteristics as previously described.

There is usually no appropriate "cure" as in the acute pain model. The acute pain has spent its usefulness in telling us "something is wrong." Acute pain medications lead to narcotic addiction. Other analgesics eventually lead to organ damage, such as analgesic hepatitis and analgesic nephropathy. Habitual use of antianxiety tranquilizers may cause and hasten reactive depression, impotence, and frigidity. Cortisone and other antiinflammatories are ineffective once tough fibrous scar tissue is laid down. Sympathy and tender loving care (TLC) may lead to reinforcement of pain behavior. Chronic pain patients are referred from doctor to doctor, even if they are fortunate to find temporary relief, the pain usually returns. Despite these obvious facts, most health care practitioners continue to use the same procedures and medications in treating both acute and chronic pain. In medical and dental schools they attended, pain management techniques were based on a rather simplistic perspective of the problem, usually in the context of acute pain.

STIMULATION-PRODUCED ANALGESIA (SPA) AND ENDOGENOUS OPIATES

Throughout the centuries mankind has attempted various methods to attenuate painful stimuli. Many of these techniques employed are what we now recognize to be counterstimulation. With the advent of chemoanesthetic agents, these techniques were superseded by either rendering the patient unconscious for acute painful experiences such as surgery or by utilizing local anesthetics to prevent noxious neural impulses from reaching higher levels of the central nervous system. Since neither of these modalities, however, is practical or effective in the treatment of chronic pain, the medical sciences are again reviewing the field of counterstimulation.

Numerous forms of counterstimulation have their roots in antiquity, ranging from cauterization of specific parts of the ear for sciatica, as described by Hippocrates and other early healers of the Mesopotamian basin, to electrical stimulation of painful conditions by Greek surgeons utilizing torpedo fish. Much of modern physical therapy may also be explained by the counterstimulation theory, but recent research suggests that more intricate mechanisms are involved.

There would appear to be at least two distinct pathways involved in the utilization of electrical stimulation of various parts of the nervous system for pain relief. The first of these provides analgesia during stimulation but has no lasting affect on termination of the stimulus. This is called non-opioid analgesia and is produced either through the peripheral or central nervous system. The analgesia obtained is *not* blocked or reversed by naloxone, a potent narcotic antagonist. The sites where this type of electrically induced analgesia has been demonstrated are listed in Table 17.5.

The second pathway for production of analgesia using SPA appears to involve an endogenous opiate system (Table 17.6).

Various researchers have demonstrated that stimulation of the central nervous system in the periaqueductal gray (PAG)

Table 17.5.
Non-opioid High Frequency Electrically Produced Analgesia

1. Peripheral stimulation
   Peripheral nerves
   Motor points
   Golgi tendon
2. Deep brain stimulation (DBS)
   Thalamus
   Internal capsule

Table 17.6
Modern History of Stimulation-Produced Analgesia

1969	Reynolds	PAG stimulation in animals
1972	Akil, Mayer, and Liebeskind	Reversal of SPA by naloxone
1973	Mainland Chinese	Cross-circulation and CSF experiments in EAC
1973	Simon et al.; Terenius, Pert, and Synder	Discover opiate receptors in CNS and ileum
1975	Hughes et al.	Discover enkephalins
1976	Bradbury et al.	Suggests β-lph in production of β-ep
1976	Li and Chung	β-ep discovered in camel pituitary
1976	Pomeranz and Chiu	Naloxone blockade of acupuncture analgesia in mice
1977	Sjölund, Terenius, and Eriksson	Increased CSF endorphins after EAC
1977	Mayer and Price	Acupuncture analgesia reversed with naloxone
1978	Akil and Richardson	50% increase in CSF enkephalins and 20–30 times increase in β-ep after PAG stimulation
1979	Hosobuchi and Adams	Pain relief with PAG stimulation and reversal with naloxone
1979	Liebeskind	Site specificity of CNS SPA and naloxone reversal
1980	Pert and Ng	Electrical auriculoacupuncture depletes brain endorphins and increases CSF endorphins
1981	Carr et al.	Physical conditioning facilitates exercise-induced secretion of β-lph and β-ep in women

Abbreviations: PAG, periaqueductal gray; SPA, stimulation-produced analgesia; EAC, electrical acupuncture; β-lph, β-lipotropin; β-ep, β-endorphin.

and periventricular gray (PVG), as well as the nucleus raphe magnus, gives rise to analgesia in both laboratory animals and man. It has also been shown to leave all other sensory and motor modalities intact and has no effect on motivational, emotional, or attentional parameters.

In contrast to the previous type of analgesia described, this analgesia outlasts the actual period of stimulation from hours to days (opioid). The analgesia can be reversed by the parenteral administration of naloxone. This has been demonstrated experimentally by reversing the effect of such noxious stimuli as electric shock, tooth pulp stimulation, radiant heat, and chemical irritants, as well as diverse clinical pain syndromes. Such findings suggested the release of an endogenous opiate at the PAG and PVG during stimulation. The isolation of several polypeptides from the cerebrospinal fluid of experimental animals which could produce similar specific analgesia and whose reaction could also be reversed by naloxone enhanced this theory. These compounds were named enkephalins (within

the brain) and led to a search for similar compounds which were to become known as the endorphins, that is, drugs produced within the body with morphine-like action.

The endorphins produced at the PAG and PVG travel to the trigeminal nucleus caudalis and to the dorsolateral funiculus (DLF). Radioactively tagged enkephalin injected into the raphe magnus has been shown to travel down the dorsolateral column and appear in the opiate receptors of lamina I, V, and, to a lesser extent, lamina II of the substantia gelatinosa at the exact level of incoming nociceptive signals. This descending pathway for modulation of pain impulses can be abolished or reduced when the DLF is sectioned above the level of noxious input. Analgesia remains above the level of sectioning and is lost below that level no matter whether analgesia is produced by electrical stimulation, morphine, or endorphin injection.

In addition to deep brain stimulation (DBS), various forms of peripheral stimulation have been shown to attenuate ex-

perimental and clinical pain with analgesia which is also reversed by naloxone
(see Table 17.6). Acupuncture and transcutaneous electrical neural stimulation
(TENS) are but two such modalities which
activate the endogenous opiates peripherally.

Recent research has demonstrated an
increase in cerebrospinal fluid levels of
endorphins following electroacupuncture
in patients with chronic low back pain.
Patients with facial pain, however, did not
consistently produce an elevation of endorphins in their cerebrospinal fluid after
successful electroacupuncture. It has
been postulated that if the fluid samples
had been taken at much higher levels, a
rise in endorphins might have been revealed.

With the presence of endorphins established, inquiring minds turned to the
source of these natural analgesics. The
fact that SPA requires some 20 to 30 minutes to produce analgesia suggested that
the endorphins were hormonal in origin.
In support of this theory was the discovery
that some of the enkephalins and endorphins which had been chemically isolated
to date were contained within the structure of a hormone of the pituitary, the β-
lipotropin (LPH). This polypeptide, consisting of some 91 amino acids, includes
within its chain:

α-Endorphin	LPH amino acids	61 to 76
β-Endorphin	LPH amino acids	61 to 91
γ-Endorphin	LPH amino acids	61 to 77
Methionine enkephalin	LPH amino acids	61 to 65

The possibility that the pituitary is the
sole producer of SPA-induced endorphins, at least in some animals, is suggested by the fact that pituitary ablation
in the rat prevents SPA analgesia being
induced.

Further understanding of the endogenous opiate system has allowed us to understand some of the negative results

achieved in several early studies by Western researchers. Many of the chronic pain
patients in these studies were receiving
exogenous opiates and opiate receptor-
like drugs (propoxyphene) for therapeutic
purposes. These would probably have in-
terfered with the endogenous opiate
mechanism and account for the failure to
produce analgesia. In the pain clinics at
the UCLA School of Medicine, the use of
these drugs is restricted during the course
of any form of SPA, thus maintaining the
availability of the opiate receptors to endogenous opiates. This is supported by
more recent research demonstrating that
electroacupuncture and TENS are more
effective when the opiate receptors are
first "flushed" with naloxone.

From this brief overview of SPA and
the endogenous opiate system, it will be
clear why many ancient techniques of
pain control have now achieved medical
and scientific respectability and why they
are now being utilized in appropriate
cases for the management of acute and
chronic pain.

STIMULATION PRODUCED ANALGESIA (SPA) IN DENTISTRY

Although chemoanesthesia, local or
general, represents the predominant
method of anesthesia in dentistry, it is
useful to know about alternative modalities that may be used when standard
methods are inadequate or inappropriate.
Acupuncture can create local analgesia
(not anesthesia) and general quiescence
and appears to stimulate the body's endogenous opiate system (endorphins and
enkephalins). Electroacupuncture has
been shown to have a more optimal clinical outcome for operative dentistry and
myofascial pain syndromes, as well as selected temporomandibular joint (TMJ)
and facial neuralgic pain syndromes.

Acupuncture in Dentistry

INTRODUCTION

Acupuncture is one of the most controversial subjects in American medicine

and dentistry. In the early 1970s, Western health care professionals received glowing reports of a "new" system of analgesia. As a result of renewed diplomatic relationships with the People's Republic of China, acupuncture came to the forefront with spectacular reports to Western scientists and lay public. Reports of surgical procedures done solely with acupuncture analgesia aroused the curiosity of scientists and clinicians involved in pain research and the clinical management of chronic and acute pain. It became apparent that more questions were raised than answered by these reports. Skepticism soon replaced curiosity as noted authorities on pain and related neuroscience openly claimed: "specious," "hypnosis," "all psychological," and "pure stoicism of Chairman Mao's captive followers." Virtually all of these "skeptics" took neither the time to learn, practice, or research acupuncture, thus evaluating it on a purely subjective basis. However, there were clinicians and scientists who did study and practice acupuncture on an experimental basis. These clinicians and scientists discovered that certain surgical procedures previously done with general or regional anesthesia were being conducted with "acupuncture analgesia." However, with little or no controlled scientific evaluation by the mainland Chinese, Western health care professionals and scientists were left in various camps of thought. It, too, became readily apparent that well-controlled scientific studies were needed to prove or dispel this notion of analgesia, which was produced by a mere twirling of solid needles in specific body loci. Two all-important questions were asked: "Is it possible?" and "What is the mechanism which achieves analgesia in the orofacial area by placing a needle in a specific point in the web space between the thumb and first finger?"

The purpose of this section is to briefly review: 1) the history of acupuncture an-

algesia, 2) its clinical efficacy, and 3) its possible role in Western dentistry.

Acupuncture is generally recognized in the Orient to be a 4- to 5,000-year-old art. The origin of acupuncture therapy has been lost in antiquity. The word "acupuncture" is derived from the Latin words *acus* (needle) and *punctura* (puncture), which is usually accomplished by insertion of very fine solid needles into specific body points (loci) and then manipulated by various techniques. The purpose of these needle insertions into the body are said to regulate the physiological functions of the body and/or to relieve pain. Traditional Oriental medicine incorporates other modalities with acupuncture, such as: diet, massage, herbs, exercise, deep breathing, and meditation. Acupuncture is seldom practiced alone in the traditional medical system. Most ancient acupuncture techniques were guarded by practitioners as family secrets and treasure; therefore, it transmitted a secretive and mystic folklore-like atmosphere to most Westerners.

The first published collective works of acupuncture appeared over 2,000 years ago in the *Huang-ti Nei Ching (The Yellow Emperor's Classic of Internal Medicine)*. These explanations of acupuncture's method of action have been largely attributed to philosophy and superstition by the Western scientific world. The magic of acupuncture's past is now being studied in terms of Western science by well-trained observers, and reports of substantial progress in understanding its mechanism of action have appeared in the Western scientific literature (Table 17.6).

These Chinese still consider acupuncture analgesia for most operative procedures experimental since its introduction in 1958 during the "Cultural Revolution." Modern acupuncture is an outgrowth of traditional Chinese acupuncture and is utilized as a modality in numerous Western countries, including: Germany, France, Austria, and the United States, where scientific investigations are also in progress. In the United States, the practice of acupuncture is still considered experimental by the AMA, ADA, and FDA, although many states now license acupuncturists as they do other health care professionals.

The State of California now has over 1400 Certified Acupuncturists (C.A.) licensed by the State Board of Medical Quality Assurance. Based on clinical studies for pain control, the Pain Management Center of the UCLA School of Medicine and its Hospital and Clinics consider acupuncture an acceptable therapeutic modality, while basic scientific investigations are being conducted to discover mechanisms of action.

Acupuncture in dentistry is currently utilized in three areas with acute and chronic pain: 1) as an analgesic for acute postoperative pain, 2) for the modulation of acute nociceptive input from operative dentistry, and 3) as frequently employed in various institutions and by individual practitioners for the treatment of chronic benign pain of orofacial origin.

In the past, in the United States, it has usually been prescribed as the treatment of last resort, but more and more practitioners are now utilizing acupuncture to modulate the pain experience before more invasive techniques are attempted.

Many recent reports on the use of acupuncture as dental analgesia, for both extraction and restorative procedures, have indicated success rates of over 90 per cent. These positive reports have been fairly consistent among reliable observers. These positive reports appear to overshadow the few studies with negative results and have, thus, encouraged further clinical use and research.

CLINICAL ACUPUNCTURE

Before describing the clinical technique of acupuncture, a neuroanatomical explanation of the acupuncture points (loci) must be discussed. Modern investigations of loci have revealed them to be of several origins, but with common anatomical and neurophysiological characteristics. Acupuncture loci are of five main types (Table 17.7).

According to ancient Chinese theoretical concepts, the acupuncture loci serve as "peeping holes" into the body and "passing holes" for energy. The traditional acupuncture system, based on a bioenergetic system that balances body energy, restores health by manipulating body energy through the various "meridians" *via* acupuncture loci. These "holes," or loci, have been investigated by use of various devices to measure galvanic skin resistance (GSR). It has been found that these loci in fact are areas of decreased electrical resistance (higher conductance) and can be measured and distinguished from adjacent nonacupuncture points. From a Western scientific viewpoint, these are electrical windows, or "holes," in the skin and do allow passage of electrical energy more readily than nonacupuncture loci.

Type I acupuncture loci have been shown to be motor points of various muscles. A motor point of a muscle is defined as a skin region where an innervated muscle is most accessible to percutaneous electrical stimulation at the lowest intensity. It is near the skin and generally lies close to the neurovascular hilum of the muscle. Large diameter neuroafferent fibers of high velocity and conduction originate from these annulospiral endings of the motor (or acupuncture) point.

If the gate control theory of pain per-

Table 17.7.
Types of Acupuncture Loci

Type I	Motor points of muscles
Type II	Loci in the midline of the body
Type III	Nerve plexuses or superficial cutaneous nerves
Type IV	Muscle tendon junctions
Type V	Trigger points
Type VI	Ear points

ception is to be considered as a possible mechanism of acupuncture's action, then these Type I_a fibers certainly fulfill the criteria for that theory. The most commonly used locus in clinical dentistry and research on orofacial pain is the locus called *Ho-ku* or Li-4. It is located in the dorsal interosseous space between the thumb and index finger and contains two points of high direct current electrical conductance. These are the motor points of the first dorsal interosseous and adductor pollicis brevis muscles. Other Type I acupuncture loci used in clinical dentistry are motor points of various dorsal extensors of the forearm and masticatory muscles.

Type II acupuncture loci are occasionally used in dentistry. They are the focal meeting points of superficial cutaneous nerves in the midline of the body, both on the abdomen and back, as well as on the head. The locus *Pai-Hue* (GV-20) is located on the vertex of the head one-half the distance from inion and nasion. This locus is supplied by the bilateral cutaneous branches of the trigeminal system and cervical nerves (C2-C3). These are mediated *via* the occipital nerves and from the supraorbital, supratrochlear, and auriculotemporal nerves of trigeminal origin.

Type III acupuncture loci generally lie over superficial nerves and nerve plexuses throughout the body. One such locus used in dentistry is *Hsia-Kuan* (ST-7) located over the deep masseter muscle, just anterior to the condyle of the mandible, where various branches of the mandibular and maxillary nerves are superficial.

Type IV acupuncture loci have recently been shown to correspond to muscle-tendon junctions. These junctions contain the Golgi tendon organs, which are diffusely located around collagen fibers of the tendon. These structures are neurally mediated *via* the large diameter afferent fibers of Type I_b classification. These Golgi tendon organs send afferent information to the central nervous system when ap-

propriately tensed, stretched, or mechanically stimulated.

Further examination of a typical locus used in clinical dentistry, such as *Ho-ku* (Li-4) reveals several other phenomena. When local anesthetic is used to block the cutaneous innervation of the overlying skin of this locus (i.e., the radial cutaneous nerve), the therapeutic affect of acupuncture analgesia is *not* lost. Nor is it lost if an arterial tourniquet is placed above the locus. The therapeutic affect *is* lost when the muscles innervated by the ulnar nerve in this dorsal interosseous space are infiltrated with local anesthetic or brachial plexus block is done. The conclusion is obvious in that the receptor in this case is not in the skin, but in muscle, and requires a functionally intact nervous system to transmit afferent information to the central nervous system. It also implies that a humoral substance is not released from the locus itself to contribute to acupuncture's analgesic properties. Although a humoral theory may in part explain acupuncture's mechanism of action, it is not released peripherally. It is apparent that the peripheral locus is involved when it is appropriately stimulated and thus activates a central mechanism of antinociception and most likely involving the endogenous analgesic peptide system.

Although approximately 20 acupuncture loci are commonly used in clinical orofacial pain (Table 17.8), the primary locus *Ho-ku* (Li-4) will be described in detail for the purpose of this presentation. In general, the other loci are utilized in a similar fashion. *Ho-ku* is located on the dorsum of the hand between the thumb and index finger. The patient extends both thumb and index finger, then places the distal phalangeal crease of the opposite thumb exactly upon the web created by the extended digits, and then rolls the tip of the thumb in a cephalad direction upon the dorsal interosseous web space. The point at which the tip of the thumb touches the skin is the *Ho-ku* point. For exact placement in actual practice, slight

Table 17.8.
Loci for Dental Acupuncture

Loci	Location	Innervation	Dental Indications
TH-17	Posterior to ear, in depression between mandible and mastoid process, when jaw is slightly opened, where lobule attaches	Superficial—greater auricular nerve Deep—facial nerve	Pain and spasms in mandible; trigeminal neuralgia; temperomandibular joint pain
GB-14	Approximately 25–30 mm above middle of eyebrow, in depression on superciliary arch	Supraorbital branch of V_1—trigeminus nerve	Trigeminal neuralgia; frontal headache; orbital neuralgia; facial nerve paralysis
GB-20	On inferior border of occiput, behind mastoid process on outer part of trapezius muscle, on a level with ear lobe	Lesser occipital nerve	Headache; throat pain; neck and shoulder pain
CV-24	Middle of mentolabial sulcus, in small depression at inferior margin of orbicularis muscle	V_3—branch of the facial nerve	Facial nerve paralysis; toothache; trismus; anterior mandibular pain; gingivitis; toothache; salivation
LI-20	Approximately 10 mm lateral to nasal ala where nasolabial fold ends	Branches of infraorbital nerve of V_2 and facial nerve	Atypical facial neuralgia; main point for the nose
ST-2	On vertical axis with pupil when eyes are looking straight ahead, at depression inferior to midpoint of infraorbital margin (over infraorbital foramen)	Infraorbital nerve of V_2 and branch of facial nerve	Trigeminal neuralgia of 2nd branch; muscle spasms of corner of mouth
ST-4	Lateral to corner of mouth, on a direct vertical axis with pupils when looking straight ahead	Cutaneous branches of V_3 (mental and buccal) and V_2 (infraorbital)	Trigeminal neuralgia; spasms or pain of oral muscles
ST-6	When jaw is clenched tightly, this point can be found in small depression of the elevated masseter muscle, just above the angle of the mandible	Branches of greater auricular, facial and masseter nerves (trigeminus), arising from C2-C3	Spasms and pain in facial muscles, lower jaw and neck; rigidity of neck; trigeminal neuralgia
ST-7	In the infratemporal fossa, immediately anterior to mandibular condyle	Zygomatico-orbital branch of auricolotemporal branch of facial (trigeminus) nerve; in deep layer: mandibular branch of trigeminus nerve	Tic douloureux; toothache; painful disorders of temperomandibular joint; facial spasms or neuralgia; headache
ST-18	Directly below external canthus on lower border of zygomatic bone, at angle formed by anterior border of masseter and inferior border of zygomatic bone	V_2 (infraorbital nerve)	Facial nerve paralysis; toothache; atypical facial pain; posterior maxillary pain
BL-2	In depression at nasal side of superciliary arch or medial margin of eyebrow, in corrugator supercilii muscle	Supratrochlear nerve of V_1—branch of trigeminus nerve	Frontal headache; forehead neuralgia

TABLE 17.8—Continued

Loci	Location	Innervation	Dental Indications
Taiyang	On temple, in small depression about 25 mm lateral to the external canthus	Auriculotemporal branch of V_2—trigeminus nerve	Headache; tic douloureux
Yintang	At glabella, midway between medial margins of eyebrow	Branches of V_1—trigeminus nerve	Forehead and frontal headache; neuralgia
LI-4	On dorsum of the hand at proximal end of crease on protuberance of muscle between first and second metacarpals	Superficial—branch of radial nerve on dorsal side of hand Deep—branch of the proper volar digital of the median nerve; ulnar nerve	All head and neck pain problems, especially headache, jaw pain and throat pain; facial paralysis; toothache
LI-11	Immediately superior to lateral epicondyle, at external end of elbow crease when elbow is flexed 90°	Superficial layer—lateral antibrachial cutaneous branch of radial nerve Deep layer—radial nerve	Headache; auxiliary locus for all head and neck pain
ST-36	On anterolateral surface of leg between tibialis anterior and extensor digitorum longus muscles; approximately 25 mm below tibial tuberosity on the lateral side of tibialis anterior muscle	Superficial layer—lateral sural cutaneous branch of saphenous nerve Deep layer—branches of deep peroneal nerve	All acute and chronic orofacial pain

circular movement of the thumb tip once it has been rolled over onto the web space in a circular fashion will reveal an area that is distinctly more tender than the adjacent muscle. This locus (Ho-ku), tender to deep pressure, is the exact anatomical location of the motor point of the first dorsal interosseous muscle. It can then be marked by a fingernail impression or appropriate marking pen. If an electronic device is utilized to locate the point, the probe is lightly run over the area until maximal electrical conductance is encountered and then marked by imprint of the probe.

The skin is then prepared with an appropriate antiseptic solution, as in venipuncture preparation. Now actual needle insertion is performed. Most health care professionals utilizing acupuncture prefer to use sterile acupuncture needles to 28 to 32 gauge rather than hypodermic needles, because less discomfort and bleeding is encountered. Tapping in the needle through a needle guide tube can be used, or other techniques can be used without a guide tube. Needle insertion at Ho-ku is done in a perpendicular fashion in a downward direction into the muscle mass until a sensory response is elicited by the patient. The appropriate response of the patient consists of a feeling of numbness, heaviness, fullness, dull ache or a tingling sensation which may radiate up or down the line of the so-called "meridian." This sensory response is called Tech'i and is generally regarded by most acupuncturists as absolutely necessary for effective acupuncture therapy.

The actual manipulation of the needle by twirling or agitation with up and down motions is done for 5 to 15 seconds and then followed by short rest periods of a few minutes in between manipulative procedures. Most Western health care professionals prefer to electrically stimulate the needles after initial insertion and manipulation. Electrical stimulation is accomplished by numerous electronic devices. Most of these devices are similar to the TENS units used in pain control.

Electroacupuncture is an innovative

method of providing continual stimulation to the locus, thus eliminating the need for manual stimulation. With these electrical devices, the degree of stimulation can be adjusted with greater accuracy as well as with a stronger degree of stimulation. After successful insertion of the needles, the clips from the stimulator are attached in pairs to complete an electrical circuit. Most acupuncture stimulators are 6 to 9 V with current flows from several hundred microamperes to not more than 2 mA. Special precaution is exercised over the chest and back when electrodes are being placed. As a general rule, no leads should cross the midline of the body, below the level of the clavicles or above the level of the L2-L3 vertebrae. This will obviate a theoretical accident of potential cardiac arrhythmia.

Most electroacupuncturists agree that a frequency of 1 to 3 Hz used on the *Ho-ku* locus is the most rewarding for generation of the opioid portion of acupuncture analgesia. Loci used on the face are usually stimulated at much higher frequencies ranging from 100 to 250 Hz but with lower intensity to attenuate the resultant muscular contraction and spasm. This appears to be non-opioid and the analgesia is not reversed with naloxone (Table 17.9).

The *Ho-ku* locus, when electrically stimulated at low frequency, will give a functional muscular contraction of the first dorsal interosseus muscle. Characteristically, the induction time for operative dental procedures is 20 to 40 minutes of continual stimulation and periodic increase of intensity as tolerance to stimulation and contraction occurs. During the course of induction for an operative procedure or for therapy, the threshold of muscular contraction and the sensation of *Techi'i* diminishes, and increased current intensity is required whenever this sensation diminishes (approximately 5 to 7 minutes).

Contraindications to electroacupuncture are cardiac pacemakers and pregnancy, as cardiac arrhythmias or uterine

Table 17.9
Point Selection for Operative Dentistry and Treatment of Chronic Orofacial Pain Syndromes

Distal points
  Li-4
  Li-10 or 11
  ST-44
  SI-3
  ST-36
Local points—high frequency (>50 Hz) and
    non-opioid in action
Mandibular anterior teeth
  CV-24   Used with low frequency
  ST-4   electrical stimulation (1–3 Hz)
  ST-5   and opiod in action
Mandibular posterior teeth
  ST-5
  ST-6
  ST-7
  TH-17
Maxillary anterior teeth
  GV-26
  LI-20
  ST-2
Maxillary posterior teeth
  ST-7
  SI-18
  TH-17

contraction may occur. Possible complication to acupuncture may include infection, needle breakage (although rare with solid stainless steel needles), dizziness and syncope as with a venipuncture vasovagal reaction, temporary nerve or organ damage (purportedly a rare occurrence), and ecchymoses at the needle site. Aseptic technique should obviate infection as well as transmission of hepatitis with appropriate sterilization. (At UCLA Pain Clinics, not one case of infection has been seen in over 40,000 patient treatments.)

If an operative procedure is to be performed, the method of stimulation is continued throughout the operative period and then discontinued at completion. Postoperative pain is minimal to nonexistent since postoperative pain control is accomplished during the induction and operative procedures. For those patients receiving acupuncture for chronic orofacial pain, the patient is disconnected from the stimulator and the needles are removed, completing that treatment session. Patients undergoing acupuncture for chronic orofacial pain are usually treated two to three times per week for a total of 10 to 12 treatments, although the duration of treatment depends upon the clinical situation.

CLINICAL EFFICACY

Several well-controlled studies of postoperative pain indicate that acupuncture analgesia has significant analgesic effect for 2 to 5 hours after completion of the operative procedure, and perhaps longer if electroacupuncture is done throughout the procedure rather than just at the termination of surgery for postoperative pain control. One of the distressing facts about electroacupuncture for operative dentistry is the incomplete or scattered analgesia in some 20 to 30 per cent of patients when compared to local or general anesthetic agents.

Other earlier investigations have claimed that acupuncture analgesia was inferior to nerve blocking or oral narcotics for producing analgesia in experimentally induced dental pain. However, it has been pointed out that pathological pain and experimental pain are not comparable when evaluating analgesic methods or drugs. Morphine for pathological pain has been demonstrated to be far superior to placebo, but may be entirely ineffective in pain which is induced in an experimental situation. Equivocal results of acupuncture analgesia have appeared in the recent literature but are difficult to properly evaluate, due to lack of appropriate techniques, patient selection and adequate controls.

Other observers using acupuncture analgesia have claimed 98 per cent success rate in various procedures from simple relief of toothache to extractions, crown and bridge reduction, periodontal surgery of soft tissue and bone, and endodontic procedures. A recent study using a counterbalanced group underwent acupuncture analgesia for a variety of Class I to Class V restorations to determine the efficacy of acupuncture analgesia with and without verbal suggestion. One group received verbal suggestion and the other no suggestion with acupuncture for the restorative procedures. Both groups were 100% successful in pain control and no local anesthetic adjunctive injections were necessary. Pain reduction was reported to be good to excellent in 81% by both patients and dentists. Ninety per cent of the patients claimed they would have acupuncture again. No significant statistical difference was noted between the group with or without verbal suggestion. Numerous factors are suggested for these similar results with both groups, and the effect of placebo is not entirely ruled out, since real acupuncture was done on both groups. Modern dental techniques and devices, including high-speed drills, may also have reduced the level of analgesia required for the success of this study. The fact remains that both groups had successful restorations with acupuncture analgesia as the only analgesic modality.

It is apparent that acupuncture analgesia for clinical use and experimental dental pain have shown true analgesic properties in these studies. The magnitude of analgesia produced for experimental pain has only been slight to moderate, contrasted to good to excellent for pathological pain. Chapman has shown acupuncture analgesia to have results similar to 33 per cent nitrous oxide in experimental pain. Also, in the testing of real acupuncture, placebo acupuncture and transcutaneous electrical nerve stimulation, real acupuncture and TENS reveal statistical significance in raising pain thresholds induced in experimental dental pain. These threshold evaluations are modest at best, but again we point out the discrepancy of pathological pain and experimental pain.

Problems with SPA in Dentistry

1. Patient acceptance
2. Induction time
3. Reliability
4. Lack of teaching programs

Indications for the Use of SPA in Dentistry

1. "Allergy" to local anesthetics
2. Psychological rejection of any drug or chemoanesthesia
3. Dislike of "numbness" of local anesthetics
4. Fear of intraoral injections
5. Avoidance of injection complications; e.g., nerve injury

Sequence of Treatment (see Table 17.8)

1. Accurate diagnosis
2. Distal points
3. Local points
4. Ear points

Bibliography

General

Bonica JJ, Albe-Fessard D: *Advances in Pain Research and Therapy,* vol 1. New York, Raven Press, 1976.

Donaldson D, Kroening R: Recognition and treatment of patients with chronic orofacial pain. *J Am Dent Assoc* 99:961–966, 1979.

Fordyce WE: *Behavioral Methods for Chronic Pain and Illness.* St. Louis, C. V. Mosby 1976.

Kroening RJ, Bresler DE: Understanding pain. In: Allen GD (ed): *Dental Anesthesia: Postgraduate Dental Handbook Series,* Littleton, Mass. Publishing Sciences Group, Inc., 1979.

Mars JL: Analgesia: how the body inhibits pain perception. *Science* 195:471, 1977.

Mayer DJ, Price DD: Central nervous system of analgesia. *Pain* 2:379, 1976.

Messing RB, Lytle DL: Serotonin-containing neurons; their possible role in pain and analgesia. *Pain* 4:1, 1977.

Sjölund B, Terenius L, Eriksson M: Increased cerebrospinal fluid levels of endorphins after electroacupuncture. *Acta Physiol Scand* 100:382, 1977.

Tilleard-Cole RR, Marks J: *The Fundamentals of Psychological Medicine,* New York, John Wiley, 1975.

Weisenberg M: Pain and pain control. *Psychol Bull* 34:1008, 1977.

Wen HL: Fast detoxification of heroin addicts by acupuncture and electrical stimulation (AES) in combination with naloxone. *Comp Med East West* V(3–4):257, 1977.

Acupuncture

Beecher HK: *Measurement of Subjective Responses: Quantitative Effects of Drugs.* New York, Oxford University Press, 1959, p 157.

Brandwein A, Corcos J: Acupuncture analgesia in dentistry. *Am J Acupuncture* 3:241, 1975.

Brennan RW, Veldhuis J, Chu R: Acupuncture anesthesia. *Lancet* 2:849, 1973.

Chapman CR, Gehrig JD, Wilson ME: Acupuncture compared with 33% nitrous oxide for dental analgesia: a sensory decision theory evaluation. *Anesthesiology* 42:532, 1975.

Chapman CR, Wilson ME, Gehrig JD: Comparative effects of acupuncture and transcutaneous stimulation of the perception of painful dental stimuli. *Pain* 2:265, 1976.

Eisenberg L, McCormack R, Taub HA, et al: Acupuncture analgesia. *Anesthesiol Rev* p 32, 1978.

Gunn CC, Ditchburn FG, King MH, et al: Acupuncture loci: a proposal for their classification according to their relationship to known neural structures. *Am J Clin Med* 4(2):183, 1976.

Kroening R, Bresler DE: *Acupuncture for Management of Facial and Dental Pain: A Syllabus.* Los Angeles, Center for Integral Medicine, 1975.

Sung YF, Kutner MH, Scerine FC, et al: Comparison of the effects of acupuncture and codeine on postoperative dental pain. *Anesth Analg* 56:473, 1977.

Taub HA, Beard MC, Eisenberg L, et al: Studies of acupuncture for operative dentistry. *J Am Dent Assoc* 95:555, 1977.

Index

Abortion, effect of nitrous oxide, 230
Accidents, 387
 vaporizers, 317
Acetaminophen, 356
Acid-base balance, 194
Acupuncture, 413
 complications, 419
 endorphins, 413
 enkephalins, 413
 experimental proof, 421
 facial pain, 419
 loci, 417
 theory of action, 411
Addiction, oral analgesics, 357
Adrenalin (see Epinephrine)
Adrenergic, β-blocking, 211
Age
 drug metabolism, 9
 elderly, selection of pain control modality, 366
 inhalation analgesia, 257
Air dilution
 leak, 250, 256
 nasal catheter/cannula, 256
Air embolus, 390
Airway
 anatomy, 199
 esophageal, 192
 head position, 196
 hypoxia, 193
 nasal mask, 244, 334
 nasopharyngeal, 244
 obstruction, treatment, 195
 oropharangeal partition, 334
 pediatric, 338, 367
 postoperative, 346
 posture and, 334
 protection, 334
Alcohol, 3, 377
 chronic alcoholic, recovery after anesthesia, 352
 oral medication, 369
Allergy, 164, 214
 chart, 6
 emergency treatment, 215
 intravenous agents, 284
 local anesthetics, 164
 subsequent risk, 214
Alphaprodine, 293
Altitude, influence on analgesia with nitrous oxide, 258
Alveolar concentration, gases, 220
Amnesia, diazepam, 299, 376
Analeptics, 11, 320
Analgesia
 acupuncture, 413
 anesthesia, difference, 301

balanced anesthesia in, 375
 hypnotic suggestion, 35
 intramuscular, 369
 intravenous techniques, 296, 370
 oral, 357
 periosteum, 261
 postoperative, establishment, 355
 safety, 254
 stimulation-produced analgesia (SPA), 411
 teeth, 260
 trancutaneous electrical nerve stimulation (TENS), 406
Anaphylactic shock, drug administration, 164
Anaphylaxis, 164, 214
Anemia, skin color, 182
Anesthesia
 analgesia, difference, 301
 balanced, 375
 general
  alternatives, 371
  clinical signs, 301
  depth, 300
  dissociative, 341
  duration, 363
  euphemisms, 372
  facilities, 365
  fatalities, 300
  halogenated agents, 305
  hazards, 373
  indications, 375
  intravenous, 317
  ketamine, 341
  local anesthesia supplement, 377
  MAC, 304
  neurolept, 340
  nitrous oxide-oxygen, signs, 261
  outpatient, 330
  planes, 302
  postoperative pain relief, 355
  previous, 4
  rectal, 378
  renal effects, 364
  requirement, 304
  selection for dental anesthesia, 360
  stages, 301
 record, 4
 safety record in dentistry, 300
 technique, vomiting, effect on, 352
 ultra-light, aspiration, 324
Anesthetic agents, blood levels, 303
Anoxia, diffusion, 218
Anticholinergics, premedication, 33, 376
Anticonvulsant, benzodiazepine, 289
Antihistamines, 164
Antihypertensive drugs, 10

423

Apnea, prolonged
    after muscle relaxant, 205
    diagnosis, 206
Apparatus, dead space, 236
Arrhythmia
    airway obstruction, 194, 210
    carbon dioxide, 192
    causes, 210
    defibrillator, 188
    diagnosis, 210
    electrolyte change, 210
    failed local anesthetic, 367
    halothane, 306
    hypoxia, 192
    incidence, 210
    intraoperative, 377
    lidocaine in, 211
    monitoring, 187
    postoperative, 349
    selection of anesthetic, 380
    treatment, 210
Aspiration
    dental anesthesia, 333
    local anesthetic, 83
    pulmonary, 204
Aspirin, 14, 27, 356
Assistants, number required, 330
Asthma, premedication, 31, 381
Ataractics, premedication, 32, 376
Atelectasis, postoperative, 349
Atropine, cardiovascular effect, 378

Barbiturates, 317
    antianalgesia, 286
    chemistry, 318
    duration of action, 285
    inactivation, 318
    laryngospasm, 201
    pharmacology, 285
    porphyria, 384
    premedication, 32, 376
    storage, 318
Baseline intravenous sedation, 296
Benadryl (see Diphenylhydramine)
Benzocaine, 64
Benzodiazepines, 33
Benzyl alcohol, 64
Blanching, 172
Blood/gas partition coefficient, 220, 225, 254
Blood loss, 336
Blood pressure, 24
    measurement, 185
Blood tests, 26
Blood volume, 214
Breathing (see Respiration)
Brevital (see Methohexital)
Bronchospasm, 203, 380
    barbiturate activity, 203
Bupivacaine, 62
Butazolidin, 14

Carbocaine (see Mepivacaine)
Carbon dioxide, 194
    absorber, 247
    arrhythmias, 210
    barbiturates, effect on, 320
    cardiovascular effects, 194, 350

hypercarbia, 194
hypocarbia, 195
monitoring, 183
peripheral effect, 23
rebreathing, 236
respiratory stimulation, 17
vascular system effects, 23
Cardiac arrest, vagal, 33
Cardiac rate, 184, 231
Cardiopulmonary resuscitation, postoperative personnel, 345
Cardiovascular system, 20
    accidents, 188, 389
    anatomical considerations, 20
    anticholinergic drugs, 33
    barbiturates, 324
    cardiac arrest, 188
    cardiac output, individual response to pain control, 24
    compromised patient and nitrous oxide-oxygen, 262, 370
    coronary blood flow, 369
    disease
        selection of pain control modality, 378
        symptomatology, 5
    effect of diazepam, 376, 371
    enflurane, 310
    epinephrine, stroke volume, change in, 368
    gallamine, 327
    halothane, effect of, 306
    hypercarbia, effects of, 194
    isoflurane, 312
    Jorgensen technique, effects of, 297
    ketamine, 375
    local anesthetics, effects of, 54
    methohexital, 320, 374
    methoxyflurane, 309
    monitoring, 184
    morphine, 375
    myocardial infarction, 212
    narcotics, 375
    nitrous oxide-oxygen
        additive drugs and posture, 264
        compared with oxygen, 264
        effects of, 263
    peripheral resistance, decrease with epinephrine, 368
    posture, 332
    pulmonary circulation, 22
    risk, 207
    Shane technique, effects of, 372
    succinylcholine, 378
Carpue, 77
Cartridge, 77
    sterility, 79
    storage, 80
Catecholamines (see Epinephrine)
Central nervous system, 188, 303
    enflurane, 311
    evaluation, 25
Cerebral blood flow, 22
Cerebrovascular accident, 213
Cervical spine, excessive movement, 394
Chart, physical evaluation and, 26
Chest pain, 5
Children (see Pediatric)
Chloral hydrate, 287

Chlordiazepoxide, 290
Chloroprocaine, 60
Chronic obstructive pulmonary disease (COPD), 381
Circuits, 236
    carbon dioxide absorption, 244
    circle absorber, 245
    classification, 237, 247
    dental anesthesia, 244
    Magill, 240
    scavenging, 248
    semiclosed, 242
    standardization, 248
    T-piece, 243
Circulation
    cardiac output, 24
    control of, 22
Citanest (see Prilocaine)
Cocaine, nasal vasoconstrictor, 54
    activity, 64
Codeine, 357
Coefficient, blood/gas solubility, 220, 254
Color coding gases, 222
Color monitoring, 182
Common cold (coryza), 380
    contraindication to inhalation analgesia, 263
    influence on selection, 4, 380
Compliance, 18
Complications
    hydroxyzine, 295, 297
    venipuncture, 272
Conjunctivitis, 353, 396
Connectors, 248
Conscious sedation (see also Analgesia)
    use with local anesthesia, 255
Contraindications
    barbiturates, 385
    curare, 384
    Innovar, 340
    meperidine, 293
    morphine, 292
    succinylcholine, 328
Convulsions, 392
Copper kettle, 316
Cough, physical examination, 5
Cricothyroid puncture, 203
Critical temperature, 218
Cyanosis, 182
Cystic fibrosis, 382

Darvon (see Propoxyphene)
Dead space
    anatomical, 17
    apparatus, 236
    physiological, 17
Death (dental office), 191
Demerol (see Meperidine)
Denitrogenation, 220
Depolarization, 58
Diabetes
    influence on operation site, 6
    pain control and, 383
Diazepam
    administration, 298
    amnesia, 299, 376
    cardiovascular effect, 371
    fasting and, 290
    intravenous sedation technique, 299

    modification, ketamine activity, 375
    respiratory effect, 376
    recovery, 290
    symptoms of sedation, 299
Diffusion, 51, 218
Digitalis, 378
Diphenylhydramine
    allergy and asthma, 31
    substitute for local anesthesia, 75
Dissociation constant, 50
Dissociative anesthesia, 341
Diuretics, 10
Dose/response relationship, nitrous oxide analgesia, 258
Droperidol, 340
Drugs
    analgesia, sedation, and hypnosis, 284
    anesthetic hazard, 7
    dependence, 3
    emergency, 191
    inactivation, 7
    interaction
        electrolyte changes, effect of, 381
        with barbiturates, 321
    metabolism, 8
    package inserts, 4
    protein binding, 9
    psychoactive, 11
    route of administration, 9
    street, influence of, 3
    tolerance, 8
    tricyclic antidepressants, 11
Dupaco, Allen T., 251
Duranest (see Etidocaine)
Dyclonine, 64
Dyspnea, 5

Ears, accidents, 396
Edema, 5
    pulmonary, 350
    subglottic, 348
Electrocardiogram, 187
    technical problems, 190, 365
    tricyclic antidepressants, 11
Electroencephalography, 188, 303
Electrolytes
    changes, drug response, 381
    replacement, 213
Emergencies, 188
    basic life support, 188, 190
    drugs, 181
    treatment of aspiration, 333, 204
Emphysema, 380
Endobronchial intubation, 388
Endocrine system
    assessment of physical status, 13
    drug metabolism, 9
        insulin, 13
    selection of pain control modality, 383
    steroid therapy, 13
    thyroid, 6
Endorphins, 413
Endotracheal anesthesia, 329
    indications, 329
    intubation accidents, 329
    mortality and morbidity, 388

Endotracheal anesthesia—*continued*
  nasal anatomy, 397
  oral, in pediatric patients, 338
Endotracheal tubes
  causes of obstruction, 388
  cuff, 388
Enflurane, 310
  analgesia, 266
  central nervous system, effect, 11
  toxic effects, 314
Enkephalins, 413
Enzyme induction, 8
  chronic toxicity and, 313
Epilepsy, 6
Epinephrine
  α and β effects, 368
  alternatives, 66, 68
  blood loss, effect on, 75
  cardiovascular disease and, 67
  contraindications, 67
  enflurane, 311
  general anesthesia and, 377
  halothane and, 308
  hazard, 368
  isoflurane, 312
  methoxyflurane and, 309
  neuroleptanesthesia, 340
  peripheral resistance, effect on, 369
  role of endogenous *vs.* exogenous, 369
Equipment
  anesthesia and analgesia, 233
  cardiopulmonary resuscitation, 190
  circuits, 247
  cleaning and sterilization, 251
  continuous flow, 240
  inhalation sedation requirements, 255
  installation, 253
  modifications, 233
  resuscitator, 202
  safety systems, 223
  valves, 243
Ethrane (see Enflurane)
Etidocaine, 63
Etomidate, 324
Evaluation, 25
  airway, 4
  cardiovascular disease, 5
  central nervous system, 25
  classification, 1
  for anesthesia and analgesia, 1
  history, 3
  musculoskeletal system, 25
  physical characteristics, 14
Excitement, postanesthetic, 351
Exodonture, operative requirement, 362
Expiratory valves, 243
  accidents, 388
  nonrebreathing, 240
Eyes
  accidents, 396
  signs of anesthesia, 301

Fainting, 110, 163, 370
  blood pressure record, 185, 379
  diagnosis, 207
  local anesthesia, 110
  treatment, 207

Fasting
  diazepam, 290
  duration prior to anesthesia, 352
  nitrous oxide analgesia, avoidance in, 257
Fatalities, 300, 191
  equipment, 317
  intravenous sedation, 371
Fentanyl, 293
Fever (see Pyrexia)
Flow, gas, 234
Flowmeter, 222, 234
Fluid balance, 213
Fluothane (see Halothane)
Foramina, 100, 102
Forane (see Isoflurane)
Full spectrum of pain control, 360

Gagging, 176, 255
Ganglion
  pterygopalatine, sphenopalatine, 98
  semilunar or gasserian, 98
Gases
  DISS, 223
  gas laws, 218
  PISS, 223
  preparation and storage, 221
  storage, 219
Gastric distension, problem of, 262
Gastrointestinal system, accidents, 352
Gland(s)
  sublingual, 103
  submandibular, 103
Guedel classification, 301

Habits, hazards to treatment, 2
Halogenated agents, properties and formula, 305
  toxicity, 313
Halothane
  copper kettle and, 316
  hangover effect, 314
  hepatitis, 314
  properties, 305
  toxicity, 313
Headache
  postanesthetic, 398
  postoperative, 353
Heart failure, 206
Hematological problems, selection of pain control modality, 382
Hematoma, 164
Hiccups, 323
Histamine release narcotics, 292
Hydroxyzine, 295
  intravenous hazard of Shane technique, 372
Hypercapnia (see Hypercarbia)
Hypercarbia, 4, 8, 192
  drug metabolism and, 8
  effects, 205
  prolonged apnea, and, 205
Hyperoxia, 193
Hypertension, 379
  causes, 209
  MAO inhibitors, 12
  under anesthesia, 209
Hyperventilation, 195

Hypnosis
  indications for, 35
  posthypnotic suggestion, 35
  problems in dentistry, 36
  relation to nitrous oxide analgesia, 47
  technique for induction, 41
  theory of action, 36
Hypocarbia, 205
  drug metabolism and, 9
  prolonged apnea and, 195
Hypotension, 207
  deliberate, 361
  MAO inhibitors, treatment, 13
  postoperative, 349
  postural, narcotics and, 292
  under anesthesia, 208
  vasopressors, 208
Hypoxia, 192
  diffusion, 228
    postoperative, 345
  during anesthesia, 228
  effect of, 193
  emergence delirium, cause of, 351

Idiosyncracy, 172
Infection, local anesthesia and, 166
Infiltration, 147
  intraosseous, 108
  intrapapillary, 145
  intrapulpal, 109
  periodontal ligament, 143
  retromolar, 159
Inhalation agents
  selection for dental anesthesia, 307
  uptake and distribution, 306, 308, 310, 312
Inhalation sedation
  equipment, 255
  patient approach, 257
  selection, 369
  signs and symptoms, 259
  volatile agents, 264
Injection
  pain, 166
  periodontal ligament, 109
  submucosal, 107
  rate, 113
  subperiosteal, 107
  technique, 112
Innovar, 340
Intraarterial injection, accidental, 373
Intramuscular injection site, 281
  response time, 369
  safety, 369
Intravenous agents
  cardiovascular effect, 297
  patient selection, 370
  uptake and distribution, 318
Intravenous sedation
  accidents, 389
  availability of oxygen, 371
  fluids, 30
  technique, 370
Intermittent flow, 254
Ionic gradient, 55
Isoflurane, 312

Jorgensen technique, 296

Ketamine, 41, 324
  analgesia, 342
  blood pressure, 375
  central nervous system, effect, 341, 374
  hallucinations, 374
  pediatric, 374
  subanesthetic dose, 342
Kidneys, general anesthesia, effect on, 364

Laboratory tests (see Blood and Urine)
Laryngospasm, 200
  barbiturates, 321
  laryngeal stridor, 200
  postoperative, 348
  treatment, 202
Larynx, 196
  anatomy, 16
Librium (see Chlordiazepoxide)
Lidocaine, 61
  antiarrhythmic effect, 62
  topical, 63
Lipoid solubility, relationship to MAC, 304
Lithium, 13
Liver
  disease, selection of pain control modality, 382
  portal blood flow, 22
Local anesthesia, 48
  agent selection, 73
  allergic reaction, 164, 170
  alternative agents, 75
  antiseptics, 77
  cartridge, 77
  chemical configuration, 61
  classification, 60
  complications, 163
  definition, 48
  dosage, 70
  duration, 73
  emotional response, 159
  epinephrine and cardiac disease, 368
  evaluation of adequacy, 153
  heating, 81
  historical aspects, 48
  inadequacy, 153
  infection, 166
  injection technique, 112
  intravascular injection, 170
  mandibular arch, 152
  margin of safety, 70
  maxillary arch, 152
  metabolism, 52
  nerve fiber, action on, 50, 54
  overdosage, 70, 170
  pain on injection, 166
  pK, 68
  preservatives, 75, 164
  pressure injectors, 90
  rate of injection too rapid, 167
  site selection, 152
  solubility, 68
  solution, 75
  structure-activity relationship, 74
  supplemental, 157
  technique, 154
  topical, 63, 107
  toxicity, 53, 171
  unwanted spread, 106, 172

Local anesthesia—*continued*
  uptake and distribution, 51
  vasoconstrictors, 64
  warming, 81
Local anesthetic
  CNS effects, 53
  effect of pH, 50
  listed, 6
  requirement, 48
  salt, 50
  systemic effects, 51
  vasoactivity, 54, 62, 69
Loma Linda technique, 296
Lung volumes, 17

MAC (see Minimum anesthetic concentration)
Malignant hyperpyrexia (hyperthermia), 215
Marcaine (see Bupivacaine)
Meperidine, 292
Mepivacaine, 62
Meprobamate, 288
Metabolic disease, selection of pain control modality, 381
Metabolism
  barbiturates, 285, 320
  benzodiazepines, 290
  halothane, 306, 313
  intravenous agents, 320
Methemoglobin
  lidocaine and, 62
  prilocaine and, 62
Methohexital, 17, 322
  blood levels, 319
  cardiovascular effect, 320
  classification, 318
  continuous infusion, 323
  contraindications, avoidance in epileptics, 383
  convulsant activity, 323
  fall in oxygen tension, 324
  minimal increment technique, 373
  Shane technique, 297
  ultra-light, 373
Methohexitone (see Methohexital)
Methoxyflurane, 308
  analgesia, 265
  blood/gas solubility, 255, 308
  delivered by Cyprane inhaler, 265
  nitrous oxide, comparison, 255
  toxicity, 314
    renal, 7
Minimal increment technique, 324
Minimum anesthetic concentration
  agents, individual, 304
  definition, 304
  inhalation agents, 304
  nitrous oxide, 376
  toxicity, relationship to, 313
Mixer dials, 236
Mongoloid (Down's syndrome), 382
Monitoring, 178
  accidents and, 387
  analgesia, 254
  blood pressure, 185
  central nervous system, 188
  EEG, 188
  electrocardiogram, 187
  muscle relaxants, 329

  pulse, 186
  respiration, 179
  responsibility, 178
Monitors (see Monitoring)
Monoamine oxidase (MAO) inhibitors, 12
Morphine, 291
Mouth, accidents, 396
Mouth prop, 335
Muscle and plate diseases, selection of pain control modality, 384
Muscle relaxants, 325
  anatomy, 326
  curare, 326
    prolonged apnea, 205
  gallamine, 327
  pancuronium, 327
  physiology, 326.
  reversal, 327
  succinylcholine, 201
    prolonged apnea, 329
  use in dentistry, 377
Muscular diseases, selection of pain control modality, 383
Musculoskeletal system, accidents, 393
Myocardial infarction, postoperative, 350

Naloxone
  electrical stimulation and, 412
  postoperative time course, 358
Narcan (see Naloxone)
Narcotic antagonist
  pentazocine, 294
  postoperative use of, 358
Narcotics, 377
  postoperative vomiting, 352
  premedication, 32, 304, 376
Nasal catheters/cannula, 245
Nasal mucosa, 196
Nasopharyngeal tubes, 334
Nausea and vomiting, 395
  emergency anesthesia, 367
  Innovar, 340
  morphine, 292
  postoperative, 352
Needles
  broken, 165
  disposal, 84
  gauge, 82
  optimum size, 72
  paresthesia, 166
  sizes, 83
  sterility, 77
  venipuncture, 275
Nembutal (see Pentobarbital)
Neostigmine, 327
Nerve(s)
  accessory innervation, 105
  axillary, 282
  buccal, 103
  cervical nerve, 2nd, 105
  chorda tympani, 104
  cross-over, 157
  facial, 103
    unwanted spread of infection, 106
  femoral, 283
  fibers, A, B, and C, 403
  glossopharyngeal, 201

incisive (see mental)
inferior alveolar, 105
infraorbital, 101
lingual, 103
mandibular, 102
maxillary, 98, 100
mental, 105
median, 268
mylohyoid, 105
nasopalatine, 100
nociceptors, 403
ophthalmic, 98
palatine, 79
peripheral, damage to, 390
peroneal, 392
pterygopalatine, 98
radial, 282, 390
sciatic, 282
sites of overlap, 105
superior alveolar
    anterior, 101
    middle, 100
    posterior, 100
supraorbital, 392
trigeminal, 98
vagus, 201
Nerve block(s), 106
    Akinosi, 142
    anterior palatine, 127
    anterior superior, alveolar infiltration, 117
    buccal, 135
    classification, 107
    equipment, 77
    Gow-Gates, 139
    inferior alveolar, 129
    infiltration, 115
    infraorbital, 122
    intraosseous, 108
    lingual, 134
    mandibular, 129
        anterior infiltration, 116
        extraoral, 151
    maxillary
        extraoral, 151
        intraoral, 148
    mental (incisive), 38
    middle superior, alveolar infiltration, 118
    nasopalatine, 125
    partial palatine, 129
    posterior superior alveolar, 121
        alveolar infiltration, 118, 120
    submucosal, 107
    subperiosteal, 107
    supraperiosteal, 107
    syringe, aspirating, 86
Nerve conduction, 55
Nerve fiber
    action potential, 54
    anatomy, 55
Nervous system
    central
        accidents, 390
        analgesia, 413
    disease, selection of pain control modality, 383
Nesacaine (see Chloroprocaine)
Neuroleptanalgesia, 374
Neuroleptanesthesia, 340

Nisentil (see Alphaprodine)
Nitrous oxide
    analgesia, dose response relationship, 258
    anesthesia and, 229
    clinical application, 231
    comparison with oxygen, 229
    concentration effect, 227
    effect on MAC, 228
    humidification, 256
    impurities, 389
    methoxyflurane, comparison, 255
    properties, 225
    second gas effect, 227
    solubility, 254
    storage, 218
    toxicity, 229
    intake and distribution, 226
    warming, 256
Nitrous oxide-oxygen analgesia
    advantage in dental office, 262
    cardiovascular response, 263
    contraindications, 262
    effect of other medications, 264
    hazards, 229
    limits, 260
    side effects, 262
    signs and symptoms, 259
    uses, 228
Nociceptors, 403
Nodes of Ranvier, 55
Nonaddictive oral analgesics, 356
Nonbarbiturate sedative-hypnotics, 284
Nordefrin, 66
Norepinephrine, 66
Nose and throat, accidents, 396
Novocaine (see Procaine)

Obesity
    anesthetic problems, 2
    anesthetic requirement, 14
    hazards, 14
    selection of pain control modality, 382
Occupation, effect on treatment, 2
Oil/gas partition coefficient
    nitrous oxide, 225
    relationship to MAC, 304
Open circuit, 247
Operative requirements
    duration, 363
    oral and maxillofacial surgery, 360
Opiates, 375
Oral medication, 369
    alcohol, 369
    promethazine, 294
Oral surgery, operative requirement, 360
Oropharangeal partition, 334
Oxygen, 193
    adequate, 183
    anemia and, 26
    hyperoxia, 193
    monitoring, 182
    preoxygenation, 225
    properties, 222
    resuscitation, 225
    toxicity, 262

Pack
  oropharyngeal
    accidents, 387
    partition, 334
  restorative dentistry, 335
Pain, 400
  acute, 410
  chronic, characteristics, 409
  definition, 401
  experimental, nitrous oxide analgesia, 260
  gate control theory, 403
  musculoskeletal, 383
  orofacial, 409
  pathways, 402
  premedication, role of, 32
  psychogenic, 406
Parenteral injection, 109
Paresthesia, 167, 390
Partial pressure, 218
Peak flow rate, 237
Peak inspiratory flow, air dilution valve, 250
Pediatric
  advantages of outpatient care, 338
  anatomical differences, 338
  anesthetic considerations, 339
  dentistry, operative requirement, 362
  postoperative problems, 348
  selection of pain control modality, 366
Pentazocine, 294
Penthrane (see Methoxyflurane)
Pentobarbital, intravenous sedation, 286
Pentothal (see Thiopental)
Permit, 26
Personnel
  alternatives to general anesthesia, 330
  postoperative care, 345
Pharmacogenetics, 9
Phenacetin, 356
Phenergan (see Promethazine)
Phenothiazines, 11, 294
Phenylephrine, 66
Physical evaluation (see Evaluation)
Physical status, 1
Physostigmine, nonspecific analeptic, 351
Poiseulle's law, 237
Pollution
  disposal of gases, 249
  equipment, 248
  factors in toxicity, 230
  health hazard to anesthesiologist, 230
  nitrous oxide, 230
  volatile agents, 315
Porphyria, 384
Position, chair
  cardiorespiratory effects, 333
  dental anesthesia, 331
  local anesthesia, 110
Positive pressure ventilation
  cause of gastric distension, 192
  laryngospasm, hazard of, 202
Postoperative period, 344
  accidents, 344
  fluid requirement, 213
  objectives, 344
  orders, 30
  pain relief, 355

  pediatric, care in, 348
Posture
  chair, 110
  child, in dental chair, 333
  influence of in inhalation analgesia, 264
  intravenous anesthetics, 331, 374
  operating position for dentistry, 331, 391
  position of safety, 347
  postoperative, 345
  postoperative cardiovascular changes, 349
  respiratory obstruction, 347
  semisupine, advantages and disadvantages, 373
  Trendelenburg, advantages and disadvantages, 373
Potassium, intracellular, 57
Pregnancy
  local anesthetics in, 52
  nitrous oxide in, 230
  selection of pain control modality, 367
Premedication, 31
  administration, 33
  alcohol, 369
  effect on MAC, 304
  in general anesthesia, 376
  intramuscular, 281, 284
  intravenous, 284
  oral, 369
  pediatric, 31
Preoperative evaluation (see Evaluation)
Preoperative orders, 29
Preservatives, 164
Pressure
  critical, of gas, 218
  gauge, 219
  partial, 218
Prilocaine, 62
Procaine, 60, 48
Promethazine, 294
Propoxycaine, 60
Propoxyphene, 357
Psychology
  depression, 405
  measures in anesthesia, 34
  methods in pain control, 367
  pain, aspects of, 404
Psychomotor effects of trace anesthetics, 231
Pulse, 186
Pyrexia, 4
  postoperative, 354

Rate/pressure product, 184
Recovery, 397
  diazepam, 290
  failure to regain consciousness, 350
  postoperative, 344
  thiopental vs. methohexital, 322
Reflex
  gag, 176, 255
  postoperative, 344
Regulators, 222
Regurgitation, 331
  postoperative, 346
Renal blood flow, 364
Renal disease, selection of pain control modality, 382
Reservoir bag, 237

Resistance, anesthetic circuits, 236
Respiration, 16
  accidents, 179
  anatomical considerations, 15
  barbiturates, 317
  classification under anesthesia, 301
  control, 16
  disease symptomatology, 18
  emergencies, 192
  inadequate, signs of, 179–184
  monitoring, 179
  narcotics, 292
Respiratory
  anatomy, 199
  management, 196
  obstruction, 182, 380
    causes, 195
    cricothyroid puncture, 203
  pattern, 241
  physiological considerations, 15
  posture, 197
  rate, 182
  tests of function, 19
Restorative dentistry, operative requirement, 362
Rubber dam, nitrous oxide analgesia, 257

Safety
  conscious sedation, 360
  inhalation analgesia, 254
Safety systems
  DISS, 223
  master regulator, 234
  PISS, 223
Scopolamine, 295
  cause of delirium 351
Secondary saturation, 221
Sedation (see Analgesia)
Sedatives, premedication, 32, 376
Selection of pain control modality, influence of disease, 378
Self-inflicted injuries, 174
Semiclosed circuit, 247
Semisupine posture, 332, 373
Sex, analgesia and chaperone, 257, 367
Shane technique
  cardiovascular effect, 297
  modification, 372
Shunt, 18, 224
Sickle cell disease, 27
Side effects, nitrous oxide-oxygen analgesia, 262
Smoking, 2
Sodium pump, 56
Solubility
  coefficient of gas, 219
  nitrous oxide and, 225
Sore throat, 354
Stroke (see Cerebrovascular accident)
Subcutaneous sedation technique, 369
Sublimaze (see Fentanyl)
Succinylcholine laryngospasm, 201
Syncope (see Fainting)
Syringe
  aspiration with cartridge, 86
  loading, 93
  p.d.l., 90
  plastic disposable, 89

Tachycardia, 23
Talwin (see Pentazocine)
Team approach, 330
Temperature
  critical, of gas, 218
  delay in recovery, 351
  monitoring, 188, 216
Teratogenetic effects of nitrous oxide, 230
Tetracaine, 63
Thiopental, 317, 321
  selection, 320
  single dose, 372
Tidal volume, 17
Tissue ischemia, 273
Topical, 63, 90
Toxic effects, 53
  chemical injury, 170
  diazepam, 290
  enflurane, 314
  factors, 315
  local anesthetics, 170
    relative and absolute, 53
  meperidine, 293, 375
  methoxyflurane, 314
  morphine, 291
  nitrous oxide, 229
  teratogenetic, 315
  volatile agents, 313
Trachea, 16
Trendelenburg position, 373
Tricyclic antidepressants, 11

Ulcer (ischemic), 168
Ultra-light anesthesia, 373
Uptake and distribution
  barbiturates, 318
  enflurane, 310
  factors affecting, 219
  halothane, 306
  isoflurane, 312
  methoxyflurane, 308
  nitrous oxide, 219
    denitrogenation and, 226
Urinary retention, 354
Urine tests, 26

Vagal stimulation, 23
Valium (see Diazepam)
Vaporization, 315
  boiling point, 305
  copper kettle, 316
Vaporizers, 316, 389
  accidents, 388
  copper kettle, 316
  Fluotec, 316
  requirements, 315
  series in, 317
  temperature controlled, 316
Vascular accidents, 393
Vasoconstrictor, 64
  blanching, 172
  cardiac patient, selection of, 67
  contraindicated, 67
  local anesthetics, 64
  rebound vasodilatation, 350
  tissue ischemia, 168
  toxicity, 65

Vasodilatation, local anesthetics and, 54
Vasopressers, mode of action, 208
Veins
  abnormalities, 267
  arm, 268
  arterial injection, 273
  difficult, 272
  hand, 272
Venipuncture
  complications, 389
  diazepam, 299
  equipment for, 275
  site selection, 269
  technique, cubital fossa, 269
Ventilation (see also Respiration)
  control, 16
  postoperative, 347

  respiratory disease, selection of pain control modality, 380
  respiratory effect of diazepam, 376
Ventilation-perfusion, 224
Verbal contact, nitrous oxide analgesia, 260
Volatile agents
  halogenated, 305
  toxicity, 313
  used for analgesia, 264
  vaporization, 315
Vomiting
  postoperative, 352
  treatment, 395

Weight, 2, 71

Xylocaine (see Lidocaine)